Microneedles

The microneedle field has been expanding exponentially with innovative designs and various applications, thus capturing the interest of academic industry and regulatory sectors.

Microneedles: The Future of Drug Delivery equips readers with a comprehensive understanding of microneedles: from percutaneous absorption to microneedles production, characterization, applications in drug delivery and diagnosis, to practical perspectives on the development, manufacturing, regulatory issues, and commercialization of microneedles. This book is written by a single author and thus provides complex information in a simple, elegant, and cohesive style.

The book is intended for graduate students, researchers, scientists, and engineers working in the pharmaceutical, medical, cosmeceutical, and biotechnology industry.

Microneedles
The Future of Drug Delivery

Hiep X. Nguyen, Ph.D.

CRC Press
Taylor & Francis Group
Boca Raton London New York

CRC Press is an imprint of the
Taylor & Francis Group, an **informa** business

Designed cover image: © Hiep X. Nguyen

First edition published 2024
by CRC Press
6000 Broken Sound Parkway NW, Suite 300, Boca Raton, FL 33487–2742

and by CRC Press
4 Park Square, Milton Park, Abingdon, Oxon, OX14 4RN

CRC Press is an imprint of Taylor & Francis Group, LLC

© 2024 Hiep X. Nguyen

ISBN: 978-0-367-26650-9 (hbk)
ISBN: 978-1-032-51408-6 (pbk)
ISBN: 978-0-429-29443-3 (ebk)

DOI: 10.1201/9780429294433

Typeset in Palatino
by Apex CoVantage, LLC

This book is dedicated to my father, NGUYỄN XUÂN LƯƠNG, my mother, NGÔ THỊ OANH,

and my family for their love, understanding, and support.

For all those who love science and technology.

Contents

Foreword

Healers have sought to breach the skin barrier for millennia to facilitate therapeutic interventions. The objective may be local therapy of skin or systemic therapy via the skin as a portal of entry. In all cases, the skin's outermost layer, called stratum corneum, provides a highly effective barrier that must be overcome for effective delivery. This can be accomplished by physical methods, such as insertion of a needle that pokes holes in the skin, or by chemical methods, like preparing formulations that increase skin permeability at the molecular scale.

Many approaches to increasing transport of material into or across the skin suffer from insufficient targeting. While the stratum corneum is comprised of cell remnants without metabolic activity, just below that layer are the viable epidermis and dermis, which are living tissues that can be damaged by physical and chemical interventions. Thus, the ideal means of increasing transport into skin is one that efficiently creates pathways across stratum corneum and minimizes damage to living tissue below.

While hypodermic needles are effective, their dimensions are larger than needed to deliver across the stratum corneum barrier. Pathways across stratum corneum should be at least tens of nanometers in width, thereby enabling transport of essentially any therapeutic compound of interest, including macromolecules, and should create a direct path across the stratum corneum. These pathways should be at least tens of micrometers long, in order to cross stratum corneum and access deeper skin tissue layers. There should be many of these pathways, with the number and density optimized to achieve sufficient delivery while minimizing tissue damage.

This analysis of skin anatomy and dimension led to the idea of microneedles for delivery to skin in the mid-20th century, and advances in microfabrication technology led to the practical application of microneedles starting in the late 20th century. Since then, the field has experienced exponential growth in interest and activity.

Interest in microneedles has been fueled by its balance between an effective means of delivery and a user-friendly format that facilitates simple and accessible administration. Microneedles are designed to be large enough to cross stratum corneum, but small enough to minimize tissue damage, avoid pain, and present in a format that is easy for healthcare providers and patients to use.

Microneedles have many designs and can be used for many purposes. Hollow microneedles are akin to hypodermic needles, but are scaled down to microscale dimensions. They are typically used for targeted injection of fluid formulations, with products already approved for clinical use, such as to target vaccine delivery to the skin or target drug delivery in the eye. Solid microneedles may be used as mechanical piercing structures, or can incorporate drug that dissolves from the microneedle in the skin. Many cosmetic products use solid microneedles, and pharmaceutical products are under clinical-stage development.

Microneedle technology is also being developed for other applications, such as slow release of drugs from detachable microneedles, collection of biomarkers from skin for diagnostics, drug release in response to physiological signals as a theranostic system, delivery of electrical pulses for electrical monitoring or electroporation, enhanced delivery of molecules into cells, and targeted delivery to diverse tissues throughout the body.

This book comprehensively presents the field of microneedles, starting with an overview that provides context on transdermal delivery and associated technologies that increase delivery to skin. This is followed by an analysis of the many microneedle designs and fabrication methods that have been developed, as well as means of characterizing the microneedles and the effects they have on skin or other tissues. The book proceeds to describe the use of microneedles for transdermal drug delivery, with specific focus on small molecules, biopharmaceuticals, and vaccines. Additional topics include uses of microneedles in cosmetics and in diagnostics, combination of microneedles with other enhancement techniques, microneedles developed for routes of administration other than skin, and laboratory techniques for microneedle research. The book ends by addressing translation and commercialization of microneedle technologies.

The simple concept of reducing the size of a needle to micrometer dimensions has proven to be compelling. The power to create transport pathways in a way that is targeted and simple to administer opens the door to increase drug efficacy, improve safety, and expand access to treatments. This book assembles the foundations of the field on which the reader can build to gain insight into microneedle science, develop new microneedle technologies, and advance them to benefit society.

Mark R. Prausnitz, Ph.D.
Regents' Professor, Regents' Entrepreneur
J. Erskine Love
Jr. Chair in Chemical & Biomolecular Engineering
Georgia Institute of Technology

Preface

For decades, transdermal drug delivery has been limited to around 20 low-molecular-weight, moderate lipophilic, and highly potent molecules due to the protective barrier function of the skin, especially the outermost lipophilic stratum corneum layer. The transdermal field possesses excellent potential to be realized owing to its numerous advantages over conventional routes of administration. The global market of transdermal products was $52 billion in 2020 and is expected to be worth $87 billion by 2030. With the advancement in the development of biopharmaceuticals (proteins, peptides, biologics, and vaccines), the applications of the transdermal system can be expanded tremendously. The global biological market is predicted to reach approximately $719.84 billion by 2030, while the global vaccine market size will be $153 billion by 2028. However, these large and hydrophilic molecules are unable to penetrate the skin by passive diffusion. Hence, several physical enhancement technologies have been developed and optimized to disrupt the skin integrity to drive these "difficult" molecules deep into the skin layers. Among these novel technologies, microneedles have recently emerged as an innovative, safe, and effective platform for transdermal and intradermal drug delivery.

Microneedles can capture the combined market of transdermal drug delivery systems, biopharmaceuticals, and vaccine sectors, thus generating an enormous demand on the market. Microneedles could effectively penetrate the skin to create microchannels to enhance the skin permeability of therapeutic agents of any size. These micrometer-sized needles have been fabricated from various low-cost materials with different designs, using scalable and inexpensive production techniques. Furthermore, researchers have employed microneedles for numerous applications, ranging from drug delivery, vaccination, and cosmetics to diagnosis, among many others.

Microneedle Types	Applications	Therapeutic Agents
Solid microneedles	Transdermal drug delivery	Hydrophilic compounds
Hollow microneedles	Vaccination	Lipophilic compounds
Coated microneedles	Cosmetical purposes	Small molecules
Dissolving microneedles	Monitoring and Diagnosis	Proteins, peptides
Swelling microneedles	Oral and ocular drug delivery	Vaccines
		Cosmeceuticals
		Particulate systems

Currently, there are over 50 active clinical trials using microneedles for therapeutic applications, while more than 10 clinical studies are conducted in the cosmetic field. There has yet to appear any commercial microneedle array-based drug delivery product on the market. However, this field has been expanding exponentially with novel designs and practical applications of microneedles. Microneedling technology captures the interest of academic, industry, and regulatory staff, e.g., the US FDA released a draft guidance, "Regulatory Considerations for Microneedling Devices," in December 2017.

Microneedles: The Future of Drug Delivery is a comprehensive book that covers all the essential and relevant information about microneedles. The book begins with the basics of percutaneous absorption, explores microneedle production and characterization, moves on to discuss the applications of microneedles in drug delivery and diagnosis, and concludes with practical views on the development and commercialization of microneedles. This book also contains a thorough discussion on microneedle application in enhanced transdermal delivery of various compounds ranging from small molecules, biopharmaceuticals, and vaccines to cosmeceuticals.

This book equips readers with a comprehensive understanding of microneedles, from fabrication, characterization, and applications in drug delivery to manufacturing and commercialization. The book also covers practical perspectives on large-scale manufacturing and regulatory issues of microneedles, as well as the latest microneedle production technologies. This book is organized into 14 chapters and contains 30 figures and 23 tables, thus serving as a ready-to-use reference for accurate information, tables, and descriptive illustrations.

This book is written by a single author and thus provides complex information in a simple, elegant, and cohesive style. The author minimizes overlap between chapters and provides extensive cross-referencing that directs the reader to the relevant parts of the book for related topics. Therefore, the book will have widespread interest to the readership in industrial companies and academic institutions in pharmaceutical, medical, cosmetic, biotechnology, and engineering or related fields.

Author Biography

Hiep X. Nguyen, Ph.D., currently holds a Scientist I position at American Regent, Inc., Ohio, USA. Dr. Nguyen also serves as the Founder and Chief Executive Officer of an international company, Novoremedy. He has many years of industry experience developing various pharmaceutical products, i.e., topical semisolids, transdermal patches, and injectable products. His research expertise covers the design, fabrication, characterization, and applications of conventional and innovative drug delivery systems and technologies in pharmaceutical sciences for various therapeutic agents (i.e., small molecules, macromolecules, and particulate drug delivery systems). He earned a Ph.D. in Pharmaceutical Sciences from Mercer University, Atlanta, Georgia, USA, a Degree of Pharmacist from Hanoi University of Pharmacy, Hanoi, Vietnam, and a Distinguished Toastmaster from Toastmaster International, USA. Dr. Nguyen was honored with Phi Kappa Phi, Rho Chi, and Sigma Xi awards during his graduate term at Mercer University. He is also the Co-Director of the Vietnamese Association of Pharmaceutical Scientists. He is currently co-advisor to one Ph.D. student and has graduated one Ph.D. student under his guidance. To date, Dr. Nguyen has published over 21 peer-reviewed journal articles in prestige journals (i.e., *Journal of Controlled Release*, *European Journal of Pharmaceutics and Biopharmaceutics*, *Pharmaceutical Research*, etc.) and four book chapters to his name. He also has several podium and poster presentations at multiple international, national, and regional conferences, with over 34 scientific abstracts to his credit. Dr. Nguyen currently serves on the Editorial Board of a pharmacy journal and as a referee for over seven drug delivery journals. He won the Hewitt T. Matthews Award (2018), the Monroe F. Swilley, Jr. Award (2018), and many other awards.

1

Percutaneous Absorption

1.1 Structure of Skin

Skin is the largest, most complex organ in the human body. It covers an area of 1.5–2.0 m^2 and accounts for 15% of total body mass. Skin is the primary barrier and first-line protection against excessive water loss and external environments such as physical and chemical assaults, microbial pathogens, and dehydration [2, 3]. The skin contains and protects internal organs and bodily fluids. Melatonin in the skin assists in the protection of the body from harmful ultraviolet radiation from sunlight [4]. Furthermore, the skin maintains homeostasis, body temperature, and humidity through the thermoregulation system and sweating mechanism [5]. The skin also serves as a communication channel to transport the sensation of heat, cold, touch, pressure, and pain to the central nervous system. In addition, many chemicals could be excreted from the skin, including xenobiotics, lipids, sodium chloride, urea, uric acid, and ammonia [6, 7]. Notably, the skin is a preferable absorption site for various therapeutic agents' transdermal and intradermal delivery.

The epidermis consists of five layers, as illustrated in Fig. 1.1. Stratum corneum is a dense skin structure of 50–20 µm thickness and impermeable to most external substances [8–10]. The stratum corneum consists of 10–15 dead keratinocytes (corneocytes) layers, intercellular lipid matrix, and corneodesmosome in a tight junction of a "bricks-and-mortar" arrangement [11]. The "bricks" represent parallel plates of keratinized corneocytes, while the "mortar" consists of a continuous interstitial lipid matrix. In actuality, corneocytes are not brick-shaped but take polygonal, elongated, and flat shape [12], while the "mortar" is also not a homogeneous matrix but take water–lipid lamellar phase arrangement with some lipid bilayers in a gel or crystalline state. Furthermore, the extracellular matrix contains intrinsic and extrinsic proteins, such as enzymes. The stratum corneum, also known as the horny layer, is formed by the cornification of dead keratinocyte cells in underlying skin layers into keratin proteins [13]. This horny layer is the final step of epidermal cell differentiation. Ceramides, cholesterols, cholesterol esters, fatty acids, squalene, wax esters, and triglycerides are only some of the many lipid components found in the stratum corneum that, when combined, form multi-lamellar bilayers [14–16]. Among those, the ceramides are the main groups of lipids, contributing to half of the total lipid mass [17], and are essential for lipid organization in the stratum corneum layer [18]. There are no phospholipids in this skin layer—a unique feature of a mammalian membrane. This lipid-enriched matrix allows only lipophilic molecules to diffuse through the skin. The lipid matrix covalently binds to the corneocytes, thus forming the skin barrier function [19]. For effective skin penetration, drugs must first permeate through this primary rate-limiting barrier of the stratum corneum layer. Interestingly, the stratum corneum continuously

DOI: 10.1201/9780429294433-1

1

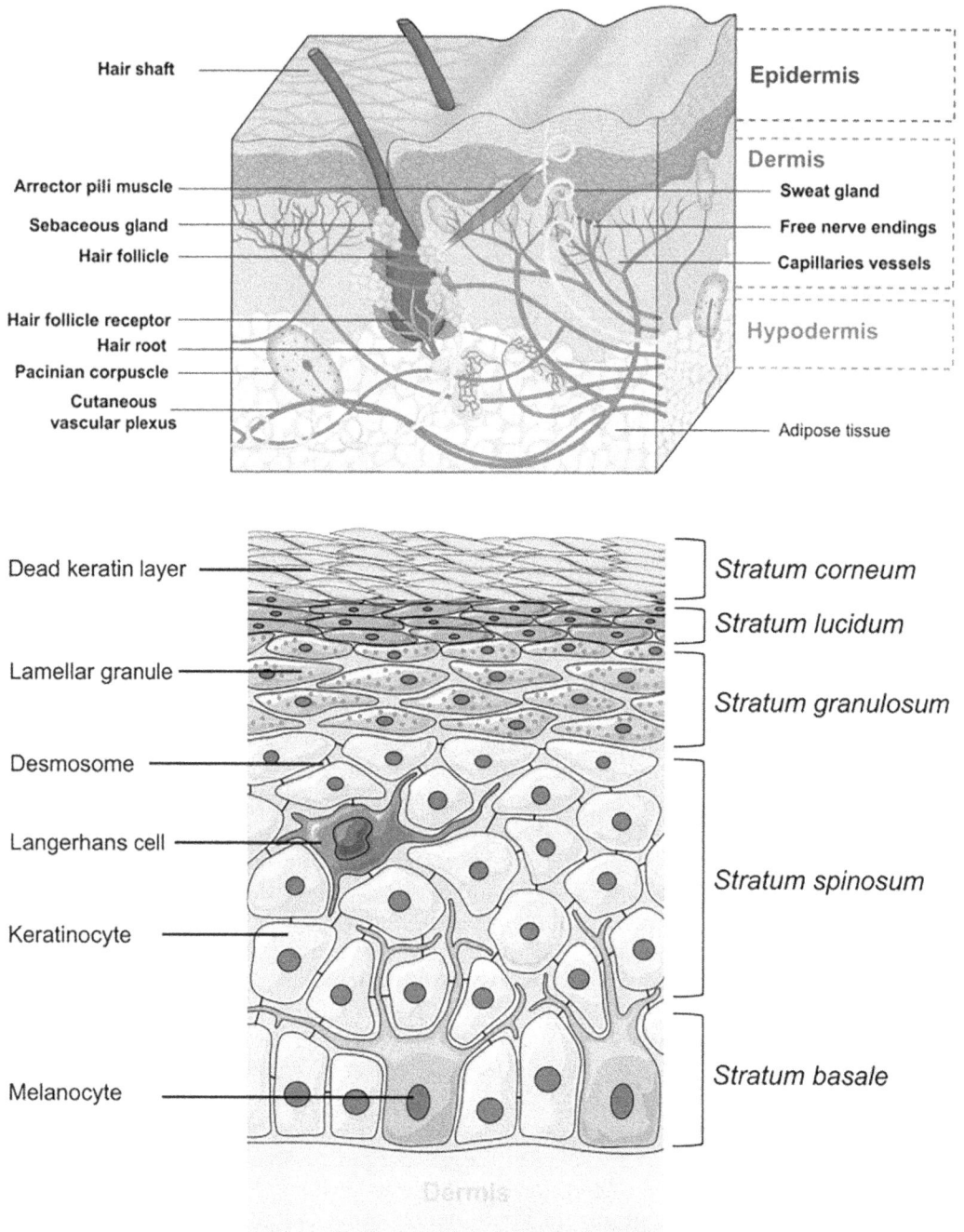

FIGURE 1.1
Representation of skin anatomy and the epidermis layer of human skin. Images reprinted with permission from [1].

regenerates every two to four weeks and can be actively resealed by cellular secretion of lamellar bodies after the barrier disruption by external insults [20–22]. The epidermal layer underneath the stratum corneum layer is called the viable epidermis, which is a cellular and avascular tissue of 130–180 μm thickness. Keratinocytes constitute most of the viable epidermis, consisting of around 40% protein, 40% water, and 15–20% lipids.

Below the stratum corneum is the thin and transparent stratum lucidum layer, which consists of two to three layers of keratinocyte cells to supply dead corneocytes for the stratum corneum. Skin cells in the stratum granulosum layer have thicker cell membranes than the upper skin layers. The granulosum is created from granules in living cells through the accumulation of keratohyalin [23]. The stratum spinosum layer or "spinny" layer consists of eight to ten keratinocyte layers which contain an abundance of Langerhans cells [24]. Desmosome serves as a connector among the cells. The deepest layer of the epidermis is the stratum basale which attaches to the dermis by collagen fibers. Skin cells in this layer proliferate and support the formation of keratinocytes in the upper layers of the epidermis [25]. Merkel functional cells of the sensory system and melanocytes are presented in this stratum basale layer [26, 27]. Stratum basale cells create a critical connection to the underlying dermis layer [28].

Below the epidermis is the dermis layer (approximately 2,000 μm thick) which consists of two layers: papillary and reticular layers. Collagen bundles, elastin strands, fibrocytes, adipocytes, blood capillaries, and lymphatic capillaries make up the top papillary layer (100–200 μm thick) [29, 30]. Moreover, water, electrolytes, plasma proteins, and polysaccharide–polypeptide complexes are all abundant in this layer. The dense reticular layer contains a large number of collagen bundles and coarse elastic fibers [28, 31]. Collagen fibers, fibrous proteins, and elastic tissue constitute the majority of the dermis layer. Collagen provides the tensile strength of the dermis layer, while fibrous elastin forms a connection between the collagen bundles to provide skin elasticity and resistance against external forces. The dermis layer contains fewer cells and more fibers than the epidermis [32]. The epidermal–dermal junction projects from the basement membrane of the epidermis into the papillary of the dermis layer [28]. This tight junction of a complex glycoprotein structure of 50 nm thickness provides significant resistance to drug permeation through skin layers [33]. Various immunological cells are located in this dermis layer, such as phagocytes, fibroblasts, leukocytes, and mast cells [29]. Furthermore, nerve fibers, nociceptors, hair follicles, and sebaceous and sweat glands are also located in the dermis [34]. Blood vessels extend from the arterial and venous systems into the skin's dermis layer without reaching into the epidermis. Thus, once drugs penetrate through the epidermal barrier to reach the dermis, they will easily and rapidly enter systemic circulation. Hair follicles, sweat glands, and apocrine and sebaceous glands are some forms of skin appendages. The hair shaft, as compacted keratinocytes, is located in a hair follicle. The sebaceous gland excrete sebum (an oil substance) to lubricate the skin and maintain the pH of the skin surface of about 5 [35]. The transfollicular path is recognized as an essential route for transdermal drug delivery. The coiled and tubular eccrine glands in the dermis layer play a crucial role in thermoregulation by the sweating mechanism. The human body contains around 3–4 million eccrine glands on the skin, which excrete up to 3 liters of sweat per hour [36]. Below the dermis layer is the hypodermis, or subcutaneous layer, which connects skin, muscles, and bones. This layer has an abundance of proteoglycans and glycosaminoglycans [37]. Also, adipose tissue in the hypodermis assists the thermal insulation function of the skin.

1.2 Immunology of Skin

Skin is a highly immunogenic organ with strong immunological function due to a large number of specialized, immunocompetent antigen-presenting cells (APCs) in the epidermal and dermal layers, which could induce robust immune responses [38, 39]. Because of strong immunocompetence and easy access, skin is an attractive target for vaccination [40–42]. Skin can produce both innate (nonspecific immune response without immunological memory) and adaptive immune responses (specific immune response with immunological memory). When entering the skin, foreign antigens are captured by APCs and presented to proximal draining lymph nodes to activate B and T lymphocytes to initiate the immune response [43]. Among the skin layers, the outermost skin layer of stratum corneum consists of dead, cornified keratinocytes, the viable epidermis contains keratinocytes and immunocompetent cells, and the dermis layer contains blood capillaries and lymphatics which circulate dermal dendritic cells, monocytes, polymorphonuclear lymphocytes, and mast cells. The primary immunological skin cells are bone-marrow-derived dendritic leukocytes named Langerhans cells in the epidermis and dermal dendritic cells in the dermis layer [44–46]. Epidermal Langerhans cells are abundantly and spatially distributed in the viable epidermis with a population of 500–1,000 cells/mm^2 (2–4% epithelial cells). Other immunological cells include monocytes, macrophages, keratinocytes, T lymphocytes, and melanocytes. Skin keratinocytes, epidermal cells, and other immune cells in the epidermis and dermis layers generate cytokines and chemokines to induce and control immunological responses. Several studies have revealed that skin vaccination results in more efficient antigen-presenting to lymph nodes than intramuscular vaccination [47–49].

1.3 Transdermal Delivery

1.3.1 History of Transdermal Products

Transdermal delivery has been developed to successfully bring several products onto the market (Table 1.1).

1.3.2 Market of Transdermal Products

Transdermal drug delivery has a significant contribution to the fields of pain control [50], hormone replacement therapy [51], central nervous system disorder [52], hypertension, cardiovascular diseases, motion sickness, and smoking cessation [53]. Forecasts show that the transdermal delivery system industry will be sizable and expanding rapidly in the following years. The leading factors for this development are technological advancement and the prevalence of chronic diseases. Prausnitz and Langer estimated the annual manufacturing volume of transdermal patches to exceed 1 billion units [8]. Currently, the market of transdermal fields is modest, with 20 molecules and 40 products approved by the FDA. Low molecular weight and high potency are two characteristics shared by all transdermally delivered drugs approved by the FDA. In dollar value, the market increased from $12.7 billion in 2005 to $21.5 billion in 2010 and $32 billion in 2015 [54–56]. Transdermal delivery captures 40% of drug moiety in the list of molecules in clinical trials and FDA approval [57, 58].

TABLE 1.1

History of Transdermal Products

Drugs	Product Name	Company	Indication	FDA Approval Year	Note
Occlusive transdermal drugs for systemic delivery in the United States					
Scopolamine	Transderm Scop™	Novartis	Travel sickness	1979	Scopolamine extended-release transdermal film. Sale of $147 million for 12 months ending August 2019
Nitroglycerin	Transderm-Nitro®	Ciba Pharmaceuticals Company	Angina pectoris	1982	5-, 10-, 15-, 20-, 30-, and 40-cm² systems deliver approximately 0.1, 0.2, 0.3, 0.4, 0.6, and 0.8 mg of nitroglycerin per hour, respectively
	Nitro-Dur®	Key Pharmaceuticals			
	Nitrodisc®	Searle Laboratories			
Clonidine	Catapres TTS®	Boehringer Ingelheim	Hypertension	1984	3.5, 7.0, and 10.5 cm² systems deliver 0.1, 0.2, and 0.3 mg of clonidine per day, respectively
Estradiol	Estraderm®	Novartis	Menopausal symptoms	1986	Transdermal patch for extended release of estradiol
Fentanyl	Duragesic™	Janssen Pharms	Chronic pain	1990	Global sale of $2 billion in 2004. Sale of >$1.2 billion in 2006 and $900 million per annum by 2009. Currently, at least six generic products
Testosterone	Testoderm®	Alza Pharmaceuticals	Testosterone deficiency (hypogonadism)	1993	The first transdermal testosterone replacement therapy
Nicotine	Harbitrol®	Sanofi-Aventis US	Smoking cessation	1996	7, 14, and 21 mg nicotine delivered over 24 h
Estradiol and norethindrone acetate	Combipatch®	Novartis	Menopausal symptoms	1996	Dose of 0.05 mg/0.14 mg or 0.05/0.25 mg per day
Ethinyl estradiol and norelgestromin	Ortho Evra™	Janssen Pharms	Female contraception	2001	Peak sales of $400 million, sales of $153 million in 2013
Ethinyl estradiol and gestodene	Apleek™	Bayer Healthcare	Contraception	2001	13 mg of ethinyl estradiol and 60 mg of gestodene per 24 h
Estradiol/ levonorgestrel	Climara Pro®	Bayer Healthcare	Menopausal symptoms	2003	A once-weekly patch containing 0.045 mg/day estradiol and 0.015 mg/day levonorgestrel
Oxybutynin	Oxytrol™	Watson	Urinary incontinence (enuresis)	2003	Sale of $30–40 million per annum
Lidocaine with tetracaine	Synera®	Galen Specialty	Local dermal analgesia	2004	Topical patch

(Continued)

TABLE 1.1 (Continued)

History of Transdermal Products

Drugs	Product Name	Company	Indication	FDA Approval Year	Note
Methylphenidate	Daytrana®	Noven Pharms, Inc.	Attention-deficit hyperactivity disorder	2006	Sales of $35 million in the first half of 2010 rose to $52 million in the first quarter of 2014
Selegiline	Emsam®	Somerset	Depression disorder	2006	Available strength of 6 mg/24 h, 9 mg/24 h, and 12 mg/24 h
Rivastigmine	Exelon™	Novartis	Alzheimer's disease (mild to moderate dementia)	2007	Combined oral and transdermal sales of Exelon™ > $1 billion in 2013 and 2014
Rotigotine	Neupro®	UCB, Inc.	Parkinson's disease and restless leg syndrome	2007 and 2012*	Approval in the United States in April 2012, in the EU in August 2012, and in Japan in December 2012. Net global sales of €59 million by October 2010, €200 million in 2014
Granisetron	Sancuso™	Prostrakan, Inc.	Chemotherapy-induced emesis	2007	US sale of $11 million in 2009
Diclofenac epolamine	Flector®	Inst. Biochem.	Acute pain	2007	10 cm × 14 cm topical patch containing 1.3% diclofenac epolamine
Capsaicin	Qutenza	Averitas	Neuropathy pain	2009	Topical system containing 8% capsaicin
Buprenorphine	Butrans™	Purdue Pharma LP	Moderate to severe pain and opioid dependence	2010	7-day patch, five different strengths: 5, 7.5, 10, 15, and 20 mcg/h patches
Menthol/methylsalicylate	Salonpas®	Hisamitsu Pharmaceutical	Minor aches and pains of the muscles/joints	2008	Topical patch containing 10% methyl salicylate and 3% menthol
Emedastine difumarate	Allesaga™ TAPE	Hisamitsu Pharmaceutical	Allergic rhinitis	2018	The first transdermal drug delivery system of emedastine difumarate, as a second-generation antihistamine
Asenapine	Secuado®	Noven Pharmaceuticals	Schizophrenia	2019	First-and-only once-daily transdermal patch formulation for the treatment of adults with schizophrenia
Ethinyl estradiol and levonorgestrel	Twirla®	Agile Therapeutics	Contraception	2020	A weekly contraceptive patch delivering a 30 mcg daily dose of estrogen and 120 mcg daily dose of progestin
Nonocclusive transdermal products approved in the United States					
Nitroglycerin	Nitroglycerin	TheraTech	Angina	1988	Ointment
Testosterone	Androgel	AbbVie	Hypogonadism	2000	Gel. US sales exceeded $2 billion in 2013. Sale of Androgel of 1.5 billion in 2013. Sale of Axiron in 2015 of $155 million

Active	Product	Company	Indication	Year	Form	Notes
Testosterone	Testim	Auxilium Pharmaceuticals, Inc.	Hypogonadism	2002		
Testosterone	Fortesta	Endo Pharmaceuticals, Inc.	Hypogonadism	2010		
Testosterone	Axiron	Eli Lilly and Company	Hypogonadism	2011		
Estradiol	Estosorb	Exeltis USA, Inc.	Female hormone replacement therapy	2003	Emulsion	
Estradiol	Estrogel	Solvay Pharmaceuticals	Female hormone replacement therapy	2004	Gel	
Estradiol	Elestrin	MEDA Pharmaceuticals, Inc.	Female hormone replacement therapy	2006	Gel	
Estradiol	Divigel	Upsher-Smith Laboratories	Female hormone replacement therapy	2007	Gel	
Estradiol	Evamist	Perrigo	Female hormone replacement therapy	2007	Spray	
Oxybutynin	Gelnique	AbbVie	Enuresis	2009	Gel	

Active topical and transdermal products approved in the United States

Active	Product	Company	Indication	Year	Notes
Lidocaine and epinephrine	Iontocaine®	IOMED, Inc.	Local anesthesia	1995	Iontophoresis. Withdrawn 2005
NA	Glucowatch®	Cygnus, Inc.	Glucose monitoring	2001	"Reverse" iontophoresis. Withdrawn 2007
Lidocaine and epinephrine	Lidosite®	Vyteris, Inc.	Local anesthesia	2004	Iontophoresis. Discontinued
Lidocaine	Sonoprep®	Sontra Medical Corporation	Local anesthesia	2004	Ultrasound. Withdrawn in 2007 due to poor commercial success
Fentanyl	Ionsys®	The Medicines Company	Pain relief	2006	Iontophoresis. Discontinued due to the risk of a fentanyl overdose. Approved again by FDA in 2015 for exclusive hospital use
Lidocaine	Zingo®	PharmaJet	Local anesthesia	2007	Needle powder injector. Withdrawn 2008, relaunched 2014
Lidocaine and tetracaine	Synera®	Nitto Denko	Local anesthesia	2005	Heated patch. Marketed
Sumatriptan	Sumavel DosePro®	Astellas Pharma US, Inc.	Migraine	2009	Needle-free liquid injector. Marketed
Sumatriptan	Zecuity®	Teva	Migraine	2013	Iontophoresis. Marketed, US launch in 2015
Influenza vaccine	Afluria®	PharmaJet	Flu	2014	Powder injectors. Withdrawn.

The global market for transdermal drug delivery products is projected to grow from $52,476.50 million in 2020 to $87,322.40 million by 2030. However, the market has been negatively and severely influenced by COVID-19. An Insight Partners market research reveals that US transdermal drug delivery market will increase from $6,063.85 million in 2019 to $8,415.04 million in 2027 with 25 FDA-approved patches and 40 products in clinical trials [59–61].

1.3.3 Pathways of Transdermal Drug Delivery

The outermost, lipophilic stratum corneum layer is the primary rate-limiting barrier to skin permeation of polar and nonpolar molecules. In general, permeants enter skin tissue via three major routes: (i) transcellular, (ii) intercellular, and (iii) transappendageal pathway. The preferred diffusion pathway of a molecule depends on the drug's physicochemical properties, the route's fractional area, and any treatment-induced disruption in the skin structure [62]. The transcellular and intercellular pathways could be combined into a group called the transepidermal route of drug delivery, which is the main absorption path for most permeants. The transcellular route is a relatively direct path in which solutes permeate across corneocytes, passing through the lipid bilayer membrane of skin cells in the stratum corneum layer. This is the preferred route of delivery for hydrophobic drugs [63]. Significant structural heterogeneity is observed in lipid bilayers, causing partial variations in partition and diffusion coefficients of permeants [64]. For the intercellular pathway, solutes diffuse through the continuous lipid matrix of the intercellular interspace between keratinocytes in the stratum corneum layer. This challenging delivery route is suitable for hydrophilic, uncharged, and small molecules [65]. Permeants must travel along a tortuous pathway around interdigitating corneocytes, diffusing within the tail group (for hydrophobic compounds) or headgroup domains (for hydrophilic compounds). Permeants can diffuse into the skin via skin appendages such as hair follicles or sweat glands (transappendageal pathway). These appendages are continuous channels across the stratum corneum whose opening diameter and follicular number volume are crucial for drug transport. This route effectively delivers polar, ionizable, hydrophilic molecules or macromolecules [66]. This route allows solutes to pass the stratum corneum and diffuse across the epidermis [19]. However, transappendageal delivery is limited due to the significantly small absorption area (approximately 0.1% of total skin area) [10].

1.3.4 Factors Affecting Transdermal Drug Delivery

Transdermal drug delivery is primarily dependent on (i) the physiology of the skin and (ii) the physicochemical properties of permeants [57]. Regarding the effect on the skin, the rate of drug absorption is affected by skin thickness, skin age and site, skin state (healthy or diseased), different species, area of application, skin contact duration, degree of skin hydration, skin treatment, amount of lipid in skin layers, and quantity of capillary blood vessels [67, 68]. The presence of skin appendages (i.e., hair follicles and sweat glands) facilitate greater drug permeation via transappendageal channels [69]. Furthermore, elevated skin temperature enhances vasodilation of skin capillaries and blood flow, thus increasing drug absorption. Also, an occlusive system leads to enhanced skin hydration, thus allowing for a greater quantity of drugs to penetrate skin tissue [70]. For the impact of the drug's properties, effective transdermal delivery is achieved in only a limited number of molecules with specific physicochemical properties (Table 1.2). Drug candidates must be moderately lipophilic with sufficient solubility in water and oil, demonstrated by a

TABLE 1.2

Physicochemical Properties of Drugs for Passive Transdermal Diffusion [79]

Drug	Product	Max. Daily Systemic Dose (mg)	Molecular Weight (Da)	Log P	Melting Point (°C)
Methylphenidate	Daytrana	30	233	2.3	224–226
Nicotine	Nicoderm	21	162	0.57	−79
Nitroglycerin	Nitro-Dur	20	227	2.2	14
Selegiline	Emsam	12	187	2.7	141–142
Rivastigmine	Exelon	9.5	250	2.1	125
Testosterone	Androderm	10	288	3.2	155
Rotigotine	Neupro	8	316	4.4	177
Oxybutynin	Oxytrol	3.9	358	5.1	186
Granisetron	Sancuso	3.1	312	1.5	210
Fentanyl	Duragesic	2.4	337	3.9	83–84
Buprenorphine	Butrans	1.7	468	2.8	209
Clonidine	Catapres-TTS	0.3	230	2.4	130
Scopolamine	Transderm Scop	0.3	303	0.76	59
Norethindrone acetate	Combipatch	0.25	341	3.8	161–162
Norelgestromin	Ortho Evra	0.15	327	4.4	112
Estradiol	VivelleDot	0.1	272	4.1	173–179
Ethinyl estradiol	Ortho Evra	0.02	296	4.1	141–146
Gestodene	Apleek	0.025	310	3.7	190–192
Levonorgestrel	Climara Pro	0.75	312	3.8	236
Lidocaine	Synera	4.5 mg/kg	234	2.4	69
Tetracaine	Synera	20	264	2.8	149
Diclofenac	Flector	150	296	2.2	156–158
Capsaicin	Qutenza	0.025 mg/kg bw/day	305	4.0	65
Methyl salicylate	Salonpas	0.5 mg/kg	152	2.1	−9
Emedastine difumarate	Allesaga™ TAPE	0.002 mg/kg/day	535	2.9	148–151
Asenapine	Secuado	20	286	4.9	141–145

log partition coefficient (log P) value of 1.0–3.0 [71]. Highly lipophilic compounds with log $P > 3$ travel along the continuous intercellular lipid matrix of the stratum corneum layer. After reaching the stratum lucidum boundary, the permeants must penetrate further into the hydrophilic viable epidermis. However, highly lipophilic drugs could not diffuse into the epidermis layer and instead form a drug reservoir in the stratum corneum [72]. For hydrophilic compounds with log $P < 1$, the transcellular path is the primary delivery route in which the drugs diffuse through hydrated corneocytes [73]. In general, hydrophilic permeants could not effectively penetrate the hydrophobic stratum corneum layer, thus being left on the skin surface. Besides, molecular weight, size, shape, and volume of drugs are critical factors for transdermal drug delivery. Ideal candidates should have a molecular weight range of 100–500 Da [74]. The smallest permeant is nicotine (molecular weight of 162 Da), while the largest is oxybutynin (molecular weight of 359 Da). Smaller compounds could diffuse into the skin more easily than larger molecules [75]. Passive transdermal diffusion also depends on drug concentration in the applied formulation [76]. The rate of drug permeation is significantly affected by its degree of ionization. Unionized compounds provide markedly greater permeation than ionizable drugs. Increasing the portion of drug in the ionized form leads to a reduction in the partition coefficient and permeability coefficient [77].

A low melting point has been found to assist in enhanced transdermal drug delivery. A lower melting point is an indicator of increased drug solubility in the stratum corneum and improved drug permeation across the skin. For effective skin diffusion, permeants must be in soluble form. A strong linear correlation was reported between the log of steady-state flux and the drug's melting point. Transdermal permeants must be highly potent with a low required daily dose of approximately 10 mg/day from a 10 cm² patch [78]. Delivering a large quantity of drugs into and across the skin is challenging.

1.3.5 Advantages and Disadvantages

Transdermal drug delivery offers numerous advantages over conventional routes such as parenteral or oral administration. Transdermal delivery of drugs through the skin has been reported to be painless, minimally invasive, or noninvasive, thus improving patient acceptability and compliance, especially in children and elderly patients [80–82]. The transdermal route allows for avoidance of first-pass hepatic metabolism; ease of application, administration, and termination; reduction in the administration frequency (one transdermal patch could deliver the drug consistently over 24–72 h); and ease of accessibility to the drug delivery site [8, 19, 74, 83–86]. This user-friendly platform requires no trained professional personnel for administration. Furthermore, transdermal delivery provides improved bioavailability, reduced overall doses, an alternative option for patients who do not prefer oral administration, and minimal risk of disease transmission. In general, hypodermic needles are not used in transdermal administration, thus preventing issues of needle phobia [19, 87]. Also, oral-related issues could be resolved, such as swallowing problems, drug absorption and degradation in the gastrointestinal tract, and interference by pH, enzymes, or intestinal bacteria [8, 61, 88–91]. Via transdermal delivery, a steady, controlled, prolonged drug concentration in blood could be achieved over an extended period [92]. This allows long-term therapy to be safe and effective without causing noticeable patient inconvenience. Transdermal delivery also enables avoidance of fluctuation in the drug plasma concentration, thereby minimizing toxicity (risk of peak-related adverse effects) and inefficacy (drug level falls below the minimum therapeutic concentration) [57]. However, for effective transdermal delivery, drugs must diffuse through the skin to a certain extent to achieve the required dose. The outermost lipophilic layer of the stratum corneum, known as the skin's primary barrier, blocks the permeation of most external chemicals. The biggest issue with transdermal delivery is circumventing the barrier function of the stratum corneum layer. Thus, only a limited range of molecules with desired physicochemical properties could be delivered across the skin.

1.4 Enhancement Methods

Several methods have been employed to enhance transdermal drug delivery. These include chemical enhancers, novel formulations, and physical enhancement technologies (Fig. 1.2). Using these techniques, enhanced transdermal absorption of a wide variety of therapeutic agents could be achieved, including hydrophilic, lipophilic drugs, vaccines, macromolecules, proteins, polypeptides, oligonucleotides, DNA, etc. In principle, transdermal drug delivery could be enhanced by (i) modifying the physicochemical properties of the drug, increasing the chemical potential of drug formulation, (ii) altering skin structure, or physically disrupting the stratum corneum to reduce its barrier function, thereby increasing drug transport through the skin, (iii) delivering vehicle-based drug-encapsulated particles directly into skin, (iv) employing a gradient field (pressure, electrical, magnetical, etc.) to induce convective flow to enhance drug delivery, and (v) physically damaging the skin, creating new pathways for drug delivery (Table 1.3). Most transdermal enhancement technologies are currently in clinical trials, with more than 1,000 studies of transdermal

TABLE 1.3

Comparison of Physical Enhancement Technologies* [19]

Delivery Method	Increased Transport	Sustained Delivery	No Pain/ Irritation	Low Cost/ Complexity
Hypodermic needle	XXX	XX	X	XXX
Chemical enhancers	X	XXX	XX	XXX
Iontophoresis	XX	XXX	XXX	X
Electroporation	XX	XXX	XX	X
Ultrasound	XX	XXX	XXX	X
Microneedles	XX	XXX	XXX	X
Jet injection	XXX	X	X	X
Thermal poration	XX	XXX	XXX	X

* Comparison is based on limited (X), moderate (XX), or good (XXX) efficacy in each category.

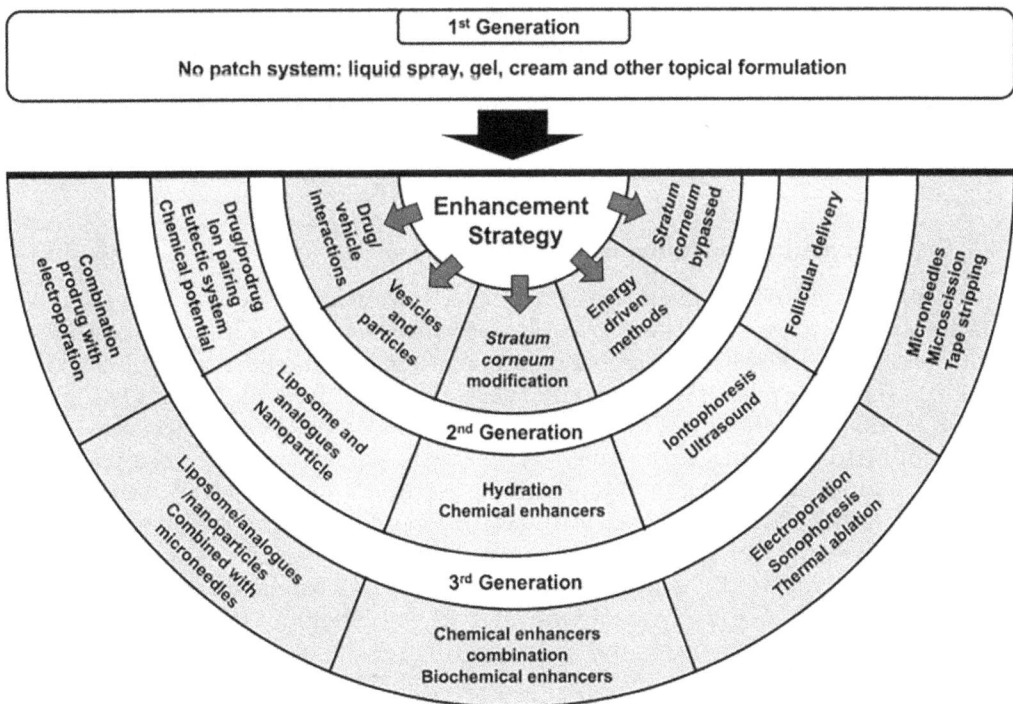

FIGURE 1.2
Technologies to enhance transdermal drug delivery. Image reprinted with permission from [1].

drug delivery listed on the US National Library of Medicine (Clinicaltrial.gov) [93]. Among those, the most investigated strategies are thermal ablation, electrically assisted techniques (iontophoresis and electroporation), and microneedles. Due to mass manufacturing and product development issues, only a few products could reach the pharmaceutical market. Noticeably, LTS is the first pharmaceutical manufacturer to obtain GMP approval for microneedle production. The developers or sellers have withdrawn most of the products from the market [94]. The failure is attributed to safety concerns or insufficient sales to remain on the market. Several companies have developed and optimized the selected technologies to an acceptable and desired level; however, they most likely fail due to business reasons. Despite those failures, enhancement technologies are still promising, given the growing market for transdermal drug delivery products [94].

Chemical penetration enhancers (i.e., alcohols, surface active agents, or fatty acids) could be included in formulation composition to improve drug permeation significantly. The type and level of penetration enhancers should be controlled to minimize the risk of skin reactions such as rash, irritation, or hypersensitivity. Novel formulations have been fabricated to enhance the skin permeability of various drugs by different mechanisms [95]. Some vehicle-based formulations (i.e., vesicles and particles, prodrugs and ion pairs, and other complexes) have been employed to enhance drug penetration. The encapsulation formulations include nanoparticles, liposomes, transferosomes, microemulsions, hydrogels, invasomes, and ethomes. Besides, physical enhancement technologies provide physical and chemical reversible disruption to skin structure, especially the skin barrier function rendered by the stratum corneum layer. These technologies include but are not limited to microneedles, sonophoresis, iontophoresis, electroporation, microwave, magnetophoresis, and lasers. These physical treatments have been found safe and effective in improving drug bioavailability and increasing transdermal drug absorption. These painless, noninvasive technologies provide more control over the drug delivery profile with significantly shorter lag time and rapid delivery onset [53, 96, 97]. Furthermore, the device and application parameters could be adjusted for individual patients. However, enhanced drug delivery has to be balanced with patient safety/compliance and cost [19].

1.4.1 Cryopneumatic and Photopneumatic Therapy

Cryopneumatic and photopneumatic technologies have recently been employed to disrupt the stratum corneum and enhance skin permeation in multiple *ex vivo* and *in vivo* permeation studies [98]. Cryopneumatic treatment creates micrometer-sized cracks on the skin surface by cycles of freezing and subsequent stretching of the skin tissue with vacuum suction. The efficacy of cryopneumatic technology has been demonstrated with fluorescent hydrophilic macromolecules (FITC and FITC-Dextran) [98]. Photopneumatic therapy combines skin stretching by negative pressure suction with broadband intense pulsed light (400–1,200 nm) to increase drug diffusion into the skin through sweat glands to effectively treat various skin conditions such as acne, keratosis pilaris, and rosacea [99, 100]. Researchers reported photopneumatic technology as a safe and effective treatment for acne vulgaris, especially in patients with severe acne conditions [101, 102].

1.4.2 Sonophoresis

Sonophoresis, also known as phonophoresis, is a novel physical enhancement technology in which an ultrasound of frequency range from 20 kHz to 16 MHz is used to disrupt the lipid bilayer arrangement, especially the interface of keratinocytes and lipids, of the stratum corneum layer [103]. Sonophoresis functions based on various mechanisms: (i) transient cavitation effect as the primary mechanism, (ii) thermal effect, (iii) mechanical effect, and (iv) induced convective transport [104]. In the cavitation effect, ultrasound works on the formation, oscillation, and collapse of cavities and bubbles in the stratum corneum. Ultrasound causes a continuous oscillation and stable cavitation, generating bubbles in the energy-application site. The inertial collapse of cavitation bubbles produces shock waves and emits acoustic microjet, penetrating the stratum corneum and collapsing near the skin surface to modify the skin's physical structure [104]. Regarding the thermal effect, ultrasound application causes an increase in the skin temperature, thus improving drug permeation into the skin. In general, increased temperature facilitates enhanced drug absorption [105]. The mechanical effect, or "acoustic pore effect," is caused by the stress and pressure variation induced by ultrasound. The high-speed ultrasonic vibration disturbs the lipid bilayer of the stratum corneum, forming pores in the cell membrane to enhance skin permeability [106].

For experimental setup, drugs are incorporated into a coupling agent (gel or cream) and placed under the frequency generator (probe). When the ultrasound is applied, the ultrasonic energy is generated from the probe and transferred through the coupling medium to the skin surface [107]. The safety and efficacy of sonophoresis depend on various factors such as frequency, intensity, ultrasound mode, application time, coupling medium, and probe-to-skin distance [108, 109]. Among those, frequency has been known to impose the most profound impact. Based on frequency, sonophoresis is divided into two classes: low-frequency sonophoresis (frequency range of 20–100 kHz) and high-frequency sonophoresis (frequency range of 0.7–16 MHz). High-frequency sonophoresis with a frequency of more than 1 MHz is regarded as therapeutic ultrasound and the popular option for ultrasound-based physical treatment [19]. In the past decade, low-frequency sonophoresis (frequency <100 kHz) has received a lot of attention [110]. Low-frequency sonophoresis has been found to be more effective in enhancing transdermal drug delivery to a greater extent than high-frequency sonophoresis. Low-frequency ultrasound causes rapid permeabilization of the skin and maintains the skin disruption state for several hours. This ultrasound forms an aqueous pathway in the disturbed lipid bilayer through cavitation to increase drug movement and penetration into the skin.

Sonophoresis offers several advantages, as described prevalently in the literature. This physical ultrasound treatment is noninvasive, causing negligible damage to the skin, thus improving patient acceptability and compliance and being user-friendly. Sonophoresis was found to effectively enhance the efficacy of topical, transdermal, and intradermal drug delivery. This technology also provides simple operation and high universality. However, several drawbacks of sonophoresis have been noted. This time-consuming treatment requires a complicated instrument and can be applied exclusively on healthy skin, thus limiting the range of application [111]. Scientists have yet to fully understand how the technology functions or evaluate its safety profile (adverse effects such as burns) [112, 113]. There are also issues with device availability, duration/exposure optimization, and treatment cycles.

There are a lot of studies showing that sonophoresis improves transdermal drug delivery. The drug candidates range from hydrophilic to hydrophobic compounds, low-molecular-weight to macromolecules, proteins, hormones, vaccines (for transcutaneous immunization), genes, liposomes, nanoparticles, biopolymers, and therapeutic agents with varying solubility, electrical properties, dissociation, and ionization constants. Sonophoresis has been employed to enhance skin delivery of ketoprofen [114], fluocinolone acetonide [115], vancomycin [116], gemcitabine hydrochloride [117], mannitol, low-molecular-weight heparin [118, 119], insulin, interferon-γ, and erythropoietin [118].

1.4.3 Iontophoresis

Iontophoresis is a novel physical enhancement technology for transdermal drug delivery where a small electrical current (0.1–1.0 mA/cm^2) is applied to drive ionized and neutral or weakly charged therapeutic agents into the skin (Fig. 1.3) [10, 120, 121]. Iontophoresis functions on different mechanisms, namely, (i) electromigration (or electrorepulsion), (ii) electroosmosis, and (iii) electroporation. First, ionized drugs could be forced and moved into skin tissue under the applied electrical repulsion. This is attributed to the electrical force in which like charges repel [121]. Specifically, in anodal iontophoresis, the positively charged electrode (anode electrode) exerts a repulsive force upon cations or neutral drugs located under the electrode to drive them into the skin. Likewise, in cathodal iontophoresis, the negatively charged electrode (cathode electrode) repels anions or negatively charged molecules into the skin. Second, electricity-induced electroosmosis assists the movement of fluid containing neutral or weakly charged molecules into the skin. Thus, electroosmosis is critical for the permeation of neutral compounds into the skin [8]. At pH > 4, skin becomes negatively charged due to the ionization of carboxylic acid groups in skin tissue. Hence, positively charged ions (i.e., Na$^+$) could permeate easily and rapidly to neutralize the negatively charged skin, thus forming an osmotic flow of water containing Na$^+$ to the cathode. This fluid flows from the positively charged electrode (anode) to the negatively charged electrode (cathode), carrying neutral molecules into the skin. Any cations under the anode always receive two forces simultaneously: repulsive force and electroosmosis force [120, 122]. Third, the electroporation effects of iontophoresis disrupt the lipid arrangement and increase the intercellular space in the stratum corneum, thus loosening skin structure and enhancing the skin's fluidity and porosity. Scientific research revealed that skin exposure to an electrical field with a transdermal voltage >1 V improved skin permeability and permeabilization of the follicular pathway. The primary pathway of permeant under iontophoresis is the transappendageal route due to its minimal electrical resistance [123].

The efficacy of iontophoresis depends on various factors such as the physicochemical properties of the drug (especially degree of drug dissociation, drug size, molecular weight, polarity, valency, and mobility), drug-loading formulation (especially pH and ionic strength, buffer concentration of the solution), application duration, instrument parameters, electrode type, current strength, and type of current [10, 121, 124, 125]. Various studies have shown that iontophoresis is more effective when the drug is more dissociated [126]. Also, higher charge and smaller molecular mass enable faster and more efficient iontophoresis-assisted drug delivery. Small and hydrophilic ions are delivered more efficiently under the application of electrical current than larger ions [19, 127, 128]. Several groups reported a strong linear correlation between the electrical current and drug delivery flux. The transdermal drug delivery is proportional to the applied current. Thus, by adjusting the electrical parameter (i.e., electrical current), the drug delivery could be easily controlled and tailored [10]. Furthermore, the modification of drug delivery is less dependent on biological variables.

Iontophoresis offers several advantages over other enhancement technologies. The merit lies in its easy application, controlled drug delivery, and high delivery-enhancement efficiency. The use of low-voltage current only causes minor effects on skin structure in short treatment duration with no pain and no severe skin irritation other than mild erythema

[129]. Several drawbacks of this technology have been reported in the literature. The electrical current is limited to only 1 mA to ensure patient compliance and minimize the risk of nonspecific vasodilation reactions [122]. Iontophoresis is more effective in delivering compounds with a molecular weight of less than 10,000 Da [130]. The application of electrical current could result in local skin irritation (i.e., burns) or current-induced skin damage when the current is applied for more than 3 min or when the current is more than 0.5 mA/cm^2 [131]. The use of continuous direct current could induce polarization effects on the skin, which could be resolved with pulsed current [10]. Also, it is challenging to predict or estimate the bioavailability of drugs. The device is expensive and complex (the requirement for instrument setup), thus affecting patient compliance. An issue with iontophoresis was reported with the corrosion of the metal component of the electrode with an aqueous gel-like adhesive during storage [132].

Various therapeutic agents have been delivered transdermally by the iontophoretic mechanism. Macromolecules such as proteins, peptides, and oligonucleotides are ideal candidates due to their charged nature at physiological pH and pH-dependent varying charge. The molecular weight and mobility of the compound have a profound impact on its permeation into the skin [134]. Iontophoresis has been employed to deliver lidocaine for pediatric anesthesia [135], diagnose cystic fibrosis by pilocarpine iontophoresis [136], monitor blood glucose levels by reverse iontophoresis [137], and deliver estradiol-encapsulated nanoparticles to increase bone mineral density for the treatment of osteoporosis [138]. Fentanyl was administered with iontophoresis for acute postoperative management in hospitalized patients. This easy and convenient delivery technique provided an equivalent analgesic effect to morphine [139, 140]. Enhanced iontophoretic delivery of various drugs has been reported, including nonsteroidal anti-inflammatory drugs (ibuprofen, aspirin, and indometacin) [126], 3-fluoroamphetamine [141], almotriptan [142], granisetron [143], sodium nonivamide acetate [144], donepezil [145], insulin [146], [^{3}H] GHRP (radiolabeled growth hormone-releasing peptide), [^{3}H] SK&F 110679 (labeled at the 5- and 7-positions of the D-tryptophan residue) [147], dexamethasone, ketorolac, luteinizing hormone-releasing hormone, calcitonin [148], and prodrug ketoprofen choline chloride [149]. Interestingly, FDA has approved several iontophoresis-based products such as pilocarpine delivery in cystic fibrosis diagnosis, tap-water delivery for hyperhidrosis treatment,

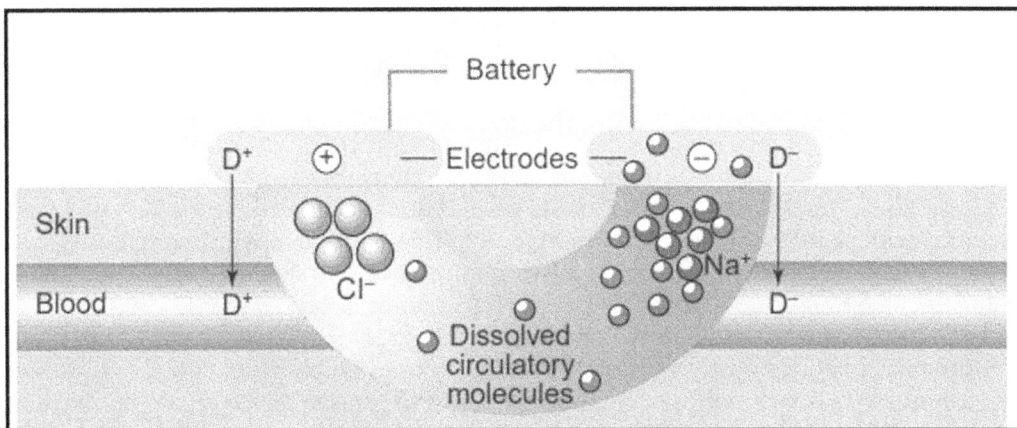

FIGURE 1.3
Principle of iontophoresis-mediated transdermal drug delivery. Image reprinted with permission from [133].

lidocaine delivery for local anesthesia (i.e., before venipuncture) [150], and extraction of interstitial fluid for monitoring blood glucose in diabetics. In 2013, the US FDA approved a low-current sumatriptan iontophoretic delivery device for the management of acute migraine. According to the pharmacokinetic analysis, the peak serum concentration was reached 15 min after system activation, at 22 ng/mL. It was also revealed that the level of current applied linearly correlated with the amount of sumatriptan administered. Devices such as Lidosite™ for lidocaine [122], Ionsys™ [151] for fentanyl, Zecuity™ for sumatriptan delivery [152], and a facial spa device by NuFace™ for face care without the need for chemicals [153] are examples of iontophoresis products now on the market. In the future, the iontophoresis drug delivery system is expected to be a user-friendly, disposable, and home-use device.

1.4.4 Electroporation

Electroporation or electro-permeabilization is a biophysical technique to apply instantaneous high-intensity and high-voltage electrical pulse on skin tissue for a short duration (microseconds to milliseconds) to induce structural perturbation and rearrangement of lipid bilayers in the stratum corneum and create aqueous microchannels in the skin [154, 155]. This treatment facilitates drug permeation into deeper skin layers. Electroporation enables the penetration of water into the lipid bilayer and the rearrangement of adjacent lipid and polar head groups. The electroporatic microchannels are miniature (<10 nm in size), transient, temporary, reversible, and sparsely distributed (approximately 0.1% skin surface area). Depending on the applied voltage, the number of pulses, and the duration of the pulses, the channels' sizes and durations of opening change accordingly. These channels are partially reversed within seconds and fully recovered minutes to hours after the electrical pulsation. By creating multiple pores in the skin, electroporation enhances transdermal drug transport by various mechanisms: (i) passive diffusion, (ii) electroosmosis, and (iii) iontophoresis in which charged molecules are repelled into the skin through the transfollicular pathway under the electrical field [156]. Electroporation has significantly reduced the lag time of transdermal drug delivery to seconds, thus demonstrating rapid response to the treatment [157]. Also, skin resistance instantaneously decreases by three orders of magnitude within seconds after the pulsation.

The safety and efficacy of electroporation depend on a variety of factors. The pulse parameters such as duration (microsecond to millisecond), pulse number and shape, the interval between pulses (a few seconds to a minute), waveform, field strength, and applied voltage (50–1,500 V) have been reported to have an impact on skin permeability and drug delivery [158–160]. The profile of the electrical field versus the time of the voltage also affects the treatment efficacy. The delivery-enhancing effect of electroporation depends on the drugs' physicochemical properties [160], the shape of the electrode, and application conditions [161]. Electroporation offers several noticeable advantages. The system is designed with closely spaced electrodes to limit the electrical field within nerve-free stratum corneum to make the treatment painless, noninvasive, and safe for the skin. The merit of this technique lies in its versatility, enabling a controlled transdermal drug delivery and offering various applications in nonselective enhanced delivery of biomacromolecules (i.e., proteins, peptides, and vaccines). However, electroporation poses several significant shortcomings. This technique requires complex and expensive devices, complicated and time-consuming treatment applications, and trained experts to operate the system. This electric pulsation could provide only a small drug delivery load, limited pore area, and low drug throughput. The use of high voltage poses the risk of cell damage, substantial cellular perturbation, cell death, heat-induced drug degradation, and denaturation of bio-macromolecules [111, 162].

Electroporation has been found to permeabilize skin tissue and enhance the transdermal delivery of various drugs by orders of magnitude. This technique effectively transports charged molecules and macromolecules through created pores [163]. Electroporation has delivered low-dose cisplatin into the skin to treat osteosarcoma [164]. Likewise, diclofenac sodium hydrogel was applied on electroporatic skin to provide anti-inflammatory and analgesic effects for arthritis treatment [165]. Electroporation has successfully enhanced the permeation of therapeutic agents with varying lipophilicity and molecular weight: small molecules, proteins, oligonucleotides, DNA, small interfering RNA, nucleic acid molecules [166], vaccines [167], insulin [168], heparin [169], microparticles [170], antiangio-genic peptides, negatively charged anticoagulant heparin, and biopharmaceuticals with molecular weights >7 kDa. Electroporation-enhanced delivery of small molecules have been reported, such as tetracaine [171], alniditan [172], fentanyl [173], timolol [174] and cal-cein [175], dextran, doxorubicin [176], mannitol, calcein, and lidocaine [177].

1.4.5 Needleless Jet Injection

Needle-free jet injection utilizes high pressure to deliver a large dose of therapeutic agents (i.e., proteins and peptides) into the skin at a high velocity [10,80]. The jet injection's high speed (120–200 m/s) creates a supersonic flow of liquid or solid particles (powders) to physically disrupt and puncture skin tissue to enhance transdermal drug delivery. The power source of jet injection is typically compressed gas or a spring [10, 178]. Needleless jet injection allows for avoidance of needles-related issues such as needle pho-bia, needlestick injuries, infection, or disease transmission, which commonly occur with improper use of hypodermic needles [179, 180]. Moreover, the pharmacokinetic profile of jet injection-based drug delivery has been reported to be equivalent to conventional needle injections. This well-tolerated technology is also painless and noninvasive, thus providing improved patient compliance, especially in patients with chronic diseases or children with diabetes [10]. Also, the induced skin damage is reversible and could recover rapidly [181]. Furthermore, controlled and targeted drug delivery to a particular skin layer could be achieved with jet injection. The jet injection-mediated drug delivery no longer depends on drug diffusion kinetics, thus superior to other physical enhancement tech-nologies such as iontophoresis and electroporation [180]. However, some shortcomings of this technique have been reported. The device is complicated, expensive, and hard-to-operate. The reusable device is bulky and inconvenient, while the convenient disposable equipment is wasteful and poses environmental concerns [182]. Also, the device's design has to be developed and optimized for controlled injection and deeper penetration into the skin tissue. Furthermore, an issue of dosing accuracy has been noted due to skin variability among different patients. The potential for long-term side effects has not been thoroughly studied.

Depending on the physical properties of the delivered formulation, the needleless jet injection could drive fluid (liquid jet injection) or solid particles (powder jet injection) into the skin. For liquid jet injection, the drug-loaded liquid formulation is compressed and pushed out of a narrow orifice (100–300 μm diameter) at a high velocity of 100–200 m/s [178]. Targeted drug delivery could be achieved by modifying the jet velocity and the ori-fice dimensions. This allows for selective drug penetration to intradermal, subcutaneous, or intramuscular areas [10, 183]. This technique is useful in delivering vaccines for large-scale immunization against measles, smallpox, cholera, hepatitis B, influenza, and polio

[184]. Some protein-delivered liquid jet injection systems are Vitajet (Bioject), Biojector (Bioject), and Medi-Jector [57]. These products are presently available on the market for the delivery of insulin, recombinant human growth hormone (hGH), and ganirelix. However, some adverse skin reactions have been reported with liquid jet injection, such as soreness, redness, or swelling [185, 186]. Besides, powder jet injection could facilitate the skin transport of drugs and vaccines, especially water-sensitive compounds. A typical powder jet injector, also known as a biolistic injector, could move dry powder, microparticles, or nanoparticles at a high speed of 600–900 m/s using a typical pressure of 200–900 psi [184, 187]. Particles of drugs are carried by the gas flow and deposited in the target tissue under the skin [80, 184]. The momentum of particles within the gas flow determines the drug penetration depth, where the flowing particles form miniature channels in the stratum corneum. The particles' velocity is governed by the physical properties such as size and density of the particles [10, 80, 184]. Specifically, the desired size of drug particles ranges from 10 to 20 µm while the size of 0.5–3 µm is appropriate for DNA vaccination. In general, larger particle size leads to reduced penetration depth. The particle density is between 1.08 and 18.2 g/cm³. Powder jet injection offers several advantages: (i) drugs and vaccines are in solid form, thus improving stability, (ii) the requirement for cold-chain or freezing storage and transportation could be avoided, thus reducing the associated cost and facilitating mass immunization, especially in developing countries [10]. The PMED® (Pfizer) device, previously known as PowderJect ™ injector, has effectively delivered testosterone, lidocaine hydrochloride, calcitonin, insulin, and vaccines [188–191].

1.4.6 Microneedles

Microneedle technology has been the most popular and promising transdermal drug delivery platform, attracting the most active research and development activities in academia and industrial fields over the past decade. This cutting-edge technology is predicted to be one of the ten leading technologies in 2020 by the World Economic Forum. Microneedles are micrometer-sized needles with a needle length ranging from 25 µm to 2,000 µm. Microneedles could porate the stratum corneum and upper skin layers to create transient and reversible hydrophilic micrometer-sized channels in the skin in a precise and controlled way. The evolution of this technology spans over 40 years.

- 1976: Gerstel and Place filed the first patent about the basic design of microneedles "Drug delivery device."
- 1996: Gross and Kelly patented the first hollow microneedle device for intradermal drug delivery.
- 1997: Jang developed a skin-perforating device.
- 1998: The first silicon solid microneedles were developed for enhanced delivery of calcein.
- 2000: Zahn invented hollow microneedles to inject drug solution into the skin.
- 2004: Cormier developed coated microneedles for transdermal delivery of desmopressin.
- 2006: Park used PLGA as the material to fabricate drug-loaded dissolving microneedles to deliver calcein and bovine serum albumin across the skin.
- 2012: Donnelly invented the most recent type of microneedles, hydrogel-forming swelling microneedles, which could absorb skin interstitial fluid and swell to create channels for drug diffusion.

Interestingly, the number of publications about microneedles has increased by 77.9% over ten years from 2004 to 2013, while the increment rate was only 14.9% since 1970. Microneedles publications contribute to 30% of all papers in transdermal delivery technologies. In the following years, greater effort is expected to be put into studying and developing microneedle-based systems. There are numerous review articles about different aspects of microneedles, such as fabrication methods [192, 193], microneedle design [194], delivery-enhancement application, clinical trials [192], ethical studies, etc. Microneedles have been found to successfully disrupt the skin barrier without reaching the dermis layer, where nerve endings and blood capillaries are located to create pain, irritation, or bleeding. Microneedles could be utilized for various purposes, such as biosignal sensing, therapeutic delivery, or cosmetic application. Enhanced transdermal delivery by microneedle treatment has been reported with a wide range of therapeutic agents such as small molecules (hydrophilic and lipophilic compounds) [195, 196], macromolecules (i.e., peptides, proteins, small interfering RNAs, oligonucleotides, and vaccines) [197–200], cosmeceuticals [201–203], and micro- and nanoparticles [204–206]. A list of microneedles-delivered compounds includes but is not limited to oligonucleotides, desmopressin, human growth hormone, insulin, DNA and protein antigens [207], and immunobiological [208]. In general, there is no size or molecular weight limit for compounds to be delivered using microneedles. Microneedles have been developed with different geometries, dimensions, designs, densities, and materials. Materials of construction of microneedles include glass [209], sugar [210], metal [211], silicon [212], solid polymer [213], aqueous hydrogel [214], and dissolving polymers [215]. Various fabrication techniques have been employed to produce microneedles, such as ion sputtering deposition [216], photolithography [217], wet and dry etching [212], photopolymerization, laser ablation, and micromoding [218, 219], layer-by-layer deposition [220], droplet-born air blowing [221], and milling [222]. Recently, novel applications of microneedles have been explored for HIV treatment, contraceptive hormones, therapeutic drug monitoring, diabetes, cosmetics, anticancer therapy, osteoporosis, and vaccination (i.e., COVID-19, etc.). The majority of microneedle use is for transdermal drug delivery [223]. Some microneedles products are commercially available on the market such as solid microneedles (Nasheng Microelectrics Co., Ltd.), 3M Microstructured transdermal system (3M), BD Libertas™ Patch injector (DB Sciences), ZP Patch (Zosano), microneedle therapy system (Clinical resolution lab), micro-Trans™ (Valeritas, Inc.), h-Patch™ (Valeritas, Inc.), Mini-Ject™ (Valeritas, Inc.), Intanza® (Sanofi Pasteur), MicronJet needle (NanoPass Technologies), Theraject (Theraject), Debioject (Debiotech), AdminPatch® (AdminMed), AdminPen™ (AdminMed), and AdminStamp™ (AdminMed).

Currently, there are five types of microneedles: solid, hollow, coated, dissolving, and swelling microneedles (Fig. 1.4). The first and foremost function of microneedles is to successfully microporate the skin to a certain penetration depth, thus disrupting the skin barrier and opening new pathways for enhanced drug delivery. Several investigations have revealed that microneedles-created channels are the preferred and primary path of drug diffusion into the skin. Solid microneedles (i.e., glass, silicon, metal, and polymeric microneedles) are inserted to puncture the skin, creating multiple microchannels after the needle's removal. Drug-loaded pharmaceutical preparations (i.e., solution, semisolid formulation, or patch) are applied on the microneedles-treated site. Then, the drug permeates through the opened, skin fluid-filled hydrophilic channels into the skin by the typical passive diffusion. Hollow microneedles, in basic concept, are downscaled micrometer-sized hypodermic needles that work on a similar mechanism as conventional needles. First, mechanically sharp microneedles are inserted to penetrate the skin tissue. Then, drug formulation (i.e., solution or formulation with controlled viscosity) is injected into the

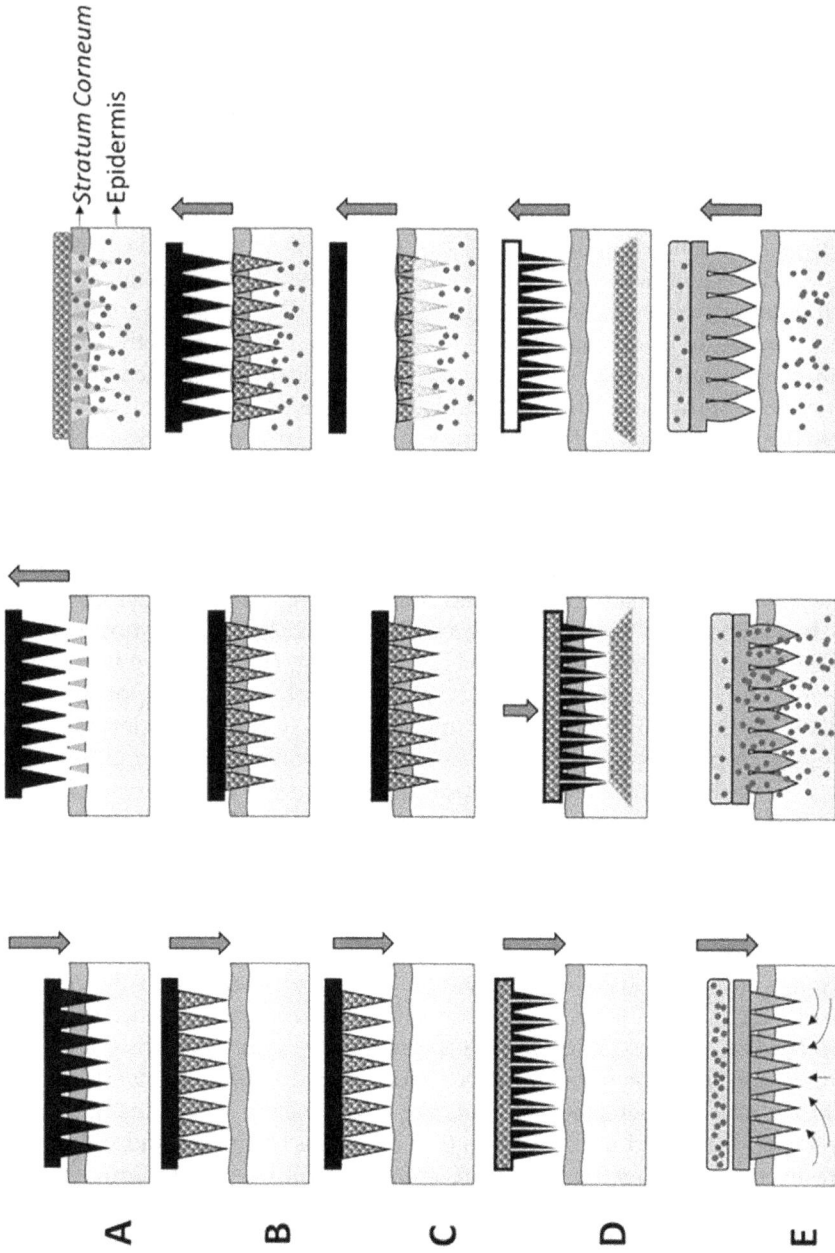

FIGURE 1.4

A representation of five types of microneedles for enhanced transdermal drug delivery. (A) Solid microneedles increase drug diffusion from topically applied formulation into the skin through microneedles-created channels. (B) Coated microneedles rapidly dissolve and release the coated drug into the skin. (C) Dissolving microneedles disintegrate and dissolve in the skin to release the drug load encapsulated within the needle matrix. (D) Hollow microneedles porate skin and enable injection of drug solution into the skin through the needle bores by infusion or diffusion. (E) Hydrogel-forming swelling microneedles absorb skin interstitial fluids and swell to create porous channels for facilitated drug permeation. Images reprinted with permission from [224].

skin through the needle bore using external pressure or passive diffusion. Maintaining a sufficient and consistent flow rate of drug injection is critical for a desired drug delivery profile. The delivery rate could be controlled by altering the level of applied pressure. Coated microneedles consist of solid microneedles and a drug-loaded coating layer on the needle surface. Upon insertion into the skin, the coated layer is separated from the needles, dissolves in skin fluid, and releases the drug into skin layers. Dissolving microneedles (i.e., polymeric microneedles) encapsulate drug load inside the needles' polymeric matrix. The needles penetrate the skin, gradually dissolve in the skin, and release the drug payload, leaving no sharp waste. Swelling microneedles are sufficiently robust to porate skin. After skin insertion, the needles absorb skin fluid and swell to form a porous hydrogel structure, allowing permeant to enter skin tissue easily.

Several advantages and disadvantages of microneedles have been reported in the literature.

Advantages of microneedles

- These short and narrow micrometer-sized needles are painless and minimally invasive, thus being less painful and more comfortable than conventional hypodermic needle injections. The needles are generally sufficiently long to penetrate skin layers but short enough to avoid nerve endings or blood capillaries embedded in the dermis layer (causing no pain stimulation or bleeding). The use of microneedles improves patients' acceptability and compliance.
- Microneedles combine the advantages of the transdermal patch and hypodermic needle injection.
- Microneedle-mediated drug delivery avoids first-pass hepatic metabolism and prevents enzymatic degradation and poor gastrointestinal absorption, thus improving the drug's bioavailability.
- Vaccine dose sparing and a wider range of immune response could be achieved for various vaccines, including IPV, seasonal influenza and rabies vaccines, influenza, rotavirus, and herpes simplex virus.
- Microneedles provide a superior immunological response, stronger antibody and cellular response, and improved protection compared to hypodermic needle injections.
- Microneedles treatment causes reversible physical skin disruption. Skin could rapidly recover after the removal of microneedles, thus minimizing the risk of skin irritation or secondary infections.
- Materials for constructing microneedles are generally safe, biocompatible, and biodegradable, hence avoiding the induction of inflammation reactions. Microneedle insertion leaves no harmful materials in the skin.
- There is no requirement for the trained healthcare provider, thus enabling self-administration of microneedles in which patients could apply the dose-loaded microneedles by themselves. Microneedles allow the vaccination campaign to move from fixed-post clinics to house-to-house campaigns with minimal involvement of trained personnel.
- Microneedles could substantially reduce vaccine wastage. Each single-use microneedle array contains one dose of vaccine whose entire vaccine quantity is administered to the skin.

- Solid drug-loaded microneedles require no reconstitution as solid, lyophilized drug powder, thus avoiding the waste of time and risk of error of reconstitution.
- Microneedles bypass the stratum corneum barrier, thus enabling sufficient transdermal delivery of "difficult" molecules (i.e., hydrophilic compounds, high-molecular-weight drugs, macromolecules, proteins, peptides, and vaccines).
- Microneedle design could be tailored for sustained or bolus drug release.
- Microneedles, especially dissolving and swelling microneedles, produce no sharp waste after the drug administration and no risk of transmission of blood-borne diseases.
- Microneedles effectively resolve all issues related to hypodermic needles, such as needlestick injuries, needle phobia, sharp waste, and the spread of blood-borne pathogens.
- With the advance in production technologies, microneedles could be manufactured at a low cost.
- When therapeutic agents are loaded in solid form in coated, dissolving, and swelling microneedles, the drug is more thermostable, thus preventing the requirement for cold-chain storage and transportation.
- Microneedles' length and penetration depth could be controlled to achieve targeted drug delivery to specific skin layers.
- The size and structure of the microneedle array could be customized to target large skin regions.
- Microneedles products provide the capacity to deliver multiple drugs simultaneously.
- The geometry, dimension, density, and material of microneedles could be changed to meet the requirement of different patient populations.
- Microneedles could be combined with other enhancement technologies to increase transdermal drug delivery further.

Disadvantages of microneedles

- Microneedles, especially coated, dissolving microneedles, could deliver a very limited dose (a few milligrams per kilogram body weight) up to a maximum of 1 mg drug transdermally.
- Microneedles could have insufficient robustness and mechanical strength to penetrate the skin barrier. When microneedle insertion force exceeds the tensile force of microneedles, these mechanically weak microneedles could be fractured or broken during skin insertion.
- Skin viscoelasticity could significantly impact microneedle penetration depth, especially for blunt and short microneedles.
- Due to skin variables (thickness, robustness, and viscoelasticity), achieving consistent and reproducible microneedle penetration depth for the required dose is challenging. Hence, an applicator is generally used to assist with microneedle insertion.
- The adverse effects of dissolved or degraded polymeric matrix in the skin should be thoroughly investigated.

- Some harsh fabrication conditions (high temperature, vacuum, etc.) could be harmful to thermosensitive drugs.
- A reverse correlation between drug load and microneedle mechanical strength has been reported. The higher the drug quantity loaded, the weaker the microneedle structure.
- Microneedle insertion requires extended application time as compared to hypodermic injection.
- Microneedles could only be fabricated from a range of biocompatible, biodegradable materials.
- The needle bore blockage has been observed frequently with hollow microneedles, affecting drug delivery and needle penetrability.
- Repetitive application of microneedles could lead to scar formation on the treatment site of the skin.
- Microneedles require a complicated controlled fabrication process.
- Microneedles application provides lower dose accuracy than hypodermic needle injections.
- It is challenging to apply microneedles at non-conformal angles. If microneedles are not inserted perpendicularly to the skin surface, this could result in dose escape and a change in skin penetration depth.
- Quality criteria of microneedle products have to be standardized to facilitate large-scale manufacturing. There is a lack of GMP manufacturing standards.
- There is a lack or absence of regulatory guidance for microneedle products, especially hollow, coated, dissolving, and swelling microneedles.
- There is currently a shortage of investment from pharmaceutical companies.

1.4.7 Magnetophoresis

Magnetophoresis enhances the penetration and passage of various compounds through biological barriers by generating a magnetic field [225]. Magnetic field intensity directly correlates with the magnitude of the increase in magnetophoretic drug delivery [225]. Research groups have reported the usage of a fixed and alternating magnetic field to improve the permeation of various compounds such as benzoic acid, salbutamol sulfate, terbutaline sulfate, and magnetic resonance imaging agents. The magnetism-based system could provide a controlled or pulsatile mode of drug delivery [226]. Also, magnetite has been encapsulated into the particulate system for effective drug delivery or imaging. Furthermore, the application of a magnetic field enables the targeted delivery of magnetoliposomes and nanoparticles to specific tissues [227]. Thus, magnetophoresis has been known as an efficient method for targeted therapies [228].

1.4.8 Pressure Waves

Pressure waves or compression waves are generated by intense laser radiation for a very short duration (nanoseconds to a few microseconds) to transiently and reversibly permeabilize the stratum corneum layer to enhance transdermal drug delivery, especially macromolecules. Pressure waves do not directly drive drugs into the skin; instead, they disrupt the skin structure to facilitate drug diffusion using concentration gradient as the driving force. The amplitude of pressure waves is hundreds of atmospheres, producing skin inter-action different from ultrasound treatment [229]. Features of pressure waves, including peak pressure, rise time, and duration, are dependent on laser parameters (wavelength, pulse duration, and fluency) and optical and mechanical properties of target materials. The conversion from light to mechanical energy is defined as the coupling coefficient, which could be used to estimate the peak pressure.

Pressure waves offer several noticeable advantages. The therapy produces no pain or discomfort, thus enhancing patient acceptability and compliance. Furthermore, treated skin can be recovered rapidly to mitigate any biosafety risk. The skin recovery can be eas-ily adjusted by changing the pressure wave parameters or using chemical enhancers, thus enabling effective control of transdermal drug delivery. This device also offers accurate control over the ablated skin depth and an excellent definition of ablated range [230]. A sin-gle pressure wave has been found to be sufficient to permeabilize the stratum corneum to enhance the skin permeation of macromolecules such as human σ-aminolevulinic acid (ALA) allergen and insulin [231].

1.4.9 Thermal Poration

Thermal poration or thermophoresis generates localized heat to selectively ablate certain areas in the stratum corneum layer to create micrometer-sized channels (50–100 µm diam-eter) in the skin to increase skin permeability [10, 19]. In principle, this therapy uses high temperatures (>100°C) to heat and vaporize skin keratin. The skin's thermal exposure lasts for a very short time (microseconds), producing a temperature gradient to selectively ablate the stratum corneum layer without damaging deeper underlying tissue. Thermal poration has effectively enhanced the transdermal delivery of various compounds ranging from small molecules to macromolecules such as proteins, DNA, and vaccines [232–236]. Since the level of skin ablation is strongly correlated to locally elevated temperature, the drug delivery could be controlled and tailored. Compared to other procedures, such as micro-dermabrasion, chemical therapy, or tape stripping, this strategy provides more precise and consistent results. Also, thermal poration's advantage lies in its minimal risk of pain, bleeding, skin irritation, or infection.

Depending on the thermal energy source, thermal ablation could be produced by laser or radiofrequency [233, 235]. For radiofrequency thermal poration, an array of microneedle-resembling metallic electrodes is placed on the skin to apply high-frequency (100–500 kHz) electrical current into the skin for a short time (a few seconds) to create ionic vibrations and localized heat in certain skin areas. This radiofrequency-induced heat leads to water evaporation and ablation of skin tissue under the filaments, thereby creating micrometer-sized channels (50 µm depth) in the skin filled with interstitial skin fluid. Several pieces of research have revealed that the ablated skin depth, size, and density of microchan-nels are proportional to drug delivery. The drug permeation profile could be controlled by changing the ablation parameters. Furthermore, this device is inexpensive and dis-posable, thus enhancing its manufacturability and usability [97]. Radiofrequency could provide sustained and enhanced delivery of a wide variety of therapeutic agents, espe-cially hydrophilic drugs and macromolecules. In addition to radiofrequency, laser light energy could be utilized as a source of thermal energy (photothermal effects). Laser light energy is absorbed by water and pigment in the skin, causing water excitation and explo-sive evaporation to selectively ablate predetermined skin areas without deep penetration into the underlying skin layer to cause pain, bleeding, or skin irritation. The degree of skin ablation, which is strongly correlated to the transdermal drug delivery profile, could be adjusted by altering various factors, including laser wavelength, pulse length, pulse number, tissue thickness, skin hydration level, absorption coefficient, and exposure duration. This painless and minimally invasive laser treatment causes controlled and minimal damage to the skin tissue, which fully recovers after a few days. The laser skin ablation leads to substantial enhancement in transdermal drug delivery and an increase in the bioavailability of various compounds, including lipophilic, hydrophilic drugs and macromolecules (i.e., peptides, proteins, vaccines, DNA, etc.) [237, 238]. The treatment also results in a shorter lag time and rapid delivery onset [239]. Laser ablation enables a reduction in the drug dose and the drug's deep penetration into underlying skin layers. However, some drawbacks have been noted, such as safety concerns about laser therapy and large specialized laser device which is inappropriate for personal use. Various laser types with different wavelengths and mechanisms have been developed, such as ruby (wavelength of 694 nm), yttrium-scandium-gallium-garnet (wavelength of 2,790 nm), erbium: yttrium-gallium-garnet (Er: YAG, the wavelength of 2,940 nm), neodymium-doped yttrium-gallium-garnet (Nd: YAG, wavelengths of 355, 532, 1,064, and 1,320 nm), and CO_2 (wavelength of 10,600 nm) lasers [240].

1.4.10 Microwave-assisted Transdermal Delivery

Recently, the microwave has received a great deal of attention as a novel technology to fluidize the skin epidermis and enhance transdermal drug delivery [241–243]. Microwave enables the movement of the lipid structure of the stratum corneum into the structureless domains [243, 244]. In general, low-intensity microwave (1 mV) is employed in skin delivery. This safe technique poses no risk of skin heating, electrical shock, or tissue damage, as illustrated in an animal study [243]. The synergistic effect of nanomedicine and microwave treatment has been demonstrated [245, 246]. The microwave was found to modify skin structure (primarily the ceramide content homogeneity) to improve skin delivery of 5-fluorouracil-encapsulated chitosan nanoparticles [245]. Harjoh et al. reported that microwaves (2,450 MHz/1 mW) facilitated greater transdermal insulin permeation than fatty acids (i.e., oleic acid and linoleic acid). Microwave treatment caused a rearrangement in the epidermal lipid/protein regions to create intercellular hydrophilic pores, thus facilitating insulin delivery and a sustained decrease in blood glucose levels *in vivo*. However, the combination of microwave and fatty acids was found to reduce the skin permeability of insulin [247]. Interestingly, the combination of microwave and penetration enhancers (pectin and pectin-oleic acid gels) hindered transdermal drug permeation [241]. Shen and colleagues reported a markedly enhanced rheumatoid arthritis treatment using methotrexate-loaded thermal-responsible flexible liposome and microwave-induced hyperthermia [248]. Microwave-based technology is regarded as a promising physical enhancement platform [249]. Further research, clinical studies, and regulatory assessment are required to explore its application and translation in the transdermal field.

1.5 Conclusion

Recently, transdermal drug delivery has attracted a lot of attention due to its several advantages over conventional oral and parenteral administration, such as avoidance of first-pass hepatic metabolism, enhanced bioavailability, improved patient compliance, etc. The US FDA has approved more than 20 transdermal products; among those, the majority of the products function based on passive diffusion. Various physical enhancement technologies have been developed to enhance transdermal drug delivery by orders of magnitude effectively. Each technology has its noted advantages and disadvantages. As a result of their dependence on the permeants' physicochemical characteristics, enhancement methods are often used only after extensive testing. The development of these novel technologies extends the application range of transdermal delivery to inappropriate transdermal candidates such as hydrophilic drugs, macromolecules, proteins, peptides, and vaccines, thus offering effective treatment options for various diseases. In the future, there will be significant unmet clinical needs, room for technological improvement, and commercialization potential for the combination of medicines, devices, artificial intelligence, and 3D printing for transdermal application.

References

[1] Ramadon D, McCrudden MTC, Courtenay AJ, et al. Enhancement strategies for transdermal drug delivery systems: current trends and applications. Drug Deliv Transl Res. 2022;12:758–791.

[2] Boer M, Duchnik E, Maleszka R, et al. Structural and biophysical characteristics of human skin in maintaining proper epidermal barrier function. Adv Dermatol Allergol. 2016;33:1–5.

[3] Kolarsick PAJ, Kolarsick MA, Goodwin C. Anatomy and physiology of the skin. J Dermatol Nurses Assoc. 2011;3:203–213.

[4] Dale Wilson B, Moon S, Armstrong F. Comprehensive review of ultraviolet radiation and the current status on sunscreens. J Clin Aesthetic Dermatol. 2012;5:18–23.

[5] Romanovsky AA. Skin temperature: its role in thermoregulation. Acta Physiol. 2014;210:498–507.

[6] Baker LB. Physiology of sweat gland function: the roles of sweating and sweat composition in human health. Temp Multidiscip Biomed J. 2019;6:211–259.

[7] Zhou S-S, Li D, Zhou Y-M, et al. The skin function: a factor of anti-metabolic syndrome. Diabetol Metab Syndr. 2012;4:15.

[8] Prausnitz MR, Langer R. Transdermal drug delivery. Nat Biotechnol. 2008;26:1261–1268.

[9] Sharma G, Alle M, Chakraborty C, et al. Strategies for transdermal drug delivery against bone disorders: a preclinical and clinical update. J Control Release. 2021;336:375–395.

[10] Zaid Alkilani A, McCrudden MT, Donnelly RF. Transdermal drug delivery: innovative pharmaceutical developments based on disruption of the barrier properties of the stratum corneum. Pharmaceutics. 2015;7:438–470.

[11] Nemes Z, Steinert PM. Bricks and mortar of the epidermal barrier. Exp Mol Med. 1999; 31:5–19.

[12] Benson HA. Transdermal drug delivery: penetration enhancement techniques. Curr Drug Deliv. 2005;2:23–33.

[13] Eckhart L, Lippens S, Tschachler E, et al. Cell death by cornification. Biochim Biophys Acta. 2013;1833:3471–3480.

[14] Goldstein AM, Abramovits W. Ceramides and the stratum corneum: structure, function, and new methods to promote repair. Int J Dermatol. 2003;42:256–259.

[15] Hamanaka S, Hara M, Nishio H, et al. Human epidermal glucosylceramides are major precursors of stratum corneum ceramides. J Invest Dermatol. 2002;119:416–423.

[16] Pappas A. Epidermal surface lipids. Dermatoendocrinol. 2009;1:72–76.

[17] Asbill CS, El-Kattan AF, Michniak B. Enhancement of transdermal drug delivery: chemical and physical approaches. Crit Rev Ther Drug Carrier Syst. 2000;17:621–658.

[18] Menon GK. New insights into skin structure: scratching the surface. Adv Drug Deliv Rev. 2002;54 Suppl 1:S3–S17.

[19] Prausnitz MR, Mitragotri S, Langer R. Current status and future potential of transdermal drug delivery. Nat Rev Drug Discov. 2004;3:115–124.

[20] Böhling A, Bielfeldt S, Himmelmann A, et al. Comparison of the stratum corneum thickness measured in vivo with confocal Raman spectroscopy and confocal reflectance microscopy. Skin Res Technol. 2014;20:50–57.

[21] Elias PM, Feingold KR. Coordinate regulation of epidermal differentiation and barrier homeostasis. Skin Pharmacol Appl Skin Physiol. 2001;14 Suppl 1:28–34.

[22] Russell LM, Wiedersberg S, Delgado-Charro MB. The determination of stratum corneum thickness: an alternative approach. Eur J Pharm Biopharm. 2008;69:861–870.

[23] Wickett RR, Visscher MO. Structure and function of the epidermal barrier. Am J Infect Control. 2006;34:S98–S110.

[24] Jaitley S, Saraswathi T. Pathophysiology of langerhans cells. J Oral Maxillofac Pathol JOMFP. 2012;16:239–244.

[25] Matsui T, Amagai M. Dissecting the formation, structure and barrier function of the stratum corneum. Int Immunol. 2015;27:269–280.

[26] Abraham J, Mathew S. Merkel cells: a collective review of current concepts. Int J Appl Basic Med Res. 2019;9:9–13.

[27] Cichorek M, Wachulska M, Stasiewicz A, et al. Skin melanocytes: biology and development. Adv Dermatol Allergol. 2013;30:30–41.

[28] Jepps OG, Dancik Y, Anissimov YG, et al. Modeling the human skin barrier-towards a better understanding of dermal absorption. Adv Drug Deliv Rev. 2013;65:152–168.

[29] Nguyen AV, Soulika AM. The dynamics of the skin's immune system. Int J Mol Sci. 2019;20:1811.

[30] Shirshin EA, Gurfinkel YI, Priezzhev AV, et al. Two-photon autofluorescence lifetime imaging of human skin papillary dermis in vivo: assessment of blood capillaries and structural proteins localization. Sci Rep. 2017;7:1171.

[31] Sorrell JM, Caplan AI. Fibroblast heterogeneity: more than skin deep. J Cell Sci. 2004;117:667–675.

[32] Igarashi T, Nishino K, Nayar SK. The appearance of human skin: a survey. Found Trends Comput Graph Vis. 2007;3:1–95.

[33] Andrews SN, Jeong E, Prausnitz MR. Transdermal delivery of molecules is limited by full epidermis, not just stratum corneum. Pharm Res. 2013;30:1099–1109.

[34] Lovászi M, Szegedi A, Zouboulis CC, et al. Sebaceous-immunobiology is orchestrated by sebum lipids. Dermatoendocrinol. 2017;9:e1375636.

[35] Singh S, Singh J. Transdermal drug delivery by passive diffusion and iontophoresis: a review. Med Res Rev. 1993;13:569–621.

[36] Dj T. Biochemistry of human skin-our brain on the outside. Chem Soc Rev. 2006;35. [Internet] [cited 2022 Aug 7]. Available from: https://pubmed.ncbi.nlm.nih.gov/16365642/.

[37] Wong R, Geyer S, Weninger W, et al. The dynamic anatomy and patterning of skin. Exp Dermatol. 2016;25:92–98.

[38] Christine B, Patrick MB, Georg S. Immune functions of the skin. Clin Dermatol. 2011;29:360–376.

[39] Kupper TS, Fuhlbrigge RC. Immune surveillance in the skin: mechanisms and clinical consequences. Nat Rev Immunol. 2004;4:211–222.

[40] Bal SM, Ding Z, van Riet E, et al. Advances in transcutaneous vaccine delivery: do all ways lead to Rome? J Control Release. 2010;148:266–282.

[41] Combadière B, Mahé B. Particle-based vaccines for transcutaneous vaccination. Comp Immunol Microbiol Infect Dis. 2008;31:293–315.

[42] Warger T, Schild H, Rechtsteiner G. Initiation of adaptive immune responses by transcutaneous immunization. Immunol Lett. 2007;109:13–20.

[43] Koutsonanos DG, Esser ES, McMaster SR, et al. Enhanced immune responses by skin vaccination with influenza subunit vaccine in young hosts. Vaccine. 2015;33:4675–4682.

[44] Huang C-M. Topical vaccination: the skin as a unique portal to adaptive immune responses. Semin Immunopathol. 2007;29:71–80.

[45] Kendall M. Engineering of needle-free physical methods to target epidermal cells for DNA vaccination. Vaccine. 2006;24:4651–4656.

[46] Lambert PH, Laurent PE. Intradermal vaccine delivery: will new delivery systems transform vaccine administration? Vaccine. 2008;26:3197–3208.

[47] Steinman RM, Banchereau J. Taking dendritic cells into medicine. Nature. 2007;449:419–426.

[48] Sugita K, Kabashima K, Atarashi K, et al. Innate immunity mediated by epidermal keratino-cytes promotes acquired immunity involving Langerhans cells and T cells in the skin. Clin Exp Immunol. 2007;147:176–183.

[49] Valladeau J, Saeland S. Cutaneous dendritic cells. Semin Immunol. 2005;17:273–283.

[50] Bajaj S, Whiteman A, Brandner B. Transdermal drug delivery in pain management. Contin Educ Anaesth Crit Care Pain. 2011;11:39–43.

[51] Abrams LS, Skee DM, Natarajan J, et al. Pharmacokinetics of a contraceptive patch (Evra™/ Ortho Evra™) containing norelgestromin and ethinyloestradiol at four application sites. Br J Clin Pharmacol. 2002;53:141–146.

[52] Frampton JE. Rotigotine transdermal patch: a review in Parkinson's disease. CNS Drugs. 2019;33:707–718.

[53] Pastore MN, Kalia YN, Horstmann M, et al. Transdermal patches: history, development and pharmacology. Br J Pharmacol. 2015;172:2179–2209.

[54] Indermun S, Luttge R, Choonara YE, et al. Current advances in the fabrication of microneedles for transdermal delivery. J Control Release. 2014;185:130–138.

[55] Margetts L, Sawyer R. Transdermal drug delivery: principles and opioid therapy. Contin Educ Anaesth Crit Care Pain. 2007;7:171–176.

[56] Paudel KS, Milewski M, Swadley CL, et al. Challenges and opportunities in dermal/transder-mal delivery. Ther Deliv. 2010;1:109–131.

[57] Alexander A, Dwivedi S, Giri TK, et al. Approaches for breaking the barriers of drug perme-ation through transdermal drug delivery. J Control Release. 2012;164:26–40.

[58] Han T, Das DB. Potential of combined ultrasound and microneedles for enhanced transdermal drug permeation: a review. Eur J Pharm Biopharm. 2015;89:312–328.

[59] Chopda G. Transdermal drug delivery systems: a review. Pharm Rev. 2006;4.

[60] Subedi RK, Oh SY, Chun M-K, et al. Recent advances in transdermal drug delivery. Arch Pharm Res. 2010;33:339–351.

[61] Tanner T, Marks R. Delivering drugs by the transdermal route: review and comment. Skin Res Technol. 2008;14:249–260.

[62] Singhal M, Lapteva M, Kalia YN. Formulation challenges for 21st century topical and trans-dermal delivery systems. Expert Opin Drug Deliv. 2017;14:705–708.

[63] Barbero AM, Frasch HF. Transcellular route of diffusion through stratum corneum: results from finite element models. J Pharm Sci. 2006;95:2186–2194.

[64] Marrink SJ, Berendsen HJ. Permeation process of small molecules across lipid membranes studied by molecular dynamics simulations. J Phys Chem. 1996;100:16729–16738.

[65] Haque T, Talukder MMU. Chemical enhancer: a simplistic way to modulate barrier function of the stratum corneum. Adv Pharm Bull. 2018;8:169–179.

[66] Barry BW. Novel mechanisms and devices to enable successful transdermal drug delivery. Eur J Pharm Sci. 2001;14:101–114.

[67] Gazerani P, Arendt-Nielsen L. Cutaneous vasomotor reactions in response to controlled heat applied on various body regions of healthy humans: evaluation of time course and application parameters. Int J Physiol Pathophysiol Pharmacol. 2011;3:202–209.

[68] Singh I, Morris AP. Performance of transdermal therapeutic systems: effects of biological fac-tors. Int J Pharm Investig. 2011;1:4–9.

[69] Verma A, Jain A, Hurkat P, et al. Transfollicular drug delivery: current perspectives. Res Rep Transdermal Drug Deliv. 2016;5:1–17.

[70] Zhai H, Maibach HI. Effects of skin occlusion on percutaneous absorption: an overview. Skin Pharmacol Appl Skin Physiol. 2001;14:1–10.

[71] Chandrashekar NS, Shobha Rani RH. Physicochemical and pharmacokinetic parameters in drug selection and loading for transdermal drug delivery. Indian J Pharm Sci. 2008;70:94–96.

[72] Funke AP, Schiller R, Motzkus HW, et al. Transdermal delivery of highly lipophilic drugs: in vitro fluxes of antiestrogens, permeation enhancers, and solvents from liquid formulations. Pharm Res. 2002;19:661–668.

[73] Williams A. Transdermal and topical drug delivery: from theory to clinical practice. London, UK: Pharmaceutical Press; 2003.

[74] Brown MB, Martin GP, Jones SA, et al. Dermal and transdermal drug delivery systems: current and future prospects. Drug Deliv. 2006;13:175–187.

[75] Gujjar M, Banga AK. Iontophoretic and microneedle mediated transdermal delivery of glycopyrrolate. Pharmaceutics. 2014;6:663–671.

[76] Bhoyar N, Giri TK, Tripathi DK, et al. Recent advances in novel drug delivery system through gels: review. J Pharm Allied Health Sci. 2012;2:21.

[77] N'Da DD. Prodrug strategies for enhancing the percutaneous absorption of drugs. Molecules. 2014;19:20780–20807.

[78] Sachdeva VK, Banga A. Microneedles and their applications. Recent Pat Drug Deliv Formul. 2011;5:95–132.

[79] Watkinson AC. A commentary on transdermal drug delivery systems in clinical trials. J Pharm Sci. 2013;102:3082–3088.

[80] Akhtar N, Singh V, Yusuf M, et al. Non-invasive drug delivery technology: development and current status of transdermal drug delivery devices, techniques and biomedical applications. Biomed Eng. 2020;65:243–272.

[81] Pires LR, Vinayakumar KB, Turos M, et al. A perspective on microneedle-based drug delivery and diagnostics in paediatrics. J Pers Med. 2019;9:E49.

[82] Ruby PK, Pathak SM, Aggarwal D. Critical attributes of transdermal drug delivery system (TDDS)-a generic product development review. Drug Dev Ind Pharm. 2014;40:1421–1428.

[83] Brogden NK, Milewski M, Ghosh P, et al. Diclofenac delays micropore closure following microneedle treatment in human subjects. J Control Release. 2012;163:220–229.

[84] Kalluri H, Banga AK. Formation and closure of microchannels in skin following microporation. Pharm Res. 2011;28:82–94.

[85] Langer R. Transdermal drug delivery: past progress, current status, and future prospects. Adv Drug Deliv Rev. 2004;56:557–558.

[86] Xie Y, Xu B, Gao Y. Controlled transdermal delivery of model drug compounds by MEMS microneedle array. Nanomedicine Nanotechnol Biol Med. 2005;1:184–190.

[87] Sachdeva V, Banga AK. Skin deep. Pharm Manufac Pack Sourcer. 2009;45:17–24.

[88] Ball AM, Smith KM. Optimizing transdermal drug therapy. Am J Health Syst Pharm. 2008;65:1337–1346.

[89] Marieb EN, Hoehn K. Human anatomy & physiology. London: Pearson Education; 2007.

[90] McAllister DV, Allen MG, Prausnitz MR. Microfabricated microneedles for gene and drug delivery. Annu Rev Biomed Eng. 2000;2:289–313.

[91] Prausnitz MR. Microneedles for transdermal drug delivery. Adv Drug Deliv Rev. 2004;56:581–587.

[92] Lutton REM, Moore J, Larrañeta E, et al. Microneedle characterisation: the need for universal acceptance criteria and GMP specifications when moving towards commercialisation. Drug Deliv Transl Res. 2015;5:313–331.

[93] Alkilani AZ, Nasereddin J, Hamed R, et al. Beneath the skin: a review of current trends and future prospects of transdermal drug delivery systems. Pharmaceutics. 2022;14:1152.

[94] Watkinson AC, Kearney M-C, Quinn HL, et al. Future of the transdermal drug delivery market-have we barely touched the surface? Expert Opin Drug Deliv. 2016;13:523–532.

[95] Caffarel-Salvador E, Donnelly RF. Transdermal drug delivery mediated by microneedle arrays: innovations and barriers to success. Curr Pharm Des. 2016;22:1105–1117.

[96] Parhi R, Suresh P, Patnaik S. Physical means of stratum corneum barrier manipulation to enhance transdermal drug delivery. Curr Drug Deliv. 2015;12:122–138.

[97] Parhi R, Mandru A. Enhancement of skin permeability with thermal ablation techniques: concept to commercial products. Drug Deliv Transl Res. 2021;11:817–841.

[98] Sun F, Anderson R, Aguilar G. Stratum corneum permeation and percutaneous drug delivery of hydrophilic molecules enhanced by cryopneumatic and photopneumatic technologies. J Drugs Dermatol. 2010;9:1528–1530.

[99] Alexiades M. Laser and light-based treatments of acne and acne scarring. Clin Dermatol. 2017;35:183–189.

[100] Rajabi-Estarabadi A, Choragudi S, Camacho I, et al. Effectiveness of photopneumatic technology: a descriptive review of the literature. Lasers Med Sci. 2018;33:1631–1637.

[101] Omi T. Photopneumatic technology in acne treatment and skin rejuvenation: histological assessment. Laser Ther. 2012;21:113–123.

[102] Wanitphakdeedecha R, Tanzi EL, Alster TS. Photopneumatic therapy for the treatment of acne. J Drugs Dermatol JDD. 2009;8:239–241.

[103] Mitragotri S, Kost J. Low-frequency sonophoresis: a review. Adv Drug Deliv Rev. 2004;56:589–601.

[104] Park D, Park H, Seo J, et al. Sonophoresis in transdermal drug deliverys. Ultrasonics. 2014;54:56–65.

[105] Azagury A, Khoury L, Enden G, et al. Ultrasound mediated transdermal drug delivery. Adv Drug Deliv Rev. 2014;72:127–143.

[106] De Cock I, Zagato E, Braeckmans K, et al. Ultrasound and microbubble mediated drug delivery: acoustic pressure as determinant for uptake via membrane pores or endocytosis. J Control Release. 2015;197:20–28.

[107] Park D, Song G, Jo Y, et al. Sonophoresis using ultrasound contrast agents: dependence on concentration. PLoS One. 2016;11:e0157707.

[108] Kumar R, Philip A. Modified transdermal technologies: breaking the barriers of drug permeation via the skin. Trop J Pharm Res. 2007;6:633–644.

[109] Machet L, Boucaud A. Phonophoresis: efficiency, mechanisms and skin tolerance. Int J Pharm. 2002;243:1–15.

[110] Merino G, Kalia YN, Guy RH. Ultrasound-enhanced transdermal transport. J Pharm Sci. 2003;92:1125–1137.

[111] Escobar-Chávez JJ, Bonilla-Martínez D, Villegas-González MA, et al. The use of sonophoresis in the administration of drugs throughout the skin. J Pharm Sci. 2009;12:88–115.

[112] Jeong WY, Kwon M, Choi HE, et al. Recent advances in transdermal drug delivery systems: a review. Biomater Res. 2021;25:24.

[113] Mitragotri S. Healing sound: the use of ultrasound in drug delivery and other therapeutic applications. Nat Rev Drug Discov. 2005;4:255–260.

[114] Herwadkar A, Sachdeva V, Taylor LF, et al. Low frequency sonophoresis mediated transdermal and intradermal delivery of ketoprofen. Int J Pharm. 2012;423:289–296.

[115] McElnay JC, Kennedy TA, Harland R. The influence of ultrasound on the percutaneous absorption of fluocinolone acetonide. Int J Pharm. 1987;40:105–110.

[116] Argenziano M, Banche G, Luganini A, et al. Vancomycin-loaded nanobubbles: a new platform for controlled antibiotic delivery against methicillin-resistant Staphylococcus aureus infections. Int J Pharm. 2017;523:176–188.

[117] Baji S, Hegde AR, Kulkarni M, et al. Skin permeation of gemcitabine hydrochloride by passive diffusion, iontophoresis and sonophoresis: in vitro and in vivo evaluations. J Drug Deliv Sci Technol. 2018;47:49–54.

[118] Mitragotri S, Blankschtein D, Langer R. Ultrasound-mediated transdermal protein delivery. Sci. 1995;269:850.

[119] Mitragotri S, Kost J. Transdermal delivery of heparin and low-molecular weight heparin using low-frequency ultrasound. Pharm Res. 2001;18:1151–1156.

[120] Ita K. Percutaneous transport of psychotropic agents. J Drug Deliv Sci Technol. 2017;39:247–259.

[121] Wang Y, Zeng L, Song W, et al. Influencing factors and drug application of iontophoresis in transdermal drug delivery: an overview of recent progress. Drug Deliv Transl Res. 2021;1–12.

[122] Dixit N, Bali V, Baboota S, et al. Iontophoresis-an approach for controlled drug delivery: a review. Curr Drug Deliv. 2007;4:1–10.

[123] Batheja P, Priya B, Thakur R, et al. Transdermal iontophoresis. Expert Opin Drug Deliv. 2006;3:127–138.

[124] Giri TK, Chakrabarty S, Ghosh B. Non-invasive extraction of gabapentin for therapeutic drug monitoring by reverse iontophoresis: effect of pH, ionic strength, and polyethylene glycol 400 in the receiving medium. Curr Pharm Anal. 2019;15:632–639.

[125] Saepang K, Li SK, Chantasart D. Effect of pH on iontophoretic transport of pramipexole dihydrochloride across human epidermal membrane. Pharm Res. 2021;38:657–668.

[126] Zuo J, Du L, Li M, et al. Transdermal enhancement effect and mechanism of iontophoresis for non-steroidal anti-inflammatory drugs. Int J Pharm. 2014;466:76–82.

[127] Chen K, Puri V, Michniak-Kohn B. Iontophoresis to overcome the challenge of nail permeation: considerations and optimizations for successful ungual drug delivery. AAPS J. 2021;23:1–15.

[128] Khan A, Yasir M, Asif M, et al. Iontophoretic drug delivery: history and applications. J Appl Pharm Sci. 2011;11–24.

[129] Schoellhammer CM, Blankschtein D, Langer R. Skin permeabilization for transdermal drug delivery: recent advances and future prospects. Expert Opin Drug Deliv. 2014;11:393–407.

[130] Vranić E. Iontophoresis: fundamentals, developments and application. Bosn J Basic Med Sci. 2003;3:54–58.

[131] Perez VL, Wirostko B, Korenfeld M, et al. Ophthalmic drug delivery using iontophoresis: recent clinical applications. J Ocul Pharmacol Ther. 2020;36:75–87.

[132] Roustit M, Blaise S, Cracowski J-L. Trials and tribulations of skin iontophoresis in therapeutics. Br J Clin Pharmacol. 2014;77:63–71.

[133] Naik A, Kalia YN, Guy RH. Transdermal drug delivery: overcoming the skin's barrier function. Pharm Sci Technol Today. 2000;3:318–326.

[134] Krishnan G, Roberts MS, Grice J, et al. Iontophoretic skin permeation of peptides: an investigation into the influence of molecular properties, iontophoretic conditions and formulation parameters. Drug Deliv Transl Res. 2014;4:222–232.

[135] Karpiński TM. Selected medicines used in iontophoresis. Pharmaceutics. 2018;10:204.

[136] Fatima T, Ajjarapu S, Shankar VK, et al. Topical pilocarpine formulation for diagnosis of cystic fibrosis. J Pharm Sci. 2020;109:1747–1751.

[137] Yengin C, Kilinc E, Der FG, et al. Optimization of extraction parameters of reverse iontophoretic determination of blood glucose in an artificial skin model. Curr Anal Chem. 2020;16:722–737.

[138] Takeuchi I, Fukuda K, Kobayashi S, et al. Transdermal delivery of estradiol-loaded PLGA nanoparticles using iontophoresis for treatment of osteoporosis. Biomed Mater Eng. 2016;27:475–483.

[139] Grond S, Radbruch L, Lehmann KA. Clinical pharmacokinetics of transdermal opioids: focus on transdermal fentanyl. Clin Pharmacokinet. 2000;38:59–89.

[140] Power I. Fentanyl HCl iontophoretic transdermal system (ITS): clinical application of iontophoretic technology in the management of acute postoperative pain. Br J Anaesth. 2007;98:4–11.

[141] Puri A, Murnane KS, Blough BE, et al. Effects of chemical and physical enhancement techniques on transdermal delivery of 3-fluoroamphetamine hydrochloride. Int J Pharm. 2017;528:452–462.

[142] Calatayud-Pascual MA, Balaguer-Fernández C, Serna-Jiménez CE, et al. Effect of iontophoresis on in vitro transdermal absorption of almotriptan. Int J Pharm. 2011;416:189–194.

[143] Cázares-Delgadillo J, Ganem-Rondero A, Quintanar-Guerrero D, et al. Using transdermal iontophoresis to increase granisetron delivery across skin in vitro and in vivo: effect of experimental conditions and a comparison with other enhancement strategies. Eur J Pharm Sci. 2010;39:387–393.

[144] Fang J-Y, Huang Y-B, Wu P-C, et al. Transdermal iontophoresis of sodium nonivamide acetate I. Consideration of electrical and chemical factors. Int J Pharm. 1996;143:47–58.

[145] Saluja S, Kasha PC, Paturi J, et al. A novel electronic skin patch for delivery and pharmacokinetic evaluation of donepezil following transdermal iontophoresis. Int J Pharm. 2013;453:395–399.

[146] Pillai O, Borkute SD, Sivaprasad N, et al. Transdermal iontophoresis of insulin. II. Physicochemical considerations. Int J Pharm. 2003;254:271–280.

[147] Ellens H, Lai Z, Marcello J, et al. Transdermal iontophoretic delivery of [3 H] GHRP in rats. Int J Pharm. 1997;159:1–11.

[148] Banga AK. Electrically assisted transdermal and topical drug delivery. London: CRC Press; 1998.

[149] Lobo S, Yan G. Improving the direct penetration into tissues underneath the skin with iontophoresis delivery of a ketoprofen cationic prodrug. Int J Pharm. 2018;535:228–236.

[150] Miller KA, Balakrishnan G, Eichbauer G, et al. 1% lidocaine injection, EMLA cream, or "numby stuff" for topical analgesia associated with peripheral intravenous cannulation. AANA J. 2001;69:185–187.

[151] Lemke J, Sardariani E, Phipps JB, et al. Fentanyl iontophoretic transdermal system (IONSYS(®)) can be safely used in the hospital environment with X-rays, computerized tomography and radiofrequency identification devices. Adv Ther. 2016;33:1649–1659.

[152] Vikelis M, Mitsikostas DD, Rapoport AM. Sumatriptan iontophoretic transdermal system for the acute treatment of migraine. Pain Manag. 2014;4:123–128.

[153] Scott JA, Banga AK. Cosmetic devices based on active transdermal technologies. Ther Deliv. 2015;6:1089–1099.

[154] Abd-Elghany AA, Mohamad EA. Ex-vivo transdermal delivery of Annona squamosa entrapped in niosomes by electroporation. J Radiat Res Appl Sci. 2020;13:164–173.

[155] Morrow DIJ, McCarron PA, Woolfson AD, et al. Innovative strategies for enhancing topical and transdermal drug delivery. Open Drug Deliv J;1. [Internet].//[cited 2022 Aug 7]. Available from: https://benthamopen.com/ABSTRACT/TODDJ-1-36.

[156] Kc S, Jia-You F, Jhi-Joung W, et al. Transdermal delivery of nalbuphine and its prodrugs by electroporation. Eur J Pharm Sci. 2003;18:63–70.

[157] Prausnitz MR, Pliquett U, Langer R, et al. Rapid temporal control of transdermal drug delivery by electroporation. Pharm Res. 1994;11:1834–1837.

[158] Charoo NA, Rahman Z, Repka MA, et al. Electroporation: an avenue for transdermal drug delivery. Curr Drug Deliv. 2010;7:125–136.

[159] Demiryurek Y, Nickaeen M, Zheng M, et al. Transport, resealing, and re-poration dynamics of two-pulse electroporation-mediated molecular delivery. Biochim Biophys Acta BBA—Biomembr. 2015;1848:1706–1714.

[160] Denet A-R, Vanbever R, Préat V. Skin electroporation for transdermal and topical delivery. Adv Drug Deliv Rev. 2004;56:659–674.

[161] Mori K, Hasegawa T, Sato S, et al. Effect of electric field on the enhanced skin permeation of drugs by electroporation. J Control Release. 2003;90:171–179.

[162] Murthy SN, Sen A, Zhao Y-L, et al. Temperature influences the postelectroporation permeability state of the skin. J Pharm Sci. 2004;93:908–915.

[163] Ita K. Perspectives on Transdermal Electroporation. Pharmaceutics. 2016;8:9.

[164] Gill KS, Fernandes P, Bird B, et al. Combination of electroporation delivered metabolic modulators with low-dose chemotherapy in osteosarcoma. Oncotarget. 2018;9:31473–31489.

[165] Hartmann P, Butt E, Fehér Á, et al. Electroporation-enhanced transdermal diclofenac sodium delivery into the knee joint in a rat model of acute arthritis. Drug Des Devel Ther. 2018;12:1917–1930.

[166] Huang D, Zhao D, Wang X, et al. Efficient delivery of nucleic acid molecules into skin by combined use of microneedle roller and flexible interdigitated electroporation array. Theranostics. 2018;8:2361–2376.

[167] Amit M, Srinivasan G, Pramod U. Needle-free, non-adjuvanted skin immunization by electroporation-enhanced transdermal delivery of diphtheria toxoid and a candidate peptide vaccine against hepatitis B virus. Vaccine. 1999;18. [Internet] [cited 2022 Aug 7]. Available from: https://pubmed.ncbi.nlm.nih.gov/10519942/.

[168] Sen A, Daly ME, Hui SW. Transdermal insulin delivery using lipid enhanced electroporation. Biochim Biophys Acta. 2002;1564:5–8.

[169] Prausnitz MR, Edelman ER, Gimm JA, et al. Transdermal delivery of heparin by skin electro-poration. Bio/Technology. 1995;13:1205–1209.

[170] Hofmann GA, Rustrum WV, Suder KS. Electro-incorporation of microcarriers as a method for the transdermal delivery of large molecules. Bioelectrochem Bioenerg. 1995;38:209–222.

[171] Hu Q, Liang W, Bao J, et al. Enhanced transdermal delivery of tetracaine by electroporation. Int J Pharm. 2000;202:121–124.

[172] Jadoul A, Lecouturier N, Mesens J, et al. Transdermal alniditan delivery by skin electropora-tion. J Control Release. 1998;54:265–272.

[173] Vanbever R, Langers G, Montmayeur S, et al. Transdermal delivery of fentanyl: rapid onset of analgesia using skin electroporation. J Control Release. 1998;50:225–235.

[174] Denet A-R, Préat V. Transdermal delivery of timolol by electroporation through human skin. J Control Release. 2003;88:253–262.

[175] Zorec B, Becker S, Reberšek M, et al. Skin electroporation for transdermal drug delivery: the influence of the order of different square wave electric pulses. Int J Pharm. 2013;457:214–223.

[176] Blagus T, Markelc B, Cemazar M, et al. In vivo real-time monitoring system of electroporation mediated control of transdermal and topical drug delivery. J Control Release. 2013;172:862–871.

[177] Wallace MS, Ridgeway B, Jun E, et al. Topical delivery of lidocaine in healthy volunteers by electroporation, electroincorporation, or iontophoresis: an evaluation of skin anesthesia. Reg Anesth Pain Med. 2001;26:229–238.

[178] Wang R, Bian Q, Xu Y, et al. Recent advances in mechanical force-assisted transdermal deliv-ery of macromolecular drugs. Int J Pharm. 2021;602:120598.

[179] Benedek K, Walker E, Doshier LA, et al. Studies on the use of needle-free injection device on proteins. J Chromatogr A. 2005;1079:397–407.

[180] Miyazaki H, Atobe S, Suzuki T, et al. Development of pyro-drive jet injector with controllable jet pressure. J Pharm Sci. 2019;108:2415–2420.

[181] Marwah H, Garg T, Goyal AK, et al. Permeation enhancer strategies in transdermal drug delivery. Drug Deliv. 2016;23:564–578.

[182] Benson HAE, Namjoshi S. Proteins and peptides: strategies for delivery to and across the skin. J Pharm Sci. 2008;97:3591–3610.

[183] Trimzi MA, Ham Y-B. A needle-free jet injection system for controlled release and repeated biopharmaceutical delivery. Pharmaceutics. 2021;13:1770.

[184] Arora A. Liquid and powder jet injectors in drug delivery: mechanisms, designs, and applica-tions. In: Nina Dragicevic, Howard I. Maibach, editors. Percutaneous penetration enhancers physical methods in penetration enhancement. New York: Springer; 2017. p. 221–230.

[185] Arora A, Prausnitz MR, Mitragotri S. Micro-scale devices for transdermal drug delivery. Int J Pharm. 2008;364:227–236.

[186] Mitragotri S. Current status and future prospects of needle-free liquid jet injectors. Nat Rev Drug Discov. 2006;5:543–548.

[187] Kale TR, Momin M. Needle free injection technology-an overview. Innov Pharm. 2014;5.

[188] Dean HJ, Chen D. Epidermal powder immunization against influenza. Vaccine. 2004;23:681–686.

[189] Mathur V, Satrawala Y, Rajput MS. Physical and chemical penetration enhancers in transder-mal drug delivery system. Asian J Pharm AJP. 2010;4.

[190] Roberts LK, Barr LJ, Fuller DH, et al. Clinical safety and efficacy of a powdered hepatitis B nucleic acid vaccine delivered to the epidermis by a commercial prototype device. Vaccine. 2005;23:4867–4878.

[191] Wolf AR, Stoddart PA, Murphy PJ, et al. Rapid skin anaesthesia using high velocity lignocaine particles: a prospective placebo controlled trial. Arch Dis Child. 2002;86:309–312.

[192] Donnelly RF, Raj Singh TR, Woolfson AD. Microneedle-based drug delivery systems: micro-fabrication, drug delivery, and safety. Drug Deliv. 2010;17:187–207.

[193] van der Maaden K, Jiskoot W, Bouwstra J. Microneedle technologies for (trans)dermal drug and vaccine delivery. J Control Release. 2012;161:645–655.

[194] Tuan-Mahmood T-M, McCrudden MT, Torrisi BM, et al. Microneedles for intradermal and transdermal drug delivery. Eur J Pharm Sci. 2013;50:623–637.

[195] Kearney M-C, Caffarel-Salvador E, Fallows SJ, et al. Microneedle-mediated delivery of donepezil: potential for improved treatment options in Alzheimer's disease. Eur J Pharm Biopharm. 2016;103:43–50.

[196] McCrudden MTC, Alkilani AZ, McCrudden CM, et al. Design and physicochemical characterisation of novel dissolving polymeric microneedle arrays for transdermal delivery of high dose, low molecular weight drugs. J Control Release. 2014;180:71–80.

[197] Chen X, Wang L, Yu H, et al. Preparation, properties and challenges of the microneedles-based insulin delivery system. J Control Release. 2018;288:173–188.

[198] Liu T, Chen M, Fu J, et al. Recent advances in microneedle-mediated transdermal delivery of protein and peptide drugs. Acta Pharm Sin B. 2021;11:2326–2343.

[199] Stinson JA, Boopathy AV, Cieslewicz BM, et al. Enhancing influenza vaccine immunogenicity and efficacy through infection mimicry using silk microneedles. Vaccine. 2021;39:5410–5421.

[200] Yin Y, Su W, Zhang J, et al. Separable microneedle patch to protect and deliver DNA nanovaccines against COVID-19. ACS Nano. 2021;15:14347–14359.

[201] Choi SY, Kwon HJ, Ahn GR, et al. Hyaluronic acid microneedle patch for the improvement of crow's feet wrinkles. Dermatol Ther. 2017;30:e12546.

[202] Mohammed YH, Yamada M, Lin LL, et al. Microneedle enhanced delivery of cosmeceutically relevant peptides in human skin. PLoS One. 2014;9:e101956.

[203] Park Y, Park J, Chu GS, et al. Transdermal delivery of cosmetic ingredients using dissolving polymer microneedle arrays. Biotechnol Bioprocess Eng. 2015;20:543–549.

[204] Niu L, Chu LY, Burton SA, et al. Intradermal delivery of vaccine nanoparticles using hollow microneedle array generates enhanced and balanced immune response. J Control Release. 2019;294:268–278.

[205] Peng K, Vora LK, Tekko IA, et al. Dissolving microneedle patches loaded with amphotericin B microparticles for localised and sustained intradermal delivery: potential for enhanced treatment of cutaneous fungal infections. J Control Release. 2021;339:361–380.

[206] Zhang D, Das DB, Rielly CD. An experimental study of microneedle-assisted microparticle delivery. J Pharm Sci. 2013;102:3632–3644.

[207] Donnelly RF, Singh TRR, Morrow DI, et al. Microneedle-mediated transdermal and intradermal drug delivery. Hoboken, New Jersey: John Wiley & Sons; 2012.

[208] Bariya SH, Gohel MC, Mehta TA, et al. Microneedles: an emerging transdermal drug delivery system. J Pharm Pharmacol. 2012;64:11–29.

[209] Martanto W, Moore JS, Kashlan O, et al. Microinfusion using hollow microneedles. Pharm Res. 2006;23:104–113.

[210] Martin CJ, Allender CJ, Brain KR, et al. Low temperature fabrication of biodegradable sugar glass microneedles for transdermal drug delivery applications. J Control Release. 2012;158:93–101.

[211] Martanto W, Davis SP, Holiday NR, et al. Transdermal delivery of insulin using microneedles in vivo. Pharm Res. 2004;21:947–952.

[212] Ji J, Tay FE, Miao J, et al. Microfabricated silicon microneedle array for transdermal drug delivery. J Phys Conf Ser. IOP Publishing; 2006. p. 1127. [Internet] Available from: http://iopscience.iop.org/article/10.1088/1742-6596/34/1/186/meta.

[213] Trautmann A, Heuck F, Mueller C, et al. Replication of microneedle arrays using vacuum casting and hot embossing. 13th Int Conf Solid-State Sens Actuators Microsyst. IEEE; 2005. p. 1420–1423.

[214] Donnelly RF, McCrudden MT, Alkilani AZ, et al. Hydrogel-forming microneedles prepared from "super swelling" polymers combined with lyophilised wafers for transdermal drug delivery. PLoS One. 2014;9:e111547.

[215] Donnelly RF, Morrow DIJ, McCrudden MTC, et al. Hydrogel-forming and dissolving microneedles for enhanced delivery of photosensitizers and precursors. Photochem Photobiol. 2014;90:641–647.

[216] Tsuchiya K, Jinnin S, Yamamoto H, et al. Design and development of a biocompatible painless microneedle by the ion sputtering deposition method. Precis Eng. 2010;34:461–466.

[217] Kochhar JS, Goh WJ, Chan SY, et al. A simple method of microneedle array fabrication for transdermal drug delivery. Drug Dev Ind Pharm. 2013;39:299–309.

[218] Aoyagi S, Izumi H, Isono Y, et al. Laser fabrication of high aspect ratio thin holes on biodegradable polymer and its application to a microneedle. Sens Actuators Phys. 2007;139:293–302.

[219] Donnelly RF, Majithiya R, Singh TRR, et al. Design, optimization and characterisation of polymeric microneedle arrays prepared by a novel laser-based micromoulding technique. Pharm Res. 2011;28:41–57.

[220] DeMuth PC, Min Y, Huang B, et al. Polymer multilayer tattooing for enhanced DNA vaccination. Nat Mater. 2013;12:367–376.

[221] Kim JD, Kim M, Yang H, et al. Droplet-born air blowing: novel dissolving microneedle fabrication. J Control Release. 2013;170:430–436.

[222] Yung KL, Xu Y, Kang C, et al. Sharp tipped plastic hollow microneedle array by microinjection moulding. J Micromechanics Microengineering. 2011;22:015016.

[223] Rejinold NS, Shin J-H, Seok HY, et al. Biomedical applications of microneedles in therapeutics: recent advancements and implications in drug delivery. Expert Opin Drug Deliv. 2016;13:109–131.

[224] Gadziński P, Froelich A, Wojtyłko M, et al. Microneedle-based ocular drug delivery systems—recent advances and challenges. Beilstein J Nanotechnol. 2022;13:1167–1184.

[225] Murthy SN, Sammeta SM, Bowers C. Magnetophoresis for enhancing transdermal drug delivery: mechanistic studies and patch design. J Control Release. 2010;148:197–203.

[226] Murthy SN. Magnetophoresis: an approach to enhance transdermal drug diffusion. Pharm. 1999;54:377–379.

[227] Arruebo M, Fernández-Pacheco R, Ibarra MR, et al. Magnetic nanoparticles for drug delivery. Nano Today. 2007;2:22–32.

[228] Medeiros SF, Santos AM, Fessi H, et al. Stimuli-responsive magnetic particles for biomedical applications. Int J Pharm. 2011;403:139–161.

[229] Doukas AG, Kollias N. Transdermal drug delivery with a pressure wave. Adv Drug Deliv Rev. 2004;56:559–579.

[230] Ogura M, Sato S, Nakanishi K, et al. In vivo targeted gene transfer in skin by the use of laser-induced stress waves. Lasers Surg Med. 2004;34:242–248.

[231] Nethercott JR. Practical problems in the use of patch testing in the evaluation of patients with contact dermatitis. Curr Probl Dermatol. 1990;2:97–123.

[232] Amnon C S, Igor K, Dorit D, et al. Radiofrequency-driven skin microchanneling as a new way for electrically assisted transdermal delivery of hydrophilic drugs. J Control Release. 2003;89. [Internet] [cited 2022 Aug 7]. Available from: https://pubmed.ncbi.nlm.nih.gov/12711453/.

[233] Amjadi M, Mostaghaci B, Sitti M. Recent advances in skin penetration enhancers for transdermal gene and drug delivery. Curr Gene Ther. 2017;17:139–146.

[234] Bramson J, Dayball K, Evelegh C, et al. Enabling topical immunization via microporation: a novel method for pain-free and needle-free delivery of adenovirus-based vaccines. Gene Ther. 2003;10:251–260.

[235] Li Y, Guo L, Lu W. Laser ablation-enhanced transdermal drug delivery: laserablationsverstärkte transdermale Medikamentenverabreichung. Photonics Lasers Med. 2013;2:315–322.

[236] Szunerits S, Boukherroub R. Heat: a highly efficient skin enhancer for transdermal drug delivery. Front Bioeng Biotechnol. 2018;6:15.

[237] Lee W-R, Hsiao C-Y, Huang T-H, et al. Post-irradiation recovery time strongly influences fractional laser-facilitated skin absorption. Int J Pharm. 2019;564:48–58.

[238] Zorec B, Škrabelj D, Marinček M, et al. The effect of pulse duration, power and energy of fractional Er: YAG laser for transdermal delivery of differently sized FITC dextrans. Int J Pharm. 2017;516:204–213.

[239] Lin C-H, Aljuffali IA, Fang J-Y. Lasers as an approach for promoting drug delivery via skin. Expert Opin Drug Deliv. 2014;11:599–614.

[240] Gao Y, Du L, Li Q, et al. How physical techniques improve the transdermal permeation of therapeutics: a review. Medicine (Baltimore). 2022;101:e29314.

[241] Khaizan AN, Wong TW. Microwave: effects and implications in transdermal drug delivery. Prog Electromagn Res. 2013;141:619–643.

[242] Moghimi HR, Alinaghi A, Erfan M. Investigating the potential of non-thermal microwave as a novel skin penetration enhancement method. Int J Pharm. 2010;401:47–50.

[243] Wong TW, Nor Khaizan A. Physicochemical modulation of skin barrier by microwave for transdermal drug delivery. Pharm Res. 2013;30:90–103.

[244] Wong TW. Electrical, magnetic, photomechanical and cavitational waves to overcome skin barrier for transdermal drug delivery. J Control Release. 2014;193:257–269.

[245] Asif N, Tin Wui W. Microwave as skin permeation enhancer for transdermal drug delivery of chitosan-5-fluorouracil nanoparticles. Carbohydr Polym. 2017;157. [Internet] [cited 2022 Jul 24]. Available from: https://pubmed.ncbi.nlm.nih.gov/27988008/.

[246] Khan NR, Wong TW. Microwave-aided skin drug penetration and retention of 5-fluorouracil-loaded ethosomes. Expert Opin Drug Deliv. 2016;13:1209–1219.

[247] Harjoh N, Wong TW, Caramella C. Transdermal insulin delivery with microwave and fatty acids as permeation enhancers. Int J Pharm. 2020;584:119416.

[248] Shen Q, Tang T, Hu Q, et al. Microwave hyperthermia-responsible flexible liposomal gel as a novel transdermal delivery of methotrexate for enhanced rheumatoid arthritis therapy. Biomater Sci. 2021;9:8386–8395.

[249] Wong TW. Use of microwave to improve nanomedicine application on skin. Expert Opin Drug Deliv. 2017;14:283–283.

2

Production of Microneedles

2.1 Introduction

Numerous patents and publications have covered extensive interest in microneedle concepts, design, and production technologies. The first patent for a microneedle-based device was filed by Gerstel and Place [1]. Initially, microneedles were manufactured simply from silicon wafers by reactive ion etching and photolithography [2–4]. The manufacturing process of microneedles was not thoroughly optimized until the 1990s, when high-precision microelectronics industrial tools became available. Since then, microneedles have been produced from silicon, glass, metal, and polymers using various fabrication techniques. Acceptable microneedles should be sharp and strong to protect the structure from forces during microneedle insertion into the skin. Transdermal and intradermal delivery of a wide variety of therapeutic agents has been mediated with the aid of microneedles in *in vitro*, *in vivo* experiments, and clinical settings.

2.2 Design and Technology

Microneedles could effectively take various shapes or geometries, including cylindrical, rectangular, pyramidal, conical, octagonal, or quadrangular [5]. Microneedle configuration has been demonstrated to markedly affect the skin permeability of various drugs (Fig. 2.1) [6]. The needle length, density, and tip dimensions could be customized for specific usage. In general, 500-μm-long microneedles have been preferential selection for microneedles design. A low-density microneedle array appears superior to dense microneedles to avoid the "bed of nails" effect, which could reduce the penetration efficiency of microneedles [7–9]. The shape and diameter of the microneedle tip are of critical importance as sharp microneedles could require less external force to penetrate skin tissue successfully. In particular, for hollow microneedles, the tip geometry significantly affects the flow rate of microneedle-assisted injection. Blunt tips compress skin more substantially, thus creating a possible risk of clogging. Therefore, hollow microneedles should be sharp tips with the bore located off-centered or on the side [10–13]. Increasing bore size could improve the flow rate but reduce the needle strength, robustness, and sharpness [13].

2.2.1 Solid Microneedles

Solid microneedles are designed to penetrate the skin to specific depths, creating micrometer-sized channels filled with interstitial fluid after the needle removal. These channels then

DOI: 10.1201/9780429294433-2

serve as the diffusion pathway for passive drug permeation from topically applied formulations (a gel, solution, or patch as the external drug reservoir). This approach has been known as "poke and patch." Compared to other types, these solid needles are easy to manufacture, robust in mechanical strength, and sharp in needle geometry [14]. Various materials could be used to fabricate solid microneedles, such as silicon, metal, glass, and polymers

2.2.1.1 Silicon Microneedles

Silicon microneedles are the first type of microneedles to be manufactured. The first design was produced from silicon wafers using photolithography and deep reactive ion etching [3, 15, 16]. These needles could be designed with various geometries and dimensions. There are two primary types of silicon microneedles: in-plane and out-of-plane. In-plane microneedles are created parallel to the silicon wafer, while out-of-plane needles are formed perpendicularly to the silicon wafer. In-plane needles offer more flexibility in the needle design and shape and the possibility to integrate biosensors and micropumps [4, 9, 13, 17–19]. Meanwhile, out-of-plane microneedles are more easily manufactured, and the needle array could be modified to apply on a large skin area [5]. Several advantages and disadvantages of silicon microneedles have been elaborated. These needles are generally sharper than other needle types, have excellent skin penetration capacity, and offer high reproducibility and accuracy on an industrial manufacturing scale. Shortcomings of silicon microneedles include the complicated multistep dry and wet etching method, expensive fabrication processes, and clean room requirements. Moreover, silicon is not a degradable, biocompatible, or FDA-approved biomaterial, thus facing significant challenges in regulatory acceptability and approval [20]. Silicon microneedles with poor mechanical strength and brittle physical nature could be easily broken in the skin, causing a significant biosafety issue.

2.2.1.2 Metal Microneedles

Metal microneedles have been commonly used to enhance transdermal and topical drug delivery. Microneedles might be fabricated from various metals, including stainless steel, titanium, palladium, palladium-cobalt alloys, nickel, and so on [21]. Different production methods have been employed to fabricate metal microneedles: electroplating, photochemical etching, and laser cutting. Gupta and coworkers fabricated stainless steel microneedles using a laser cutting technique with the aid of AutoCAD software for microneedles design (shape and dimensions) [22]. Stainless steel microneedles could be formed from stainless steel sheets using photolithographic wet-etching [23]. Several reports revealed the advantages of metal microneedles which include low cost, excellent mechanical strength, easy skin penetration, minimal risk of needle fracture in the skin, and biocompatibility for certain metals. However, a drawback is reported as metal microneedles could potentially induce an immuno-inflammatory response.

2.2.2 Hollow Microneedles

A hollow microneedles device is generally designed with a chamber as a drug reservoir and hollow micrometer-sized needles [24]. Fluid infusion of liquid formulation could be delivered via the bore on hollow microneedles. In the simplest configuration, therapeutic agents could be driven into skin layers by passive diffusion without any external stimulus.

This delivery rate is slow due to the small interfacial area of the microneedle bore and back pressure imposed by dense skin tissue. More frequently, a force is applied to pump drug liquid formulation from the reservoir into the skin, thus providing a steady infusion rate. This is regarded as an active delivery system. The applied pressure could be tailored to adjust the flow rate and drug delivery rate. For the most basic fabrication method, hollow microneedles could be made by assembling the 30-gauge or 31-gauge most miniature available hypodermic needles with a controlled length of needle exposure on a supporting substrate [25]. This way offers ease of manufacturing; however, it poses several drawbacks. There is a limited design of microneedles with varying needle lengths, widths, and densities. Also, these needles are used the same way as solid microneedles (poke and patch approach), in which the bore plays no critical role. Generally, hollow microneedles have been produced from metal tubing using laser machining, electrochemical etching, or electrode discharge machining [3]. Hollow microneedles could be made from silicon, metal, glass, carbon nanotubes, polyimide, or polymers.

Interestingly, hollow microneedles are the only design of microneedles that enable the administration of large doses or volumes of drug formulation [26]. The delivery of large molecules and particle systems is also effectively assisted. Hollow microneedles provide continuous, tunable, and controlled drug release over a certain period [27]. The formulation composition and properties dictate the delivery rate: high drug concentration provides burst release, while matrix-based formulation delivers the drug in a steady and long-lasting way [28]. Several shortcomings of hollow microneedles have been discussed in a plethora of publications. These needles are relatively weak, thus causing a possibility of needle breakage in the skin. Another issue is with the high cost and complex fabrication method. Hollow microneedles are generally more sophisticated than solid microneedles. Technical issues have been reported in needle design, insertion technique, drug leakage, and clogging during the injection [29, 30]. This device also requires the integration of a drug reservoir with the needles.

2.2.3 Coated Microneedles

Coated microneedles are solid microneedles coated with the drug solution. Generally, coated microneedles could contain a small quantity of a drug depending on the coating layer's thickness [31]. The effectiveness of coated microneedles is significantly impacted by the reliable coating process of a controlled coating layer [32]. Numerous therapeutic agents could be loaded into coated microneedles, such as hydrophilic/lipophilic molecules, macromolecules, DNA, RNA, proteins, peptides, vaccines, and particle systems [7, 32–37]. Coated microneedles provide several advantages over hollow and solid microneedles. The coating process is typically performed at ambient conditions (i.e., temperature and humidity). Moreover, the drug in solid form in coated microneedles is more stable than in liquid formulation [32, 35, 38]. The loaded drug in coated needles could release rapidly into skin layers within seconds or minutes after the needle insertion. Furthermore, the drug release kinetics could be tailored by modifying the coating composition. However, several drawbacks have been noted. The remaining drug on the needle tip after removal of the needles from the skin could infect other people [39]. The minute quantity of drug coated on the needles reduces the drug delivery efficiency [34, 40–42]. If more drug is required to be incorporated, the coating layer will be markedly thicker, thus decreasing the needles' sharpness and causing a possible high drug loss. Hence, the coating strategy is generally used for enhanced transdermal delivery of potent compounds which require a low dose for therapeutic effectiveness, such as vaccines, proteins, or peptides [7, 8, 36].

2.2.4 Dissolving Microneedles

The first design of dissolving microneedles came into existence in 2005 [29]. These needles are fabricated from water-soluble, safe, inert, inexpensive, biocompatible, and biodegradable materials such as sugars and polymers, which facilitate effective mass production [43]. To date, the most commonly used method to produce dissolving microneedles is the micromolding technique [29]. As the latest design of microneedles, dissolving microneedles offer several advantages over other microneedle types. The needles could dissolve rapidly with a limited volume of interstitial skin fluid and provide a burst release of drug (i.e., macromolecules) within a short time. The application of dissolving microneedles is just a one-step process. This so-called poke and release approach provides easy and convenient administration and improves patient compliance and acceptability. The needle array is applied on the skin in a similar way as for conventional transdermal patches. The embedded needles then absorb water in the skin and quickly disintegrate to release the drug load within minutes. Moreover, these needles have less shear-caused breakage due to the physical properties of their polymeric composition [8, 11, 19, 44, 45]. Multiple aspects of this system could be customized to provide a desired controlled drug delivery, such as material composition, needle dimensions, geometry (i.e., length, base size, needle density), and applied pressure during needle insertion. Since the drug is encapsulated into the polymeric matrix, a higher drug quantity could be loaded into dissolving microneedles, thus delivering a larger dose. Also, the drug exists in the solid form; hence, it provides excellent stability as compared to liquid formulation. The majority of drug is incorporated into the needles, especially the needle tips. Therefore, the drug wastage is minimized, which is particularly meaningful for high-cost pharmaceutical active ingredients. Furthermore, no concern has been raised about unexpected particles being detached from coated microneedles [46]. An advantage of dissolving microneedles lies in the ease, convenience, and efficiency of micromolding fabrication technique using low-cost, readily available polymeric materials [20]. Ideally, the manufacturing process should be quick with minimal steps, cost-effective, and reproducible. Formulation flexibility could be exploited to include various excipients with desired physicochemical properties. Moreover, there is no sharp waste, reuse, disposability issue, and risk of leaving biohazardous sharp waste in the skin as commonly reported with silicon, glass, and metal microneedles [44, 47–49]. Despite all these advantages, dissolving microneedles impose several noticeable drawbacks. Researchers should monitor the risk of skin irritation or inflammation when the skin is exposed to microneedles or the array substrate over a certain period. Dissolving microneedles have been demonstrated to have compromised mechanical strength, weaker than silicon or metal solid microneedles. Dissolving microneedles' mechanical properties and robustness depended on the drug load's quantity and location: the higher the drug loaded, the weaker the needles. The impact of drug load on the mechanical properties of microneedles also depends on the geometries and dimensions of the needles. Dissolving microneedles were reported to be capable of delivering only 1 mg of drug transdermally [45, 50]. Similarly, when the drug encapsulation is localized closer to the needle tips, the possibility of compromising the needle sharpness and failing the needle insertion is significantly more. Besides, biomolecules could easily degrade upon exposure to harsh conditions (i.e., high temperature) of the manufacturing process [45, 51].

2.2.5 Swellable Microneedles

Recently, there emerged a novel design of microneedles—swellable microneedles. Upon the skin insertion, the needles absorb interstitial fluid in skin tissue and swell to release

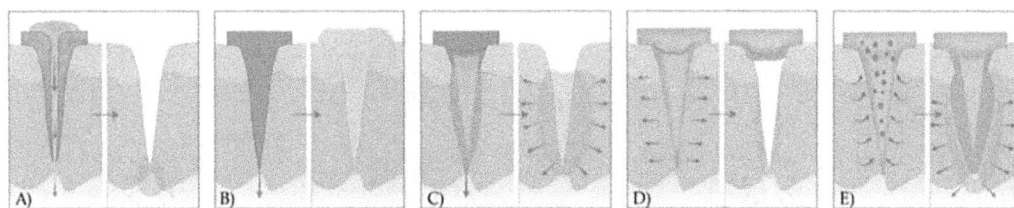

FIGURE 2.1
A schematic representation of different types of microneedles. (A) Hollow microneedles. (B) Solid microneedles. (C) Coated microneedles. (D) Dissolving microneedles. (E) Hydrogel microneedles. Images reprinted with permission from [55].

therapeutic agents through newly formed conduits in the swollen needles into skin layers [52, 53]. The needles effectively serve two roles: (i) to penetrate the skin barrier and (ii) to control drug release and permeation. This type of microneedle offers several advantages. The delivered dose could be significantly larger than coated or dissolving microneedles. The drug delivery quantity is no longer restrained to the amount loaded inside the needles. Also, the needles could be designed with various patch sizes and geometries. It has been reported that sterilization is easy and convenient for swellable microneedles. The swelling function of this needle type prevents the issue of pore closure, as commonly observed in solid and dissolving microneedles. Furthermore, the needles could be removed intact from the skin, leaving no traces of polymeric materials in skin tissue, thus alleviating the risk of biosafety complications [54].

2.3 Production Materials

Various materials have been used in the construction of microneedles. These materials should be biodegradable, nonirritant, nonallergenic, nontoxic, biocompatible, readily available, and cost-effective. The ideal properties of microneedle materials include ease of production, sterilization, mechanical strength or robustness, and physicochemical stability under different environmental conditions [49]. Materials should be carefully selected to facilitate microneedle manufacturability, which is accurate, reproducible, and robust. Material selection, the ratio of material combination, and the level of crosslinking are tailored to meet the specific requirement of the fabricated needles. The fundamental function of microneedles is to penetrate and disrupt the skin barrier, especially the stratum corneum layer, known as the primary barrier to skin permeability. The materials should have sufficient physical strength to contribute to the mechanical robustness of the microneedle product. Weak materials would pose a significant risk of failure of microneedle insertion into the skin tissue. Furthermore, materials with high Young's modulus would mitigate the risk of microneedles failure by buckling [56, 57], while those with high yield strength reduce the possibility of failure by fracture or tip deformation (Fig. 2.2). Material selection would markedly affect the manufacturing condition, which in turn poses the risk of degradation of thermosensitive compounds. Besides, microneedles materials could be selected and engineered to provide a controlled drug release rate. Material selection is dependent on the microneedle types. In particular, solid microneedles could be made from silicon,

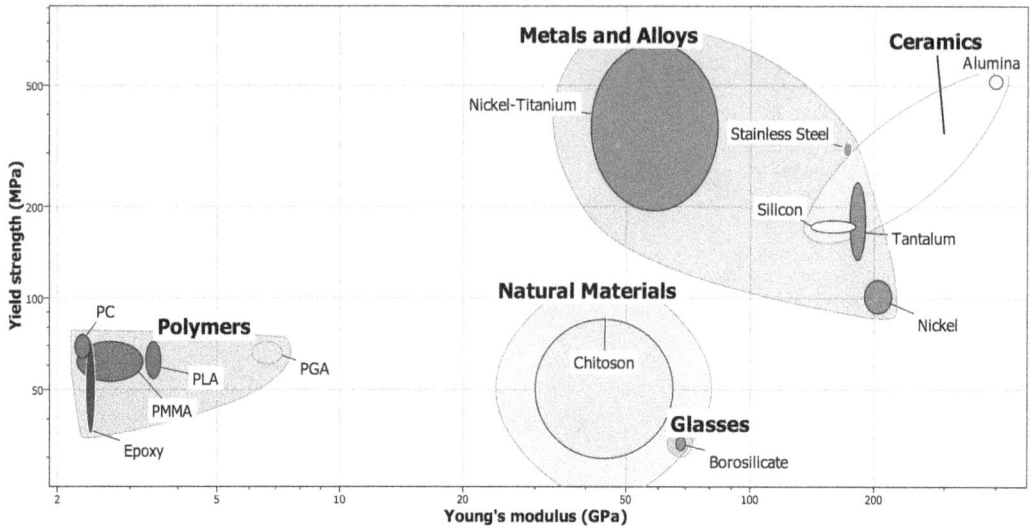

FIGURE 2.2
Yield strength and Young's modulus of various microneedles materials. Images reprinted with permission from [62].

titanium, stainless steel, nickel-iron, glass, or ceramics [58–60]. Polymeric microneedles have been fabricated from water-soluble polymers and various biodegradable polymers [61]. Interestingly, dissolving microneedles are effectively manufactured from different sugars, including maltose, dextran, and galactose.

2.3.1 Silicon

Silicon was first used to fabricate microneedles in the 1990s [63]. Different types of microneedles could be made from silicon, such as solid, hollow, and coated microneedles. Silicon material offers ease and flexibility of manufacturability with various dimensions and geometries. However, microneedle production could be time-consuming and costly [64]. This type of microneedle could be easily broken and fractured in the skin, thus causing a severe biosafety issue [65].

2.3.2 Metal

Metal microneedles were one of the early designs of microneedles. These needles were initially fabricated from stainless steel, followed by other kinds of metal, such as titanium. Solid, coated, and hollow microneedles have all been made using different metals. Metal microneedles are biocompatible and mechanically robust, with excellent fracture resistance [66, 67]. However, these needles could induce allergic reactions upon insertion into the skin [68].

2.3.3 Ceramic

Microneedles have been fabricated from ceramic materials such as alumina, calcium sulfate dihydrate, calcium phosphate dihydrate, and so on [24]. These needles possess excellent chemical properties and compression resistance but have low tensile strength. The conventional micromolding technique could easily and conveniently fabricate ceramic microneedles. The production process could be scaled up at a relatively low cost [69].

2.3.4 Polymers

Polymer appears as a commonly used and superior material for microneedle fabrication. Polymer is a promising alternative to other materials to fabricate all types of microneedles, namely, dissolving, swellable, solid, coated, and hollow microneedles. Various therapeutic agents, including small molecules, macromolecules, and particulate systems, have been encapsulated in the polymeric matrix of microneedles [70]. Polymers must meet specific requirements to be selected and used as the material of construction for microneedles. The preferred polymers must be biocompatible, nontoxic, nonallergenic, noncarcinogenic, nonmutagenic, nonharmful to fertility, and inexpensive with low-cost supply [71]. The biocompatibility of polymers could be examined using the International Organization for Standardization (ISO) and USP 30-NF25. Being biodegradable, the polymers should degrade and be eliminated rapidly from the human body after drug administration. Currently, FDA-approved biomaterials are preferred; however, these materials must possess sufficient mechanical strength and physical hardness to ensure successful skin microporation of fabricated microneedles. Also, the polymers should be compatible with the encapsulated drug and other components in the matrix. The polymer shall be carefully selected to achieve the desired drug release kinetic, i.e., for the needles to dissolve rapidly, polymers with high water solubility would be feasible options so that the needles would absorb the limited quantity of moisture in the skin and degrade quickly to release the drug load. Microneedles are typically made from the following polymers: polycarbonate, poly(methyl methacrylate), poly-L-lactic acid, poly-glycolic acid, and poly-lactic-*co*-glycolic acid, cyclic-olefin copolymer, poly(vinyl pyrrolidone), and sodium carboxy methyl cellulose. Various micromold-based techniques have been employed to produce polymeric microneedles, such as casting, hot embossing, injection molding, investment molding, laser, and X-ray methods.

2.4 Production Methods of Microneedles

2.4.1 Microelectromechanical Systems

The MEMS process involves three precise and controlled steps: deposition, patterning, and etching of material [72]. It has been reported that this method could produce complex micrometer-sized 3D structures. The technique has been employed to fabricate solid and hollow microneedles as well as micromold (i.e., photolithography to make PDMS mold) for the production of dissolving microneedles [73]. An advantage of MEMS is the ease of scaling up and mass manufacturability [49]. In the etching process, a strong acid or caustic chemical is applied to remove or etch out the uncovered portion of the substrate to create a pattern on the material surface. Wet etching and dry etching are the two most common techniques. The etched-out material waste is removed by immersing the material substrate in a chemical liquid in wet etching. The dry etching is performed with a vapor phase or plasma etcher. There are two major types of dry etching: reactive ion etching and ion-beam milling.

2.4.2 Micromolding Technique

Micromolding has been known as the most common technique of microneedle fabrication, especially dissolving microneedles [74]. Using this technique, microneedles could be designed with different geometries and dimensions, thus changing the release kinetics of encapsulated drug. The shape and size of microneedles have been found to affect needle manufacturability significantly. The geometry of the finished microneedles product primarily depends on the geometry of the mold in which the needles closely follow the shape and size of the female mold. In some cases, during the solvent evaporation process, the polymeric matrix could shrink dramatically to create shorter, thinner, and sharper microneedles. The most commonly used mold is polydimethylsiloxane (PDMS) due to its inert, stable, and flexible properties. PDMS mold could be reused more than 100 times, making it a cost-effective method of microneedle fabrication. The mold is an accurate inverse replicate of the master structure, which is often a silicon or metal microneedle array. For the process of making a mold, PDMS solution or mixture is first poured into the master structure. To prevent adhesion between the mold material and the master structure, the master structure is usually sputter-coated with platinum. All entrapped air is eliminated using a vacuum or centrifugation; then, the mold is cured at controlled conditions. Finally, the solid and flexible mold is manually peeled off the master structure [75].

The mold is subsequently utilized to manufacture microneedles. First, the liquefied polymeric mixture with active pharmaceutical ingredients is cast on the clean, dry mold. The mixture is pulled into the mold cavity, and any entrapped air is removed using an external force such as vacuum, pressure, or centrifugation [76, 77]. Subsequently, the matrix is solidified using heat (at a specific temperature in an oven or desiccator) or solvent evaporation [68]. If the polymeric mixture is a liquid monomer, then *in situ* polymerization could be used to crosslink the monomers to form a solid microneedle structure. For ceramic microneedles, a ceramic slurry (i.e., alumina slurry) is cast and filled on the mold before the structure sintering [78].

Various types of materials could be used to fabricate microneedles using this micromolding technique. These include dextran [79], carboxymethyl cellulose [80], dextrin [3], polyvinyl pyrrolidine [3], chondroitin sulfate [81], polyvinyl alcohol [82], fibroin [83], poly(lactic-*co*-glycolic) acid [45], ceramics, and sugars [84]. The materials must be biodegradable and biocompatible to improve biosafety and manufacturability.

The micromolding technique provides several advantages, such as a low-cost process, ease of scaling-up and mass manufacturability, ease of use, low surface energy, and thermal stability [85]. Furthermore, thermolabile drugs, macromolecules, and vaccines could be incorporated into drug-excipient solutions before the drying step at mild conditions. Also, microneedles have been produced with various geometries and dimensions. The drug could be loaded in different locations within a microneedle array, such as needle tip and array substrate, thus enabling a controlled and tailored release of drug payload. However, polymeric microneedles fabricated by the micromolding technique pose some shortcomings. When the drug payload on these needles increases, the mechanical properties of the needles may be impaired. A critical requirement for successfully fabricating these microneedles is to ensure sufficient mechanical strength of the needles so that the needles can microporate skin tissues. These polymeric needles have limited drug-loading capacity. The polymer matrix has been reported to affect these needles' depth of penetration and insertion efficiency.

2.4.3 Additive Manufacturing

Additive manufacturing is a novel and innovative method of building 3D objects. This technique works on depositing or fusing selected materials layer-by-layer to form the desired object as designed by a computer-aided design program (CAD). The object design is first built on CAD, converted to an STL file, and transferred to a 3D printer with printing setup parameters. A 3D printing could be executed using various materials such as ceramics, liquids, thermoplastic, plastic, photopolymer, and powders. Several advantages of additive manufacturing have been revealed, including (i) flexibility in the object design with the capacity to build complex geometries or modify the original design, (ii) reduction of processing time [86], (iii) simplicity of manufacturing process, (iv) cost-effectiveness, and (v) fabrication of patient-individualized device [87, 88].

2.4.3.1 Fused Deposition Modeling

A fused deposition modeling printer has been commonly utilized to build 3D structures. The geometries and dimensions of microneedles are designed and optimized on CAD software. Thermoplastic material is fed into the printer as filament at a specific diameter. This filament is heated beyond the glass transition temperature T_g to melt the material effectively. After that, the molten and softened material is extruded through the printer head or nozzle and deposited on a building plate layer-by-layer, corresponding to the CAD design. Following the printing step, the 3D structure is cooled and solidified rapidly. Regarding the printing direction, the printer head moves in the x- and y-axes while the platform is moved to the z-axis to create the 3D structure [87]. Various thermoplastic filaments could be used in FDM printing, including acrylonitrile butadiene styrene, PLA, PVA, high-impact polystyrene, polyethylene terephthalate glycol-modified, and nylon. The general diameter of the commercially available filament is 1.75 mm or 2.85–3 mm [89]. Several processing parameters of FDM printing could be modified and optimized: (i) printer nozzle diameter, (ii) material feeding rate, (iii) temperature of printer nozzle and building plate, (iv) printing speed, (v) height of printing layer, (vi) structure-building orientation [87, 90]. Even though the advantages of being versatile and inexpensive, FDM only provides limited printing resolution, making it challenging to fabricate micrometer-sized structures such as microneedles with sharp and miniature tips.

2.4.3.2 Stereolithography

Stereolithography (SLA) works by photopolymerization and solidification of a mixture of liquid resin and photoactive monomers under exposure to high-energy ultraviolet (UV) light. The design and pattern of microneedles are created by shedding a laser beam on the resin surface. Then, the excessive resin residue is removed by washing the structure in an alcohol bath. The 3D structure is cured in a controlled UV chamber [89, 91, 92]. SLA has been known as the most commonly used technique to manufacture microneedles due to its fine resolution (10 μm), high accuracy, and ability to form a smooth surface of the finished product. However, notable drawbacks include its slow printing speed, high cost, and limited range of suitable materials [93].

2.4.3.3 Digital Light Processing

The mechanism of digital light processing (DLP) is photopolymerization, in which a projection of light is used to polymerize photosensitive polymeric materials. This technique sheds light on the whole cross section of the object to create a volumetric pixel, thus making the process faster and more efficient than SLA [94].

2.4.3.4 Photon Polymerization

The layer-by-layer printing process of two-photon-polymerization (2PP) works on photopolymerization using the temporal and spatial overlap of photons [95]. A liquid resin droplet is exposed to a focused laser to polymerize the 3D structure of microneedles [94, 96]. Several advantages of 2PP have been reported: cost-effectiveness, versatile printing materials (solid, liquid, or powder precursors), high flexibility, scalable and fine resolution, excellent control over the printing structure's geometries, and ease of manufacturing in conventional facilities [94, 96]. Prausnitz group has fabricated drug-loaded poly(vinyl pyrrolidone) dissolving microneedles using this photopolymerization method [97]. The authors modified the needle dissolution kinetics by incorporating methacrylic acid as a copolymer during the polymerization process, which improved the needle fracture resistance/strength and reduced the drug release rate. Likewise, Ovsianikov and colleagues employed the 2PP method to fabricate in-plane and out-of-plane hollow microneedles using a chemically modified ceramic, Ormocer®, as the printing substrate [98]. A femtosecond laser was focused on a small photosensitive resin and moved in 3D direction to cleave the chemical bonds to create the desired 3D structure of microneedles.

2.4.4 Atomized Spraying Technique

Atomized spraying technique applies pressure from an air source to push liquid formulation through a nozzle as an atomized spray. This spray is then filled into a micromold, and the resulting needles are dried at room temperature. Various materials could be used to fabricate dissolving microneedles using this atomized spraying technique, including sugars (i.e., trehalose, fructose, and raffinose) and polymers (i.e., PVA, PVP, CMC, HPMC, and sodium alginate). This method overcomes technical issues with surface tension and viscosity of liquid formulation as a vacuum or pressure is generally required to fill the formulation into the mold. Furthermore, this technique enables the production of laminate-layered and horizontal-layered microneedle designs and ease of mass manufacturing [99].

2.4.5 X-ray Technique

Researchers have employed deep X-rays to fabricate 3D microneedle structures efficiently. For the first time, Moon and Lee proposed this technique to fabricate high-aspect-ratio microneedles with sharp tips. The manufacturing process includes vertical exposure and an inclined exposure to deep X-ray. An alteration to the inclined angle and the gap between the mask and the substrate causes a difference in the needle design. This method is more accessible, convenient, and efficient than silicon-based etching techniques, enabling the fabrication of a long needle shank that can be used in blood extraction from skin [100]. These needles could be used for drug delivery and blood sampling. Similarly, Perennes and coworkers employed this deep X-ray lithography method to fabricate PMMA hollow microneedles with sharp, beveled needle tips [101].

2.4.6 Laser Technique

The laser-based technique has been explored due to its ability to produce microneedles with a high aspect ratio and density [102]. Various types of laser have been utilized in microneedle fabrication; among those, carbon dioxide and neodymium:YAG are the most common. A pulsed excimer laser has also been used to selectively remove the material by disturbing the chemical bonds in the material structure. Several factors, including material type, pulse duration, and laser intensity, influence the total amount of material ablated.

2.4.6.1 Laser Cutting

The laser cutting method has been commonly used to manufacture solid metal microneedles. First, a computer-aided design (CAD) program is employed to customize the geometries and dimensions of desired microneedles. After that, an infrared laser is set up to cut sheets of stainless steel or titanium, following the CAD design. The sheet is then cleaned with hot water, and needles are bent 90°, perpendicular to the base substrate (the metal sheet). The needles are then sharpened, electropolished, finished, washed, and dried under compressed air. This technique enables the production of a single row of microneedles of various geometries and dimensions, multiple rows of microneedles, hollow microneedles [103], and micromold for subsequent fabrication of dissolving microneedles [104].

2.4.6.2 Laser Ablation

A high-energy, high-intensity, focused laser beam has been used to ablate material on a substrate to create the 3D structure of microneedles. Suited laser types include CO_2 [105], UV excimer [106], and femtosecond laser [107]. Laser ablation has been demonstrated as a rapid and efficient method for microneedle fabrication, taking only 10–100 ns to reach the burning point in the substrate material [71]. This noncontact processing applies only a low heat load on the material sheet and could shape any type of metal. Some shortcoming of this technique has been noted. The thermal effects on the cutting surface could modify the structure of mechanical properties of fabricated microneedles, causing cracking, or compromise with the needles' mechanical resistance [108, 109]. Furthermore, laser usage is expensive and unsuitable for mass manufacturing [71, 108].

2.4.7 Droplet-born Air Blowing

Kimet and colleagues first proposed this novel method to rapidly and efficiently manufacture dissolving polymeric microneedles (Fig. 2.3) [110]. This method enables the fabrication of dissolving microneedles simply from a polymeric droplet under mild and gentle conditions [44]. The principle of this technique is to elongate a droplet of a polymeric formulation and eventually separate and shape it into two microneedles which are dried under air blowing. For the fabrication process, droplets of a specific size are dispensed on a plate. The physical properties (i.e., surface tension, viscosity, polymer concentration) and dimensions of the droplet will dictate the size and shape of fabricated microneedles. The upper plate is then moved down to contact the droplets for proper adhesion and interaction. The two plates are separated at a predetermined speed to elongate the droplets consistently. While the plates are moving, controlled air at a specific temperature, humidity, composition, speed, and direction is blown through the droplets to remove residual water and solidify the microneedles structure [110, 111]. The physical features of microneedles

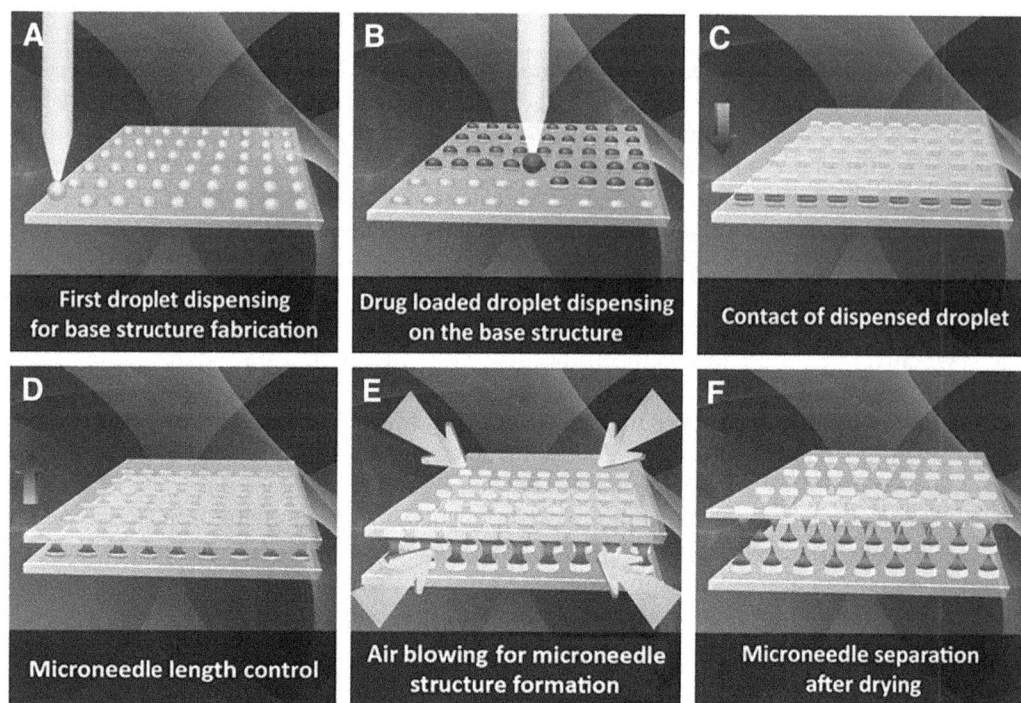

FIGURE 2.3
Schematic illustration of dissolving polymeric microneedles fabricated by droplet-born air blowing technique. Images reprinted with permission from [110].

(i.e., dimensions, geometries, sharpness) and the loaded drug's chemical stability depend on the pulling speed of the plates and the controlled air blowing. It has been stated that this approach offers many benefits. The fabrication process is fast; microneedles can be produced within 10 min. Furthermore, researchers could control the droplet size and the drug concentration and quantity of the drug load while minimizing possible drug loss. Moreover, there is no UV irradiation or heat usage during the fabrication process, thus reserving the chemical stability of the loaded compound and avoiding the risk of interaction between different ingredients in the formulation composition [69]. However, there is a specific limit to the shape, length, and sharpness of microneedles fabricated by this method. This novel technique has been commonly used to fabricate microneedles for cosmetic purposes. In the pharmaceutical field, insulin-encapsulated microneedles have been produced using this droplet-born air blowing method. The needles could effectively reduce blood glucose level in diabetic mice [110].

2.4.8 Drawing Lithography

The drawing lithography technique uses extensional deformation and capillary self-thinning to extend planar 2D viscous polymeric substrate material into a 3D structure of microneedles. This technique could produce hollow, dissolving, and hybrid electro-microneedles. The continuous drawing technique has been employed to fabricate hollow microneedles with ultrahigh aspect ratio, while the stepwise controlled drawing method enables the production of dissolving microneedles. The drawing with antidromic isolation could successfully make a hybrid electro-microneedle array. The manufacturing process relies on the glass transition history of the materials [5]. Researchers have revealed that the drawing lithography technique could provide precise geometries and smooth vertical sidewalls of microneedles [71]. Various materials have been explored, such as glass, metals, sugars, ceramics, and plastics [112]. For instance, maltose has been commonly used due to its triple states (liquid, glassy, and solid) and changing viscosity with temperature manipulation [113].

2.4.9 Pulling Pipettes

Pulling pipette is a simple and convenient method to fabricate hollow glass microneedles. Fire-polished borosilicate glass pipettes are pulled out using a micropipette and beveled at a certain speed and high temperature [12, 114]. Hollow glass microneedles fabricated by the pulling pipettes technique have been used to assist transdermal delivery of various compounds, enabling the injection of milliliters of liquid formulation into the skin [12]. These needles effectively delivered a bolus insulin dose to patients with type 1 diabetes [114] or injected 6-aminoquinolone and Rose Bengal into the eye for minimally invasive and enhanced intraocular drug delivery [115].

2.4.10 Microinjection Molding

Microinjection molding relies on a simple principle where a thermoplastic material is heated to a high temperature beyond its melting point to melt the material into a thin molten liquid. This low-viscosity liquid is injected into a closed mold with a defined shape and size. After that, the fabricated microneedles are separated from the mold. The processing parameters, such as clamping force, shot size, injection velocity, packing pressure, and temperature, could be modified to obtain the desired reproducibility. This injection molding technique offers several advantages, such as high repeatability, precise dosing, and high injection flow rate [116]. This is also a promising technique for large-scale manufacturing of solid microneedles with miniature tip diameters. However, some shortcomings are noted, such as the requirement to control the small shot size with the dimension of the conventional screw of 15–150 mm, and the high initial cost/investment in the manufacturing equipment [117]. Furthermore, this technique uses high temperatures during the injection process, which could induce significant drug degradation. Lhernould and coworkers employed this microinjection molding method to fabricate hollow polymeric microneedles arrays from polycarbonate material. The needles were reported to resist high mechanical pressure and deliver multiple injections without blunting the needle tips [118]. Researchers could employ this technique in another investigation to produce solid microneedles to effectively deliver hydrophilic macromolecules [14].

2.4.11 Coating Techniques

The coating has been popularly used to coat a layer of drug-loaded formulation (solution or suspension) onto the surface of solid microneedles, which could be silicon, metal, or polymeric microneedles. The coating process parameters could be customized to control the contact area between the microneedles and the coating formulation. This way, the coating layer could cover the needle shafts only or both the needle shafts and the base substrate of the array. The coating process could be selective and optimized to minimize drug loss, control drug dosage, and improve drug delivery efficiency. An advantage of coated microneedles is in the rapid release profile of the drug payload [119]. Once coated microneedles are inserted, the coating layer is easily separated from the needles and quickly disintegrates in skin tissue [120]. Furthermore, these needles are fabricated based on sharp and mechanically strong solid microneedles; thus, these coated microneedles have excellent mechanical toughness, which can withstand high external force during skin insertion. Also, the coating formulation has a negligible effect on the needles' mechanical strength. This is an advantage of coated microneedles over dissolving microneedles, whose mechanical robustness could be significantly influenced by the polymeric formulation. Moreover, various polymers have been used to formulate the coating layer to efficiently deliver therapeutic agents of any size. Also, the coated drug is in a solid coating layer, thus enhancing the drug stability and bypassing the requirement for cold-chain storage. However, the drug release profile depends on the microneedle structure, geometries, and dimensions. Generally, the drug load in coated microneedles is very limited due to the small surface area of the needles. Coated microneedles possess several technical issues, such as drug stability during the drying step and the uniformity of the coating thickness, which markedly impact the accurate dosing, coating consistency, reproducibility of the manufacturing process, and substantial drug loss. There are several coating techniques, including layer-by-layer assembly, electrohydrodynamic atomization, dip-coating, drop-coating, gas-jet drying, spray coating, and piezoelectric inkjet printing. To improve the coating efficiency, scientists have performed precoating of the surface of the microneedle with SiO_2, PLGA, polyvinylpyrrolidone [35], or chitosan [42]. Also, polyelectrolyte coatings with microencapsulation properties have been executed with poly[di(carboxylatophenoxy) phosphazene] [121, 122], chitosan, and carboxymethyl cellulose [123]. This precoating step could improve the coating consistency, uniformity, and efficiency; enhance drug delivery; and increase drug stability.

2.4.11.1 Immersion Coating

Immersion coating is the first coating technique reported in the literature and has been commonly used by many research groups [124–127]. For the process, the entire array is immersed in the coating formulation; thus, the whole needle array, including micronee-dles shafts, and the front and back sides of the base substrate are all coated. Although this is a simple and convenient coating method, substantial drug loss has been reported. Also, this coating method leads to the variable thickness of the coating layer [34, 40].

2.4.11.2 Dip-coating Method

Dip-coating has been regarded as a simple, convenient, and cost-effective method to coat microneedles. In general, the needle shafts are selectively coated without coating the base substrate from which the drug could not enter the skin and is considered a loss. First, a coating formulation (i.e., aqueous solution, organic solvent-based liquid, or molten fluid) is prepared at a predetermined viscosity and surface tension. The solid needles are immersed into the drug formulation for proper adhesion of a liquid film on the surface of the needles. After this dip, the needles are elevated, removed from the coating liquid, and dried to form a solid film on the needles. These dip-and-lift steps could be repeated until the desired coating thickness is achieved [119, 128]. Two critical parameters of the coating liquid are viscosity and surface tension, which could significantly affect the coating thick-ness and level for a selective coating on the needle shafts. This selective coating could be obtained using masked or thin-film dip-coating. In masked dip-coating, the base substrate is masked or covered to avoid interacting with the coating formulation [129]. To prevent the coating formulation from rising and touching the array substrate, thin-film dip-coating typically uses coating liquids with thicknesses that are shorter than the needle length [128]. The loaded drug quantity depends on the coating layer's thickness, which varies depending on various factors, such as the physical properties of the coating formulation and the drying time between the dips [120]. A thicker coating layer or greater drug load could be attained by increasing the speed of microneedles exiting the coating formulation, increasing the formulation viscosity, or increasing the number of dips. In many studies, surfactants were added to the coating formulation to reduce the surface tension of the coating formulation, thereby improving the coating consistency and uniformity. Several drawbacks of the dip-coating technique have been revealed: (i) slow drying could cause a significant drug loss, (ii) the inherent surface tension of the coating liquid could cause an issue with the coating uniformity, especially for adjacent microneedles which are closely located on the array [128].

2.4.11.3 Layer-by-layer Coating

Layer-by-layer (LbL) assembly is a modified dip-coating method in which electrostatic interaction deposits an ultrathin coating layer on the needle surface. The mechanism of the LbL assembly/coating technique is the deposition of interacting species on a substrate with the intervening step of rinsing the structure [130]. Multiple nano-sized layers of microneedles are formed by alternately coating positively and negatively charged polyelectrolytes on the structure [131]. The LbL technique allows for control over the nanoscale structure, multiple loaded therapeutic agents, and released materials. This method protects and stabilizes encapsulated agents by occlusions against impacts from environmental conditions. This method enables the fabrication of thermostable solid coated microneedles, which could be stored without refrigeration or a cold chain [69]. This delicate fabrication process suits thermosensitive compounds such as biologics, macromolecules, proteins, DNA, and vaccines [132, 133]. Due to the thin coating layer (about 100 nm), microneedles' original shape and sharpness are well-maintained [33, 42, 132–134]. For DNA and proteins, the coating formulation consists of DNA or proteins with a negative charge and a selected polymer with a positive charge, thus forming a polyelectrolyte multilayer coating on the surface of the needles. DeMuth and colleagues employed the layer-by-layer assembly method to coat poly(lactide-*co*-glycolide) (PLGA) microneedles with multiple layers of cationic poly(β-amino ester) and negatively charged interbilayer-crosslinked multi-lamellar lipid vesicles loaded with the protein antigen ovalbumin (OVA) and the adjuvant monophosphoryl lipid A [135]. The fabricated needles could penetrate the skin and rapidly release the drug load into skin tissue within 5 min. This group also used the LbL method to fabricate coated microneedles loaded with immune-stimulatory RNA and DNA in biodegradable polymeric multilayer films to achieve rapid delivery and enhanced vaccination [136].

2.4.11.4 Drop-coating Method

Drop-coating is a modified dip-coating technique. The coating liquid is dropped onto the microneedle array, covering all the needles rather than dipping the array into the coating formulation. This way, the coating liquid will cover all needles and the base substrate's front side without coating the substrate's back side. When the solvent or water evaporates, the remaining solid coats the needles and base substrate uniformly. However, due to the slow evaporation rate at ambient conditions, the coating becomes nonuniform; the coating liquid is separated from the needle tip and accumulates primarily on the substrate between the needles. Thus, conformal and uniform coating is not achieved [33, 137]. This issue could be addressed by increasing the solvent evaporation rate under heat [138] or vacuum application [139]. Accelerated drying could be obtained by using gas jet–assisted drying. Rapid solvent evaporation could result in conformal coating on microneedle shafts; however, it could not completely avoid coating the base substrate.

2.4.11.5 Spray Coating

The spray coating technique uses fluid pressure to generate fine droplets (smaller than 280 μm) deposited and coated on a microneedles array. For the process, atomization under high pressure is first performed to produce droplets. These droplets are then deposited and adhered to the surface of the microneedles. Then, the droplets are outspread and merged to form a conformal coating film on the needle shaft and base substrate. A conformal coating is governed by the coalescence of the droplets on the needle surface, which is influenced by the viscosity and surface tension of the coating formulation, as well as the size of the droplets [137, 140]. Several factors are found to affect the coating efficiency. The droplet deposition is dictated by spray velocity and density [140]. The coating fluid's physicochemical qualities (i.e., concentration, viscosity, surface tension, and density), as well as the spraying parameters (i.e., air-to-liquid mass ratio, spraying duration, atomization air pressure, gun-to-surface distance, and air cap setting), have a significant impact on the droplet size.

2.4.11.6 Electrohydrodynamic Atomization

Electrohydrodynamic atomization (EHDA) is a modified spray coating technique. Instead of using fluid pressure to create droplets, this technique uses electrical potential to produce atomized droplets. This method has been used to prepare nano- and microscaled coating [141]. For the system setup, the microneedles array (specifically metal microneedles) is grounded to an electrode while the liquid nozzle is connected to a high voltage. When the voltage reaches a critical level, the coating liquid spurts out of the spraying nozzle to create droplets. This electrical field creates a charge inside the droplets. The droplets are then deposited on the grounded microneedle array positioned at a certain distance from the nozzle [142]. EHDA could produce particles (electrospraying) or fibers (electrospinning). Khan et al. [141] employed this technique with a sacrificial insulating mask to selectively coat the needles shafts and prevent the coating of the base substrate. This selective coating approach still causes a significant drug loss on the mask [143]. EHDA enables the coating of a single needle (formulation injection through a single nozzle), coaxial coating (immiscible fluids are injected through separate nozzles), or multiplexed coating (formulation injected through a single or coaxial nozzle array) [144]. Physical properties of the droplets (i.e., size, porosity, shape, surface charge) are determined by the flow rate, voltage, nozzle-to-collector distance, viscosity, and surface tension of the coating liquid. The most critical requirement for the EHDA process is the low electrical conductivity of the solvent [143].

2.4.11.7 Gas-jet Drying

Gas-jet drying employs a gas-jet applicator to turn a drug suspension coating formulation into the gas form [145]. This technique enables fast drying of coating formulation, thus preventing the movement of the coating layer, the change in the coating thickness, and the alteration in the dose accuracy. Hence, gas-jet drying is preferable to coat short, dense, or curved microneedles for which the conventional wet coating faces technical issues of coating consistency, uniformity, and drug loss [144]. Another advantage is noted as gas-jet drying provides uniform distribution of the coating liquid and selective coating on microneedles shafts [33]. For example, coating formulation including methylcellulose, surfactant, and the drug was successfully coated on solid silicon microneedles. The drying step was carried out using a gas jet at 6–8 m/s and incident angle at 20° horizontally. The thickness of the resulting coated layer was 5 μm. The coating liquid was coated selectively and dried rapidly on the needle shaft surface without migrating to the base substrate.

2.4.11.8 Piezoelectric Inkjet Printing

Piezoelectric inkjet printing enables a controlled and accurate coating with fine droplets ejected from a piezo-driven nozzle [92, 146, 147]. This technique could use various aqueous or solvent-based formulations. Formulation composition with a low viscosity is required to prevent the risk of clogging the jetting nozzle and to facilitate the generation of tiny droplets [147]. This method deposits several small-sized drops to cover and coat the needle surface. Inkjet printing can only coat one side of the needles at a time in a unidirectional way. A second coating cycle is needed to have all sides of the needles coated. To simultaneously coat multiple needles, several nozzles have to work at the same time. If the spacing of the needles is small, then it will be difficult to arrange the nozzles. This piezoelectric inkjet printing technique provides improved accuracy, reproducibility, lesser waste, scalability, and capacity for continuous manufacturing. A shortcoming of this method is the limited surface area of microneedles that could be targeted for printing [148]. A modified piezoelectric inkjet printing is thermal inkjet printing in which the droplets are created by raising the formulation temperature above its boiling point [149]. The pressure pulse in the ink compartment distorts piezoelectric crystal and causes the ejection of droplets from the printing nozzle. The coating efficiency primarily depends on the nozzle size, applied voltage, and pulse duration [147].

2.5 Applicators for Microneedle Insertion

2.5.1 Introduction of Applicators

Due to the inherent viscoelasticity and irregular surface of the skin, it is challenging to insert microneedles into skin tissue with high precision, accuracy, reproducibility, and minimal inter-individual variability. It is common consent that microneedles require an external force to be inserted to the desired depth. Initially, in feasibility studies, manual insertion was regarded as a reliable method for microneedle penetration [60, 150]. Qualified and trained researchers performed this insertion. However, the scenario is significantly different with untrained patients and healthcare givers who execute the drug administration. Patients would indeed require some training for reproducible microneedles application. Thus, the development of applicators is inevitable for the use of microneedles to assist transdermal drug delivery. For patients to receive reliable, consistent, and accurate doses, microneedles should porate the skin to reproducible depths without breaking or bending [49]. This enables patients to take the dose independently and improves patient and healthcare professional acceptability. So far, there is no universal applicator available on the market. The design of the applicator depends on the geometry, design, sharpness, and density of microneedles, the device's accuracy, ease of fabrication and handling, intended use, and manufacturing cost [49]. In particular, an impact-insertion applicator is used to insert high-density or blunt microneedles to the desired depth in the skin. In contrast, a manual handheld applicator is generally used for sharp microneedles [5]. The ideal applicator should be inexpensive, reusable, portable, and easily handled regardless of users' age, gender, and educational background. The use of an applicator makes microneedles a simple, user-friendly, and low-cost medical device. Numerous simple custom-made applicators have been reported in the literature to be utilized in laboratories. There are many different kinds of applicators available, such as those with a syringe built right into the array of microneedles [151], those with the array of microneedles affixed to the plunger of a syringe [152], those made from an inverted plastic syringe whose plunger surface has been smoothed to remove any protrusions [153], those made from a cylinder of aluminum covered with one or more of the following: soft rubber, elastic band rubber, hard rubber, foam, or rubber cushion [153]. Other applicator designs include a customized pen-like device [154], a spring-loaded applicator [33, 80, 155], an electrically driven applicator [150, 156], and a handheld applicator for manual application [157]. Several pharmaceutical companies have designed innovative applicator devices for microneedle drug delivery systems, including 3M, Clinical Resolution Laboratory, Corium, BD, Alza Corporation, and NanoBioSciences. BD Soluvia™ employs a syringe integrated into a single microneedle for both microneedles insertion and delivery of fluid. Numerous applicator designs have been disclosed in recent patents, some in the development stage, and some are available on the market.

2.5.2 Features of Applicators

There are several critical features of applicators. A reliable applicator should cause no pain and no risk of microneedles breaking or bending [7, 8, 34, 150, 153, 158, 159]. The primary use of applicators is to ensure an effective, reproducible, and controlled penetration depth of microneedles into the skin tissue. The device should be easy to use or handle by patients of different ages, genders, and educational backgrounds. Manual applicators generally require thumb pressure, semiautomatic applicators require some adjustment before use, while fully automated applicators should be actuated automatically and reliably at a particular stimulus. The applicator should not cause any reaction or irritation on the skin. The cost of a microneedle device consists of the constituting costs of the applicator, microneedle array, and active pharmaceutical ingredient. Thus, a low price is also an essential feature of an applicator, facilitating widespread use and acceptability among patients and healthcare professionals. Besides, the applicator can be disposed of safely at a reasonable expense. Nondegradable microneedles such as silicon, metal, and glass microneedles generate sharp waste after usage, thus adding up to the economic cost of sharp disposal. On the other hand, biodegradable polymeric microneedles could be disposed of safely and efficiently.

There are numerous designs of applicators. A direct manual application relying on impact insertion is commonly used in the simplest configuration. Despite its simplicity, this design possesses several drawbacks. Low accuracy and limited reproducibility in microneedle penetration have been noted. Due to the inherent viscoelasticity and irregular surface of the skin, the skin tends to fold around the needles to cause partial and incomplete penetration of microneedles (only around 30% of microneedle length effectively penetrates the skin). Also, the application force could vary significantly among users, thus leading to significant inter- and intra-individual variability, especially in old-aged patients. A simple manual stretching of the skin has been revealed to circumvent and reduce skin elasticity. Also, reduced elasticity could be achieved by applying reduced pressure or adhering to a thin film or membrane over the application site [150]. Applicators could function based on mechanical or electromechanical force to deliver a defined pressure to insert microneedles into the skin. The device could be triggered by a push-button system, a pressure/distance sensor, or an electrical control. The design of impact-insertion applicators varies from handheld applicators, in which microneedles are manually or mechanically inserted into the skin, to complex electrically driven applicators [47, 150].

Applicators could be designed for single use or multiple uses. For single use, the applicator could be included in the sterile package of the product, as proposed by Yeshurun et al. [160]. The single-use applicator could be disposed of after use. A mechanically driven design is suitable for single use from the economic perspective [5]. Besides, applicators could be designed for multiple uses. The applicator could be packed with a certain number of microneedles arrays for multiple uses in repeated doses or various patients. This applicator should preferably deliver electrically driven force that is conveniently adjustable and remains consistent over the device's lifetime. Such a device should be calibrated regularly to confirm its accuracy, reliability, and reproducibility.

In a two-step application system, a microneedle array is first applied onto the skin in the same way as a conventional transdermal patch. Then, the applicator is activated to deliver a specific force on the path to achieve the desired penetration depth of microneedles. This simple design could provide reliable microneedles-assisted drug delivery. Also, the applicator device could be reused for multiple microneedle patches. However, this two-step process is inconvenient and could cause errors due to misarrangement between the microneedles patch and the applicator. A microneedle patch could be integrated into the applicator device to address this issue. This way, when the applicator is activated, the microneedles are inserted into the skin simultaneously to deliver the drug load. This one-step application process is more reliable, accurate, and convenient.

The size and shape of microneedles applicators should be carefully designed, taking into consideration the ease of handling and storage. Portable devices called "pen injectors" have been used to accurately deliver variable doses of insulin and hormone [160]. This design could be applied to a microneedle applicator device to improve handling and portability. Significantly, a measure to ensure successful microneedle penetration should be developed. Markers or indicators can reveal microneedle penetration into the skin tissue. These signal demonstrators include audible prompts (popping, clicking, snaping), visible markers, electrical signals, or specific indicators. This way, patients and healthcare providers gain confidence that the microneedle-mediated dose has been properly administered. Interestingly, several research groups have reported the "push-out" phenomenon of microneedles from the skin after the removal of the applicator due to the skin's viscoelasticity. This reduces the penetration depth of microneedles, partially closes microneedles-created microchannels in the skin, and lowers drug delivery. Thus, microneedles should be kept and secured in the skin tissue by applying a pressure-sensitive adhesive on the backing layer of the microneedle array. The adhesive could be pressed manually or included as an add-on device within the applicator [161]. Dissolving, coated, and swelling microneedles should be kept in the skin for a certain period for the needles to disintegrate and release the drug load. Therefore, the ideal adhesive should be sufficiently strong to secure the needles in the skin for such a drug-releasing period.

2.5.3 Packaging of Microneedles

Packaging of microneedles should be appropriately designed to preserve the physical and chemical integrity of microneedles products during transport and storage, especially in harsh conditions such as warm temperatures and high humidity. Under high temperatures, encapsulated drugs could be degraded rapidly, rendering the microneedles ineffective. Under high humidity, the needles could absorb moisture and lose their sharpness and strength, thus failing the skin insertion. The controlled packaging is critical for coated, dissolving, and hydrogel microneedles. Hydrogel microneedles could swell and become unusable in a high-moisture environment. The sharpness of dissolving microneedles could be compromised as the needle tips absorb moisture quickly. Patients could generally carry small-sized microneedle packages in a purse or pockets [49]. Hence, the package should be sufficiently robust to prevent contamination, damage, or accidental drug release during storage [162]. For the packaging components, a suitable desiccant should be included in the package to reduce the moisture content. Furthermore, a cushion or protective cover should protect the fragile needle tips. Besides, clear, legible, and easy-to-follow labeling should be present on the package to assist in patient handling of the product.

References

[1] Gerstel MS, Place VA. Drug delivery device. 1976. [Internet]. Available from: https://patents.google.com/patent/US3964482A/en.

[2] Henry S, McAllister DV, Allen MG, et al. Micromachined needles for the transdermal delivery of drugs. Elev Annu Int Workshop Micro Electro Mech Syst 1998 MEMS 98 Proc. 1998. p. 494–498.

[3] Smart WH, Subramanian K. The use of silicon microfabrication technology in painless blood glucose monitoring. Diabetes Technol Ther. 2000;2:549–559.

[4] Gardeniers HJ, Luttge R, Berenschot EJ, et al. Silicon micromachined hollow microneedles for transdermal liquid transport. J Microelectromechanical Syst. 2003;12:855–862.

[5] van der Maaden K, Jiskoot W, Bouwstra J. Microneedle technologies for (trans)dermal drug and vaccine delivery. J Control Release. 2012;161:645–655.

[6] Davidson A, Al-Qallaf B, Das DB. Transdermal drug delivery by coated microneedles: geometry effects on effective skin thickness and drug permeability. Chem Eng Res Des. 2008;86:1196–1206.

[7] Bal SM, Ding Z, van Riet E, et al. Advances in transcutaneous vaccine delivery: do all ways lead to Rome? J Control Release. 2010;148:266–282.

[8] Banga AK. Microporation applications for enhancing drug delivery. Expert Opin Drug Deliv. 2009;6:343–354.

[9] Sivamani RK, Liepmann D, Maibach HI. Microneedles and transdermal applications. Expert Opin Drug Deliv. 2007;4:19–25.

[10] Bodhale DW, Nisar A, Afzulpurkar N. Structural and microfluidic analysis of hollow side-open polymeric microneedles for transdermal drug delivery applications. Microfluid Nanofluidics. 2010;8:373–392.

[11] Luttge R, Berenschot EJW, de Boer MJ, et al. Integrated lithographic molding for microneedle-based devices. J Microelectromechanical Syst. 2007;16:872–884.

[12] Martanto W, Moore JS, Kashlan O, et al. Microinfusion using hollow microneedles. Pharm Res. 2006;23:104–113.

[13] Stoeber B, Liepmann D. Design, fabrication and testing of a MEMS syringe. Proc Solid-State Sens Actuator Workshop. 2002. p. 2–7.

[14] Nair KJ. Micro-injection moulded microneedles for drug delivery. Bradford: University of Bradford; 2016.

[15] Henry S, McAllister DV, Allen MG, et al. Microfabricated microneedles: a novel approach to transdermal drug delivery. J Pharm Sci. 1998;87:922–925.

[16] McAllister DV, Allen MG, Prausnitz MR. Microfabricated microneedles for gene and drug delivery. Annu Rev Biomed Eng. 2000;2:289–313.

[17] McAllister DV, Wang PM, Davis SP, et al. Microfabricated needles for transdermal delivery of macromolecules and nanoparticles: fabrication methods and transport studies. Proc Natl Acad Sci. 2003;100:13755–13760.

[18] Paik S-J, Byun S, Lim J-M, et al. In-plane single-crystal-silicon microneedles for minimally invasive microfluid systems. Sens Actuators Phys. 2004;114:276–284.

[19] Reed ML, Lye W-K. Microsystems for drug and gene delivery. Proc IEEE. 2004;92:56–75.

[20] Caffarel-Salvador E, Donnelly RF. Transdermal drug delivery mediated by microneedle arrays: innovations and barriers to success. Curr Pharm Des. 2016;22:1105–1117.

[21] Verbaan FJ, Bal SM, van den Berg DJ, et al. Assembled microneedle arrays enhance the transport of compounds varying over a large range of molecular weight across human dermatomed skin. J Control Release. 2007;117:238–245.

[22] Gupta J, Gill HS, Andrews SN, et al. Kinetics of skin resealing after insertion of microneedles in human subjects. J Control Release. 2011;154:148–155.

[23] Kim M-C, Lee JW, Choi H-J, et al. Microneedle patch delivery to the skin of virus-like particles containing heterologous M2e extracellular domains of influenza virus induces broad heterosubtypic cross-protection. J Control Release. 2015;210:208–216.

[24] Waghule T, Singhvi G, Dubey SK, et al. Microneedles: a smart approach and increasing potential for transdermal drug delivery system. Biomed Pharmacother. 2019;109:1249–1258.

[25] Hilt JZ, Peppas NA. Microfabricated drug delivery devices. Int J Pharm. 2005;306:15–23.

[26] Cheung K, Das DB. Microneedles for drug delivery: trends and progress. Drug Deliv. 2015;1–17.

[27] Davis SP, Martanto W, Allen MG, et al. Hollow metal microneedles for insulin delivery to diabetic rats. IEEE Trans Biomed Eng. 2005;52:909–915.

[28] Donnelly RF, Morrow DIJ, McCrudden MTC, et al. Hydrogel-forming and dissolving microneedles for enhanced delivery of photosensitizers and precursors. Photochem Photobiol. 2014;90:641–647.

[29] Dang N, Liu TY, Prow TW. Nano-and microtechnology in skin delivery of vaccines. In: Micro nanotechnology in vaccine development. Amsterdam, NL: Elsevier; 2017. p. 327–341.

[30] Zhang P, Dalton C, Jullien GA. Design and fabrication of MEMS-based microneedle arrays for medical applications. Microsyst Technol. 2009;15:1073–1082.

[31] Li J, Zeng M, Shan H, et al. Microneedle patches as drug and vaccine delivery platform. Curr Med Chem. 2017;24:2413–2422.

[32] Gill HS, Prausnitz MR. Coated microneedles for transdermal delivery. J Control Release. 2007;117:227–237.

[33] Chen X, Prow TW, Crichton ML, et al. Dry-coated microprojection array patches for targeted delivery of immunotherapeutics to the skin. J Control Release. 2009;139:212–220.

[34] Cormier M, Johnson B, Ameri M, et al. Transdermal delivery of desmopressin using a coated microneedle array patch system. J Control Release. 2004;97:503–511.

[35] Gill HS, Prausnitz MR. Coating formulations for microneedles. Pharm Res. 2007;24:1369–1380.

[36] Prausnitz MR, Gill HS, Park J-H. Microneedles for drug delivery. In: Michael J. Rathbone, Jonathan Hadgraft, Michael S. Roberts, Majella E. Lane, editors. Modified-release drug delivery technology. Boca Raton, Florida: CRC Press; 2008. p. 323–338.

[37] Zhang Y, Brown K, Siebenaler K, et al. Development of lidocaine-coated microneedle product for rapid, safe, and prolonged local analgesic action. Pharm Res. 2012;29:170–177.

[38] Chen X, Fernando GJ, Crichton ML, et al. Improving the reach of vaccines to low-resource regions, with a needle-free vaccine delivery device and long-term thermostabilization. J Control Release. 2011;152:349–355.

[39] Kwon KM, Lim S-M, Choi S, et al. Microneedles: quick and easy delivery methods of vaccines. Clin Exp Vaccine Res. 2017;6:156–159.

[40] Matriano JA, Cormier M, Johnson J, et al. Macroflux® Microprojection array patch technology: a new and efficient approach for intracutaneous immunization. Pharm Res. 2002;19:63–70.

[41] Widera G, Johnson J, Kim L, et al. Effect of delivery parameters on immunization to ovalbumin following intracutaneous administration by a coated microneedle array patch system. Vaccine. 2006;24:1653–1664.

[42] Xie Y, Xu B, Gao Y. Controlled transdermal delivery of model drug compounds by MEMS microneedle array. Nanomedicine Nanotechnol Biol Med. 2005;1:184–190.

[43] González-Vázquez P, Larrañeta E, McCrudden MT, et al. Transdermal delivery of gentamicin using dissolving microneedle arrays for potential treatment of neonatal sepsis. J Control Release. 2017;265:30–40.

[44] Park J-H, Allen MG, Prausnitz MR. Biodegradable polymer microneedles: fabrication, mechanics and transdermal drug delivery. J Control Release. 2005;104:51–66.

[45] Park J-H, Allen MG, Prausnitz MR. Polymer microneedles for controlled-release drug delivery. Pharm Res. 2006;23:1008–1019.

[46] Corrie SR, Fernando GJ, Crichton ML, et al. Surface-modified microprojection arrays for intradermal biomarker capture, with low non-specific protein binding. Lab Chip. 2010;10:2655–2658.

[47] Bal SM, Caussin J, Pavel S, et al. In vivo assessment of safety of microneedle arrays in human skin. Eur J Pharm Sci. 2008;35:193–202.

[48] Prausnitz MR, Langer R. Transdermal drug delivery. Nat Biotechnol. 2008;26:1261–1268.

[49] Sachdeva VK, Banga A. Microneedles and their applications. Recent Pat Drug Deliv Formul. 2011;5:95–132.

[50] Miyano T, Tobinaga Y, Kanno T, et al. Sugar micro needles as transdermic drug delivery system. Biomed Microdevices. 2005;7:185–188.

[51] Donnelly RF, Morrow DIJ, Singh TRR, et al. Processing difficulties and instability of carbohydrate microneedle arrays. Drug Dev Ind Pharm. 2009;35:1242–1254.

[52] Donnelly RF, McCrudden MT, Alkilani AZ, et al. Hydrogel-forming microneedles prepared from "super swelling" polymers combined with lyophilised wafers for transdermal drug delivery. PLoS One. 2014;9:e111547.

[53] Jin T. Phase-transition polymeric microneedles. 2016. [Internet] [cited 2022 Nov 9]. Available from: https://patents.google.com/patent/US9320878B2/en?q=Phase-transition+polymeric+microneedles&oq=Phase-transition+polymeric+microneedles.

[54] Donnelly RF, Singh TRR, Garland MJ, et al. Hydrogel-forming microneedle arrays for enhanced transdermal drug delivery. Adv Funct Mater. 2012;22:4879–4890.

[55] Tucak A, Sirbubalo M, Hindija L, et al. Microneedles: characteristics, materials, production methods and commercial development. Micromachines. 2020;11:961.

[56] Davis SP, Landis BJ, Adams ZH, et al. Insertion of microneedles into skin: measurement and prediction of insertion force and needle fracture force. J Biomech. 2004;37:1155–1163.

[57] Park J-H, Prausnitz MR. Analysis of mechanical failure of polymer microneedles by axial force. J Korean Phys Soc. 2010;56:1223.

[58] Martanto W, Moore JS, Couse T, et al. Mechanism of fluid infusion during microneedle insertion and retraction. J Control Release. 2006;112:357–361.

[59] Doddaballapur S, others. Microneedling with dermaroller. J Cutan Aesthetic Surg. 2009;2:110.

[60] Li W-Z, Huo M-R, Zhou J-P, et al. Super-short solid silicon microneedles for transdermal drug delivery applications. Int J Pharm. 2010;389:122–129.

[61] Arora A, Prausnitz MR, Mitragotri S. Micro-scale devices for transdermal drug delivery. Int J Pharm. 2008;364:227–236.

[62] Cahill EM, O'Cearbhaill ED. Toward biofunctional microneedles for stimulus responsive drug delivery. Bioconjug Chem. 2015;26:1289–1296.

[63] Sharma D. Microneedles: an approach in transdermal drug delivery: a Review. PharmaTutor. 2018;6:7–15.

[64] Donnelly RF, Singh TRR, Larrañeta E, et al. Microneedles for drug and vaccine delivery and patient monitoring. New Jersey: John Wiley & Sons; 2018.

[65] O'Mahony C. Structural characterization and in-vivo reliability evaluation of silicon microneedles. Biomed Microdevices. 2014;16:333–343.

[66] Monteiro-Riviere NA. Toxicology of the skin. Florida: CRC Press; 2010.

[67] Niinomi M, Nakai M. Titanium-based biomaterials for preventing stress shielding between implant devices and bone. Int J Biomater. 2011;2011.

[68] Donnelly RF, Singh TRR, Morrow DI, et al. Microneedle-mediated transdermal and intradermal drug delivery. New Jersey: John Wiley & Sons; 2012.

[69] Indermun S, Luttge R, Choonara YE, et al. Current advances in the fabrication of microneedles for transdermal delivery. J Control Release. 2014;185:130–138.

[70] Hong X, Wei L, Wu F, et al. Dissolving and biodegradable microneedle technologies for transdermal sustained delivery of drug and vaccine. Drug Des Devel Ther. 2013;7:945–952.

[71] Jeggy C. Micro-injection moulding: from process to modelling. Belgium: Presses univ. de Louvain; 2004.

[72] Lall D, Naim MJ, Rathore S. An emerging transdermal drug delivery system: fabrication and characterization of natural and biodegradable polymeric microneedles transdermal patch. J Pharm Res Int. 2021;46–54.

[73] Kim Y-C, Park J-H, Prausnitz MR. Microneedles for drug and vaccine delivery. Adv Drug Deliv Rev. 2012;64:1547–1568.

[74] Kim MJ, Park SC, Rizal B, et al. Fabrication of circular obelisk-type multilayer microneedles using micro-milling and spray deposition. Front Bioeng Biotechnol. 2018;6:54.

[75] Ita K. Transdermal delivery of drugs with microneedles-potential and challenges. Pharmaceutics. 2015;7:90–105.

[76] Donnelly RF, Majithiya R, Singh TRR, et al. Design, optimization and characterisation of polymeric microneedle arrays prepared by a novel laser-based micromoulding technique. Pharm Res. 2011;28:41–57.

[77] McCrudden MTC, Alkilani AZ, McCrudden CM, et al. Design and physicochemical characterisation of novel dissolving polymeric microneedle arrays for transdermal delivery of high dose, low molecular weight drugs. J Control Release. 2014;180:71–80.

[78] Bystrova S, Luttge R. Micromolding for ceramic microneedle arrays. Microelectron Eng. 2011;88:1681–1684.

[79] Fukushima K, Ise A, Morita H, et al. Two-layered dissolving microneedles for percutaneous delivery of peptide/protein drugs in rats. Pharm Res. 2011;28:7–21.

[80] Raphael AP, Prow TW, Crichton ML, et al. Targeted, needle-free vaccinations in skin using multilayered, densely-packed dissolving microprojection arrays. Small. 2010;6:1785–1793.

[81] Ito Y, Hasegawa R, Fukushima K, et al. Self-dissolving micropile array chip as percutaneous delivery system of protein drug. Biol Pharm Bull. 2010;33:683–690.

[82] Wendorf JR, Ghartey-Tagoe EB, Williams SC, et al. Transdermal delivery of macromolecules using solid-state biodegradable microstructures. Pharm Res. 2010;28:22–30.

[83] You X, Chang J, Ju B-K, et al. Rapidly dissolving fibroin microneedles for transdermal drug delivery. Mater Sci Eng C. 2011;31:1632–1636.

[84] Martin CJ, Allender CJ, Brain KR, et al. Low temperature fabrication of biodegradable sugar glass microneedles for transdermal drug delivery applications. J Control Release. 2012;158:93–101.

[85] Griffiths CA. Micro injection moulding: tooling and process factors. Cardiff: Cardiff University; 2008.

[86] Johnson AR, Procopio AT. Low cost additive manufacturing of microneedle masters. 3D Print Med. 2019;5:1–10.

[87] Goole J, Amighi K. 3D printing in pharmaceutics: a new tool for designing customized drug delivery systems. Int J Pharm. 2016;499:376–394.

[88] Wu M, Zhang Y, Huang H, et al. Assisted 3D printing of microneedle patches for minimally invasive glucose control in diabetes. Mater Sci Eng C. 2020;117:111299.

[89] Jamróz W, Szafraniec J, Kurek M, et al. 3D printing in pharmaceutical and medical applications—recent achievements and challenges. Pharm Res. 2018;35:176.

[90] Prasad LK, Smyth H. 3D Printing technologies for drug delivery: a review. Drug Dev Ind Pharm. 2016;42:1019–1031.

[91] Kim HR, Kim IK, Bae KH, et al. Cationic solid lipid nanoparticles reconstituted from low density lipoprotein components for delivery of siRNA. Mol Pharm. 2008;5:622–631.

[92] Pere CPP, Economidou SN, Lall G, et al. 3D printed microneedles for insulin skin delivery. Int J Pharm. 2018;544:425–432.

[93] Ngo TD, Kashani A, Imbalzano G, et al. Additive manufacturing (3D printing): a review of materials, methods, applications and challenges. Compos Part B Eng. 2018;143:172–196.

[94] Economidou SN, Lamprou DA, Douroumis D. 3D printing applications for transdermal drug delivery. Int J Pharm. 2018;544:415–424.

[95] Gittard SD, Ovsianikov A, Chichkov BN, et al. Two-photon polymerization of microneedles for transdermal drug delivery. Expert Opin Drug Deliv. 2010;7:513–533.

[96] Nagarkar R, Singh M, Nguyen HX, et al. A review of recent advances in microneedle technology for transdermal drug delivery. J Drug Deliv Sci Technol. 2020;59:101923.

[97] Sullivan SP, Murthy N, Prausnitz MR. Minimally invasive protein delivery with rapidly dissolving polymer microneedles. Adv Mater. 2008;20:933–938.

[98] Ovsianikov A, Chichkov B, Mente P, et al. Two photon polymerization of polymer–ceramic hybrid materials for transdermal drug delivery. Int J Appl Ceram Technol. 2007;4:22–29.

[99] McGrath MG, Vucen S, Vrdoljak A, et al. Production of dissolvable microneedles using an atomised spray process: effect of microneedle composition on skin penetration. Eur J Pharm Biopharm. 2014;86:200–211.

[100] Moon SJ, Lee SS, Lee HS, et al. Fabrication of microneedle array using LIGA and hot embossing process. Microsyst Technol. 11:311–318.

[101] Pérennès F, Marmiroli B, Matteucci M, et al. Sharp beveled tip hollow microneedle arrays fabricated by LIGA and 3D soft lithography with polyvinyl alcohol. J Micromechanics Microengineering. 2006;16:473.

[102] Donnelly RF, Garland MJ, Morrow DI, et al. Optical coherence tomography is a valuable tool in the study of the effects of microneedle geometry on skin penetration characteristics and in-skin dissolution. J Control Release. 2010;147:333–341.

[103] Aoyagi S, Izumi H, Isono Y, et al. Laser fabrication of high aspect ratio thin holes on biodegradable polymer and its application to a microneedle. Sens Actuators Phys. 2007;139:293–302.

[104] Albarahmieh E, AbuAmmouneh L, Kaddoura Z, et al. Fabrication of dissolvable microneedle patches using an innovative laser-cut mould design to shortlist potentially transungual delivery systems: in vitro evaluation. AAPS PharmSciTech. 2019;20:215.

[105] Tu K-T, Chung C-K. Fabrication of biodegradable polymer microneedle array via CO_2 laser ablation. 10th IEEE Int Conf NanoMicro Eng Mol Syst. IEEE; 2015. p. 494–497.

[106] Chen Y-T, Ma K-J, Tseng AA, et al. Projection ablation of glass-based single and arrayed microstructures using excimer laser. Opt Laser Technol. 2005;37:271–280.

[107] Zheng HY, Lam YC, Sundarraman C, et al. Influence of substrate cooling on femtosecond laser machined hole depth and diameter. Appl Phys A. 2007;89:559–563.

[108] Lutton REM, Larrañeta E, Kearney M-C, et al. A novel scalable manufacturing process for the production of hydrogel-forming microneedle arrays. Int J Pharm. 2015;494:417–429.

[109] Zaied M, Miraoui I, Boujelbene M, et al. Analysis of heat affected zone obtained by $CO2$ laser cutting of low carbon steel (S235). AIP Conf Proc. American Institute of Physics; 2013. p. 323–326.

[110] Kim JD, Kim M, Yang H, et al. Droplet-born air blowing: novel dissolving microneedle fabrication. J Control Release. 2013;170:430–436.

[111] Huh I, Kim S, Yang H, et al. Effects of two droplet-based dissolving microneedle manufacturing methods on the activity of encapsulated epidermal growth factor and ascorbic acid. Eur J Pharm Sci. 2018;114:285–292.

[112] Tran KT, Nguyen TD. Lithography-based methods to manufacture biomaterials at small scales. J Sci Adv Mater Devices. 2017;2:1–14.

[113] Lee K, Lee CY, Jung H. Dissolving microneedles for transdermal drug administration prepared by stepwise controlled drawing of maltose. Biomaterials. 2011;32:3134–3140.

[114] Gupta J, Felner EI, Prausnitz MR. Minimally invasive insulin delivery in subjects with type 1 diabetes using hollow microneedles. Diabetes Technol Ther. 2009;11:329–337.

[115] Mahadevan G, Sheardown H, Selvaganapathy P. PDMS embedded microneedles as a controlled release system for the eye. J Biomater Appl. 2013;28:20–27.

[116] Demir YK, Akan Z, Kerimoglu O. Characterization of polymeric microneedle arrays for transdermal drug delivery. PLoS One. 2013;8:e77289.

[117] Juster H, van der Aar B, de Brouwer H. A review on microfabrication of thermoplastic polymer-based microneedle arrays. Polym Eng Sci. 2019;59:877–890.

[118] Lhernould MS, Deleers M, Delchambre A. Hollow polymer microneedles array resistance and insertion tests. Int J Pharm. 2015;480:152–157.

[119] Duarah S, Sharma M, Wen J. Recent advances in microneedle-based drug delivery: special emphasis on its use in paediatric population. Eur J Pharm Biopharm. 2019;136:48–69.

[120] Ingrole RSJ, Gill HS. Microneedle coating methods: a review with a perspective. J Pharmacol Exp Ther. 2019;370:555–569.

[121] Andrianov AK, DeCollibus DP, Gillis HA, et al. Poly[di(carboxylatophenoxy)phosphazene] is a potent adjuvant for intradermal immunization. Proc Natl Acad Sci U S A. 2009;106:18936–18941.

[122] Andrianov AK, Marin A, DeCollibus DP. Microneedles with intrinsic immunoadjuvant properties: microfabrication, protein stability, and modulated release. Pharm Res. 2011;28:58–65.

[123] Marin A, Andrianov AK. Carboxymethylcellulose–Chitosan-coated microneedles with modulated hydration properties. J Appl Polym Sci. 2011;121:395–401.

[124] Chandler CE, Harberts EM, Laemmermann T, et al. In vivo intradermal delivery of bacteria by using microneedle arrays. Infect Immun. 2018;86:e00406–418.

[125] Raja WK, Maccorkle S, Diwan IM, et al. Transdermal delivery devices: fabrication, mechanics and drug release from silk. Small. 2013;9:3704–3713.

[126] van der Maaden K, Varypataki EM, Romeijn S, et al. Ovalbumin-coated pH-sensitive microneedle arrays effectively induce ovalbumin-specific antibody and T-cell responses in mice. Eur J Pharm Biopharm. 2014;88:310–315.

[127] Zeng Q, Gammon JM, Tostanoski LH, et al. In vivo expansion of melanoma-specific T cells using microneedle arrays coated with immune-polyelectrolyte multilayers. ACS Biomater Sci Eng. 2017;3:195–205.

[128] Ita K. Transdermal delivery of drugs with microneedles: strategies and outcomes. J Drug Deliv Sci Technol. 2015;29:16–23.

[129] Caudill CL, Perry JL, Tian S, et al. Spatially controlled coating of continuous liquid interface production microneedles for transdermal protein delivery. J Control Release. 2018;284:122–132.

[130] Ariga K, Yamauchi Y, Rydzek G, et al. Layer-by-layer nanoarchitectonics: invention, innovation, and evolution. Chem Lett. 2014;43:36–68.

[131] Su X, Kim B-S, Kim SR, et al. Layer-by-layer-assembled multilayer films for transcutaneous drug and vaccine delivery. Acs Nano. 2009;3:3719–3729.

[132] DeMuth PC, Su X, Samuel RE, et al. Nano-layered microneedles for transcutaneous delivery of polymer nanoparticles and plasmid DNA. Adv Mater. 2010;22:4851–4856.

[133] Saurer EM, Flessner RM, Sullivan SP, et al. Layer-by-layer assembly of DNA-and protein-containing films on microneedles for drug delivery to the skin. Biomacromolecules. 2010;11:3136–3143.

[134] Ameri M, Daddona PE, Maa Y-F. Demonstrated solid-state stability of parathyroid hormone PTH (1–34) coated on a novel transdermal microprojection delivery system. Pharm Res. 2009;26:2454–2463.

[135] DeMuth PC, Moon JJ, Suh H, et al. Releasable layer-by-layer assembly of stabilized lipid nanocapsules on microneedles for enhanced transcutaneous vaccine delivery. ACS Nano. 2012;6:8041–8051.

[136] DeMuth PC, Min Y, Huang B, et al. Polymer multilayer tattooing for enhanced DNA vaccination. Nat Mater. 2013;12:367–376.

[137] Vrdoljak A, McGrath MG, Carey JB, et al. Coated microneedle arrays for transcutaneous delivery of live virus vaccines. J Control Release. 2012;159:34–42.

[138] Gittard SD, Chen B, Xu H, et al. The effects of geometry on skin penetration and failure of polymer microneedles. J Adhes Sci Technol. 2013;27:227–243.

[139] DeMuth PC, Li AV, Abbink P, et al. Vaccine delivery with microneedle skin patches in nonhuman primates. Nat Biotechnol. 2013;31:1082–1085.

[140] McGrath MG, Vrdoljak A, O'Mahony C, et al. Determination of parameters for successful spray coating of silicon microneedle arrays. Int J Pharm. 2011;415:140–149.

[141] Khan H, Mehta P, Msallam H, et al. Smart microneedle coatings for controlled delivery and biomedical analysis. J Drug Target. 2014;22:790–795.

[142] Nikolaou M, Krasia-Christoforou T. Electrohydrodynamic methods for the development of pulmonary drug delivery systems. Eur J Pharm Sci. 2018;113:29–40.

[143] Haj-Ahmad R, Rasekh M, Nazari K, et al. EHDA spraying: a multi-material nano-engineering route. Curr Pharm Des. 2015;21:3239–3247.

[144] Haj-Ahmad R, Khan H, Arshad MS, et al. Microneedle coating techniques for transdermal drug delivery. Pharmaceutics. 2015;7:486–502.

[145] Lim D-J, Vines JB, Park H, et al. Microneedles: a versatile strategy for transdermal delivery of biological molecules. Int J Biol Macromol. 2018;110:30–38.

[146] Boehm RD, Jaipan P, Skoog SA, et al. Inkjet deposition of itraconazole onto poly(glycolic acid) microneedle arrays. Biointerphases. 2016;11:011008.

[147] Uddin MJ, Scoutaris N, Klepetsanis P, et al. Inkjet printing of transdermal microneedles for the delivery of anticancer agents. Int J Pharm. 2015;494:593–602.

[148] Tarbox TN, Watts AB, Cui Z, et al. An update on coating/manufacturing techniques of microneedles. Drug Deliv Transl Res. 2018;8:1828–1843.

[149] Boehm RD, Miller PR, Daniels J, et al. Inkjet printing for pharmaceutical applications. Mater Today. 2014;17:247–252.

[150] Verbaan FJ, Bal SM, van den Berg DJ, et al. Improved piercing of microneedle arrays in dermatomed human skin by an impact insertion method. J Control Release. 2008;128:80–88.

[151] Yuzhakov VV. The AdminPen™ microneedle device for painless & convenient drug delivery. Drug Deliv Technol. 2010;10:32–36.

[152] Yan G, Warner KS, Zhang J, et al. Evaluation needle length and density of microneedle arrays in the pretreatment of skin for transdermal drug delivery. Int J Pharm. 2010;391:7–12.

[153] Haq MI, Smith E, John DN, et al. Clinical administration of microneedles: skin puncture, pain and sensation. Biomed Microdevices. 2009;11:35–47.

[154] Patel SR, Lin AS, Edelhauser HF, et al. Suprachoroidal drug delivery to the back of the eye using hollow microneedles. Pharm Res. 2011;28:166–176.

[155] Crichton ML, Ansaldo A, Chen X, et al. The effect of strain rate on the precision of penetration of short densely-packed microprojection array patches coated with vaccine. Biomaterials. 2010;31:4562–4572.

[156] Ding Z, Verbaan FJ, Bivas-Benita M, et al. Microneedle arrays for the transcutaneous immunization of diphtheria and influenza in BALB/c mice. J Control Release. 2009;136:71–78.

[157] Mikszta JA, Sullivan VJ, Dean C, et al. Protective immunization against inhalational anthrax: a comparison of minimally invasive delivery platforms. J Infect Dis. 2005;191:278–288.

[158] Donnelly RF, Raj Singh TR, Woolfson AD. Microneedle-based drug delivery systems: microfabrication, drug delivery, and safety. Drug Deliv. 2010;17:187–207.

[159] Wang PM, Cornwell M, Hill J, et al. Precise microinjection into skin using hollow microneedles. J Invest Dermatol. 2006;126:1080–1087.

[160] Yeshurun Y, Levin Y, Hefetz M, et al. Microneedle adaptor for dosed drug delivery devices. 2009. [Internet] [cited 2022 Jul 9]. Available from: https://patents.google.com/patent/US20090 247953A1/en.

[161] Tobinaga Y, Sugiyama S. Applicator for applying functional substances into human skin. 2013. [Internet] [cited 2022 Jul 9]. Available from: https://patents.google.com/patent/US8353861B2/ en.

[162] Donnelly RF, Mooney K, Caffarel-Salvador E, et al. Microneedle-mediated minimally invasive patient monitoring. Ther Drug Monit. 2014;36:10–17.

3

Characterization of Microneedles

3.1 Introduction

Micrometer-sized needles (microneedles) are designed to porate the SC and generate aqueous channels for drug delivery through the skin. Microneedles are classified as solid, coated, hollow, dissolving, and swellable microneedles. These needles may be made from various materials and used to perform diverse functions employing mechanisms particular to the specific design: (i) porating the skin with solid microneedles and then applying the dosage form at the treatment site, (ii) coating the microneedles with the drug and inserting the coated needles into the skin; drug dissolution and release occur within the skin, (iii) drug loaded within polymeric biodegradable microneedles and then they are inserted into the skin for controlled drug release, and (iv) injecting drug solution into the skin by hollow microneedles. Several review publications have described microneedle technology in terms of design, geometry, fabrication and production techniques, clinical studies, and safety issues [1]. Nevertheless, the research is scant on the characterization studies of microneedles. Characterization provides a qualitative and quantitative evaluation of microneedles to acquire a more suited design structure.

Numerous investigations should be performed to characterize microneedles (Table 3.1). Evaluation of microneedle formulation and fabrication technique is required to achieve effective microneedle penetration. Drug solubility, drug-excipient compatibility, stability, homogeneity, and rheological properties should be assessed. SEM, cryoSEM, bright-field stereomicroscope, brightfield/epi-fluorescence microscopy, and AFM are routinely employed to characterize microneedle surface morphology and geometry. Microneedles' length, base dimensions, tip radius, wall thickness, and body profile govern their mechanical properties. The mechanical strength of microneedles should be studied to achieve the effective penetration of microneedles in the skin. Factors affecting microneedle dissolution and drug release kinetics include insertion time, physicochemical and mechanical characteristics of the microneedle polymer matrix, dissolution of the loaded drug and microneedle component, skin tissue (thickness and water content), and microneedle dimensions (size, length, and geometry). Drug quantification and distribution are critical for drug stability, dosage consistency, drug delivery, and encapsulation efficiency. Penetration efficiency is a vital performance characteristic of a microneedle system. Microneedles should uniformly and consistently microporate skin tissue without bending or breakage. The microneedles' hygroscopic properties and water content should be evaluated to determine the appropriate storage conditions.

DOI: 10.1201/9780429294433-3

TABLE 3.1

Summary of the Different Instruments and Methodologies to Evaluate Various Characteristics of Microneedles

Major Parameters Evaluated/Variables	Techniques/Equipment	Relevance and Value	References
Drug solubility in the polymer mixture	Differential scanning calorimetry	Examine the level of drug solubility in the polymer matrix	[2]
Drug–polymer interactions	Fourier transform infrared spectroscopy	Inspect any physical or chemical interaction between the drug and the polymer	[3]
Stability and uniformity of drug in the formulation	Addition of stabilizers	Improve the drug's chemical stability and ensure the drug's uniform distribution in the microneedle formulations	[4–6]
Physical characterization of polymers	Differential scanning calorimetry	Examine any modification in the polymer structure	[2]
Geometry and radius of curvature, needle length, base dimensions, tip diameter, sharpness, angles, needle-to-needle spacing, interior structure, and surface morphology Reproducibility, precision, and accuracy of the fabrication process	Microscopy techniques: CryoSEM, Brightfield stereomicroscope, Brightfield/ epi-fluorescence microscopy, and atomic force microscopy Stereomicroscopy Scanning electron microscope	Examine microneedles geometry and morphology Evaluate the reproducibility of the fabrication process in manufacturing microneedles and microneedles' uniform geometry and tip sharpness	[7–10]
Microneedle insertion and fracture force	Bose™ Electroforce™ 3100 mechanical testing stage TA-XT with a texture analyzer Displacement–force test station Axial compression test Nanoindentation	Mechanical strength Fracture force Determine if the microneedle possesses sufficient mechanical strength to withstand deformation during handling and skin insertion	[11–14]
Microneedles dissolution and drug release kinetics	Fluorescent microscopy or microscopic imaging of dye or drug-loaded microneedles Dissolution of microneedles *in vitro* Change in microneedle tip length after skin insertion Histological sectioning followed by imaging under a bright field and fluorescence microscope OCT imaging of *in situ* dissolution Immunohistochemistry Multiphoton microscopy	Investigate microneedles dissolution and drug release	[11, 15]
Drug content	Drug extraction, followed by analysis with analytical tools	Evaluate drug loading and quantification	[16, 17]

TABLE 3.1 *(Continued)*

Summary of the Different Instruments and Methodologies to Evaluate Various Characteristics of Microneedles

Major Parameters Evaluated/Variables	Techniques/Equipment	Relevance and Value	References
Drug/fluorescently labeled drug distribution pattern	Fluorescent microscopy Dissolution and quantification of separated tip and backing layer	Visualize and quantify the localization and distribution of loaded molecules in a microneedle array	[18–20]
Insertion capability	Parafilm M® insertion.	Provides a predictive value of the microneedle length capable of insertion into the skin	[21–23]
Formation of microchannels	TEWL, electrical impedance/ resistance measurement Microchannel staining *Ex vivo* and *in vivo* (porcine, rodent, murine, and human volunteer) skin insertion	Skin penetration/insertion efficiency	[24, 25]
The penetration depth of microchannels	Histological cryosectioning and staining Confocal microscopy OCT imaging	Measure the depth of microneedles-created channels	[26–28]
Moisture content	Measurement of microneedle weight at different time intervals (exposed to controlled humidity) Thermogravimetric analyzer Karl Fischer Moisture balance Endpoint water content determination with water activity analyzer	Examine the hygroscopicity of microneedles	[11, 14, 29]
Morphology of microneedles after skin insertion or contact with buffer solution	Microneedle microscopic imaging (SEM, OCT) after contact with buffer or insertion into the skin at different time intervals	Study swelling behavior of swellable microneedles	[30, 31]
The integrity of drugs and biopharmaceuticals	Circular dichroism analysis, dynamic light scattering, solubility measurement, fluorescence microscopy, and electrophoresis Forced (elevated humidity and temperature) and real-time stability testing	Evaluate the drug's physicochemical stability	[32, 33]
Safety and toxicity Skin irritation	Biophysical characterization techniques: laser doppler flowmetry, TEWL, high-frequency ultrasound, capacitance reflectance spectroscopy, changes in the skin color by chromameter, Draize test for skin irritation, and visual scoring	Evaluate biological safety and potential to induce any significant skin irritation or dermatological adverse effects	[34–36]

(Continued)

TABLE 3.1 *(Continued)*

Summary of the Different Instruments and Methodologies to Evaluate Various Characteristics of Microneedles

Major Parameters Evaluated/Variables	Techniques/Equipment	Relevance and Value	References
Skin recovery	TEWL Transepidermal electrical resistance	Determine the duration required for the skin to recover or for microchannels to close	[37, 38]
Sterility testing	Ph. Eur Method 2.6	Investigate the sterility of the finished product of microneedles	[39]

3.2 Microneedle Formulations

Before casting onto the molds, microneedles formulation must be evaluated for drug or antigen solubility, drug–polymer interactions, stability, and homogeneity. To ensure uniform drug distribution in the microneedles, the drug must be completely dissolved in the polymer matrix, thus preventing drug precipitation and instability. Stabilizers (i.e., trehalose) may be used with microfabricating materials (i.e., sodium carboxymethyl cellulose) to retain the immunogenicity of vaccines [15, 40]. Insights into the chemical interactions between the active ingredient and polymeric compositions are essential to predict the formulation's stability, uniformity, and drug release. Dangol et al. employed Fourier transform infrared spectroscopy to study the chemical bonding between capsaicin and biodegradable polymers in dissolving microneedles [3]. Differential scanning calorimetry has also been utilized to investigate the solid-state properties of drugs and excipients, the solubility of the drug in the polymeric matrix, the amorphous state of polymers, and the impact of additive solvents on microneedles crystallinity [41]. The rheological and interfacial properties of microneedle formulations (i.e., kinematic viscosity and contact angle) would significantly impact the mechanical strength of the fabricated needles and the efficiency of the mold-filling process [42]. The components' concentrations were controlled to obtain the expected viscosity. For example, the polymeric solution viscosity should be 1 mPa·s for sugar solutions and 22 mPa·s for carboxymethylcellulose solution for the atomized spray to fill the mold [42]. Several formulation strategies might be explored to fabricate microneedles with suitable dissolving characteristics. Milewski et al. [43] reviewed several formulations for maximizing drug delivery via microchannels.

3.3 Microneedle Geometry and Morphology

Microscopic techniques such as scanning electron microscopy (SEM), cryoSEM, brightfield stereomicroscope, brightfield/epi-fluorescence microscopy, and atomic force microscopy are often used to study the shape, geometry, surface morphology, and sharpness of microneedles [7–10]. Microscopy may also be employed during product development to examine the distribution of fluorescent-labeled antigens in microneedles. This technique allows observing the morphology of coated layers on microneedles, inspecting any damage in microneedles, characterizing microneedle dimensions (needle length, base dimensions, tip diameter, tip sharpness, tip angles, needle-to-needle spacing, interior structure, width, thickness), and evaluating the reproducibility, precision, and accuracy of microneedle fabrication process [9, 41, 44].

The repeatability and reproducibility of microneedles manufactured by the micromolding method with a master structure are determined by measuring the diameters of at least one-third of the needles on an array [45, 46]. Microneedle performance is determined by many interdependent elements, including the materials used to fabricate microneedles, the manufacturing process, parameters, and the design and architecture of microneedle arrays. The radius of microneedle curvature is an essential characteristic that determines the array's insertion efficiency in the skin [21, 47]. Any variation in the microneedle design may result in the device's insufficient penetration into the skin [48]. Davis et al. [49] were the first to demonstrate the critical importance of hollow microneedle tip design and geometry in microneedle insertion. They discovered that by reducing the tip radius from 80 μm to 30 μm, they could obtain a more effective penetration with insertion force decreasing from 3.04 N to 0.08 N per needle. Aoyagi et al. [50] elucidated how tip geometry affects microneedle insertion by comprehensively investigating the influence of tip angle and needle width on the performance of biodegradable microneedles.

For hollow microneedles, the microneedle tip's geometry significantly affects the flow rate; for example, the flow from a blunt-tip microneedle supports less flow than that from a bevel-tip microneedle since the blunt-tip compresses the skin more extensively, increasing the likelihood of clogging [51, 52]. It may be advantageous to have very sharp microneedles with the bore of the microneedle off-centered or to the side [52–23]. While increasing the bore size may result in increased flow rates, it also decreases microneedle strength and sharpness [23].

3.3.1 Pre-insertion Assessment of Microneedle Geometry

Before skin insertion, microneedles are characterized to study the needle dimensions and geometries and assess the uniformity of needles in the array. SEM has been used to observe microneedle array and to quantify needle dimensions, including needle length, tip diameter, needle-to-needle distance, and base size. SEM images also revealed the surface morphology of microneedles and the distribution of drugs or nanoparticles inside or coated on the needles [56, 57]. Zhen et al. demonstrated that the dimensions of the microneedle collected by SEM might be used to determine the microneedle volume and delivery dose [58]. Researchers observed and measured the needle geometry, consistency, and distribution on the array using a stereomicroscope or brightfield microscope [9, 10]. A program such as ImageJ should be utilized to obtain an accurate measurement of the tip diameter of microneedles. To precisely measure the needle length, a microneedle array with a flat base must be carefully fixed on a 90° angle on the sample holder. This measurement only counts the first line of the array. Yan et al. reported that the needle length of the master structure was 218 μm, whereas the length of fabricated sodium carboxymethylcellulose needles was 165 ± 3 μm, a loss of 24% in length owing to the contraction and solidification of the material after drying [44]. Using SEM, Kim et al. studied the surface morphology of hyaluronic acid microneedles and reported that the surface of retinyl retionate-encapsulated microneedles was rougher than ascorbic acid-loaded microneedles [56]. Bing Cai et al. employed SEM to determine bioceramic microneedles' length, edge, and tip. The needles appeared sharp, with a 5 µm tip radius and clean edges. Among all dimensions, the sharpness of the needles was found to be the most important for effective microneedle penetration. Dissolving microneedles might have the same geometry and dimensions as the master structure or a slightly smaller size due to the shrinkage of the polymer matrix during the drying process. Vrdoljak and coworkers captured and reported the images of dissolving microneedles in their respective characterization study (Fig. 3.1) [59].

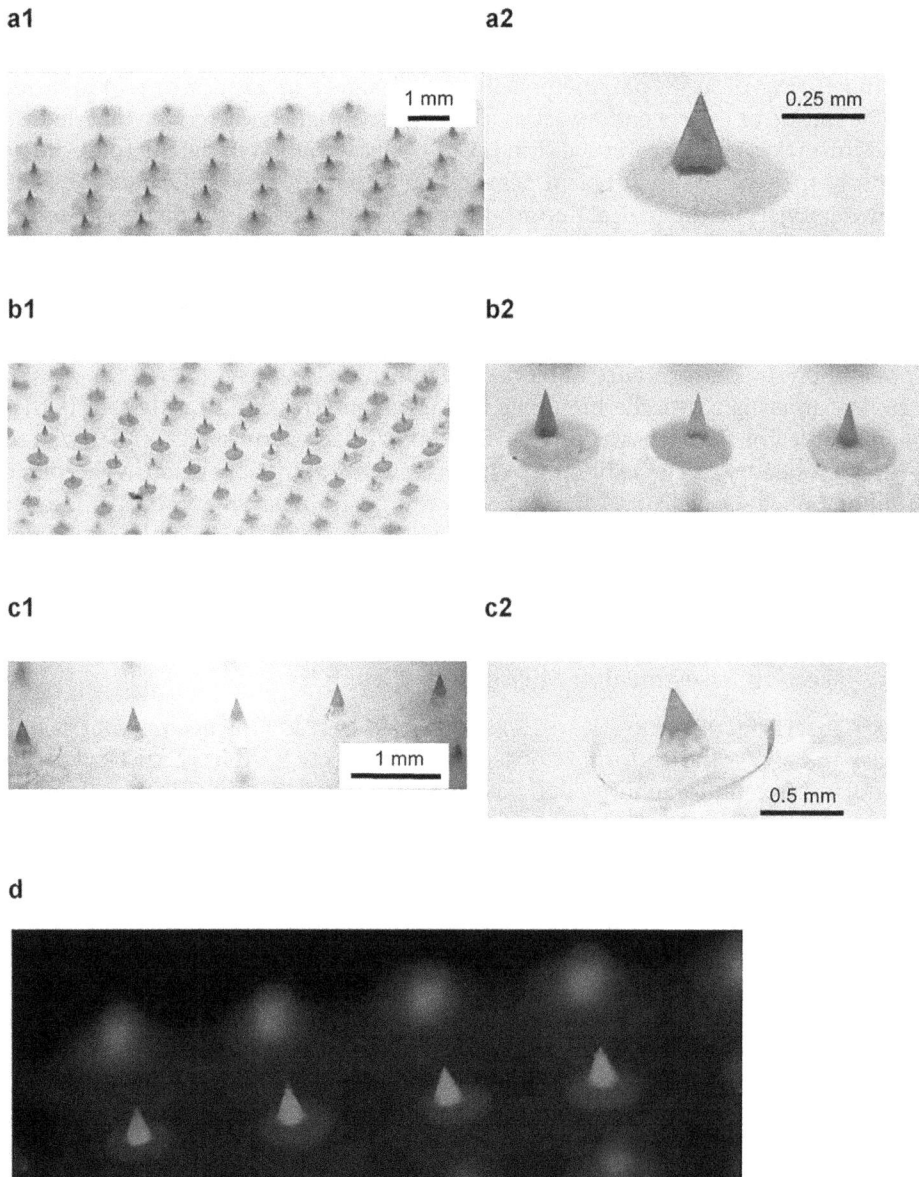

FIGURE 3.1
Microscopic images of dissolving microneedle patches. (a1) Homogeneous microneedle array. (a2) One needle. (b1) Heterogeneous array of microneedles fabricated from two different formulations. (b2) Three needles. (c1 and c2) Microneedles with formulation localized in the needle tip. (d) Fluorescent microscopic images of Congo red–loaded microneedles. Images reprinted with permission from [59].

3.3.2 Post-insertion Assessment of Microneedle Geometry

The geometry of dissolving microneedles after skin insertion provides insights into microneedle dissolution and drug release [56]. Analysis of post-insertion solid microneedles assists in determining the extent of damage to the needles or needle residues remaining in the skin and the feasibility of reusing the needles. Solid microneedles such as silicon [60], stainless steel [61], and bioceramic [62] microneedles were found to maintain the original morphology and geometry after skin penetration: none of the needles were bent or fractured, and no residues were found in the skin after the insertion. Characterization of dissolving microneedles post-insertion allows for examining the needle dissolution and drug release in skin tissue. This then provides evidence for the estimated treatment duration for efficient drug administration. Trehalose microneedles lost their sharp tip after the skin treatment, which became rounded and smooth needle tips due to the instantaneous dissolution of the microneedle upon contact with the skin [42]. Similarly, by visualizing hydrogel-forming microneedles embedded in rat skin at different intervals, the authors found that the needles dissolve gradually in the skin to release the encapsulated drug [63]. In general, solid and hollow microneedles are expected to remain intact after the skin insertion so as to prevent any residues in the skin. However, dissolving microneedles should disintegrate and dissolve in skin fluid at a predetermined rate to release the drug load into skin layers. Swellable microneedles absorb skin fluid and swell and should be removed entirely from the skin in the swollen state, leaving a minimal residue of polymer in skin tissue. Using a cryoSEM, Crichton et al. observed no fracture of Nanopatch silicon microneedles in the skin [60]. Wermeling et al. found no bending or breakage of stainless steel microneedles and no microneedle residue pieces in the skin after the insertion [61]. After 4 h of drug release from bioceramic microneedles, Bing Cai et al. observed the complete dissolution of the needle with no needle residues on the array [62].

3.4 Mechanical Properties of Microneedles

3.4.1 Introduction of Mechanical Properties

As the skin is viscoelastic and nonuniform, various stresses are applied to microneedles during insertion and removal, and the skin structure could reduce the penetration efficiency of microneedles [37]. These forces could cause bending, fracture, and buckling of microneedles [64]. To penetrate the stratum corneum without bending or breakage, microneedles must possess the required intrinsic mechanical and tensile strength, toughness, and hardness; also, the force applied to the microneedle array should be greater than the shear skin forces. Microneedle mechanical strength depends on the tip sharpness, skin tension, microneedle materials, and geometry (i.e., height, base diameter, tip radius, wall thickness, and needle density) [65]. Microneedles must be sufficiently strong to prevent fracture and buckling failure under an applied force during skin insertion [66]. The optimal microneedle design would require minimal insertion force and maximal fracture force to obtain the greatest margin of safety. Insertion is facilitated by a miniature tip radius and sufficient length to bypass the skin's physical resistance, while mechanical strength is boosted by increasing the needle wall thickness, base diameter, and Young's modulus. For certain microneedle geometries, the failure force may be predicted using an elastic buckling model [32]. A variety of mechanical tests should be performed on the microneedle for characterization. The axial force, transverse force, base strength, and insertion force all are examples of these tests. According to Lutton et al., no single test can accurately imitate and examine the mechanical properties of the needle and the skin penetration of microneedles *in vivo* [24]. The correlation between mechanical qualities and microneedle production factors has been investigated [67]. Different testing systems have been employed to characterize the mechanical properties of microneedles, such as a universal testing machine, a texture analyzer, nanoindentation, Instron testing, and a Bose™ Electroforce™ 3100 mechanical testing stage. For microneedles' mechanical robustness, the standard practice is axial compression testing, often referred to as the needle failure assessment [68]. In the experiment, a force is applied perpendicularly to the microneedles base plate. The displacement and force are recorded as microneedles are moved at a predetermined speed and pressed against a flat hard metallic block [46, 65]. An abrupt discontinuity in the force–displacement curve is denoted as the mechanical failure of microneedles [49, 65]. A greater failure force suggested that the needles have superior mechanical qualities. Increases in the base diameter of polymeric needles and Young's modulus of the polymer material increased the failure force [65]. However, the sudden fracture discontinuity was rarely observed in silicon microneedles. Instead, these microneedles fail by gradual "grinding" mechanism [69]. Microneedles were visualized under a microscope pre- and post-mechanical test to examine the breaking model. Buckling is most likely to be the primary source of mechanical failure for slender, high-aspect-ratio microneedles [70]. The brittleness of microneedles could be estimated from the slope of the force–distance curve: the steeper the curve, the more brittle the microneedles [22]. Microneedle mechanical strength is typically expressed in terms of "force per needle." This value is obtained by dividing the greatest force measured with the texture analyzer by the number of needles in the array, presuming that all microneedles fracture concurrently at the maximum applied force due to the same failure mechanism. This may falsify the result since heterogeneity may occur within the same microneedle patch. During a compression test, the applied force is expected to be distributed evenly across the needles on the array, resulting in the "bed of nails effect," which is absent in a single needle compression test. Romgens et al. [71] recently stressed the necessity of determining microneedle mechanical strength using a single needle rather than an entire microneedle patch. Combining the two tests—nanoindentation for a few microneedles and mechanical compression test for the entire array—may be an acceptable strategy to characterize the microneedle mechanical properties [72]. The failure force of microneedles must exceed the force required for successful microneedle penetration in skin. To penetrate the stratum corneum, an insertion force of as low as 0.03 N/needle may suffice [73]. Mechanically, polymeric microneedles are weaker than metal, silicon, or glass needles, thus polymeric microneedles should be designed properly to achieve a sufficient mechanical strength for successful skin insertion. Solid metal microneedles are generally strong and robust, while hollow microneedles may fracture if not constructed appropriately, and polymer microneedles generally fail due to plastic deformation [65, 70]. The microneedles' breakage is negligible when the microneedles are inserted gently. The amount of force needed to insert a microneedle into the body reduces in direct proportion to the tip's sharpness [49]. The inability to make direct comparisons of microneedle mechanical properties is attributed to the vast variety of microneedle geometrical dimensions, the diversity of test techniques, and mechanical equipment. Consolidating tests and implementing a consistent mechanical testing would be beneficial for microneedles characterization in this case [24]. Sawutdeechaikul et al. employed a universal testing machine (Shimadzu EZ-S) to measure the compressive force (applied axial force) of dissolving microneedle array in its dependence on displaced distance. The force–displacement graph is displayed in Fig. 3.2 [74].

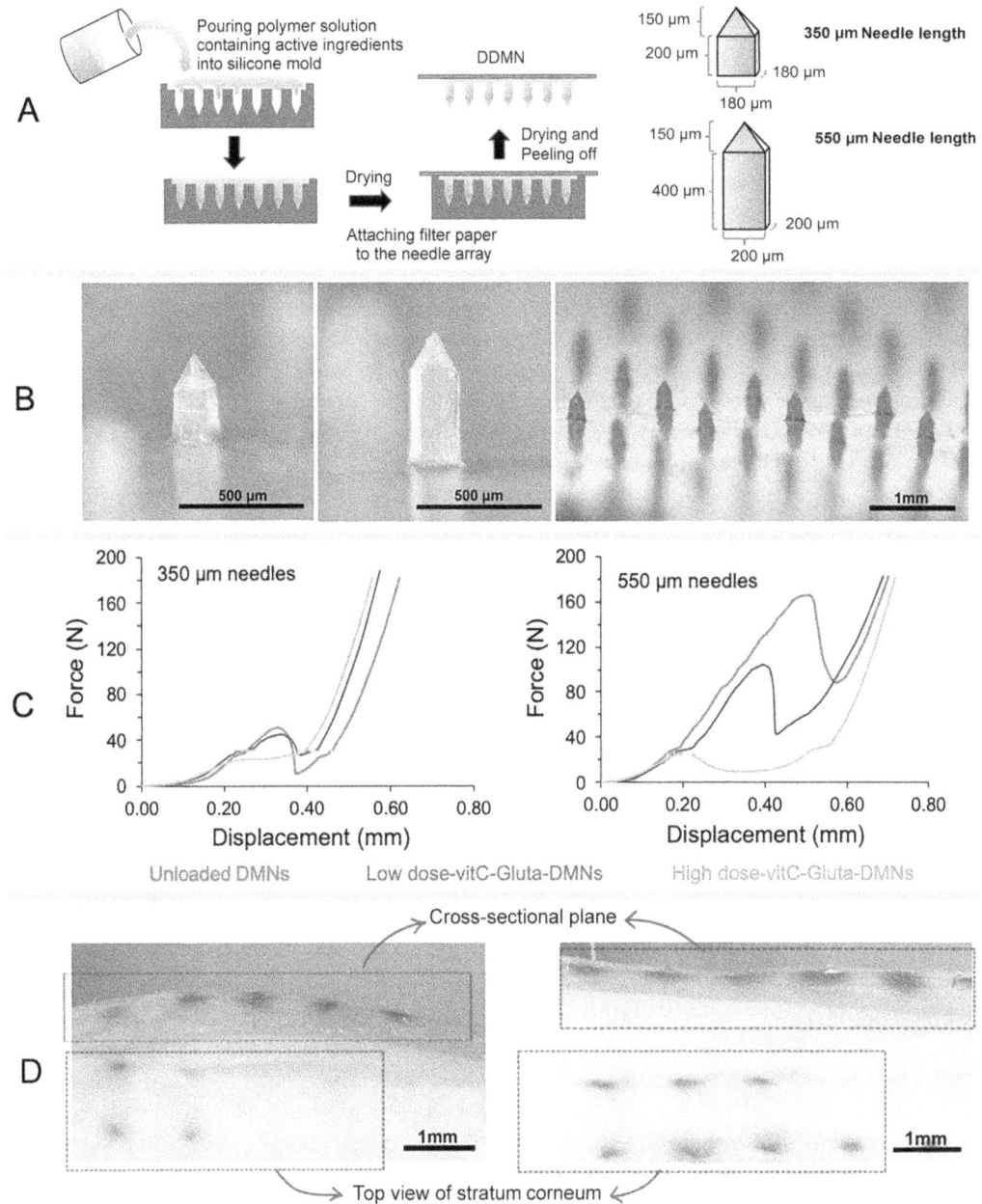

FIGURE 3.2

Fabrication, dimensions, morphology, mechanical property, and skin insertion of detachable dissolvable microneedle. (A) Fabrication and dimensions of microneedles. (B) Microscopic images of the vitamin C- glutathione-loaded microneedles and red dye-spiked microneedles. (C) Force–displacement curve of mechanical test of microneedles. (D) Microscopic images of porcine ear skin after the insertion of red dye-spiked microneedles. Images reprinted with permission from [74].

3.4.2 Factors Affecting the Mechanical Strength of Microneedles

The mechanical characteristics of microneedles are affected by various parameters such as their geometry, height, base diameter, tip radius, wall thickness, aspect ratio, the material of construction, and physicochemical properties of loaded drugs, with the aspect ratio being a significant determinant in needle mechanical strength [49, 65, 75]. For example, a pyramidal shape was mechanically stronger for chitosan microneedles than a conical shape [75]. Under compressive loadings, slender microneedles were shown to be weaker than bullet-type microneedles. Slender microneedles are ideal when the microneedle material is strong enough to tolerate mechanical stress during insertion. However, when the compressive force is increased upon insertion, microneedles of the standard or bullet design of microneedles become more suited [41]. Loizidou et al. manufactured several types of sugar microneedles and discovered that carboxymethylcellulose/maltose microneedles outperform carboxymethylcellulose/trehalose and carboxymethylcellulose/sucrose microneedles in terms of mechanical strength and drug delivery capabilities. Buckling was anticipated to be the primary cause of microneedle physical failure, and the order of buckling was shown to be strongly associated with Young's modulus values of each microneedle's sugar ingredients [76].

The mechanical strength of microneedles may be improved in several ways. Adding a metal coating on microneedles increases their strength but reduces their sharpness [64, 77]. Thus, more acceptable geometrical designs and materials are required: a needle with a tiny tip radius and a long needle length effectively penetrates the skin. A lower aspect ratio might strengthen mechanically fragile polymeric needles such as chitosan microneedles [32]. With the same aspect ratio, needle mechanical characteristics were not influenced by varied dimensions [75]. To improve the mechanical strength of silk protein microneedle arrays, Raja et al. loaded silk microparticles in the needles [44]. Yan et al. reported that adding 5% layered double hydroxide nanoparticles to generally weak dissolving sodium carboxymethylcellulose microneedles substantially increased microneedles' mechanical strength without affecting skin dissolution kinetics [78]. Mechanical properties of microneedles materials could also be influenced by varied drying conditions [10]. Methacrylic acid was copolymerized with vinyl pyrrolidone to fabricate poly(vinylpyrrolidone-*co*-methacrylic acid) microneedles with improved mechanical strength [79]. Weak microneedles composed only of carboxymethyl cellulose deformed significantly even when the minimal weight of 5 N was applied. Adding amylopectin to the polymeric matrix enhanced the mechanical strength of microneedles [32]. Both carboxymethyl cellulose and amylopectin are biocompatible carbohydrates with a high Young's modulus and high water solubility enabling fast dissolution. Furthermore, increasing amylopectin content in carboxymethyl cellulose microneedles led to an increase in microneedles' mechanical strength and a reduction in deformation. In all ratios examined, microneedles containing amylopectin preserved over 90% of their initial height. When the amylopectin percentage was greater than 1:2.3, the microneedles were excessively stiff and brittle, causing microneedle breakage during mold removal or skin application [80]. Carboxymethylcellulose was often combined with sugars to enhance storage profiles and provide stiffer material composition, to fabricate mechanically stronger microneedles [76, 81]. Similarly, the compression resistance of silk firoin microneedles increased from 23 g/needle to 49 g/needle by altering the exposure duration of the material to methanol [5].

However, several factors could lead to weaker mechanical properties of microneedles. The inclusion or encapsulation of drug molecules could weaken the structural polymer mechanically in a concentration-dependent way [11, 82]. For instance, the failure force of poly(lactide-*co*-glycolide) needles decreased from 163 mN per needle to 91 mN and 40 mN per needle when the content of loaded calcein increased from 0% to 2% and 10% [82]. The effect of drug loading also differs from one drug to another since it is dictated by the physicochemical qualities of the encapsulated molecule. The loading of 5 μg exenatide reduces the failure force of sodium hyaluronate needles from 28.14 N to 25.19 N [11], while it took only 17.5 N/cm² to fail a hyaluronic microneedle with bovine insulin [29]. This could be explained by the drug particles' low mechanical strength and poor interaction between the drug and the polymer matrix [82]. Similarly, the less mechanical strength of microneedles was observed with greater collagen concentrations in PVP microneedles [9].

3.4.3 Case Studies of Mechanical Strength of Microneedles

Davis et al., for the first time, studied the mechanical properties of microneedles by measuring the force required for fracture, insertion, and their ratio (the margin of safety). The fracture force to insertion force ratio should be larger than 1, indicating needles that will not break when inserted into the skin. They rendered a displacement–force test to quantify the force exerted on a single microneedle with varying wall thickness, angle, and tip radius. The applied force of 0.1–3 N is required for successful microneedle insertion in the skin. This range of force could be achieved by finger insertion [49]. Insertion forces are linearly related to needle tip interfacial area but not wall thickness. The fracture force increased dramatically with an increase in wall thickness and increased modestly with wall angle and tip radius. Using needles with a small tip radius reduces insertion force, while a large wall thickness increases strength and fracture force [49]. In another research [65], Park et al. investigated the mechanical strength of microneedles made from polylactic, polyglycolic, and polylactic-*co*-glycolic acids. They revealed that the force needed to trigger microneedle failure by axial loading increased by lowering microneedle length, increasing base diameter, or employing microneedles with higher Young's modulus (a measure of stiffness of materials). A higher microneedle needed greater force to break with the same needle tip and base diameter. The transverse load necessary to cause microneedle failure was also measured. In the case of microneedles with identical shapes and materials, the transverse failure force is typically lower than the axial failure force. Substantial transverse stress from erroneous axial insertion causes microneedles to bend. To minimize axial force failure, microneedles with Young's modulus above 3 GPa and a length-to-diameter proportion below 12:1 were recommended [70]. The fabricated lidocaine-loaded microneedle patch had a fracture force of 28 N. Microneedle patch with varied lidocaine concentrations (2.2%, 15%, 21% w/w) had greater than 90% penetration efficiency at 10–30 N force. At 10–30 N, more than 95% of the microneedles remained intact on the patch containing 21% lidocaine. At force above 30 N, 10–20% of the microneedles were broken [2]. Skin insertion test also demonstrated microneedle strength. Microneedles composed of sucrose and PVP exhibited enough strength to penetrate porcine skin [58].

3.4.3.1 Axial Force Mechanical Tests

An axial force is frequently measured to evaluate the mechanical strength of the microneedle array. In the experiment, compression force is applied perpendicular to the microneedles' base [12]. The test station records the force and displacement changes while microneedles are axially pressed against a solid metallic block at a predetermined rate [46, 65]. Initially, the applied force increased with the displacement. Then, the force–displacement curve shows the abrupt reduction in the force during microneedle breakdown, which is commonly assumed to represent a microneedle failure force [46, 49, 65]. This mechanical test determines the needles' failure force, which indicates the safety point to offer an estimated range of needle insertion force [65]. The failure force of microneedles must be higher than the force of skin penetration to be considered safe for use.

Equipment and calculating techniques have been used to calculate the microneedles' failure force. Demir and associates utilized a universal testing system (Instron® Model 5969) [46], while Khanna and colleagues employed a compression load cell and motorized actuators (Z600 series Thorlabs Motorized Actuators) to study axial fracture [83]. Donnelly et al. used a TA-XT2 Texture Analyzer (Stable Microsystems) and a GXMGE-5 digital microscope (Laboratory Analysis Ltd.) [84], while Park and Prausnitz used a displacement–force test station (Tricor System) [70] to perform mechanical compression testing. In a microneedle failure force test, a dissolving hyaluronic acid microneedle was separated from a cosmetic microneedle patch. The axial fracture force was calculated as the concentration of the loaded active ingredient (retinyl retinoate and ascorbic acid) increased. Drug concentration in microneedles was found to affect the fracture force. Increasing the drug content led to a reduction in the microneedle axial fracture force [56].

The failure force of a microneedle array is not the same as that of a single microneedle due to the impact of needle density on the distributed force. Furthermore, the force applied to microneedles during the compression test does not precisely match the forces experienced following microneedle insertion into the skin. When microneedles are compressed against a rigid metallic surface, the entire force is focused on the microneedle tip contact surface [24]. The applied force is dispersed across a larger microneedle as the flexible and viscoelastic skin wraps around the microneedle area [67].

3.4.3.2 Transverse Failure Force Testing

Partial microneedle insertion and transverse failure of microneedles result from the skin's irregular surface. Thus, determining the transverse fracture force would be required to characterize the mechanical properties of microneedles. The transverse force mechanical test employs the same test station as the axial force test. Using a rigid metallic probe, the force is applied transversely to the microneedle array, parallel to the microneedle base plate, until microneedle fracture is achieved [24]. The force–displacement curve of microneedles demonstrates their mechanical strength. A limitation of this test is to manually align the metal probe with a specific length of the microneedle or defined distance from the base plate [24]. Due to the microneedle's miniature dimensions, this alignment may create experimental inconsistencies, albeit a microscope camera may help to a certain extent [46]. It took greater force to fracture the needle at 100% needle height than at 60% needle height [13]. A sudden decline in the force–displacement curve represents the microneedle's transverse failure force [12, 46]. The transverse force is applied on a row of microneedles on the array rather than a single microneedle.

Donnelly et al. used the Stable Micro Systems TA.XT-plus Texture Analyzer to determine the transverse failure force of microneedle arrays [12]. Force–displacement equipment and a microscope were used in the study by Park and colleagues to measure the transverse force [85]. Demir et al. measured the microneedle's transverse force by employing a micromechanical tester (Instron® Model 5969) [46]. Even with a low aspect ratio, the transverse force of nanopatch microneedles was significantly greater than the axial force [60]. O'Mahony et al. [69] observed a similar behavior in silicon microneedles, with a transverse failure force ranging from 0.3 N to 0.5 N. They found that the fracture often occurred along the material's weaker crystallographic plane of the crystal orientation. Khanna et al. [86] emphasized the requirement of characterizing shear fractures caused by lateral stresses on microneedle arrays. They explored the influence of geometry on the strength of microneedle shear fractures. This research compared the shear strength of silicon microneedles with an "I-shaped" lumen with those with a circular lumen. As predicted, the lateral shear fracture of "I-shaped" microneedles was consistently greater than those of circular microneedles.

3.4.3.3 Base Strength

The success of microneedle insertion into the skin depends on the mechanical properties of both microneedles and the base plate. With a rigid base, the microneedle array would face the "bed of nail" effect caused by the skin viscoelasticity, which reduces the microneedle penetration efficiency [62]. Regardless of the microneedle's robustness, breaking the base plate on the patient application is unacceptable [24]. Besides, the base plate must be sufficiently flexible to adhere to the irregular skin topography. Employing a mechanical test, Donnelly et al. [12] evaluated the strength and flexibility of polymeric base plates. The base plate was fixed between two aluminum blocks, and a metal probe of a Texture Analyzer moved toward the base plate at a speed of 2 mm/s, with a maximum travel distance of 5 mm. The maximum force found in the force–distance curve indicated the force required to fracture the base plate (2.38 ± 0.54 N). The bending angle of the base plate was captured to study its flexibility (1.28° ± 0.21°) [24].

3.4.4 Skin Puncture Force

Several studies have investigated the force microneedles require to successfully porate skin tissue. Crichton et al. employed micrometer-scale probes to measure the required force for microneedles to penetrate the ear skin of C57/Black 6 mice. On the graph, the force dramatically reduced at the puncture point. They found no significant difference in the insertion force for probes of varied tip diameters (1 or 2 μm). The puncture force of the skin was 34.97 ± 20.64 and 8.03 ± 4.74 MPa for 1 and 2 μm probes, respectively. The puncture force of the stratum corneum layer was 2 mN [60]. The stiff corneocytes of the stratum corneum and the composite-plate-like surface of the skin can disperse the applied force, even distributing highly localized stresses at miniature scales. Thus, determining a single skin failure stress is challenging [60, 87]. Davis et al. found that depending on the geometry, their microneedles needed 0.08–3.04 N to penetrate the skin [49]. O'Mahony [69] reported a maximum skin insertion stress of 4 MPa imposed on microneedles. Kendall et al. [88] estimated failure stress of 13 MPa, and Wildnaur et al. [89] documented the stratum corneum failure at 17 MPa. The probe shape and size likely affect this variation in the measurement results.

3.5 Dissolution and Drug Release

3.5.1 Introduction of Microneedle Dissolution and Drug Release

It is critical to characterize the drug release kinetics from microneedles to guarantee their effective delivery into the skin or systemic circulation. Generally, dissolving microneedles need to be inserted and kept in skin tissue for 5 min for complete dissolution. Multiple methods have been used to shorten the time required for microneedles to dissolve. For the controlled-release degradation of biodegradable polymeric microneedles, microneedles must penetrate and stay in the skin for several days [82]. Hydrogel microparticles-loaded microneedles were intended to successfully disintegrate microneedles in less than 1 h after injection into the skin [78]. A crucial characteristic of dissolving microneedles is the ability to penetrate and dissolve in the skin at an expected rate. For a vaccine-loaded microneedle patch, the needles should dissolve immediately after skin insertion to avoid the reuse of the product. Dissolution might take seconds or hours, depending on microneedle length, skin thickness, and formulation release time.

3.5.2 Factors Affecting Microneedle Dissolution and Drug Release

The dissolution kinetics of microneedles in skin and drug release process depends on several factors, including duration of needle treatment, chemical and mechanical characteristics of the polymer matrix [90], the dissolution kinetics of the loaded drug and microneedle ingredients, microneedle type, skin properties (skin model, thickness, and viscoelasticity), and microneedle dimensions (length, size, geometry). The release of drugs from dissolving microneedle arrays is primarily controlled by the dissolution of the microneedle matrix [91]. Using different polymer types caused markedly different polymer dissolution and drug release profiles [90]. For example, the dissolution rate of microneedles might be controlled by altering the carboxymethyl cellulose to amylopectin mixing ratio within a specified range. Using a 1:1 mixture of carboxymethyl cellulose and amylopectin, it took 8 min to dissolve half of the microneedle in the skin and 30 s in PBS [80]. Fast microneedle dissolution leads to a bolus dose of encapsulated drug, whereas delayed dissolution allows for sustained release. The polymer matrix's physical state significantly affects microneedles' dissolution profile. McGrath et al. fabricated dissolving microneedles with the majority of trehalose in amorphous form and a minor proportion of crystalline trehalose. This benefit accelerated microneedle dissolution and drug release [42]. Bing Cai et al. [62] reported sustained release of clonidine from bioceramic microneedles. Also, microneedle geometry had negligible effect on drug release kinetics. Drug-coated microneedles released drug load more rapidly than drug-encapsulated needles. This was explained by the polymer breakdown before drug release. The mechanism of drug release from microneedles is dependent on drug diffusion and microneedle degradation. In general, the drug diffusion rate relies on the total contact area between microneedles and skin fluid. The mechanism of drug release from various microneedle types should be studied.

3.5.3 Tests of Microneedle Dissolution and Drug Release

Microneedle dissolution and drug release kinetics are studied *in vivo* and *in vitro*. Studies have used biological tissues or artificial membranes that mimic human skin. Drug-loaded microneedles were inserted into porcine, mice, or rat skin and photographed periodically (using light microscopy, stereomicroscopy, bright field, and fluorescence microscopy) to monitor microneedle degradation and drug release [10, 92, 93]. To study microneedle dissolution *in vitro*, microneedles are immersed in PBS solution (simulate body fluid) at 32°C, the buffer is sampled at certain intervals, and the drug content is analyzed [41, 90]. Immunohistochemistry may also track the therapeutic agents' permeation pathways (lateral and vertical) [94]. Multi-photon microscopy can monitor the release of fluorescent molecules after microneedle penetration [95]. Optical coherence tomography (OCT) may also assess *in situ* disintegration of microneedles in the skin. Based on microneedle length after specific insertion durations, the best application time for dissolving microneedles in the skin may be calculated [32, 96, 97]. The dissolution of carboxymethyl cellulose microneedles was studied in phosphate-buffered saline (PBS, pH 7.0). In the experiment, the microneedle array was immobilized in a container with just the microneedle tips immersed in the buffer solution. A series of microscopic images of microneedle tips were taken at different intervals to measure the changes in microneedle length [80].

Since temperature and humidity conditions are challenging to duplicate in *ex vivo* experiments, it is vital to investigate microneedle dissolution in preclinical and early clinical trials. Furthermore, preclinical testing does not entirely replace clinical testing of microneedle dissolution. It is conceivable that the characteristics of the skin (i.e., thickness, viscoelasticity, moisture levels, etc.) have a significant impact on the kinetics of microneedle dissolution and drug release; hence this topic deserves further investigation. Biological tissue is commonly used in published studies into microneedle dissolution [98]. However, biological tissue cannot be standardized and reproduced; thus, the tissue cannot be used for quality control. Therefore, a controllable artificial membrane that simulates skin tissue is required [24]. Drug release from microneedle arrays was also tested using silicone membranes [98, 99]. For Silescol® membranes, the elasticity of the membrane made the microneedle array retract after the insertion, resulting in incomplete drug release profiles. Parafilm, however, does not have this constraint. In this case, the microneedle tips are located within micropores without retraction [90]. Drug release from hydrogel-forming microneedles was investigated by Larraeta et al. A TA.XT Plus Texture Analyzer in compression mode was used to insert microneedle arrays into a single parafilm layer of Parafilm M®. The microneedle array substrate or base plate was then wrapped with parafilm and thermally sealed, forming a hermetic "pouch." This closed parafilm and microneedles array system was submerged in PBS at 32°C. Samples were taken and analyzed to study the drug release from microneedles. Water diffusion causes controlled swelling of microneedle arrays, forming *in situ* hydrogel conduit to release the drug load. The authors also observed the dissolution of microneedles under a Leica EZ4 D digital microscope, a Keyence VHX-700F digital microscope with a VH-Z20R lens, and an EX1301 OCT microscope [90]. The USP "Paddle over Disk" method [100] has been employed to study the drug release from the transdermal patch. This test measures the drug release from the entire patch surface. However, dissolving microneedle arrays works differently. The needles reside on the surface of the array. The loaded drug is released after the microneedle polymeric matrix dissolves or degrades in the vial skin layers [91]. Thus, the USP performance test does not accurately represent the microneedle mode of action. Besides, researchers employed Franz diffusion cells to analyze drug release from microneedles inserted into various skin models [101]. Raja et al. fabricated silk protein microneedle arrays and utilized 3D collagen gel and human cadaver skin to study the drug release [44]. Tsioris devised 10–20% gelatin hydrogel to mimic skin layers to study microneedle penetration. The gelatin hydrogel and polymer film membrane enhanced experimental control of drug release kinetics compared to *in vivo* or cadaver skin models [102].

3.5.4 Case Studies

Microneedle dissolution and drug release have been performed in numerous studies. Kim et al. studied the release of an R18-labeled virus from a solid coated microneedle array into human cadaver skin for 10 min. The skin tissue with embedded needles was frozen before the needle removal from the skin. The skin was then sectioned and visualized under a bright field and fluorescence microscope to track the coating release [15]. In research performed by Zhu et al., a fluorescent microplate reader was utilized to determine the release rate and drug content (sulforhodamine-B) provided by a rapidly separable microneedle array. A stereomicroscope was used to capture images of the microneedles and cadaver skin before and after microneedle insertion. At 30 min after sulforhodamine B-loaded microneedles insertion, the authors observed fading red color and drug diffusion in the skin. Within 10 s of insertion, the dissolution of the polymeric matrix in the skin caused the polylactic acid microneedles to lose roughly 20% of their initial length and release about 57% drug load into the skin. Gradually, with the increasing insertion time, the needle kept dissolving, leaving less drug in the remaining microneedle patch. Nonetheless, rapidly separating microneedles with a PVA/sucrose matrix tip delivered most of the drug (approximately 91%) more quickly and efficiently into the skin [10]. Most sulforhodamine B was driven into porcine cadaver skin for rapidly separating microneedles within 10 s. No drug was left on the microneedle patch after 30, 60, and 120 s insertion into the porcine skin, demonstrating complete dissolution of the top dissolving microneedles in the skin [10]. *In situ* dissolution of dissolving microneedles is investigated using human cadaver skin for qualitative and quantitative estimation. Nguyen and colleagues studied *in situ* dissolution of maltose microneedles after 1, 2, 3, 4, and 5 min. At the predetermined time points, microneedles were analyzed under an SEM to identify changes in microneedle geometry and dissolution [103]. The inclusion of nanomaterials (layered double hydroxide nanoparticles) in a weak polymer (sodium carboxymethylcellulose) improves the mechanical strength of microneedles without affecting the microneedle dissolution rate in the skin. The nanocomposite polymeric microneedles dissolved in the skin to release the drug load within 1 min [44]. Differently, methacrylic acid (MAA) was copolymerized with vinyl pyrrolidone (PVP) to enhance the mechanical strength of the microneedles. However, the inclusion of methacrylic acid significantly slows down the microneedle dissolution rate. Specifically, PVP-MAA microneedles (25% MAA) dissolved in 2 h, while pure PVP microneedles dissolved in just 15 min [79]. The stereomicroscope was used to record the dissolution kinetics of PVP microneedles (1% rhodamine-labeled collagen). As a result, the microneedles disintegrated within 15 sec of insertion into porcine skin. After 5 min, the microneedles dissolved almost completely. After 15 min in porcine skin, most of the microneedle base also dissolved. These PVP microneedle patches dissolve quickly, allowing collagen delivery to the skin [9]. The dissolution profile of insulin-encapsulated poly-γ-glutamic acid microneedles was investigated using porcine cadaver skin. At certain intervals, the microneedle patch was removed, and tape stripping was performed to analyze the quantity of drug delivered into the skin. After 4 min of contact with the skin's fluid, all polyglutamic acid needles dissolved completely in the skin and released the loaded insulin [16]. Lee J. discovered that extended methanol treatment slowed down the release of rhodamine B from silk fibroin microneedles. The microneedle samples with varying methanol treatment durations had the greatest difference during the initial burst release (0–16 h). This treatment inhibited the early burst release of rhodamine B from the microneedles. The effect of methanol treatment on drug release rate decreased in mid-stage and became insignificant in late-stage [104].

The dissolution kinetics of dissolving microneedles was tested on cadaver pig skin. Microneedles with trehalose tips containing Congo red dye and PVP base loading with methylene blue dye were applied on pig skin for 1 s, 10 min, and 60 min. Most of the formulation is released within a few minutes, and the formulation is completely released in the skin in 10–60 min [59]. Matsuo et al. used a stereomicroscope to investigate the dissolution of fabricated sodium hyaluronate microneedles (MicroHyala®) in skin tissue. The tips of 200- or 300-µm-long sodium hyaluronate microneedles dissolve in 5 min, and the entire needles dissolve in 1 h in mice's or rats' skin. Microneedles of 800 µm length dissolved 50% in 5 min and vanished in 1 h [92]. Bediz et al. fabricated microneedles from a combination of carboxymethylcellulose, polyvinylpyrrolidone (PVP), and maltodextrin in various ratios. They reported that a higher level of PVP resulted in a delayed release of ovalbumin load [45]. Separable arrowhead microneedles were designed to disintegrate the drug-loaded shaft seconds after skin insertion. Altering the arrowhead's composition would modulate the drug release [105]. Sulforhodamine-encapsulated dissolving microneedles made of CMC and amylopectin dissolved in 5 min, delivering 0.04 µg drug. Sulforhodamine-loaded base plate made of a swellable hydrogel provided sustained drug release of up to 1 mg in 72 h [32]. Donnelly et al. fabricated hydrogel microneedles that swell when inserted into the skin. The microneedles were made of crosslinked poly(methyl vinyl ether/maleic acid) (PMVE/MA) and poly(ethylene glycol) (PEG) or glycerol. The needles act as hydrogel conduits for drugs to enter skin tissue from the reservoir in the backing layer. Crosslinking density regulates the delivery rate. This system allows for sustained and controlled insulin release over 16 days [106]. Trehalose microneedles made by atomized spraying method dissolve quickly in *ex vivo* porcine skin within 30 s of insertion in the skin, resulting in rounded and smooth needles tip. The dissolution of microneedles is most distinguishable in the needle tips [42]. For swellable microneedles, the needles and base plate could be designed to swell at a different rate, facilitating the needle separation from the array after skin insertion. After removing the base plate, the needles are left in skin for continuous drug delivery [62]. Calcein-loaded microneedles were applied to skin to assess microneedle penetration, needle dissolution, and drug diffusion in skin tissue. Microneedle-treated skin was observed under a fluorescence microscope, revealing that calcein was kept inside the channels without quick dispersion into adjacent skin [58]. Sucrose or PVA/sucrose microneedles provide rapid dissolution and drug release [107]. The dissolution of hyaluronan microneedles was studied by applying the needle to the skin for certain intervals and measuring the remaining needle length and polymer or drug deposition in the skin [33]. Consequently, more than 50% and 65% of the needle tip's length disappeared after 1 and 10 min, respectively. The microneedles tip underwent negligible changes when removed from the skin instantaneously after skin insertion. Thus, the insertion time determines microneedle disintegration in the skin. Furthermore, the reduction in the needle length was attributed to the needle dissolution, not the mechanical change during skin insertion. The IgG content of IgG-encapsulated hyaluronan microneedles had insignificant impact on the needle dissolution rate. Due to the skin's limited moisture content, the dissolution rate of microneedles in buffer and skin differed markedly [33]. Lee et al. reported that their fabricated carboxymethyl cellulose microneedles dissolved half of the needle length within 1 min embedded in porcine skin [32]. Ross et al. discovered that coated microneedles with different polymer matrix released insulin differently [101]. *In vitro* release efficiency of interferon-α-2b-loaded dissolving microneedles was reproducibly at 49.2% [108]. Controllable drug dosage and reproducible release efficiency are essential for accurate drug administration. Dissolving microneedles made of chondroitin sulfate or dextran release practically all loaded drug within 1 h of skin insertion [109, 110].

3.6 Drug Loading and Distribution in Microneedles

It is critical to quantify the drug level in a microneedle array as this affects the encapsulation efficiency, drug stability, and delivery dose. In general, microneedles can only deliver a limited quantity of drugs ranging from micrograms to milligrams drug levels [1]. The deliverable dose of dissolving microneedles was calculated by microneedle volume and concentration of drug loading [33]. Chen reported a strong correlation between drug dose and volume of drug formulation applied to the PDMS mold during the manufacturing process [108]. The uniformity of drug distribution within microneedles and among needles on an array governs consistent dosing. The complete solubilization of the drug could achieve this uniformity within the polymer matrix before microneedle fabrication. The homogeneity of the coating layer on coated microneedles might indicate uniform drug distribution [94, 111]. If visualization of drugs in microneedles is difficult, alternative fluorescence-exhibiting agents such as calcein dye, blue-dextran, rhodamine-B, indocyanine green (ICG), red fluospheres, etc. can substitute them as the drug model to investigate drug distribution [16]. It has been shown that using fluorescently labeled molecules and dyes aids in identifying molecules that have been effectively integrated into the microneedle patch [18–20]. The distribution and location of these fluorescent molecules in microneedle arrays could be inspected under confocal laser scanning microscopy or fluorescent microscopy. Also, this inspection indicates the reproducibility and consistency of drug encapsulation in microneedles. The most commonly used method to quantify the encapsulated drug is to dissolve the microneedle array in a suited media and analyze the drug levels using a quantitative analysis method such as high-performance liquid chromatography, immunoassay, stereomicroscopy, fluorescence microscopy, and so on. Before the fabrication process (i.e., mold casting and filling), techniques such as differential scanning calorimetry could be used to examine the complete drug solubilization in a polymer matrix [2].

The quantity of drug loaded in microneedles and drug distribution in microneedle array are affected by the drug concentration, drug properties, polymer matrix (molecular weight and concentration of polymer, polymer type, and viscosity of polymer solution), excipients, and manufacturing methods. Also, mold filling is significantly affected by the polymer solution's viscosity and physicochemical properties. The concentration of polymers or ingredients in the polymeric matrix has to be optimized to avoid the nonuniformity of microneedles fabricated by the centrifugation process [44]. The quantity of drug concentrated in microneedle tips varies depending on the distance between the needle array and the centrifuge's center. For the fabrication method using vacuum application, the drug load is often pulled to the substrate rather than the needle tips [44]. The viscosity of the polymer matrix controls the efficiency of mold casting and filling as well as drug migration and diffusion during the fabrication process [33].

For instance, hyaluronan microneedles (10 kDa) manufactured by the micromolding technique could contain 500 mg/mL, while the drawing lithography method could allow for the fabrication of hyaluronan microneedles (29 kDa) loaded with only 20 mg/mL IgG [17]. In another study, Monkare et al. found that drug loading content (IgG) in 2% and 10% hyaluronan microneedles varied insignificantly across arrays in various places in the centrifuge. A fluorescently labeled compound and confocal laser scanning microscopy were employed to analyze IgG distribution in a microneedle array. The authors revealed a uniform distribution of hyaluronan and IgG in the microneedle array, which was not affected by the IgG mass ratio. However, the drying and centrifugation steps caused the variation in IgG distribution within a needle array [33]. Confocal fluorescence microscopy was used to analyze Type-I collagen distribution inside polyvinylpyrrolidone microneedles. The researchers scanned 1% rhodamine-labeled Type-I collagen microneedles and found homogeneous collagen distribution throughout the horizontal plane. However, vertical sections revealed a greater collagen content near the needle tips [9]. Brambilla et al. demonstrated that indocyanine green (ICG) was distributed consistently in PVP solid matrix microneedles at a particular ICG–PVP ratio without drug aggregation. Thus, PVP could retain the fluorescent signal of ICG and prevent ICG from aggregating in solid form. However, hyaluronic acid microneedles displayed decreased fluorescence (15- to 20-fold lower than PVP microneedles), indicating ICG aggregation [7]. To determine insulin encapsulation in poly-γ-glutamic acid microneedles, Chen et al. completely dissolved the needle array in a buffer at 4°C for one day and analyzed the solution sample. They also used blue dextran as a drug model to observe a homogeneous drug distribution in microneedles [16]. Ma et al. determined the loading of doxorubicin in coated microneedles by dissolving the drug-loaded needles in NaOH solution [57]. The uniformity of the coating layers on coated microneedles has been visualized under a fluorescence microscope, stereo zoom microscope, and light stereomicroscope. Red fluospheres and fluorescence microscopy were used to examine the drug distribution in multilayer microneedles fabricated by atomized spraying method [42]. Bing Cai employed rhodamine B as a drug model to investigate drug distribution in microneedles, revealing a homogeneous distribution of the fluorescent dye from tip to base of microneedles [62]. This technique has been commonly used to evaluate drug distribution in a microneedle array.

3.7 Skin Penetration/Insertion Efficiency

3.7.1 Introduction of Microneedle Penetration

Microneedle penetration into the skin is crucial for drug delivery into and across the skin. Microneedle penetration depth is the essential predictor of drug permeability efficiency. Assuring effective drug delivery requires microneedles to penetrate the skin to an appropriate depth. Microneedles should generally bypass the stratum corneum and viable epidermis to approach the superficial dermis layer [71]. Microneedle penetration in the skin has always been required to evaluate successful skin insertion. Incomplete penetration has been recognized as a frequent concern for microneedle application, especially mechanically weak dissolving polymeric microneedles [10]. In addition, the penetration depth should not exceed the threshold of 800 μm due to the blood capillary networks' location at around 1 mm depth in the papillary dermal area [112, 113]. Thus, this threshold allows for the avoidance of disturbing the blood vessels and nerve fibers. To deliver proteins and peptides, the desired microneedles must be long enough to bypass the epidermal layer and the basement membrane at the epidermal–dermal junction [90].

3.7.2 Factors Affecting Microneedle Penetration

The microneedle tip's sharpness is critical for skin penetration: sharper microneedles are more capable of penetrating skin tissue [65]. Microneedle penetration force is defined as the force at which a sudden reduction in the applied force is observed, indicating skin disruption [49]. Due to needle alignment and uneven skin surface, it was challenging to have all needle tips break the skin's stratum corneum simultaneously. For an accurate measurement, all needles must remain straight and simultaneously puncture the skin barrier. The penetration depth of microneedles depends on the microneedle tip's diameter, microneedle design (length and density), substrate materials, and microneedle insertion method (force, speed, and duration). The penetration depth varies from 10% to 80% of microneedle length [71, 114] due to the deformation, indentation, viscoelasticity, and irregular surface of skin tissue [115]. Microneedle design and insertion technique may determine whether a microneedle can penetrate the skin completely, partly, or not at all. The depth to which microneedles penetrate the skin significantly depends on their length. Longer microneedle or low-density microneedle array could easily overcome skin deformation for an effective penetration [116]. Pressure from a thumb or an applicator might be used to apply microneedles. Derma roller with protruding microneedles attached on a cylindrical roller was rolled on the skin surface for microneedle penetration. Microneedle tip dimensions were discovered to have a marked effect on the insertion process. The application force directly impacts microneedle penetration depth, affecting drug delivery into the skin [117]. Other critical aspects that need to be addressed for effective needle insertion include the skin's moisture content and relative humidity, the intended site of insertion, and dermatoglyphics in different populations. Histology or video frame analysis may be used to determine the depth of microneedle penetration. The penetration depth, determined by video frames, was significantly more than the actual insertion depth [71]. According to Romgens et al., the penetration process of microneedles, especially those with sharp tips, was smooth and did not result in a detectable decrease in the applied force. However, larger needle tips led to an abrupt increase in penetration after initial insertion. The skin was indented to a certain degree before being pierced [71]. In addition, the compression of skin under the needles affected the insertion force. Also, Romgens et al. [71] compared the penetration test of a single needle and an array of needles.

3.7.3 Test Methods

Ex vivo human or excised animal skin or artificial gel layers might be used to study microneedle penetration into the skin. Microneedle insertion depth is classified into two categories: real depth and approximated depth. The penetration of a single microneedle into the skin layers may be investigated in detail by analyzing histological cross sections of skin. However, this is a more time-consuming procedure and unsuitable for regular examination [32, 118, 119]. Pore staining, transepidermal water loss, skin electrical resistance, confocal microscopy, and fluorescence microscopy were also used to determine microneedle penetration. Confocal microscopy, X-ray transmission computational tomography, and optical coherence tomography (OCT) are noninvasive diagnostic procedures that reveal real depth, while histology and pore staining only provide an estimate of microneedle penetration depth. Skin tissue, with the stratum corneum pointing upward, is mounted on a flat surface of parafilm layers or a wooden board to mimic the underlying soft tissue. After gently stretching the chosen treatment spot to level out any skin folds, microneedles are manually inserted into the skin. After inserting and removing the microneedles, the investigator will apply a dye to the treatment site (e.g., gentian violet, methylene blue, or trypan blue). If microneedles effectively penetrate the skin, the dyed channels will be visible. The percentage of successful microneedle poration could be calculated by counting the number of dye-stained sites and dividing that number by the array's total microneedle count [22]. Kochhar et al. [120] discovered variations in *in vitro* microneedle penetration between human, porcine, and murine skins. The research underscored the critical nature of the array substrate when it comes to skin insertion. Additionally, owing to interspecies variances, care should be taken when extrapolating findings from animal to human skin. Additionally, microneedle penetration into *ex vivo* human skins does not correspond to true microneedle penetration *in vivo* utilizing human volunteers [26]. Thus, the capacity of OCT to photograph and quantify actual microneedle penetration in the skin *in vivo* offers a way to overcome the low correlation between *ex vivo* and *in vivo* microneedle penetration in humans [72]. The penetration profile of microneedles was studied using computerized X-ray tomography. This nondestructive technology employs a series of X-ray scans taken at various rotation angles to obtain 3D volumetric data that enables 3D imaging of microneedle insertion. However, such approaches are limited by the necessity for microneedle materials with X-ray contrast qualities and the difficulty of differentiating the precise layers of skin (stratum corneum, epidermis, and dermis) that have been penetrated by the microneedles [72]. Larraeta et al. [121] devised a straightforward and reliable microneedle insertion model employing a thermoplastic sheet consisting of an olefin-type polymer (Parafilm M®). They multiply the number of layers pierced by the microneedle with the thickness of each Parafilm M® layer to get the insertion depth. Parafilm M® may be utilized as a skin simulant for microneedle insertion, as shown by its excellent concordance with findings obtained using excised pig skin, which is a suitable model for human skin. This simple, quick, and reliable insertion test may be performed for quality control purposes or to conduct comparative formulation studies. The utilization of several human or animal skin models at various locations for microneedle assessment is critical due to its therapeutic relevance. To conduct a skin penetration test, researchers must first establish the skin models, the force and speed of microneedle application, the machine and probe to be used, the methodology to be used, and the appropriate penetration depth for a particular array or needle to achieve maximum drug cargo delivery [24]. Furthermore, microneedles should not break when in contact with the skin; this is less critical for dissolving microneedles but critical for solid microneedles with a high degree of fragility and biocompatibility, such as silicon. It is essential to ascertain how the microneedle will deliver the drug on time and at an appropriate level. Swelling must be adequate for hydrogel microneedles, depending on the degree of crosslinking. Dissolution or disintegration tests should be required for dissolving microneedles [24]. The requirements for drug delivery for different microneedle types vary according to the route of administration. For coated needles [91], some drug release research will be required. For hollow microneedles that need a separate delivery system or injector [115], tests to examine the microneedle channels for possible obstruction will be required in addition to the separate injector system. Effective drug delivery is a test that will certainly be included in the criteria adapted to various microneedle types.

3.7.4 Effect of Applicators

Paustnitz et al. have patented several device designs that minimize skin deformation and maximize microneedle penetration at the application location [122]. These device designs are built on three principles: (i) limiting skin elasticity or wrinkles, (ii) assisting the device in adapting to the elasticity, and (iii) providing other methods for controlled microneedle insertion into the skin. Methods such as applying a membrane or a film to the application site before insertion, chilling the stratum corneum with chemicals or liquefied gas, or utilizing ring/clamping devices have been suggested to reduce skin elasticity. Other options include the use of a flexible substrate, changing the height of the microneedles in an array, applying the microneedles rapidly, and using a device with extensions or gaps between the microneedles. In addition, the usage of microneedles coupled with a piezoelectric transducer has been suggested to improve needle penetration owing to vibration. The authors found a 70% decrease in the insertion force due to vibration actuation [123]. The use of applicators is predicted to improve microneedle penetration, particularly for short microneedles. To enable microneedle insertion into the skin, a vibratory actuator assisted microneedles in penetrating the skin with less pressure [123–125], while an electrically powered applicator ensured microneedle penetration to improve skin permeability [115]. A spring-loaded applicator has been widely utilized to ensure the speed, depth of penetration, and quantity of drug delivered from microneedles [114]. Microneedle insertion through drilling allowed for excellent control of the needle insertion depth [126]. Wang and Praustnitz also invented a microneedle drilling device that utilizes rotating motion to enable smooth, stable, and effective microneedle insertion up to a specified depth (500–1,000 µm). If the device could be automated to detect the skin thickness of specific patients and alter the drilling depth suitably, this design might provide significant advantages in terms of individualization of microneedle device-based treatment for various patients. Lastovich et al. recommended the use of an outlet port (luer lock collar for syringe attachment) to draw a vacuum from the microneedle application site to enable better contact and microneedle penetration. Along with penetration, the vacuum would minimize needle movement relative to the skin during the injection, lowering the risk of needle breakage. Apart from that, the insertion force, the insertion velocity, and the height above the skin from which microneedles are placed all contribute to determining the length of microneedles required to accomplish the desired insertion [122].

3.7.5 Case Studies for Microneedle Penetration

Lee et al. demonstrated that a 1.5 N force could be used to insert a pyramidal microneedle into full-thickness cadaver pig skin [32]. Utilizing a movable cylindrical probe, Donnelly and coworkers applied a microneedle array onto piglet skin [84]. Similarly, Khan et al. used a texture analyzer to apply varying microneedle pressures on a newborn pig skin in order to determine the insertion depth [127]. Davis et al. [49] conducted several insertion test experiments on three Caucasian male skins, utilizing Tricor Systems. Another research scanned the penetration depth of microneedles in human skin using optical coherence tomography (OCT) technology [128]. Zhu et al. discovered that the dissolving portion of rapidly separating microneedles formed around 500-µm deep channels in pig cadaver skin that were comparable in length to the dissolving microneedles. Sulforhodamine B's fluorescent region remained roughly 150 µm from the skin's surface, showing that the drug-loaded points were entirely embedded in the skin [10]. The researchers noticed that when a silicon microneedle (280 µm in length) is inserted into the skin and examined using OCT, the microneedles penetrate roughly 61–64% of their length [129]. Research employing Trypan blue staining and TEWL to determine the association between microneedle length and skin penetration demonstrated that manual insertion of short (300-µm-long) microneedles failed to penetrate the stratum corneum. Microneedles with a length of 550 µm or more were required to penetrate the skin's viscoelasticity and resistance. An effective insertion was accomplished by moving an electrical applicator at a rate of 1 or 3 m/s. Bal et al. [130] showed that microneedle design and application speed affected the depth and shape of created channels in human participants. The penetration effectiveness of hyaluronan microneedles loaded with IgG was reported to be between 80% and 88% [33]. Additionally, almost 80% of solid microneedle arrays effectively penetrate skin [131]. Martanto et al. investigated the relationship between the retraction distance of a hollow microneedle and the flow rate after skin insertion. Consequently, a greater retraction distance results in a greater flow rate. Furthermore, the effect of infusion pressure, microneedle tip bevel angle, and microneedle tip opening size on the flow rate was also examined [54]. Wang et al. were able to insert microneedles to specified depths under controlled and repeatable procedures using rotary drilling and glass hollow microneedles [126]. Drilling insertion was projected to result in less skin deformation than direct piercing, allowing for more reproducible microneedle insertion. Yang et al. (2012) demonstrated reliable microneedle penetration in the skin by applying 5 N thumb pressure, which resulted in penetration of almost half of the microneedle's length (800 µm), as determined by histological sectioning [132]. Larraneta et al. (2014) described the effective insertion of polymeric microneedles into excised neonatal pig skin utilizing thumb pressure for 30 s. Moreover, the average force applied to the microneedle by 20 human volunteers (10 men and 10 females) selected for this investigation was determined to be roughly 20 N [121]. This force was seen to be adequate to penetrate every microneedle in an array successfully, implying that the use of an applicator may be unnecessary since microneedle insertion may be accomplished with thumb pressure.

3.8 Safety Test

3.8.1 Biological Safety

Assurance of the safety and efficacy of this innovative microneedle-based drug delivery technology by a more thorough study would result in widespread patient acceptance. To achieve microneedle biological safety goals, it is essential to understand the mechanics of pore closure, the risk of infection and bleeding, local adverse reactions at the treatment site (irritation, itching, erythema, redness, bruising, or edema), remaining drug on the skin, needle fracture, the biocompatibility of needle material with the skin, the likelihood of blood vessel rupturing and unwanted injuries, thermal stability of components, the potential for and complications associated with reuse, the safe disposability of used devices, and the influence of external factors on delivery [56, 122]. These characteristics can address microneedle safety: microbial limits, sterility, particulate matter, extractables, osmolarity, and antimicrobial preservative content. Given the fact that microneedles stay in touch with skin layers, it is critical to assess the irritation potential of the polymers used to fabricate microneedles, the loaded drug, and excipients [34]. Local irritation or erythema (reddening) of the skin may be a concern for specific individuals. It is crucial to determine if frequent microneedle usage results in an immunological response to the drug or microneedle excipients.

Microneedle biological safety test shows microneedles to be safe for skin application. The safety and toxicity of microneedles can be determined using various physicochemical characterization methods, including laser Doppler flowmetry, TEWL, high-frequency ultrasound, capacitance reflectance spectroscopy, changes in skin color measured with a chromameter, the Draize skin irritation test, and visual scoring [34–36]. Numerous microneedle-based investigations have been published in the literature demonstrating the lack or moderate and insignificant incidence of localized skin reactions after microporation in human trials or animal models [133–136]. Modepalli et al. evaluated the safety and toxicity of hydrogel-forming microneedles incorporating ferric pyrophosphate on human skin cell lines. They reported that ferric pyrophosphate loaded into microneedles is a better source of iron for cutaneous delivery and exhibited no toxicity in human skin fibro-blast cell lines [63]. The MTT test was used to assess the cytotoxicity of the microneedle construction polymer using the HaCaT and HEK293 cell lines. The findings indicated that cell viability was more than 87% after three days [3]. Another research found that each component of hydrogel-forming microneedles and wafers examined had endotoxin levels less than the FDA's established limits for medical devices in close contact with cardiovas-cular or lymphatic tissue [39].

The sterility of microneedles for medicinal uses is a legitimate issue that has sparked debate. Sterility testing and endotoxin analysis of microneedle devices might be beneficial in determining their biological safety and expediting the regulatory approval and com-mercialization processes for microneedle-based products [39, 137]. Furthermore, sterility tests in compliance with Ph. Eur Method 2.6. were conducted to identify the growth of microorganisms and bioburden in manufactured microneedle devices [39]. Different ster-ilization techniques, such as aseptic processing and terminal sterilization, are documented in the literature [138]. According to some researchers, sterility is unnecessary since it is no more disruptive than a scratch on the skin [137]. Nevertheless, microneedle sterility is likely to be questioned if an application for FDA approval for a microneedle system is filed. This may be accomplished by the use of ethylene oxide gas sterilization, aseptic process-ing, or another type of sterilization [137]. Ameri and coworkers [138] examined the stabil-ity of parathyroid hormone-loaded coated microneedles following aseptic manufacturing and terminal sterilization. They revealed that terminal sterilization using γ-irradiation or an e-beam elevated oxidation of the active ingredient in the product, which could be minimized by adjusting the irradiation doses and temperature for the lowest oxidation. Assembly under a laminar flow hood, accompanied by ethylene oxide sterilization, was recommended by Wermeling and colleagues as a means of ensuring sterility during the integration of stainless steel solid microneedles into a patch system [61]. In another study, there was no signs of microbial development in any of the hydrogel-forming microneedle samples across the 14-day experiment in either soya bean casein or thioglycolate envi-ronments. All sterility tests were performed under aseptic conditions in line with Ph. Eur Method 2.6.1. There was no evidence of bioburden in any of the hydrogel-forming microneedle or lyophilized wafer formulations examined, and endotoxin levels were very minimal [39]. Sterilization of microneedles and associated products is a crucial challenge that warrants further investigation [137].

3.8.2 Skin Irritation and Recovery Studies

Erythema and edema are indeed the features of skin irritation. Skin reactions such as irrita-tion, erythema, redness, bruising, or edema at the injection site are frequently documented with conventional hypodermic needles. Researchers should consider the probability of such reactions at the microneedle-porated area [122]. This will be critical in determin-ing the technology's acceptance among patients. The most often seen adverse reaction to microneedle insertion is moderate, temporary erythema at the application site. To evalu-ate skin irritation, biophysical characterization techniques such as transepidermal water loss, laser Doppler flowmetry, high-frequency ultrasound, and visual scoring may be per-formed [34]. The likelihood of such skin irritation varies according to various parameters, including the microneedle dimension, the materials utilized to produce the microneedles, and the kind of formulation injected through microneedles [72]. The critical component contributing to irritation development is the material used to construct microneedles. Researchers could assess the microneedles' safety and tolerability by measuring the intensity of skin reactions. No patients developed allergic or irritating contact dermatitis. Dissolving microneedle patches containing retinyl retinoate and ascorbic acid exhibited no significant adverse effects and were considered safe for cosmetic applications [56]. Liu et al. [36] conducted a primary skin irritation test following microneedle penetration using the Draize dermal scoring criteria; the slight redness reported was related to physical compression of the microneedles, which indicated that irritation and skin injuries caused by the microneedle were negligible.

Numerous researchers have confirmed the safety and efficacy of microneedles. Previous microneedle-based investigations have verified the lack or insignificant incidence of local skin irritation after microporation. These evaluations may include basic dermatoscopic observation or stereomicroscopy, which enables the identification of any localized erythema and symptoms of irritation that may have emerged during or after microneedle insertion [10]. Several authors have found that redness and minor itching subside a few minutes or hours after microneedle microporation [94]. These are minor concerns, particularly given the magnitude of local skin responses generated by hypodermic needles. Skin irritation possibly depends on the pore closure. The kinetics of microneedle pore sealing are very diverse and greatly depend on the kind of skin (animal versus human) and experimental design employed (*ex vivo* versus *in vivo*). The kinetics of microneedle pore sealing are very diverse and greatly depend on the kind of skin (animal versus human) and experimental design employed (*ex vivo* versus *in vivo*).

Matsuo et al. observed that sodium hyaluronate microneedles fully dissolved in the skin fluid and posed no risk of remaining components in the skin, rendering dissolving microneedles safer than metal solid microneedles arrays [92]. Kaushik et al. demonstrated the absence of redness, swelling, irritation, or other unwanted effects after microneedle penetration in clinical research utilizing silicon microneedles (array of 400 µm microneedles of 150 µm length) [139]. Shirkhanzadeh reported no skin reactions in human participants after applying porous calcium phosphate-coated stainless steel microneedles (500 µm long, implanted to a depth of 100–300 µm) [136]. Miyano et al. stated that they employed dissolving and biodegradable maltose microneedles (500 µm) encapsulating ascorbate-2-glycoside on human subjects and that the microneedles did not produce any dermatological concerns [107]. Daddona et al. showed that human volunteers tolerated the drug-coated microneedle patch systems (Macroflux® transdermal delivery system) well in all phase I and phase II clinical studies [134]. Daddona demonstrated a similar safety profile during placebo-wearing investigations. The application areas exhibited no or minimal erythema and no indications of skin infection during or after the application of microneedle system [140]. Sathyan et al. revealed that coated titanium microneedles (Macroflux® transdermal delivery system) were safe for the delivery of desmopressin in hairless guinea pigs and human subjects, with no to moderate topical reactions [141, 142]. Ameri et al. verified the safety of using similar coated needles to administer erythropoietin transdermally in hairless guinea pigs [133]. Burton et al. [143] examined the microneedle insertion area on hairless guinea pigs and swine skin using a simple visual and touch evaluation. *In vivo*, the researchers observed the appearance of a white ring and blotch after microneedle application. Kusamori et al. [144, 145] sought to assess the degree of skin irritation caused by microneedle application using the Draize technique. The severity of erythema and edema on the skin was scored. This technique enables the quantitative evaluation of the effects of microneedle insertion on skin irritation. However, the Draize method is very subjective and may differ according to the investigators. More research is required to determine the possibility of developing skin reactions and other undesirable outcomes due to the usage of microneedles.

3.9 Physicochemical Stability

3.9.1 Hygroscopicity

Moisture absorption may reduce the sharpness of the needles, weakening their mechanical strength and the ability to penetrate the skin effectively. Hygroscopicity tests were conducted to determine the moisture content of the microneedles absorbed from their surroundings. Prior to the experiment, all microneedles were stored in a dry desiccator to maintain comparable conditions for all samples. Microneedles are typically incubated with saturated salt solutions in desiccators at ambient conditions to determine their hygroscopicity. Adjusting the relative humidity of the environment requires varying ratios of saturated potassium acetate, potassium carbonate, magnesium chloride, and sodium chloride solutions [11, 29]. The needles were then removed, and microneedles' weights may be recorded using electronic balances at specified time intervals, followed by a calculation of the percentage increase in weight moisture absorption. A water activity analyzer may also be utilized to determine the endpoint water level [16, 14]. Sugar-based microneedles encapsulated with biomacromolecules may exhibit stability issues owing to their intrinsic hygroscopic properties, resulting in poor storage at ambient relative humidity conditions. Combining multiple substituents with variable degrees of elasticity and hardness is one strategy to increase the long-term stability of sugar microneedles [76]. Analysis of the effect of moisture content on the mechanical qualities of exenatide-encapsulated sodium hyaluronate-based microneedles revealed that an increase in the water level decreases the physical robustness of microneedles [11]. In an environment with relative humidity levels of more than 50%, maltose microneedles were reported to dissolve spontaneously owing to the hydrolysis mechanism. When the needles were subjected to an environment with less than 40% humidity, no hydrolysis or alteration in the geometry was noticed for up to three months [107]. Since gamma polyglutamic acid (γ-PGA) is a hygroscopic and hydrophilic polypeptide, it is difficult to maintain the hardness and sharpness of γ-PGA microneedles due to their proclivity for absorbing moisture from the surrounding environment. γ-PGA hydrogels were included in the microneedles formulation to minimize hygroscopicity and improve stability. These covalently crosslinked hydrogels preserved the mechanical integrity of the microneedle during moisture exposure and provided resistance to microneedle deformation. The effect of adding various amounts of γ-PGA hydrogel (0, 25, 50, and 75 wt%) on the hygroscopicity and mechanical strength of microneedles was studied. Thus, increasing the hydrogel proportion significantly decreased the water uptake. The addition of hydrogel to the microneedles (at a 50 wt% concentration) was found to increase their resistance to moisture [16]. PVP microneedles have long been known for their hygroscopic characteristics. It assisted in smoothing the surface of microneedles; nevertheless, it may impair the strength of microneedle, which is why PVP microneedle must be kept in a vacuum or with desiccant [9].

3.9.2 Swelling Behavior

For swellable microneedles, the swelling behavior of the needles is critical for drug release and delivery into the skin tissue. PBS is often used as the swelling medium to investigate the swelling capabilities of microneedles since it is assumed to mimic interstitial skin fluid [30, 39, 146]. Microneedles constructed from polyvinyl alcohol (PVA) swell as body fluids are absorbed, forming pathways for the release of encapsulated medicines via diffusion. The swelling capabilities of the needles were determined by inserting them into the arms of human subjects and observing the swelling at various time intervals. The authors found that microneedles swelled 1 and 3 h after patch application and removal [41]. Different polymers may be incorporated to control the swelling level and deliver the drug immediately or sustainably. Carboxymethylcellulose disintegrates, creating negatively charged long chains with wide spaces for water to be absorbed. Polymers, including polyvinylpyrrolidone and dextran, function as diluents for crosslinking. Kim et al. examined the swelling behavior of PLGA microneedles loaded with hydrogel microparticles for their mechanical strength upon contact with PBS or after penetration into pig skin at various intervals. Within 10 s of contact with PBS, the swollen hydrogel microparticles on the surface of the microneedle began to fracture, while the microneedles began to break after 30 s of contact. Within 60 s, all microneedles demonstrated mechanical failure. A SEM photograph of the PLGA microneedles containing hydrogel microparticles demonstrates that the microneedles began to fracture and the majority of them were broken after 15 min of insertion and separation from the pig skin [78]. Donnelly et al. reported the fabrication of hydrogel-forming microneedle arrays using a "super swelling" combination of Gantrez, polyethylene glycol, and sodium carbonate [30]. They evaluated the swelling of the microneedle arrays *in situ* using OCT at various time points following the microneedle insertion into neonatal pig skin until 3 h.

3.9.3 Stability

Drugs and biopharmaceuticals incorporated in microneedles should maintain their integrity and bioactivity throughout the production process and intended storage duration. Drug stability analysis is critical because many stresses are imparted to the molecules during microneedle manufacturing, particularly heating, drying, and interaction with other ingredients, which may affect protein integrity and cause the drugs to degrade [82, 33]. The protein stability can be affected by formulation, polymer matrix, high temperature, extreme pHs, and drug–polymer interaction [33]. Drug recovery after microneedle fabrication studies must be performed to evaluate the amount of drug remaining. The reduction in vaccine stability may be due to drying during solid microneedle coating or loading into dissolving microneedles [1]. Elevated temperatures, in particular, may promote protein denaturation or aggregation. The stability of the protein in microneedle formulation was reported elsewhere [45, 109, 147, 148]. It has been shown that maintaining proteins in the solid form throughout thermal manufacturing procedures improves stability [82]. Production of dissolving microneedles demands technical knowledge to load the drug or antigen into the polymeric matrix of the microneedle material using gentle techniques that do not deteriorate the antigen or impair the material's strength [149]. The stability of antigens and vaccine-loaded microneedles seems to have attracted considerable attention since they can be stored and distributed at temperatures exceeding those required for conventional cold-chain conditions [58, 150]. This eliminates the storage constraints associated with the cold chain [58]. Microneedle-based solid-state vaccine delivery offers improved antigen stability and may obviate the requirement for cold-chain storage [58, 151]. Microneedles have been manufactured using carbohydrates that act as lyoprotectants in substitute of water, efficiently shielding antigens against physiochemical breakdown throughout the production and storage processes [58].

In published research, protein integrity has been investigated using a variety of techniques, including circular dichroism analysis, dynamic light scattering, solubility testing, fluorescence microscopy, and electrophoresis [32, 33]. Spectroscopic methods such as circular dichroism [32] and fluorescence spectroscopy [33] may be employed to determine the conformation of proteins. SDS-PAGE may also be used to determine the integrity of the protein backbone [152]. To examine the DNA supercoiling and effectiveness in dissolving microneedles, agarose gel electrophoresis and *in vitro* transfection could be used [153]. Furthermore, protein stability is evaluated by determining the degree of protein recovery or measuring the level of retained bioactivity [16, 33]. Numerous techniques can be used to scrutinize the aggregation of protein antigens or particulate vaccines, including size exclusion chromatography, asymmetrical flow field–flow fractionation, micro-flow imaging, transmission electron microscopy, dynamic light scattering, and nanoparticle tracking analysis. For live attenuated or vector vaccines, virus or bacterium viability may be adequate since the antigen replicates upon vaccination, and thus the vaccine potency may be assessed by measuring the titer of live antigen [154]. Immunogenicity testing is essential in determining vaccination efficacy [155]. Antigen stability should be evaluated during microneedle manufacture [156] and after storage periods [14, 97].

The stability of vaccines may be compromised during coating on solid microneedles or encapsulation inside dissolving microneedles, mainly owing to the drying process [1]. Numerous vaccine compositions have been explored for coating influenza vaccines on metal microneedles, and it was determined that the inclusion of trehalose was crucial for maintaining vaccine antigenicity [15, 157]. After seven weeks of storage on coated microneedles at ambient conditions, the BCG vaccine lost roughly 30% of its viability. The use of trehalose, in addition to surfactants, was essential for the stabilization of the BCG vaccine on coated microneedles [158]. The biological activity of insulin loaded in poly-γ-glutamic acid microneedles was determined for untreated insulin, insulin entrapped in microneedles dissolved after one day and one month of storage at 37°C, and insulin thermally exposed to 80°C for 1 h or after one month of storage at –20°C, 4°C, 25°C, and 37°C. There was no statistical difference between the insulin activity of the untreated insulin solution and that of encapsulated insulin in polyglutamic acid microneedles after storage at 37°C for one day. Moreover, after one month of storage at 37°C, the insulin activity of the microneedle group reduced only modestly. Encapsulating insulin inside poly-γ-glutamic acid microneedles did not substantially affect its biological activity; also, these microneedles were stable at 25°C and 37°C for at least one month, a feature that may lessen the necessity of cold-chain storage and transportation [16]. Zhen et al. developed liposome-encapsulated microneedles that contained vaccines. Sucrose was incorporated into the composition as a lyoprotectant to prevent disturbance to the antigens' physicochemical attributes during the production and storage of microneedles. They reported minimal effect on the liposomes-loaded PVP microneedle after six months at 40°C, two weeks at 25°C, or three days at 40°C [58]. Several studies have employed trehalose to improve drug stability. Trehalose creates large hydration spheres, which has been linked to trehalose's assistance in increasing stability for macromolecules [159, 160]. To preserve antigenicity, trehalose is required to produce coated metal microneedles for influenza vaccines [2, 158]. The storage stability of dissolving microneedles encapsulating human interferon α-2b was investigated for 30–90 days at temperatures of 4°C, 25°C, and 40°C. After 30 days of storage at various temperatures, a negligible decrease was noticed. After 90 days, the stability of all groups of microneedles manufactured from various materials decreased dramatically, averaging 46.1%. Stability analysis revealed that the manufacturing process (micromolding at ambient conditions) of human interferon α-2b-loaded microneedles had no influence on the interferon α-2b's activity. There was a discrepancy in the thermal stability profile of the drug among various polymer matrixes (chondroitin sulfate, polyvinylpyrrolidone, and hyaluronic acid); the polymer materials heavily governed the drug stability. While hyaluronic acid inhibited interferon α-2b activity, chondroitin sulfate and polyvinylpyrrolidone did not [108]. In another study, Sullivan and colleagues employed a photopolymerization technique to fabricate microneedles without impairing β-galactosidase activity.

Numerous research has examined vaccine stability in dissolving microneedles in a systematic way. Mistilis et al. demonstrated that the buffer composition and manufacturing processes (e.g., drying temperature) must be adjusted appropriately to preserve the vaccine stability of the subunit influenza vaccine [161]. Specifically, ammonium acetate buffer (pH 7.0) and HEPES exhibited significantly more antigenicity in solution and dry form than phosphate buffers. Moreover, surfactants adversely affected the antigen, particularly in the liquid composition before the fabrication of dissolving microneedles, and the surfactants may result in crystallization of the microneedles matrix, causing antigen degradation [161]. Antigen encapsulation also contributes to antigen stability. Antigen-specific CD8+ proliferative responses to OVA-PLGA nanoparticles in dissolving microneedles were comparable before and after ten weeks of storage at ambient temperatures [162]. T-cell responses were considerably lower in those injected with monomeric OVA in dissolving microneedles that had been kept for ten weeks than those treated with monomeric OVA that had not been preserved [162]. This observation indicates the protective effect of PLGA nanoparticles on OVA stability. Sun W et al. investigated the stability of Type-I collagen loaded in polyvinylpyrrolidone microneedles following e-beam sterilization. The ELISA method was used to assess the amount of functional collagen in PVP microneedles. Around 80–90% of protein maintained active of the collagen retrieved from PVP microneedles. At 1%, 2%, and 4% collagen levels, there is an insignificant, minor reduction in functional collagen concentration after e-beam therapy [9]. SDS-PAGE and CD analysis reveal that over 80% of collagen remained stable and active inside the PVP microneedles and that integration shielded collagen against e-beam destruction [9].

Similarly, the stability of indocyanine green in PVP microneedles was assessed using spectroscopy after six-month storage. Despite indocyanine green having poor chemical stability in the solution, it was stable for at least six months when incorporated in PVP microneedles [7]. Vrdoljak et al. manufactured dissolving microneedles encapsulating adenovirus and inactivated influenza vaccine using an innovative microfluidic drop dispensing technique and reported that the vaccine contained in microneedles remained stable for more than six months at 40°C. Subunit vaccines embedded inside dissolving microneedles markedly enhanced their stability outside cold-chain conditions [59]. Biodegradable PLGA polymer microneedles were fabricated to enclose bovine serum albumin. High-temperature exposure for less than 10 min during microneedle production had no noticeable effect on protein stability, whereas thermal stress of more than 20 min triggered protein aggregation [82]. Carboxymethylcellulose-based dissolving microneedles containing lysozyme and human growth hormone were effectively fabricated and kept stable for 2 and 15 months, respectively, at ambient temperature [32]. Insulin, low-molecular-weight heparin, and desmopressin were similarly encapsulated in dissolving microneedles and preserved their activity for at least one month, even at temperatures as high as 40°C or as low as −80°C [109, 163, 164]. Likewise, horseradish peroxidase was successfully coated on microneedles and retained a substantial portion of its enzymatic activity after one month at 70°C [111]. PTH coated on solid microneedles maintained its bioactivity for up to 18 months at ambient temperature and 60% relative humidity. Terminal sterilization of PTH-loaded microneedles using γ-irradiation or e-beam irradiation led to PTH oxidation, which may be mitigated by reducing the irradiation intensity and temperature, as well as by limiting moisture and oxygen levels in the container. Nevertheless, aseptic processing was employed due to the inability of these methods to ensure product performance for a two-year shelf life at room temperature [138]. PVP microneedles fabricated by UV polymerization technique were observed to maintain the immunogenicity of inactivated influenza vaccine [155]. Although microneedles coated with an inactivated influenza vaccine and kept at ambient temperature for one month lost nearly 20% of their antigenicity *in vitro*, mice immunized with these microneedles generated comparable IgG responses *in vivo* to those taking unstored microneedles [40]. In another study, after six months of storage, an influenza subunit vaccine coated on solid microneedles elicited antibody responses in mice comparable to those induced by newly coated microneedles [165]. Likewise, IgG recovery from hyaluronan microneedles was reported to be 82% of the initial IgG level, and the IgG load's tertiary structure remained unchanged. No aggregation or complex formation occurred between hyaluronan and IgG. Without complexation with hyaluronan, IgG was predominantly monomeric in the microneedle matrix [33].

3.9.4 Water Content

The moisture content of microneedles must be evaluated since it considerably affects the microneedles' mechanical strength, drug stability, dissolution kinetics, and performance. Researchers have examined the influence of moisture content on the mechanical properties of microneedles [29]. The water content of freeze-dried vaccines is typically advised to be less than 3% w/w, which might also be used as a guideline for dissolving microneedles. Since dissolving microneedles are in dry form, it is critical to determine their moisture content using Karl Fischer titration (a coulometric or volumetric titration), thermogravimetric analysis, or moisture balance [161]. Researchers have observed that the concentration of IgG in dissolving microneedles had no impact on the moisture content of the needles [33]. In another study, the moisture level of hyaluronan microneedles was determined to be 18.5% (using an equilibrium relative humidity analysis) [14], 1.6% (using an electronic moisture balance) [11], and 11.9–12.8% (using thermogravimetric analysis) [33]. The effect of water content on the mechanical properties of sodium hyaluronate microneedles loaded with exenatide was examined, and increasing the water content was observed to reduce the microneedle hardness [11]. Also, when insulin-encapsulated hyaluronic acid-based microneedles were incubated at 75% relative humidity, the softening behavior of the needles was seen as a consequence of the increased weight of the microneedles owing to moisture absorption [29]. Hiraishi et al. investigated the influence of humidity on the mechanical strength of sodium hyaluronate microneedle patch. One week of storage at 75% relative humidity increased the water activity from 18.5% to 59.1%. In addition, the mechanical failure force for microneedle patches with 59.1% water activity was 0.14 N/needle, which was 50% less than the failure force for dry microneedle patches (with 18.5% water activity) [14]. Another research discovered that maltose microneedles disintegrate immediately due to the hydrolysis in an environment with a relative humidity of more than 50%. However, no hydrolysis or physical deformation was detected when the needles were exposed to less than 40% humidity for up to three months [107].

3.9.5 Solid State of Microneedles

The solid state of microneedles has been found as a critical characteristic that affects microneedle performance. In a study, SEM and DSC analyses were performed to determine the effect of methanol treatment on the degree of crystallinity of silk fibroin microneedles. The study revealed that the degree of crystallization is most significant on the surface of silk fibroin microneedles and decreases with depth in the microneedle matrix. When the microneedles were exposed to methanol for a longer time, the morphological alterations on the surface of the microneedles were more pronounced. The crystallinity of silk fibroin microneedles increased when the methanol treatment period was increased [41]. Similarly, the DSC was used to perform thermal testing on microneedles encapsulated with lidocaine. The thermograms of the unloaded microneedle and microneedle loaded with 21% lidocaine were comparable. Furthermore, the absence of endothermic drug peaks indicated that the drug was in an amorphous state inside the microneedle matrix. Due to the amorphous property of lidocaine in the microneedle, the drug was entirely diffused and dissolved in the polymer matrix [2]. Differential scanning calorimetry (DSC) and powder X-ray diffraction were employed to characterize trehalose dihydrate raw material and trehalose microneedles. The study revealed that trehalose is in an amorphous form, which is preferable for the stability of protein-based medicines and vaccines [42].

3.10 Conclusions

Microneedles have been studied extensively for various purposes, including drug administration, diagnosis, and monitoring. Patient-centered care-driven research combined with the advancement of microfabrication technologies has created innovative and intelligent microneedle systems. The rigorous characterization of microneedles is critical for determining the drug delivery system's capacity to penetrate the skin and deliver therapeutic agents efficiently and safely. These assessment methods should be capable of assessing the geometry and dimensions of microneedles at the micrometer scale, thereby providing researchers with information about the repeatability and reliability of microfabrication procedures. Furthermore, these tests should demonstrate the microneedle device's capacity to penetrate the target tissue, which is often the skin. Moreover, the microneedle system's potential to deliver the drug load with the required release profile must be illustrated *in vitro* and *in vivo*. Even though there are no standardized methods for characterizing microneedles, it is anticipated that the presentation of current techniques in the area would prepare the way for the future establishment of standardized procedures for microneedle assessment. If microneedle-based delivery systems become more widely used and marketed, this level of standardization will guarantee consistency, effectiveness, and patient safety.

References

[1] Kim Y-C, Park J-H, Prausnitz MR. Microneedles for drug and vaccine delivery. Adv Drug Deliv Rev. 2012;64:1547–1568.

[2] Kathuria H, Li H, Pan J, et al. Large size microneedle patch to deliver lidocaine through skin. Pharm Res. 2016;1–15.

[3] Dangol M, Yang H, Li CG, et al. Innovative polymeric system (IPS) for solvent-free lipophilic drug transdermal delivery via dissolving microneedles. J Control Release. 2016;223:118–125.

[4] Andrianov AK, Decollibus DP, Marin A, et al. PCPP-formulated H5N1 influenza vaccine displays improved stability and dose-sparing effect in lethal challenge studies. J Pharm Sci. 2011;100:1436–1443.

[5] Marin A, DeCollibus DP, Andrianov AK. Protein stabilization in aqueous solutions of poly-phosphazene polyelectrolyte and non-ionic surfactants. Biomacromolecules. 2010;11:2268–2273.

[6] Quan F-S, Kim Y-C, Yoo D-G, et al. Stabilization of influenza vaccine enhances protection by microneedle delivery in the mouse skin. PLoS One. 2009;4:e7152.

[7] Brambilla D, Proulx ST, Marschalkova P, et al. Microneedles for the noninvasive structural and functional assessment of dermal lymphatic vessels. Small. 2016;12:1053–1061.

[8] Park J-H, Choi S-O, Kamath R, et al. Polymer particle-based micromolding to fabricate novel microstructures. Biomed Microdevices. 2007;9:223–234.

[9] Sun W, Inayathullah M, Manoukian MAC, et al. Transdermal delivery of functional collagen via polyvinylpyrrolidone microneedles. Ann Biomed Eng. 2015;43:2978–2990.

[10] Zhu DD, Wang QL, Liu XB, et al. Rapidly separating microneedles for transdermal drug delivery. Acta Biomater. 2016;41:312–319.

[11] Zhu Z, Luo H, Lu W, et al. Rapidly dissolvable microneedle patches for transdermal delivery of exenatide. Pharm Res. 2014;31:3348–3360.

[12] Donnelly RF, Majithiya R, Singh TRR, et al. Design, optimization and characterisation of poly-meric microneedle arrays prepared by a novel laser-based micromoulding technique. Pharm Res. 2011;28:41–57.

[13] Donnelly RF, Singh TRR, Alkilani AZ, et al. Hydrogel-forming microneedle arrays exhibit antimicrobial properties: potential for enhanced patient safety. Int J Pharm. 2013;451:76–91.

[14] Hiraishi Y, Nakagawa T, Quan Y-S, et al. Performance and characteristics evaluation of a sodium hyaluronate-based microneedle patch for a transcutaneous drug delivery system. Int J Pharm. 2013;441:570–579.

[15] Kim Y-C, Quan F-S, Compans RW, et al. Formulation and coating of microneedles with inactivated influenza virus to improve vaccine stability and immunogenicity. J Control Release. 2010;142:187–195.

[16] Chen M-C, Ling M-H, Kusuma SJ. Poly-γ-glutamic acid microneedles with a supporting structure design as a potential tool for transdermal delivery of insulin. Acta Biomater. 2015;24:106–116.

[17] Lee SG, Jeong JH, Lee KM, et al. Nanostructured lipid carrier-loaded hyaluronic acid microneedles for controlled dermal delivery of a lipophilic molecule. Int J Nanomedicine. 2014;9:289–299.

[18] Donnelly RF, Morrow DIJ, Fay F, et al. Microneedle-mediated intradermal nanoparticle delivery: potential for enhanced local administration of hydrophobic pre-formed photosensitisers. Photodiagnosis Photodyn Ther. 2010;7:222–231.

[19] Liu S, Wu D, Quan Y, et al. Improvement of transdermal delivery of exendin-4 using novel tip-loaded microneedle arrays fabricated from hyaluronic acid. Molecular Pharmaceutics. 2016;13:272–279.

[20] Zhao X, Li X, Zhang P, et al. Tip-loaded fast-dissolving microneedle patches for photodynamic therapy of subcutaneous tumor. J Control Release. 2018;286:201–209.

[21] Kolli CS, Banga AK. Characterization of solid maltose microneedles and their use for transdermal delivery. Pharm Res. 2008;25:104–113.

[22] Jeong H-R, Kim J-Y, Kim S-N, et al. Local dermal delivery of cyclosporin A, a hydrophobic and high molecular weight drug, using dissolving microneedles. Eur J Pharm Biopharm. 2018;127:237–243.

[23] Gill HS, Denson DD, Burris BA, et al. Effect of microneedle design on pain in human volunteers. Clin J Pain. 2008;24:585–594.

[24] Lutton REM, Moore J, Larrañeta E, et al. Microneedle characterisation: the need for universal acceptance criteria and GMP specifications when moving towards commercialisation. Drug Deliv Transl Res. 2015;5:313–331.

[25] Quinn HL, Kearney M-C, Courtenay AJ, et al. The role of microneedles for drug and vaccine delivery. Expert Opin Drug Deliv. 2014;11:1769–1780.

[26] Coulman SA, Birchall JC, Alex A, et al. In vivo, in situ imaging of microneedle insertion into the skin of human volunteers using optical coherence tomography. Pharm Res. 2011;28:66–81.

[27] Coffey JW, Meliga SC, Corrie SR, et al. Dynamic application of microprojection arrays to skin induces circulating protein extravasation for enhanced biomarker capture and detection. Biomaterials. 2016;84:130–143.

[28] Kochhar JS, Anbalagan P, Shelar SB, et al. Direct microneedle array fabrication off a photomask to deliver collagen through skin. Pharm Res. 2014;31:1724–1734.

[29] Liu S, Jin M, Quan Y, et al. The development and characteristics of novel microneedle arrays fabricated from hyaluronic acid, and their application in the transdermal delivery of insulin. J Control Release. 2012;161:933–941.

[30] Donnelly RF, McCrudden MT, Alkilani AZ, et al. Hydrogel-forming microneedles prepared from "super swelling" polymers combined with lyophilised wafers for transdermal drug delivery. PLoS one. 2014;9:e111547.

[31] Donnelly RF, Morrow DIJ, Singh TRR, et al. Processing difficulties and instability of carbohydrate microneedle arrays. Drug Dev Ind Pharm. 2009;35:1242–1254.

[32] Lee JW, Park J-H, Prausnitz MR. Dissolving microneedles for transdermal drug delivery. Biomaterials. 2008;29:2113–2124.

[33] Mönkäre J, Reza Nejadnik M, Baccouche K, et al. IgG-loaded hyaluronan-based dissolving microneedles for intradermal protein delivery. J Control Release. 2015;218:53–62.

[34] Bal SM, Caussin J, Pavel S, et al. In vivo assessment of safety of microneedle arrays in human skin. Eur J Pharm Sci. 2008;35:193–202.

[35] Kalluri H, Banga AK. Formation and closure of microchannels in skin following microporation. Pharm Res. 2011;28:82–94.

[36] Liu S, Jin M, Quan Y, et al. Transdermal delivery of relatively high molecular weight drugs using novel self-dissolving microneedle arrays fabricated from hyaluronic acid and their characteristics and safety after application to the skin. Eur J Pharm Biopharm. 2014;86:267–276.

[37] Nguyen HX, Banga AK. Enhanced skin delivery of vismodegib by microneedle treatment. Drug Deliv Transl Res. 2015;5:407–423.

[38] Gomaa YA, El-Khordagui LK, Garland MJ, et al. Effect of microneedle treatment on the skin permeation of a nanoencapsulated dye. J Pharm Pharmacol. 2012;64:1592–1602.

[39] McCrudden MTC, Alkilani AZ, Courtenay AJ, et al. Considerations in the sterile manufacture of polymeric microneedle arrays. Drug Deliv Transl Res. 2015;5:3–14.

[40] Kim Y-C, Quan F-S, Compans RW, et al. Stability kinetics of influenza vaccine coated onto microneedles during drying and storage. Pharm Res. 2011;28:135–144.

[41] Lee J, Park SH, Seo IH, et al. Rapid and repeatable fabrication of high A/R silk fibroin microneedles using thermally-drawn micromolds. Eur J Pharm Biopharm. 2015;94:11–19.

[42] McGrath MG, Vucen S, Vrdoljak A, et al. Production of dissolvable microneedles using an atomised spray process: effect of microneedle composition on skin penetration. Eur J Pharm Biopharm. 2014;86:200–211.

[43] Milewski M, Brogden NK, Stinchcomb AL. Current aspects of formulation efforts and pore lifetime related to microneedle treatment of skin. Expert Opin Drug Deliv. 2010;7:617–629.

[44] Yan L, Raphael AP, Zhu X, et al. Nanocomposite-strengthened dissolving microneedles for improved transdermal delivery to human skin. Adv Healthc Mater. 2014;3:555–564.

[45] Bediz B, Korkmaz E, Khilwani R, et al. Dissolvable microneedle arrays for intradermal delivery of biologics: fabrication and application. Pharm Res. 2014;31:117–135.

[46] Demir YK, Akan Z, Kerimoglu O. Characterization of polymeric microneedle arrays for transdermal drug delivery. PLoS One. 2013;8:e77289.

[47] Lee HS, Ryu HR, Roh JY, et al. Bleomycin-coated microneedles for treatment of warts. Pharm Res. 2017;34:101–112.

[48] Raphael AP, Crichton ML, Falconer RJ, et al. Formulations for microprojection/microneedle vaccine delivery: structure, strength and release profiles. J Control Release. 2016;225:40–52.

[49] Davis SP, Landis BJ, Adams ZH, et al. Insertion of microneedles into skin: measurement and prediction of insertion force and needle fracture force. J Biomech. 2004;37:1155–1163.

[50] Aoyagi S, Izumi H, Fukuda M. Biodegradable polymer needle with various tip angles and consideration on insertion mechanism of mosquito's proboscis. Sensors and Actuators A: Physical. 2008;143:20–28.

[51] Arora A, Prausnitz MR, Mitragotri S. Micro-scale devices for transdermal drug delivery. Int J Pharm. 2008;364:227–236.

[52] Luttge R, Berenschot EJW, de Boer MJ, et al. Integrated lithographic molding for microneedle-based devices. J Microelectromech Syst. 2007;16:872–884.

[53] Bodhale DW, Nisar A, Afzulpurkar N. Structural and microfluidic analysis of hollow side-open polymeric microneedles for transdermal drug delivery applications. Microfluid Nanofluidics. 2010;8:373–392.

[54] Martanto W, Moore JS, Kashlan O, et al. Microinfusion using hollow microneedles. Pharm Res. 2006;23:104–113.

[55] Stoeber B, Liepmann D. Design, fabrication and testing of a MEMS syringe. Proceedings of Solid-State Sensor and Actuator Workshop. 2002. p. 2–7.

[56] Kim M, Yang H, Kim H, et al. Novel cosmetic patches for wrinkle improvement: retinyl retinoate- and ascorbic acid-loaded dissolving microneedles. Int J Cosmet Sci. 2014;36:207–212.

[57] Ma Y, Boese SE, Luo Z, et al. Drug coated microneedles for minimally-invasive treatment of oral carcinomas: development and in vitro evaluation. Biomed Microdevices. 2015;17:44.

[58] Zhen Y, Wang N, Gao Z, et al. Multifunctional liposomes constituting microneedles induced robust systemic and mucosal immunoresponses against the loaded antigens via oral mucosal vaccination. Vaccine. 2015;33:4330–4340.

[59] Vrdoljak A, Allen EA, Ferrara F, et al. Induction of broad immunity by thermostabilised vaccines incorporated in dissolvable microneedles using novel fabrication methods. J Control Release. 2016;225:192–204.

[60] Crichton ML, Archer-Jones C, Meliga S, et al. Characterising the material properties at the interface between skin and a skin vaccination microprojection device. Acta Biomater. 2016;36:186–194.

[61] Wermeling DP, Banks SL, Hudson DA, et al. Microneedles permit transdermal delivery of a skin-impermeant medication to humans. Proc Natl Acad Sci. 2008;105:2058–2063.

[62] Cai B, Xia W, Bredenberg S, et al. Bioceramic microneedles with flexible and self-swelling substrate. Eur J Pharm Biopharm. 2015;94:404–410.

[63] Modepalli N, Shivakumar HN, McCrudden MTC, et al. Transdermal delivery of iron using soluble microneedles: dermal kinetics and safety. J Pharm Sci. 2016;105:1196–1200.

[64] Zahn JD, Talbot NH, Liepmann D, et al. Microfabricated polysilicon microneedles for minimally invasive biomedical devices. Biomed Microdevices. 2000;2:295–303.

[65] Park J-H, Allen MG, Prausnitz MR. Biodegradable polymer microneedles: fabrication, mechanics and transdermal drug delivery. J Control Release. 2005;104:51–66.

[66] Khann P, Silv H, Bhansali S. Variation in microneedle geometry to increase shear strength. Procedia Eng. 2010;5:977–980.

[67] Gittard SD, Chen B, Xu H, et al. The effects of geometry on skin penetration and failure of polymer microneedles. J Adhes Sci Technol. 2013;27:227–243.

[68] Larrañeta E, Lutton REM, Brady AJ, et al. Microwave-assisted preparation of hydrogel-forming microneedle arrays for transdermal drug delivery applications. Macromol Mater Eng. 2015;300:586–595.

[69] O'Mahony C. Structural characterization and in-vivo reliability evaluation of silicon microneedles. Biomed Microdevices. 2014;16:333–343.

[70] Park J-H, Prausnitz MR. Analysis of mechanical failure of polymer microneedles by axial force. J Korean Phys Soc. 2010;56:1223.

[71] Römgens AM, Bader DL, Bouwstra JA, et al. Monitoring the penetration process of single microneedles with varying tip diameters. J Mech Behav Biomed Mater. 2014;40:397–405.

[72] Sabri AH, Kim Y, Marlow M, et al. Intradermal and transdermal drug delivery using microneedles–Fabrication, performance evaluation and application to lymphatic delivery. Adv Drug Deliv Rev. 2020;153:195–215.

[73] Donnelly RF, Singh TRR, Garland MJ, et al. Hydrogel-forming microneedle arrays for enhanced transdermal drug delivery. Adv Funct Mater. 2012;22:4879–4890.

[74] Sawutdeechaikul P, Kanokrungsee S, Sahaspot T, et al. Detachable dissolvable microneedles: intra-epidermal and intradermal diffusion, effect on skin surface, and application in hyper-pigmentation treatment. Sci Rep. 2021;11:24114.

[75] Chen M-C, Ling M-H, Lai K-Y, et al. Chitosan microneedle patches for sustained transdermal delivery of macromolecules. Biomacromolecules. 2012;13:4022–4031.

[76] Loizidou EZ, Williams NA, Barrow DA, et al. Structural characterisation and transdermal delivery studies on sugar microneedles: experimental and finite element modelling analyses. Eur J Pharm Biopharm. 2015;89:224–231.

[77] Choi S-O, Kim YC, Park J-H, et al. An electrically active microneedle array for electroporation. Biomed Microdevices. 2010;12:263–273.

[78] Kim M, Jung B, Park J-H. Hydrogel swelling as a trigger to release biodegradable polymer microneedles in skin. Biomaterials. 2012;33:668–678.

[79] Sullivan SP, Murthy N, Prausnitz MR. Minimally invasive protein delivery with rapidly dissolving polymer microneedles. Adv Mater. 2008;20:933–938.

[80] Park Y-H, Ha SK, Choi I, et al. Fabrication of degradable carboxymethyl cellulose (CMC) microneedle with laser writing and replica molding process for enhancement of transdermal drug delivery. Biotechnol Bioprocess Eng. 2016;21:110–118.

[81] Bachy V, Hervouet C, Becker PD, et al. Langerin negative dendritic cells promote potent CD8+ T-cell priming by skin delivery of live adenovirus vaccine microneedle arrays. Proc Natl Acad Sci. 2013;110:3041–3046.

[82] Park J-H, Allen MG, Prausnitz MR. Polymer microneedles for controlled-release drug delivery. Pharm Res. 2006;23:1008–1019.

[83] Khanna P, Luongo K, Strom JA, et al. Axial and shear fracture strength evaluation of silicon microneedles. Microsyst Technol. 2010;16:973–978.

[84] McCrudden MTC, Alkilani AZ, McCrudden CM, et al. Design and physicochemical characterisation of novel dissolving polymeric microneedle arrays for transdermal delivery of high dose, low molecular weight drugs. J Control Release. 2014;180:71–80.

[85] Park J-H, Yoon Y-K, Choi S-O, et al. Tapered conical polymer microneedles fabricated using an integrated lens technique for transdermal drug delivery. IEEE Trans Biomed Eng. 2007;54:903–913.

[86] Khanna P, Strom JA, Malone JI, et al. Microneedle-based automated therapy for diabetes mellitus. J Diabetes Sci Technol. 2008;2:1122–1129.

[87] Crichton ML, Chen X, Huang H, et al. Elastic modulus and viscoelastic properties of full thickness skin characterised at micro scales. Biomaterials. 2013;34:2087–2097.

[88] Kendall MA, Chong Y-F, Cock A. The mechanical properties of the skin epidermis in relation to targeted gene and drug delivery. Biomaterials. 2007;28:4968–4977.

[89] Wildnauer RH, Bothwell JW, Douglass AB. Stratum corneum biomechanical properties I. Influence of relative humidity on normal and extracted human stratum corneum. J Invest Dermatol. 1971;56:72–78.

[90] Larrañeta E, Stewart S, Fallows SJ, et al. A facile system to evaluate in vitro drug release from dissolving microneedle arrays. Int J Pharm. 2016;497:62–69.

[91] Prausnitz MR. Microneedles for transdermal drug delivery. Adv Drug Deliv Rev. 2004; 56:581–587.

[92] Matsuo K, Yokota Y, Zhai Y, et al. A low-invasive and effective transcutaneous immunization system using a novel dissolving microneedle array for soluble and particulate antigens. J Control Release. 2012;161:10–17.

[93] Matsuo K, Hirobe S, Yokota Y, et al. Corrigendum to "Transcutaneous immunization using a dissolving microneedle array protects against tetanus, diphtheria, malaria, and influenza" [J. Control. Release 160 (2012) 495–501]. J Control Release. 2014;184:18–19.

[94] Laurent PE, Bonnet S, Alchas P, et al. Evaluation of the clinical performance of a new intradermal vaccine administration technique and associated delivery system. Vaccine. 2007;25:8833–8842.

[95] Chen X, Prow TW, Crichton ML, et al. Dry-coated microprojection array patches for targeted delivery of immunotherapeutics to the skin. J Control Release. 2009;139:212–220.

[96] Thakur RRS, Tekko IA, Al-Shammari F, et al. Rapidly dissolving polymeric microneedles for minimally invasive intraocular drug delivery. Drug Deliv Transl Res. 2016;6:800–815.

[97] Zhu Z, Ye X, Ku Z, et al. Transcutaneous immunization via rapidly dissolvable microneedles protects against hand-foot-and-mouth disease caused by enterovirus 71. J Control Release. 2016;243:291–302.

[98] Garland MJ, Migalska K, Tuan-Mahmood T-M, et al. Influence of skin model on in vitro performance of drug-loaded soluble microneedle arrays. Int J Pharm. 2012;434:80–89.

[99] Donnelly RF, Singh TRR, Tunney MM, et al. Microneedle arrays allow lower microbial penetration than hypodermic needles in vitro. Pharm Res. 2009;26:2513–2522.

[100] Ueda CT, Shah VP, Derdzinski K, et al. Topical and transdermal drug products. Pharmacopeial Forum; 2009. p. 750–764. [Internet] [cited 2016 Sep 4]. Available from: www.triphasepharmaso lutions.com/Resources/USP%20Topical%20and%20Transdermal%20Products.pdf.

[101] Ross S, Scoutaris N, Lamprou D, et al. Inkjet printing of insulin microneedles for transdermal delivery. Drug Deliv Transl Res. 2015;5:451–461.

[102] Tsioris K, Raja WK, Pritchard EM, et al. Fabrication of silk microneedles for controlled-release drug delivery. Adv Funct Mater. 2012;22:330–335.

[103] Nguyen HX, Banga AK. Fabrication, characterization and application of sugar microneedles for transdermal drug delivery. Ther Deliv. 2017;8:249–264.

[104] Gerstel MS, Place VA. Drug delivery device. Google Patents; 1976. [Internet] [cited 2016 Aug 23]. Available from: www.google.com/patents/US3964482.

[105] Chu LY, Prausnitz MR. Separable arrowhead microneedles. J Control Release. 2011;149:242–249.

[106] Peng Q, Sun X, Gong T, et al. Injectable and biodegradable thermosensitive hydrogels loaded with PHBHHx nanoparticles for the sustained and controlled release of insulin. Acta Biomater. 2013;9:5063–5069.

[107] Miyano T, Tobinaga Y, Kanno T, et al. Sugar micro needles as transdermic drug delivery system. Biomed Microdevices. 2005;7:185–188.

[108] Chen J, Qiu Y, Zhang S, et al. Dissolving microneedle-based intradermal delivery of interferon-α-2b. Drug Dev Ind Pharm. 2016;42:890–896.

[109] Fukushima K, Ise A, Morita H, et al. Two-layered dissolving microneedles for percutaneous delivery of peptide/protein drugs in rats. Pharm Res. 2011;28:7–21.

[110] Ito Y, Yoshimitsu J-I, Shiroyama K, et al. Self-dissolving microneedles for the percutaneous absorption of EPO in mice. J Drug Target. 2006;14:255–261.

[111] Andrianov AK, Marin A, DeCollibus DP. Microneedles with intrinsic immunoadjuvant properties: microfabrication, protein stability, and modulated release. Pharm Res. 2011;28:58–65.

[112] Gupta J, Felner EI, Prausnitz MR. Minimally invasive insulin delivery in subjects with type 1 diabetes using hollow microneedles. Diabetes Technol Ther. 2009;11:329–337.

[113] Tuan-Mahmood T-M, McCrudden MT, Torrisi BM, et al. Microneedles for intradermal and transdermal drug delivery. Eur J Pharm Sci. 2013;50:623–637.

[114] Crichton ML, Ansaldo A, Chen X, et al. The effect of strain rate on the precision of penetration of short densely-packed microprojection array patches coated with vaccine. Biomaterials. 2010;31:4562–4572.

[115] Verbaan FJ, Bal SM, van den Berg DJ, et al. Improved piercing of microneedle arrays in dermatomed human skin by an impact insertion method. J Control Release. 2008;128:80–88.

[116] Yan G, Warner KS, Zhang J, et al. Evaluation needle length and density of microneedle arrays in the pretreatment of skin for transdermal drug delivery. Int J Pharm. 2010;391:7–12.

[117] Olatunji O, Das DB, Garland MJ, et al. Influence of array interspacing on the force required for successful microneedle skin penetration: theoretical and practical approaches. J Pharm Sci. 2013;102:1209–1221.

[118] Chen M-C, Huang S-F, Lai K-Y, et al. Fully embeddable chitosan microneedles as a sustained release depot for intradermal vaccination. Biomaterials. 2013;34:3077–3086.

[119] Chu LY, Choi S-O, Prausnitz MR. Fabrication of dissolving polymer microneedles for controlled drug encapsulation and delivery: bubble and pedestal microneedle designs. J Pharm Sci. 2010;99:4228–4238.

[120] Kochhar JS, Quek TC, Soon WJ, et al. Effect of microneedle geometry and supporting substrate on microneedle array penetration into skin. J Pharm Sci. 2013;102:4100–4108.

[121] Larrañeta E, Moore J, Vicente-Pérez EM, et al. A proposed model membrane and test method for microneedle insertion studies. Int J Pharm. 2014;472:65–73.

[122] Sachdeva VK, Banga A. Microneedles and their applications. Recent Pat Drug Deliv Formul. 2011;5:95–132.

[123] Yang M, Zahn JD. Microneedle insertion force reduction using vibratory actuation. Biomedical Microdevices. 2004;6:177–182.

[124] Daugimont L, Baron N, Vandermeulen G, et al. Hollow microneedle arrays for intradermal drug delivery and DNA electroporation. J Membr Biol. 2010;236:117–125.

[125] Sun L, Wang H, Chen L, et al. A novel ultrasonic micro-dissection technique for biomedicine. Ultrasonics. 2006;44:e255–e260.

[126] Wang PM, Cornwell M, Hill J, et al. Precise microinjection into skin using hollow microneedles. J Invest Dermatol. 2006;126:1080–1087.

[127] Khan S, Minhas MU, Tekko IA, et al. Evaluation of microneedles-assisted in situ depot forming poloxamer gels for sustained transdermal drug delivery. Drug Deliv Transl Res. 2019;9:764–782.

[128] Ripolin A, Quinn J, Larrañeta E, et al. Successful application of large microneedle patches by human volunteers. Int J Pharm. 2017;521:92–101.

[129] Enfield J, O'Connell M-L, Lawlor K, et al. In-vivo dynamic characterization of microneedle skin penetration using optical coherence tomography. J Biomed Opt. 2010;15:046001.

[130] Bal SM, Kruithof AC, Zwier R, et al. Influence of microneedle shape on the transport of a fluorescent dye into human skin in vivo. J Control Release. 2010;147:218–224.

[131] van der Maaden K, Sekerdag E, Jiskoot W, et al. Impact-insertion applicator improves reliability of skin penetration by solid microneedle arrays. The AAPS Journal. 2014;16:681.

[132] Yang S, Feng Y, Zhang L, et al. A scalable fabrication process of polymer microneedles. Int J Nanomed. 2012;7:1415–1422.

[133] Ameri M, Peters EE, Wang X, et al. Erythropoietin (EPO) coated microprojection transdermal system: pre-clinical formulation, stability and delivery. AAPS J. 2009;11:T2245.

[134] Daddona PE, Matriano JA, Mandema J, et al. Parathyroid hormone (1–34)-coated microneedle patch system: clinical pharmacokinetics and pharmacodynamics for treatment of osteoporosis. Pharm Res. 2011;28:159–165.

[135] Gardeniers HJ, Luttge R, Berenschot EJ, et al. Silicon micromachined hollow microneedles for transdermal liquid transport. J Microelectromech Syst. 2003;12:855–862.

[136] Shirkhanzadeh M. Microneedles coated with porous calcium phosphate ceramics: effective vehicles for transdermal delivery of solid trehalose. J Mater Sci Mater Med. 2005;16:37–45.

[137] Kalluri H, Banga AK. Transdermal delivery of proteins. AAPS PharmSciTech. 2011;12:431–441.

[138] Ameri M, Wang X, Maa Y-F. Effect of irradiation on parathyroid hormone PTH(1–34) coated on a novel transdermal microprojection delivery system to produce a sterile product-adhesive compatibility. J Pharm Sci. 2010;99:2123–2134.

[139] Kaushik S, Hord AH, Denson DD, et al. Lack of pain associated with microfabricated microneedles. Anesthesia & Analgesia. 2001;92:502–504.

[140] Daddona P. Macroflux® transdermal technology development for the delivery of therapeutic peptides and proteins. Drug Deliv Tech. 2002;2.

[141] Sathyan G, Sun YN, Weyers R, et al. Macroflux® desmopressin transdermal delivery system: pharmacokinetics and pharmacodynamic evaluation in healthy volunteers. AAPS J. 2004;6:665.

[142] Sathyan G, Weyers R, Daddona P, et al. Apparatus and method for transdermal delivery of desmopressin. 2006. [Internet] [cited 2022 Nov 8]. Available from: https://patents.google.com/patent/US20060093658A1/en.

[143] Burton SA, Ng C-Y, Simmers R, et al. Rapid intradermal delivery of liquid formulations using a hollow microstructured array. Pharm Res. 2011;28:31–40.

[144] Kusamori K, Katsumi H, Abe M, et al. Development of a novel transdermal patch of alendronate, a nitrogen-containing bisphosphonate, for the treatment of osteoporosis. J Bone Miner Res. 2010;25:2582–2591.

[145] Kusamori K, Katsumi H, Sakai R, et al. Development of a drug-coated microneedle array and its application for transdermal delivery of interferon alpha. Biofabrication. 2016;8:015006.

[146] Singh TRR, McCarron PA, Woolfson AD, et al. Investigation of swelling and network parameters of poly (ethylene glycol)-crosslinked poly (methyl vinyl ether-co-maleic acid) hydrogels. Eur Polym J. 2009;45:1239–1249.

[147] Lee JW, Choi S-O, Felner EI, et al. Dissolving microneedle patch for transdermal delivery of human growth hormone. Small. 2011;7:531–539.

[148] Sun W, Araci Z, Inayathullah M, et al. Polyvinylpyrrolidone microneedles enable delivery of intact proteins for diagnostic and therapeutic applications. Acta Biomater. 2013;9:7767–7774.

[149] Hirobe S, Okada N, Nakagawa S. Transcutaneous vaccines-current and emerging strategies. Expert Opin Drug Deliv. 2013;10:485–498.

[150] Zipursky S, Djingarey MH, Lodjo J-C, et al. Benefits of using vaccines out of the cold chain: delivering meningitis a vaccine in a controlled temperature chain during the mass immunization campaign in Benin. Vaccine. 2014;32:1431–1435.

[151] Gill HS, Prausnitz MR. Coated microneedles for transdermal delivery. J Control Release. 2007;117:227–237.

[152] Guo L, Chen J, Qiu Y, et al. Enhanced transcutaneous immunization via dissolving microneedle array loaded with liposome encapsulated antigen and adjuvant. Int J Pharm. 2013;447:22–30.

[153] Arya JM, Dewitt K, Scott-Garrard M, et al. Rabies vaccination in dogs using a dissolving microneedle patch. J Control Release. [Internet]. [cited 2016 Aug 13]; Available from: www.sciencedirect.com/science/article/pii/S0168365916305144.

[154] Edens C, Collins ML, Goodson JL, et al. A microneedle patch containing measles vaccine is immunogenic in non-human primates. Vaccine. 2015;33:4712–4718.

[155] Sullivan SP, Koutsonanos DG, Del Pilar Martin M, et al. Dissolving polymer microneedle patches for influenza vaccination. Nat Med. 2010;16:915–920.

[156] Kommareddy S, Baudner BC, Oh S, et al. Dissolvable microneedle patches for the delivery of cell-culture-derived influenza vaccine antigens. J Pharm Sci. 2012;101:1021–1027.

[157] Kim Y-C, Quan F-S, Compans RW, et al. Formulation of microneedles coated with influenza virus-like particle vaccine. AAPS PharmSciTech. 2010;11:1193–1201.

[158] Hiraishi Y, Nandakumar S, Choi S-O, et al. Bacillus Calmette-Guérin vaccination using a microneedle patch. Vaccine. 2011;29:2626–2636.

[159] Ekdawi-Sever N, de Pablo JJ, Feick E, et al. Diffusion of sucrose and α, α-trehalose in aqueous solutions. J Phys Chem A. 2003;107:936–943.

[160] Lerbret A, Bordat P, Affouard F, et al. How homogeneous are the trehalose, maltose, and sucrose water solutions? An insight from molecular dynamics simulations. J Phys Chem B. 2005;109:11046–11057.

[161] Mistilis MJ, Bommarius AS, Prausnitz MR. Development of a thermostable microneedle patch for influenza vaccination. J Pharm Sci. 2015;104:740–749.

[162] Zaric M, Lyubomska O, Touzelet O, et al. Skin dendritic cell targeting via microneedle arrays laden with antigen-encapsulated poly-D,L-lactide-co-glycolide nanoparticles induces efficient antitumor and antiviral immune responses. ACS Nano. 2013;7:2042–2055.

[163] Ito Y, Hagiwara E, Saeki A, et al. Feasibility of microneedles for percutaneous absorption of insulin. Eur J Pharm Sci. 2006;29:82–88.

[164] Ito Y, Murakami A, Maeda T, et al. Evaluation of self-dissolving needles containing low molecular weight heparin (LMWH) in rats. Int J Pharm. 2008;349:124–129.

[165] Chen X, Fernando GJ, Crichton ML, et al. Improving the reach of vaccines to low-resource regions, with a needle-free vaccine delivery device and long-term thermostabilization. J Control Release. 2011;152:349–355.

4

Characterization of Microchannels

4.1 Introduction

Scanning electron microscope (SEM), cryogenic SEM, and other microscopes could be employed to evaluate the microchannels' geometry, dimensions, and morphology. Skin electrical resistance measurements provide insight into the penetrating force, the effectiveness of skin penetration, and the channel closing features. In multiple studies, the skin resistance value is inversely related to drug permeability and is closely associated with needle dimensions. Besides, transepidermal water loss (TEWL) is a reliable measure of the skin's barrier function and capability to close pores and recover the structure. The TEWL assessment may be performed using vaporimeters or evaporimeters. Furthermore, histological sectioning and dye binding studies may be used to demonstrate the successful creation of microchannels or the disruption of skin integrity. The former could be used to quantify the amount of fluid delivered through hollow microneedles. A confocal laser scanning microscope has been commonly used to measure the penetration depth of microchannels. This method requires neither physical sectioning nor alteration to the microchannels. It is critical to assess the uniformity of the created channels to achieve effective and consistent drug transport. This study is performed primarily using calcein imaging and the calculation of pore permeability index values. Pore sealing has a marked effect on the rate of drug transport and could be measured using skin resistance and TEWL measurements, as well as optical coherence tomography (OCT) and calcein imaging. Microneedling technology is a viable platform for skin delivery of various drugs, vaccines, macromolecules, bioactive, and particulate systems. While the merits of microneedles have been shown beyond any reasonable doubt, some challenges, including sterilization and stability, must be resolved before microneedle products may complete clinical trials and achieve commercialization. Further studies will likely concentrate on constructing, refining, and standardizing various characterization methodologies for evaluating microneedles and microchannels formed in the skin (Table 4.1).

4.2 Characterization of Microchannels

4.2.1 Morphology

SEM has been commonly used to examine the dimensions and morphology of microchannels created in the skin and investigate modifications in microneedle surface structure

DOI: 10.1201/9780429294433-4

TABLE 4.1

Summary of Characterization Studies for Microchannels

Product Attributes	Testing Methods	References
Microchannel morphology, geometry, and dimensions (diameter, surface area)	Optical microscopy, scanning electron microscopy, and cryogenic scanning electron microscopy	[1–4]
Skin integrity and barrier function	Skin resistance/impedance measurement TEWL measurement (vapometers such as Dermalab TEWL probe, Tewameter® TM 210 probe, Tewameter® TM 300, or Cyberderm evaporimeter) Optical coherence tomography imaging of skin compression	[5–7, 8, 9, 10, 11, 12]
Changes in the histology of the skin layers to confirm the creation and measure the depth of the microchannel	Histological sectioning, staining, and imaging	[13, 14–16]
Number of channels, pore density, microneedle insertion ratio, pore-to-pore distance	Dye binding studies to visualize the stained microchannels	[17, 18]
Depth and surface area of microchannels	Confocal laser scanning microscopy	[17, 19, 20]
Pore uniformity	Calcein staining, imaging, and analysis to determine Pore Uniformity Index values	[21, 22, 17]
Pore closure kinetics	Transepidermal water loss, optical coherence tomography, calcein imaging	[11, 19, 23, 24]

post-skin insertion [1–4]. Skin samples are frozen, dissected, and coated before being observed under SEM [25–27]. Furthermore, cryoSEM offers a high-quality analysis of skin deformation due to microneedle penetration [2]. Sliced skin tissue with an affixed nano-patch microneedle array was inspected under cryoSEM, revealing that the needles penetrated the skin to the depth of approximately two-thirds of the needle length [26].

Similarly, field emission SEM is employed with a measuring instrument to observe microchannels in the skin [1, 21]. Microneedles-porated skin is treated with glutaraldehyde solution, cleaned, and dried in a vacuum oven. After mounting the dried skin tissue on an SEM metallic sample holder, the skin is covered with a thin gold or palladium layer and observed under the microscope. A primary beam voltage is used to acquire photographs of secondary ions. Numerous researchers have also taken images of microneedles-porated skin areas using a digital or video microscope [21–29]. Microchannels are anticipated to have a similar shape and geometry as microneedles. Specifically, pyramidal maltose microneedles were found to generate corresponding V-shaped microchannels [30, 31].

4.2.2 Skin Resistance Measurement

While the microneedles penetrate the skin, the skin tissue generates certain resistive stresses. Thus, the pressure required to drive the microneedles must be greater than the physical resistance of the skin in order to puncture the skin successfully. As the skin is porated, the applied force reduces dramatically [32]. Besides, the measurement of skin electrical resistance is helpful in evaluating the skin's capability to reseal microchannels [5–7] and the penetration force of skin tissue [5, 33, 34]. This method utilizes the electrical insulating properties of the stratum corneum layer [13]. A basic configuration for measuring skin resistance comprises putting an electrode on skin sites and completing the electrical circuit with a counter electrode positioned at the other side of the skin [5–7]. It has been revealed that the skin's moisture content has a noticeable impact on the sensitivity and reliability of this method [5]. The technique has also been associated with intersubject variability in skin electrical resistance levels [7]. Silver and silver chloride electrodes in tandem with a digital multimeter are suited for this measurement [8]. To determine the impedance of the skin, electrodes are attached to an impedance meter that generates an alternating current at a 30 Hz frequency [3]. An investigation revealed that a physical treatment with Derma stamp microneedles significantly reduced skin resistance [8]. Skin resistance values have been evaluated with regard to skin occlusion and microneedles geometry and dimensions [3, 35]. To meet these objectives, microneedles of varying lengths, densities, thickness, and width, as well as study conditions (occlusive and nonocclusive), were investigated and compared to positive (conventional hypodermic needle) and negative (no treatment) controls. The findings indicated that both microneedles and hypodermic needle insertions resulted in considerably lower impedance than the untreated control. However, no statistically significant variation was detected between treatments using microneedles of various shapes [3]. Furthermore, OCT imaging of skin compression during needle treatment was employed to characterize skin resistance [9]. Skin electrical resistance has been shown to be inversely related to drug permeation in multiple experiments [36, 37], while the resistance is directly related to stratum corneum thickness [38] and microneedle length [9].

The pressure reduction necessary to inject transdermal products into the skin using hollow microneedles depends on the needle geometry, the viscosity of the injected fluid, and the density of the fluid [39]. It is essential to effectively estimate fluid flow in hollow microneedles to prevent complications such as fluid leakage during the injection. Khumpuang and colleagues [40] estimate that a 10 kPa inlet pressure is adequate to enable microneedles to transfer fluids into the skin. This pressure is an expected level based on commercially available micropumping devices. Lhernould and Delchambre [41] reveal that the flow rate of the fluid is mainly dictated by the applied pressure and the dimension of the hole opening. Since the skin is not flat or uniform, each needle has a variable hydrodynamic resistance, resulting in nonuniform injections through hollow microneedles. Martanto et al. [42] report that partial retraction, higher insertion depth, increased applied pressure, employment of a beveled needle tip, and the inclusion of hyaluronidase enhanced flow rate by circumventing resistance induced by needle compression. The injection flow rate will also improve if the infusion pressure is elevated. The flow rate is faster with a beveled tip than with a blunt tip. Dense dermal tissues may be the most significant constraint for microneedle applications. Flow resistance is reduced significantly when fluid flows parallel to the dermal fibers. However, injecting fluid via hollow microneedles requires that the needles be applied perpendicular to the skin. Compression and compaction of the dense coiled fiber occur as a result of the perpendicular insertion, leading to a rise in pressure and flow resistance. It is challenging to quantify the backpressure imposed by compressed dense tissues during microneedle insertion and product injection. Moreover, the backpressure depends on the injection location, the patient's age, and ethnicity.

4.2.3 Transepidermal Water Loss Measurement

Microchannel creation [1, 22, 43] and resealing kinetics [11, 44] may be evaluated by monitoring TEWL, a skin integrity indicator [7, 17]. TEWL has been measured using various vaporimeters, including the Dermalab TEWL probe, the Tewameter® TM 210 probe [10–12], the Tewameter® TM 300 probe, or the Cyberderm evaporimeter. These instruments are equipped with sensors that monitor the relative humidity and output a measurement that corresponds to TEWL (g/m^2h) [23]. The TEWL value may be measured both *in vitro* using permeation cells and *in vivo* on animal or human skin [11]. TEWL values are obtained pre– and post–microneedle insertion. Prior to microneedle treatment, the probe is placed and kept on the intact skin until a reliable reading is recorded. This is a baseline value that implies intact skin integrity. The TEWL values are then measured instantaneously after the microneedle insertion and removal. Numerous studies have reported increased transepidermal water loss upon microneedle penetration [36, 44, 45]. Several experiments have shown that altering the length of the microneedles has a marked effect on the TEWL values [36, 44, 46]. Moreover, tracking TEWL values at various intervals during a 24-h period following microneedle insertion reveals the time required for the skin to restore its typical barrier function [47, 48]. One research on hairless rat skin porated with maltose microneedles demonstrated a more than 150% rise in TEWL values after microneedle insertion and a considerable drop within the first 5 min after microneedle removal. The TEWL readings rapidly decreased to baseline levels after 4 h, demonstrating that the skin recovered its barrier function. The impact of occlusion on pore sealing was also monitored by determining TEWL 24 and 72 h after the occlusion. For the occluded samples, TEWL values remained as high after 24 h as they were instantly after microporation, suggesting that occlusion retarded the closing of pores [23]. Moreover, a significant relationship between pore count and TEWL has been demonstrated [45, 49]. The impact of the number of micropores on TEWL values was investigated using a 26G hypodermic needle and maltose microneedle array. As a positive control, the TEWL value was measured and recorded after tape stripping as the complete disruption of the stratum corneum layer [49]. The findings of this research revealed that TEWL rose to a certain level but did not grow further when the number of pores created by a hypodermic needle or the microneedle array increased. The TEWL value obtained after tape stripping was observed to be substantially greater than that following other needle insertions. Variation in the experimental procedure may lead to differing TEWL values even with the same microneedle patch but different skin tissues. Also, TEWL levels could be influenced by environmental temperatures and the skin's moisture content [45, 50].

4.2.4 Histological Analysis

Microneedles' capacity to penetrate the skin has been thoroughly researched using histological sectioning [30, 37, 51, 52]. The microneedles-treated skin area is removed from the skin piece. The isolated skin section is placed in the optimal cutting medium and frozen with dry ice or liquid nitrogen [7, 17, 23]. In a cryostat, frozen skin tissue is subsequently sectioned into slices of varying thickness. Following that, hematoxylin and eosin (H&E) or methylene blue are used to stain the acquired skin slices [13, 14–16]. The slices are mounted on a glass microscope slide and covered with cytoseal 60. A microscope equipped with a digital camera is employed to observe the microscopic structure of skin tissue [53–55]. The ability of metal and maltose microneedles to penetrate hairless rat skin was demonstrated by the histology study in a research published by Li and coworkers [28]. Furthermore, histological evaluations have been performed to measure the penetration depth of microneedles [17, 51, 56]. Kalluri and Banga conducted histological sectioning experiments to verify the formation and depth of the maltose microneedles-created channels in hairless rat skin [23]. Lahiji et al. conducted a histological examination of porcine skin porated by a Microlancer dissolving microneedle system to measure the skin insertion depth of microneedles (Fig. 4.1) [57]. Similarly, Nguyen and Banga executed a histology study to prove the successful formation of microchannels by PLGA microneedles on dermatomed pig ear skin *in vitro* [58]. Interestingly, Coffey et al. revealed dye diffusion and permeation into skin tissue using histology staining [2]. Besides, the histological evaluation may be utilized to determine the volume of sample delivered through hollow microneedles [59] and to evaluate the impact of microneedle composition on skin penetration and disruption [48]. Nevertheless, measuring pore dimensions using histological investigations may result in an overvaluation of pore depth and width due to the physical distortion of the channels [9, 60].

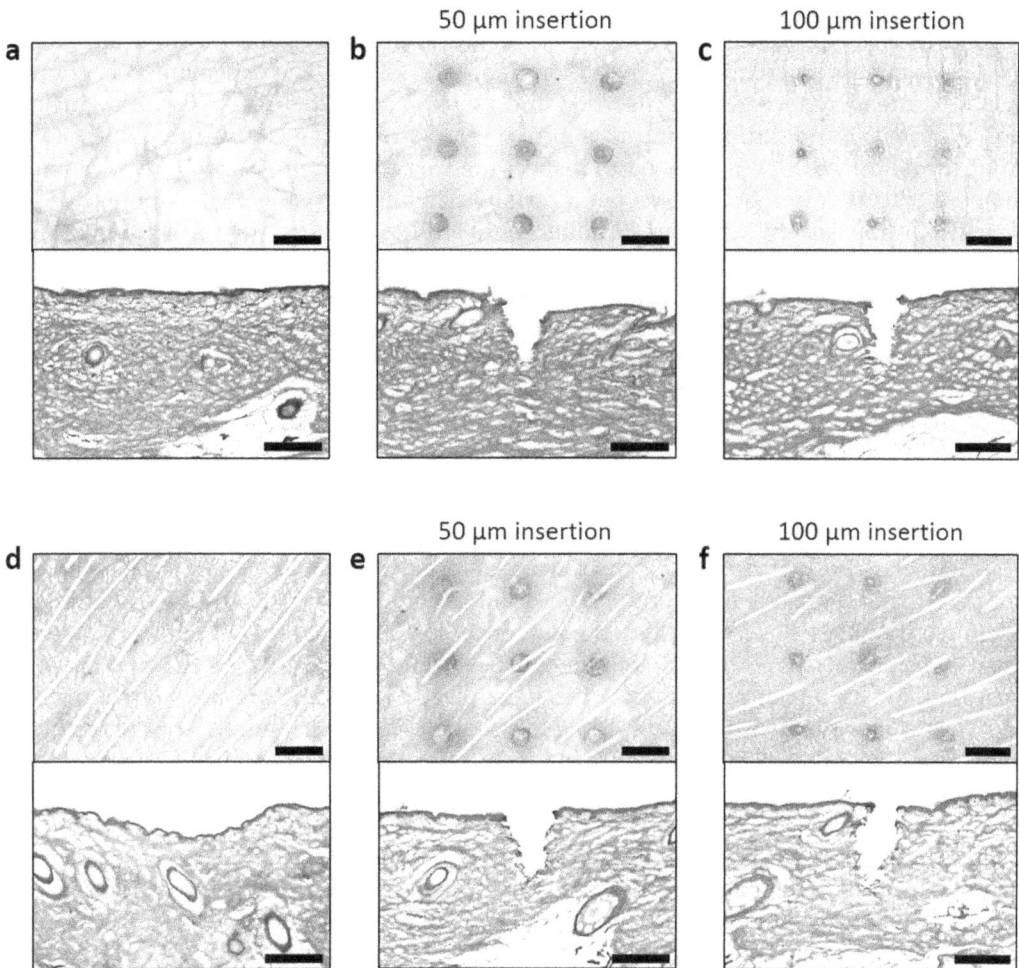

FIGURE 4.1
Histological and microscopic analyses of hairy and hairless porcine cadaver skin. (a) Hairless porcine skin prior to microneedle application. (b) 50 μm insertion of 600-μm-long microneedles penetrated to 650 μm depth in skin tissue. (c) 100 μm insertion of microneedles penetrated to 700 μm depth in skin tissue. (d) Hairy porcine skin prior to microneedle application. (e) Inserting microneedles at a depth of 50 μm into hairy skin exhibited a similar visual appearance as inserting them into hairless skin. (f) 100 μm insertion of microneedles penetrated to 700 μm depth in hairy porcine skin. Images reprinted with permission from [57].

4.2.5 Dye Binding Studies

A commonly used characterization method is dye binding, which may be used to determine the effectiveness of skin penetration or the creation of microchannels by microneedles [61–63]. Moreover, this method has been employed to investigate the uniformity of the channels [64], to examine the influence of microneedle insertion force on microchannels [65], and to analyze drug release patterns [7, 66]. This method employs hydrophilic dyes that rapidly diffuse into the aqueous, skin interstitial fluid-filled microchannels produced by microneedle insertion, allowing for precise visualization of the dyed pores. Thus, this visualization allows reliable channel counting and calculation of microneedle insertion ratio [17, 67, 18]. The insertion ratio is determined as the ratio of observable spots (successful creation of channels by microneedle treatment) to the total number of needles on the array [10, 62], and this provides information about the hardness and physical properties of microneedles [68]. Histological analysis after dye-binding staining allows the assessment of microneedle penetration depth [17, 23, 69]. The dye solution is applied instantly after the microneedle insertion and removal from the skin. After allowing the dye to permeate the skin for around 5 min, the remaining dye is carefully wiped away. After that, a microscope is utilized to inspect the treated skin area [17, 18]. In addition to the pore density (number of pores per a certain skin area) [23], the pore-to-pore distance may also be measured [70]. Interestingly, several studies describe the penetration of dye-incorporated microneedles into the skin rather than applying dye after skin microporation [18, 23, 67]. Furthermore, Kalluri and Banga estimated a penetration depth of 160 ± 20 μm for the microchannels generated by 560-μm-long maltose microneedles using methylene blue staining and histological sectioning analysis [23]. The method of dye staining to determine skin perforation and pore dimension may not be reliable since hydrophilic dyes may diffuse into the vicinity of the channels, resulting in false results [7, 60, 71].

4.2.6 Microchannel Depth

The diameters or surface area of microneedles-formed channels in the skin have been accurately measured using confocal laser scanning microscopy [19, 17, 20]. After inserting and removing the microneedles, the microneedle-treated site is stained with a fluorescent dye solution (Fluoresoft® [31]) or microparticles (Fluospheres® [17, 19]). Then, a confocal microscope is used to observe the skin piece at a preset wavelength. Confocal laser microscopy provides a noninvasive and reliable technique for measuring the depth of channels in the skin [19] and the surface dimensions of the channels [17] by capturing a collection of microphotographs of fluorescence at varying depths. This precise and efficient method collects images *ex vivo*, *in vivo*, and *in vitro* without the need for fixation, staining, or sectioning, which might affect the channel geometry [31]. This method provides several advantageous qualities, particularly when microneedles (metal, glass, silicon, or other solid microneedles) are removed before the application of the formulation. Unfortunately, the confocal laser can only reach a particular depth in the skin (200–250 μm below the skin's surface at the maximum). This aspect complicates the investigation of the penetration depth of deeper pores created by lengthier microneedles [9, 72]. A strong correlation between microneedles height and penetration depth was presented by Donnelly et al. [9]. Likewise, the actual depth of microchannels might be strongly impacted by the microscope's detection limit [49, 73]. A notable disadvantage of this method is the underestimation of pore dimensions caused by microneedles removal and the skin's intrinsic viscoelastic properties [7, 60].

4.2.7 Pore Uniformity

The uniformity of microneedles-created microchannels is critical for optimizing and controlling transdermal drug delivery [19]. This is determined by analyzing the pore permeability index (PPI) values using the calcein imaging technique [19, 17, 74]. This evaluation may be conducted in the lab (*in vitro*) [17] or in animal models (*in vivo*) [74].

In most cases, a fluorescent calcein dye is employed for the experiment. Following the penetration and removal of microneedles from the skin, the treated site is covered with calcein dye solution for around 1 min. After removing the excess dye, two-dimensional fluorescent photographs of the stained area are recorded using a digital camera. The image analysis software (fluoropore) is then employed to evaluate the relative skin permeability [21, 17, 23]. Each photograph is calibrated with standards based on its quality. The microchannels are then chosen separately, and the software converts the pixel density (which represents the calcein intensity inside and around the pores) to a number known as the pore permeability index (PPI) [21, 22, 17], which indicates the relative calcein flux through each channel. PPI values enable precise and ratiometric assessments of the flux flowing through individual pores [21, 17]. If the range of PPI values for microchannels formed by microneedle insertion is narrowly distributed, this indicates the creation of uniform channels [21].

4.2.8 Micropore Closure Kinetics

The rate at which drugs are delivered through the skin is strongly influenced by the rate at which the skin heals after microneedle-induced disruption [6, 75, 76]. To attain extended transdermal drug transport through microneedles-treated skin, it is vital to identify the period that the formed pores stay open before being resealed by the skin's natural healing processes. Disruption of the stratum corneum triggers lamellar body secretions and lipid production, which contribute to the restoration of its barrier function [6, 23]. Pore closure kinetics may be determined using various techniques, including skin impedance measurement, TEWL, OCT, and microscopic imaging [11, 19, 24, 31].

Impedance spectroscopy is a recently developed technology that has been used to investigate the closure kinetics of microchannels in animal models and human subjects [48, 77]. This is derived from the finding that microporation leads to a decrease in the skin's electrical impedance [3, 8], which rises as the skin recovers and the pores seal. It entails the use of an impedance setup that includes an impedance meter, resistor, and electrodes. Impedance evaluation was used to investigate the impact of microneedle dimensions and occlusive condition, pH, and the presence of cations (i.e., calcium and magnesium) on pore closure kinetics after microneedle treatment [6, 77]. Occlusion has been shown to retard pore resealing [77]. Calcein imaging is often employed to directly evaluate pore closure in microneedle-porated skin. The treated skin is stained with calcein, and photographs are taken at various time points to determine the closure rate [19, 23]. Banga et al. studied the impacts of microneedle length and occlusion on the pore resealing kinetic in hairless rats *in vivo* and revealed an inverse relationship between these factors. Furthermore, it was reported that occlusion rendered by a vapor-impermeable plastic sheet or a solution postponed pore closure to 72 h [19, 23]. Moreover, the impact of occlusion, microneedle dimensions, and pH on pore sealing has been investigated using TEWL and various imaging methods [23, 59, 78].

4.3 Future Perspectives

With the speedy development of transdermal delivery products for current pharmaceuticals, the global transdermal product market will likely continue growing consistently. The subject of transdermal delivery is no longer restricted to low-molecular-weight and moderate lipophilic compounds but has substantially extended to include therapeutic agents with large sizes and high molecular weight. Meanwhile, the vaccination industry has grown tremendously. A sizable number of publications in the area attest to the expansion in the transdermal and vaccine markets. Because of this increased interest and demand, microneedles are the most favorable technological platform for drug administration and vaccination. Among the numerous varieties of microneedles, dissolving microneedles provide a wealth of advantages, including the avoidance of sharp waste, the stability of the drug inside the polymeric structure, and the diminution of drug waste. While the merits of microneedles-based systems have been shown beyond any reasonable doubt, some difficulties must be resolved before microneedle systems may complete clinical trials and reach the stage of commercialization. The future study will emphasize building, improving, and standardizing various characterization methods for evaluating microneedles and microneedles-created microchannels in the skin. Special consideration would need to be devoted to the mechanical performance, drug loading, sterilization, and physical and biological safety of the needles.

4.4 Conclusion

Microneedle technology is a compelling platform for enhancing and controlling therapeutic drug delivery through transdermal and intradermal pathways. In many research studies, microneedle treatment is safe and effective in enhancing drug delivery. Multiple pharmaceutical manufacturers are developing and improving large-scale manufacturing processes for microneedles. Characterization tests, optimization, and validation are required to ensure the quality and performance of microneedles products. Several strategies for evaluating microneedle-formed microchannels in the skin are presented in this chapter. These offer scientists a range of tools for screening microneedle formulations and attributes to ensure their suitability and performance for transdermal drug delivery.

References

[1] Badran MM, Kuntsche J, Fahr A. Skin penetration enhancement by a microneedle device (Dermaroller®) in vitro: dependency on needle size and applied formulation. Eur J Pharm Sci. 2009;36:511–523.

[2] Coffey JW, Meliga SC, Corrie SR, et al. Dynamic application of microprojection arrays to skin induces circulating protein extravasation for enhanced biomarker capture and detection. Biomaterials. 2016;84:130–143.

[3] Coulman SA, Anstey A, Gateley C, et al. Microneedle mediated delivery of nanoparticles into human skin. Int J Pharm. 2009;366:190–200.

[4] Park J-H, Choi S-O, Seo S, et al. A microneedle roller for transdermal drug delivery. Eur J Pharm Biopharm. 2010;76:282–289.

[5] Brogden NK, Milewski M, Ghosh P, et al. Diclofenac delays micropore closure following microneedle treatment in human subjects. J Control Release. 2012;163:220–229.

[6] Gupta J, Gill HS, Andrews SN, et al. Kinetics of skin resealing after insertion of microneedles in human subjects. J Control Release. 2011;154:148–155.

[7] Lutton REM, Moore J, Larrañeta E, et al. Microneedle characterisation: the need for universal acceptance criteria and GMP specifications when moving towards commercialisation. Drug Deliv Transl Res. 2015;5:313–331.

[8] Ma Y, Boese SE, Luo Z, et al. Drug coated microneedles for minimally-invasive treatment of oral carcinomas: development and in vitro evaluation. Biomed Microdevices. 2015;17:44.

[9] Donnelly RF, Garland MJ, Morrow DI, et al. Optical coherence tomography is a valuable tool in the study of the effects of microneedle geometry on skin penetration characteristics and in-skin dissolution. J Control Release. 2010;147:333–341.

[10] Chen M-C, Ling M-H, Kusuma SJ. Poly-γ-glutamic acid microneedles with a supporting structure design as a potential tool for transdermal delivery of insulin. Acta Biomater. 2015;24:106–116.

[11] Haq MI, Smith E, John DN, et al. Clinical administration of microneedles: skin puncture, pain and sensation. Biomed Microdevices. 2009;11:35–47.

[12] Milewski M, Yerramreddy TR, Ghosh P, et al. In vitro permeation of a pegylated naltrexone prodrug across microneedle-treated skin. J Control Release. 2010;146:37–44.

[13] Roxhed N, Gasser TC, Griss P, et al. Penetration-enhanced ultrasharp microneedles and prediction on skin interaction for efficient transdermal drug delivery. J Microelectromech Syst. 2007;16:1429–1440.

[14] Choi S-O, Kim YC, Park J-H, et al. An electrically active microneedle array for electroporation. Biomed Microdevices. 2010;12:263–273.

[15] Chu LY, Prausnitz MR. Separable arrowhead microneedles. J Control Release. 2011;149:242–249

[16] Loeters PWH, Duwel RF, Verbaan FJ, et al. Measuring the insertion of microfabricated microneedles into skin with a penetration sensor. 8th International Conference on Micro Total Analysis Systems, µTAS 2004. 2004;296:497–499.

[17] Li G, Badkar A, Kalluri H, et al. Microchannels created by sugar and metal microneedles: characterization by microscopy, macromolecular flux and other techniques. J Pharm Sci. 2010;99:1931–1941.

[18] Zhu Z, Luo H, Lu W, et al. Rapidly dissolvable microneedle patches for transdermal delivery of exenatide. Pharm Res. 2014;31:3348–3360.

[19] Kalluri H, Kolli CS, Banga AK. Characterization of microchannels created by metal microneedles: formation and closure. AAPS J. 2011;13:473–481.

[20] Alvarez-Román R, Naik A, Kalia YN, et al. Visualization of skin penetration using confocal laser scanning microscopy. Eur J Pharm Biopharm. 2004;58:301–316.

[21] Kolli CS, Banga AK. Characterization of solid maltose microneedles and their use for transdermal delivery. Pharm Res. 2008;25:104–113.

[22] Singh N, Kalluri H, Herwadkar A, et al. Transcending the skin barrier to deliver peptides and proteins using active technologies. Crit Rev Ther Drug Carrier Syst. 2012;29:265–298.

[23] Kalluri H, Banga AK. Formation and closure of microchannels in skin following microporation. Pharm Res. 2011;28:82–94.

[24] Matsuo K, Yokota Y, Zhai Y, et al. A low-invasive and effective transcutaneous immunization system using a novel dissolving microneedle array for soluble and particulate antigens. J Control Release. 2012;161:10–17.

[25] Chen X, Prow TW, Crichton ML, et al. Dry-coated microprojection array patches for targeted delivery of immunotherapeutics to the skin. J Control Release. 2009;139:212–220.

[26] Crichton ML, Archer-Jones C, Meliga S, et al. Characterising the material properties at the interface between skin and a skin vaccination microprojection device. Acta Biomater. 2016;36:186–194.

[27] Prow TW, Chen X, Prow NA, et al. Nanopatch-targeted skin vaccination against west nile virus and chikungunya virus in mice. Small. 2010;6:1776–1784.

[28] Li G, Badkar A, Nema S, et al. In vitro transdermal delivery of therapeutic antibodies using maltose microneedles. Int J Pharm. 2009;368:109–115.

[29] Matriano JA, Cormier M, Johnson J, et al. Macroflux® Microprojection array patch technology: a new and efficient approach for intracutaneous immunization. Pharm Res. 2002;19:63–70.

[30] Bai Y, Sachdeva V, Kim H, et al. Transdermal delivery of proteins using a combination of iontophoresis and microporation. Ther Deliv. 2014;5:525–536.

[31] Nguyen HX, Banga AK. Enhanced skin delivery of vismodegib by microneedle treatment. Drug Deliv Transl Res. 2015;5:407–423.

[32] Frick TB, Marucci DD, Cartmill JA, et al. Resistance forces acting on suture needles. J Biomech. 2001;34:1335–1340.

[33] Davis SP, Landis BJ, Adams ZH, et al. Insertion of microneedles into skin: measurement and prediction of insertion force and needle fracture force. J Biomech. 2004;37:1155–1163.

[34] Forvi E, Soncini M, Bedoni M, et al. A method to determine the margin of safety for microneedles arrays. Proceedings of the World Congress on Engineering; 2010. p. 1150–1154.

[35] Römgens AM, Bader DL, Bouwstra JA, et al. Monitoring the penetration process of single microneedles with varying tip diameters. J Mech Behav Biomed Mater. 2014;40:397–405.

[36] Yan G, Warner KS, Zhang J, et al. Evaluation needle length and density of microneedle arrays in the pretreatment of skin for transdermal drug delivery. Int J Pharm. 2010;391:7–12.

[37] Zhang W, Gao J, Zhu Q, et al. Penetration and distribution of PLGA nanoparticles in the human skin treated with microneedles. Int J Pharm. 2010;402:205–212.

[38] Kong XQ, Zhou P, Wu CW. Numerical simulation of microneedles' insertion into skin. Comput Methods Biomech Biomed Engin. 2011;14:827–835.

[39] Martanto W, Moore JS, Couse T, et al. Mechanism of fluid infusion during microneedle insertion and retraction. J Control Release. 2006;112:357–361.

[40] Khumpuang S, Maeda R, Sugiyama S. Design and fabrication of a coupled microneedle array and insertion guide array for safe penetration through skin. MHS2003 Proceedings of 2003 International Symposium on Micromechatronics and Human Science (IEEE Cat No 03TH8717). IEEE; 2003. p. 233–237.

[41] Sausse Lhernould M, Delchambre A. Innovative design of hollow polymeric microneedles for transdermal drug delivery. Microsystem technologies. 2011;17:1675–1682.

[42] Martanto W, Moore JS, Kashlan O, et al. Microinfusion using hollow microneedles. Pharm Res. 2006;23:104–113.

[43] Ding Z, Verbaan FJ, Bivas-Benita M, et al. Microneedle arrays for the transcutaneous immunization of diphtheria and influenza in BALB/c mice. J Control Release. 2009;136:71–78.

[44] Bal SM, Caussin J, Pavel S, et al. In vivo assessment of safety of microneedle arrays in human skin. Eur J Pharm Sci. 2008;35:193–202.

[45] Gomaa YA, Morrow DI, Garland MJ, et al. Effects of microneedle length, density, insertion time and multiple applications on human skin barrier function: assessments by transepidermal water loss. Toxicol In Vitro. 2010;24:1971–1978.

[46] Verbaan FJ, Bal SM, van den Berg DJ, et al. Assembled microneedle arrays enhance the transport of compounds varying over a large range of molecular weight across human dermatomed skin. J Control Release. 2007;117:238–245.

[47] Daddona P. Macroflux® transdermal technology development for the delivery of therapeutic peptides and proteins. Drug Deliv Tech. 2002;2.

[48] McGrath MG, Vucen S, Vrdoljak A, et al. Production of dissolvable microneedles using an atomised spray process: effect of microneedle composition on skin penetration. Eur J Pharm Biopharm. 2014;86:200–211.

[49] Loizidou EZ, Williams NA, Barrow DA, et al. Structural characterisation and transdermal delivery studies on sugar microneedles: experimental and finite element modelling analyses. Eur J Pharm Biopharm. 2015;89:224–231.

[50] Elmahjoubi E, Frum Y, Eccleston GM, et al. Transepidermal water loss for probing full-thickness skin barrier function: correlation with tritiated water flux, sensitivity to punctures and diverse surfactant exposures. Toxicol In Vitro. 2009;23:1429–1435.

[51] Cai B, Xia W, Bredenberg S, et al. Bioceramic microneedles with flexible and self-swelling substrate. Eur J Pharm Biopharm. 2015;94:404–410.

[52] Ye Y, Yu J, Wang C, et al. Microneedles integrated with pancreatic cells and synthetic glucose-signal amplifiers for smart insulin delivery. Adv Mater. 2016;28:3115–3121.

[53] Brambilla D, Proulx ST, Marschalkova P, et al. Microneedles for the noninvasive structural and functional assessment of dermal lymphatic vessels. Small. 2016;12:1053–1061.

[54] Deng Y, Chen J, Zhao Y, et al. Transdermal delivery of siRNA through microneedle array. Sci Rep. 2016;6:21422.

[55] Zhu DD, Wang QL, Liu XB, et al. Rapidly separating microneedles for transdermal drug delivery. Acta Biomater. 2016;41:312–319.

[56] Park J-H, Choi S-O, Kamath R, et al. Polymer particle-based micromolding to fabricate novel microstructures. Biomed Microdevices. 2007;9:223–234.

[57] Lahiji SF, Dangol M, Jung H. A patchless dissolving microneedle delivery system enabling rapid and efficient transdermal drug delivery. Sci Rep. 2015;5:7914.

[58] Nguyen HX, Banga AK. Delivery of methotrexate and characterization of skin treated by fabricated PLGA microneedles and fractional ablative laser. Pharm Res. 2018;35:1–20.

[59] Wang PM, Cornwell M, Hill J, et al. Precise microinjection into skin using hollow microneedles. J Invest Dermatol. 2006;126:1080–1087.

[60] Coulman SA, Birchall JC, Alex A, et al. In vivo, in situ imaging of microneedle insertion into the skin of human volunteers using optical coherence tomography. Pharm Res. 2011;28:66–81.

[61] Kim M, Yang H, Kim H, et al. Novel cosmetic patches for wrinkle improvement: retinyl retinoate- and ascorbic acid-loaded dissolving microneedles. Int J Cosmet Sci. 2014;36:207–212.

[62] Sun W, Inayathullah M, Manoukian MAC, et al. Transdermal delivery of functional collagen via polyvinylpyrrolidone microneedles. Ann Biomed Eng. 2015;43:2978–2990.

[63] Widera G, Johnson J, Kim L, et al. Effect of delivery parameters on immunization to ovalbumin following intracutaneous administration by a coated microneedle array patch system. Vaccine. 2006;24:1653–1664.

[64] Häfeli UO, Mokhtari A, Liepmann D, et al. In vivo evaluation of a microneedle-based miniature syringe for intradermal drug delivery. Biomed Microdevices. 2009;11:943–950.

[65] Pearton M, Saller V, Coulman SA, et al. Microneedle delivery of plasmid DNA to living human skin: formulation coating, skin insertion and gene expression. J Control Release. 2012;160:561–569.

[66] Lee JW, Park J-H, Prausnitz MR. Dissolving microneedles for transdermal drug delivery. Biomaterials. 2008;29:2113–2124.

[67] Ling M-H, Chen M-C. Dissolving polymer microneedle patches for rapid and efficient transdermal delivery of insulin to diabetic rats. Acta Biomater. 2013;9:8952–8961.

[68] Yang S, Feng Y, Zhang L, et al. A scalable fabrication process of polymer microneedles. Int J Nanomed. 2012;7:1415–1422.

[69] Burton SA, Ng C-Y, Simmers R, et al. Rapid intradermal delivery of liquid formulations using a hollow microstructured array. Pharm Res. 2011;28:31–40.

[70] Birchall J, Coulman S, Pearton M, et al. Cutaneous DNA delivery and gene expression in ex vivo human skin explants via wet-etch microfabricated microneedles. J Drug Target. 2005;13:415–421.

[71] Kochhar JS, Quek TC, Soon WJ, et al. Effect of microneedle geometry and supporting substrate on microneedle array penetration into skin. J Pharm Sci. 2013;102:4100–4108.

[72] Rossetti FC, Depieri LV, Bentley MVLB, et al. Confocal laser scanning microscopy as a tool for the investigation of skin drug delivery systems and diagnosis of skin disorders. Confocal

Laser Microscopy—Principles and Applications in Medicine, Biology, and the Food Sciences. IntechOpen; 2013. [Internet] [cited 2022 Nov 8]. Available from: www.intechopen.com/state. item.id.

[73] Mortensen LJ, Glazowski CE, Zavislan JM, et al. Near-IR fluorescence and reflectance confocal microscopy for imaging of quantum dots in mammalian skin. Biomed Opt Express. 2011;2:1610–1625.

[74] Gujjar M, Banga AK. Iontophoretic and microneedle mediated transdermal delivery of glycopyrrolate. Pharmaceutics. 2014;6:663–671.

[75] Brogden NK, Banks SL, Crofford LJ, et al. Diclofenac enables unprecedented week-long microneedle-enhanced delivery of a skin impermeable medication in humans. Pharm Res. 2013;30:1947–1955.

[76] Wermeling DP, Banks SL, Hudson DA, et al. Microneedles permit transdermal delivery of a skin-impermeant medication to humans. Proc Natl Acad Sci. 2008;105:2058–2063.

[77] Ghosh P, Brogden NK, Stinchcomb AL. Effect of formulation pH on transport of naltrexone species and pore closure in microneedle-enhanced transdermal drug delivery. Mol Pharm. 2013;10:2331–2339.

[78] Enfield J, O'Connell M-L, Lawlor K, et al. In-vivo dynamic characterization of microneedle skin penetration using optical coherence tomography. J Biomed Opt. 2010;15:046001.

5

Microneedle-mediated Transdermal Drug Delivery

5.1 Introduction

Microneedle technology has emerged as a promising drug delivery platform, as described in numerous studies in the literature. Solid microneedles have been the subject of most research articles (35%). Coated microneedles were well-reported in the early literature, but they have since been substituted by dissolving microneedles, which were discussed in nearly as many publications (25%) as hollow microneedles. Approximately half (49%) of the publications dealt with *in vivo* (nonhuman) investigations, 25% were associated with *in vitro* studies, 17% related to human subjects, and the remainder, 9%, involved only with the production and characterization of the microneedles [1].

Originally, microneedles were designed to substitute hypodermic needles to deliver different drug formulations into the skin. Comparatively, microneedles have several benefits over hypodermic needles. Standard hypodermic needles have several limitations, including (i) the pain associated with injections (needle phobias), (ii) the necessity for a qualified healthcare professional to administer the dose, (iii) the possibility of accidental needlestick injuries, and (iv) the generation of biohazardous sharp waste. Furthermore, microneedle-based transdermal drug delivery offers several benefits over the oral route, including avoiding hepatic first-pass metabolism, zero-order drug delivery, fewer adverse effects, and lower required doses.

Microneedles are micrometer-sized needles generally extending from a flat rigid or flexible substrate to administer the drug payload into the targeted tissue. A multitude of various-sized molecules may be delivered into the tissue by microneedle penetration, generating numerous microchannels which serve as the drug delivery pathway. A significant quantity of drug solution might be slowly infused into the skin using hollow microneedles. The drug payload carried by coated and dissolving microneedles may be little, but it would be formulated in a dry and stable condition. In addition, there is no risk of sharp hazards with dissolving microneedles since, once inserted, they dissolve in the skin fluid, discharging the loaded drug into the tissue. To prevent bleeding and pain, microneedles are designed to cause no disruption to blood capillaries and nerve fibers. There may be a significantly higher rate of skin absorption of drugs administered using microneedles. Compared to hypodermic needles or prefilled syringes, microneedle patches are more cost-effective and convenient since they may be self-administered at home [1]. Recently, a multitude of research indicates that microneedle-based devices can administer molecules of any size. Experiments differ substantially regarding the drug compound, skin models, formulation composition, and microneedle insertion strategy. Furthermore, the types of microneedles might vary considerably regarding composition, design, dimensions, tip radius, and needle density. A substantial collection of information favors microneedles

DOI: 10.1201/9780429294433-5

application to deliver hydrophilic compounds. Typically, microneedle penetration into the skin leads to the creation of transient hydrophilic micrometer-sized channels. These channels are magnitudes larger than any therapeutic agent's molecular size and, thus, should effortlessly facilitate the absorption of even large molecules. The increased permeability of pharmaceuticals of different molecular weights and size is extensively recognized. Nevertheless, other physicochemical properties, including the ionization degree and solubility, have not been thoroughly investigated.

For the most part, research on microneedles has been published in the context of transdermal delivery of macromolecules (i.e., peptides and proteins). The skin delivery of these difficult molecules is practically the "Holy Grail" of microneedles-based drug delivery, and every research that advances this endeavor is to be embraced with great zeal. However, biopharmaceutical molecules are not the only sector where microneedles research may and should be conducted. Drugs with a low molecular weight would also greatly benefit from microneedles-assisted transdermal delivery.

There may be significant commercial interest in microneedle-mediated transdermal and intradermal delivery of compounds with low molecular weight. Previous research often used microneedles made of metal or silicon. The possibility for microneedles' broken pieces to be left in the skin is the primary biosafety issue with these types of microneedles. Recent years have noticed intensive research and development of biodegradable dissolving microneedles made from carbohydrates or polymers that are safe for human use. There could be numerous benefits to using such drug delivery systems. Drugs may be encapsulated into the polymeric matrix, enabling a simple, one-step method of drug delivery. Furthermore, adjusting the polymer material characteristics may alter the drug release kinetics. Many of these materials may be handled at room temperature, allowing for the manufacturing of pharmaceutical products with thermosensitive drugs at a reduced cost. As an additional benefit, these dissolving microneedles systems may disable themselves, indicating no further steps must be taken when disposing of them. Various criteria need to be considered to load a therapeutic agent within the polymeric matrix of microneedles. If the polymer has to be processed at high temperatures, this might affect the drug's stability. The addition of a drug might alter the polymer's physical properties. For instance, the mechanical robustness of microneedles might be affected. The state of the loaded drug must also be assessed. Recently, most research has only investigated how microneedles effectively deliver drug models into and across skin tissue. Fundamental research characterizing the interaction between the microneedles material and therapeutic agent are essential to properly understand and improve the safety and efficacy of these microneedles-based drug delivery systems.

A handful of safety issues must be resolved before microneedles drug delivery systems can realize their full potential. Microneedles treatment is widely perceived as non-painful and noninvasive [2], even though it physically disturbs the skin's protective barrier. Consequently, delivery systems considered for treating chronic illnesses must undergo safety studies that assess the impact of long-term usage. Evidence that microchannel formation is safe, reversible, and does not pose the risk of microbial infection must be provided and validated in clinical trials. Another critical issue is whether the microneedles-delivered dose is consistent among different patients. An external pressure must be utilized for microneedles to penetrate the skin deeply enough during microneedles application. The results of a manual application may vary dramatically across patients and even different skin areas on the same subject. One strategy to resolve this issue is using an applicator device that produces a consistent force on microneedles. The mechanical qualities of the microneedles should be considered appropriately. The miniature size of a microneedle's tip makes breaking a realistic possibility. To reduce these risks, new methods of packaging and application are necessary. Increasing evidence suggests that transdermal drug delivery with the use of microneedles is efficient. These systems can potentially expand the variety of therapeutic agents that can be delivered percutaneously. Nevertheless, this capacity cannot be realized without thoroughly assessing and addressing concerns about safety and application.

5.2 Factors Affecting Microneedle-mediated Drug Delivery

Various factors were found to significantly affect microneedle-mediated drug delivery into and across the skin. Drug permeation into skin tissue was shown to be most dependent on microneedle dimensions, penetration depth, and microneedle density [3, 4].

5.2.1 Limited Drug Loading

The quantity of medications that can be delivered using microneedles is restricted by their minute size and loading capacity. Consequently, their use becomes more challenging when a high dose or sustained drug release is desired. Multiple microneedles patches applied at once or regular replacement of the microneedle patch both are viable options for getting around the limitation of the drug payload. Research into improving the drug dose that can be loaded in microneedles is, nevertheless, necessary for broadening the applications of microneedles [5].

5.2.2 Drug Solubility

An essential technique in addressing the issue of microneedles is the ability to solubilize poorly soluble drugs. A drug has to be sufficiently soluble in an aqueous media to be loaded into microneedles. However, only a small fraction of drugs can be administered with microneedles since numerous compounds have limited aqueous solubility [6]. It is possible to incorporate greater quantities of drugs into smaller delivery devices like microneedles by improving the solubility of a poorly soluble drug. One common strategy is to use prodrugs to enhance the solubility of drugs. There has also been ongoing study into the efficacy of employing surfactants or liposomes, the salt form of the drug, pH modification, and micro/nanoparticle technologies to increase the solubility of various drugs [5].

5.2.3 Sustained Drug Delivery

While microneedles are useful for administering a single dose of a medication, they cannot be used for sustained drug delivery due to their small size. Separable microneedles have been designed to exhibit the capacity of microneedle-based continuous drug release. Researchers have investigated microneedle designs that can be disassembled, with the goal of shortening the duration a microneedles patch must be worn [7–10]. Further, efficient drug delivery may be achieved for a wide variety of therapeutic agents via the development and optimization of formulation for long-term drug delivery. It is also crucial to create an adhesive patch that is safe to apply for extended periods using a microneedle patch [5].

5.2.4 Microneedle Production Technology

Microneedle molds, used to fabricate the microscopic needle tips, are often produced using the deep reactive ion etching technique because of their incredible precision and repeatability. There is a significant obstacle to entering the area of microneedle production due to the high cost of the equipment and its complicated operation; thus, large-scale manufacturing technology has only been accessible to a few companies.

5.2.5 Regulations

Currently, microneedle product approval is handled on a case-by-case basis (product-specific approval) rather than on the basis of the microneedle technology as a whole. Consequently, there is a lag in the regulatory approval of microneedle devices, which is a barrier preventing the widespread use of these products. Microneedle regulations that specify the microneedle's geometries, composition, sterilization, and packaging are expected to deal with this issue. Building a microneedle regulation system based on quality by design to facilitate the mass production of microneedle devices requires the harmonization of current good manufacturing practices and quality control systems [5].

5.2.6 Advances in Digital Technology

Currently, microneedles primarily function as drug delivery systems, but with the assistance of advanced information technologies, they may be transformed into digital medicine. Strategies may be designed to offer information about drug loading quantity, patch change interval, and programmed drug release kinetics. Convergence technology can potentially expand the uses of microneedles in drug administration and provide novel product lines [5].

Microneedle-mediated drug delivery could vary, depending on the design and types of microneedles. Each type of microneedles (solid, coated, hollow, dissolving, and swelling) has unique properties, advantages, and disadvantages. Various factors affecting microneedles drug delivery have been reported widely in the literature.

5.2.7 Solid Microneedles

Historically, the "poke and patch" method has been used to deliver various drugs through the skin. This method employs solid microneedles for enhancing transdermal drug delivery. Microneedles are first inserted into the skin. The microneedles are then removed, and a drug-loaded formulation (i.e., a patch) is placed over the area where the microneedles were inserted previously [11–13]. After solid microneedles are inserted into the skin, temporary open skin fluid-filled microchannels are formed. The drug is delivered locally or systemically by passive diffusion (vertical or lateral) from the applied formulation into the microneedles-created microchannels. The drug diffusion via microchannels depends on the pore dimensions (surface area and depth) and pore number, as well as the drug concentration in the formulation, which is regarded as the driving force for drug permeation into the skin. The "poke and patch" method with solid microneedles has been employed to enhance transdermal and intradermal delivery of various molecules, as reported in *in vitro* and *in vivo* studies [11, 14–17]. When using solid microneedles for drug delivery, removing the needles after the skin insertion is preferable rather than leaving them in the skin during the delivery duration. Previous attempts have been to produce solid microneedles for drug administration in various geometries, dimensions, and from various materials (i.e., glass, silicon, metal, and polymers).

Advantages

- Improved mechanical strength or robustness and efficient skin penetration
- Manufactured in a variety of geometries and dimensions
- Technically simple in microneedles and formulation designs
- Potential for sustained drug delivery
- Drug delivery based on passive diffusion (vertical and lateral diffusion) through microchannels

Disadvantages

- Complicated production processes require expensive clean room facilities
- Biosafety issues of microneedle fracture in skin
- Possible error in the two-step application process
- No precise drug dosing
- Concerns about sharp wastes

5.2.8 Hollow Microneedles

The "poke and flow" method uses hollow microneedles to administer drug solution to the skin. A hollow microneedle's functioning is identical to that of a hypodermic needle, despite the latter being considerably larger in dimensions. The drug solution could flow slowly but steadily into the skin via the microneedle's channels [18]. The drug-loaded formulation is typically a fluid, and the microneedle serves as a path for drug delivery. As with the traditional syringe and needle, the microneedles are inserted into the skin and then transported the fluid formulation from the reservoir to the treated skin area [19]. When using hollow microneedles for transdermal drug delivery, keeping the flow rate consistent without sacrificing the needles' mechanical properties is crucial. The compression of the dense skin tissue surrounding the needle tip after insertion is the primary factor influencing the flow rate [20].

When compared to solid microneedles, hollow microneedles have the potential to accelerate the fluid flow, which in turn increases drug delivery rates [11, 12, 21]. Hollow microneedles enable the administration of a large volume of drug solution, which is markedly greater than the quantity delivered by other types of microneedles. Furthermore, lab-on-chips systems could be integrated into hollow microneedle devices. Precise dosing could be achieved by controlling the amount or volume of the injected drug solution. Also, minimal reformulation is required since most therapeutic agents should be formulated in solution form. In addition, the dosage of the required medicine in solution may be adjusted more precisely to meet the patient's requirements. Hollow microneedles enable drug injection at a precise depth in the skin and rapid onset of drug delivery. Passive permeation of the drug formulation via the microneedle's bore is the cornerstone of this technique [22, 23]. There are additional active delivery systems in which the drug solution is pumped into the skin via the microneedle's bore. The force-driven drug delivery necessitates some kind of pressured driving force, either a syringe, pump, or pressurized gas combined with a microneedle injection applicator [21, 24–27]. Moreover, a microneedle device may incorporate a microfluidic chip [28] or a micropump to govern the drug delivery from the reservoir into the skin [29]. Connecting the drug reservoir with a controlled heater might cause the drug solution to expand and be forced into the skin due to bubble creation [30]. Pushing a flexible drug reservoir manually by fingers may also cause the drug solution to be released onto the skin and facilitate transdermal drug delivery [31]. The system's simplicity of production and low cost make it the most competitive option available.

A low injection flow rate (50–300 nL/min) is a common drawback of the "poke and flow" method with hollow microneedles [23, 25, 27]. High flow rates of up to 18.8 μL/min could be achieved, however, by partially retracting the needles or by including hyaluronidase in the drug formulation, which degrades the hyaluronic acid inside the skin's collagen fibers to diminish the pressure from the dense skin tissue [25]. Interestingly, iontophoresis, a physical enhancement technology that applies an electrical driving force to transport drugs into the skin, may be used in conjunction with hollow microneedles to improve the effectiveness of transdermal drug delivery [11]. But when an intense electrical current is employed, the skin could be irritated because a high level of electricity flows through the micropores, which have the lowest electrical resistance [32].

Hollow microneedles could also provide the benefit of their capacity to withdraw a small volume of blood or interstitial fluid below the skin, allowing for monitoring of the amounts of certain substances in the body, such as blood glucose [33]. The next step in the evolution of this technology is refining the microneedles' dimensions and design to achieve the desired level of extraction rate [34].

A critical factor that has been investigated and modified is the flow rate within the hollow needles [35]. Though hollow microneedles allow for precise control over drug infusion rates, a key drawback is that these microneedles may be obstructed by compressed dense skin tissue, which prevents the intended dose from being administered. If the applied pressure is excessively high, the drug solution will leak out of the needle and onto the skin surface. Also, significant back pressure hinders the drug infusion rate. Research has also been performed to optimize the process of inserting microneedles and applied pressure during the drug delivery process since the miniature size of hollow microneedles makes insertion and injection more challenging. In a similar vein, if the microneedles were to break into the skin unexpectedly, the drug solution may leak out or be released too quickly [36]. Hollow microneedles generally have weaker mechanical robustness than solid microneedles, especially those made from silicon. Notably, a large needle tip diameter could cause poor needle insertion into the skin. Besides, hollow microneedles offer no further advantages over hypodermic needles in terms of sharp waste elimination, improved drug stability, or requirement for cold-chain storage.

5.2.9 Coated Microneedles

Solid microneedles are coated with the drug formulation and inserted into the skin for drug delivery; this procedure is known as the "coat and poke" of coated microneedles [37, 38]. Microneedles coated with a polymer-based formulation of potent drugs are inserted into the skin, where they perforate the skin. Then the coated layer dissolves, releasing the drug into skin layers. After the microneedles have been safely removed from the skin, the therapeutic coating layer remains under the skin [39]. These coated microneedles will be preferable to solid microneedles because a one-step method for skin poration and drug delivery will prevent the risk of error during self-administration [19]. Many therapeutic agents (small molecules, macromolecules, DNA, viruses, and proteins) may be effectively delivered into the skin using coated microneedles [40]. Selecting a reliable drug-coating method is crucial for optimizing drug delivery with these microneedles. For effective coating of the microneedles, various coating formulations, procedures, and stability-related parameters will need to be evaluated [19]. When developing a drug formulation, choosing the suitable drug form, solvent system, buffering system, and polymeric materials is critical. A coated microneedle array could carry as much as 1 mg of the drug, with the actual quantity dependent on the coating efficiency, coating length, needle surface area, and needle density [41, 42]. To prevent the coated layer from coming off the microneedle during storage or administration, the drying process (duration, temperature, humidity) must be carried out properly. To prevent physical, chemical, or biological degradation of the coated component during drying, optimal drying conditions are required. Since the whole microneedles do not penetrate skin due to the skin viscoelasticity, the coating's height on the needles must be controlled. This will also aid in preventing undesired surface contamination and possible drug loss [40]. Another crucial factor is the long-term stability of the drug coating on the microneedles. Stability issues may also emerge if the drug reacts unfavorably with the microneedle material or is stored for an extended period. Therefore, real-time and accelerated stability tests are required to evaluate the stability of the finished coated microneedles product [43].

The primary benefit of this "coat and poke" approach is that the excellent mechanical robustness of the microneedles is maintained throughout drug delivery. Solid microneedles serve as the strong and sturdy frame for the product, thus preventing issues related to microneedles' mechanical properties. A noted benefit of employing coated microneedles is enhanced bioavailability and effective drug delivery [19]. The coated drug is deposited to a precise depth in the skin. Also, this device does not require a separate drug reservoir or microfluidics component. The simple and convenient application of coated microneedles resembles the conventional transdermal patch.

Some drawbacks of coated microneedles have been reported in the literature [40]. The success of enhanced drug delivery and the finished product's performance depends on the coating formulation and processes. Furthermore, the quantity of coated drugs is limited; hence this platform is only suitable for potent compounds which require a low therapeutic dose. The excessive coating could lead to compromised needle sharpness, thus affecting the needle insertion efficiency.

5.2.10 Dissolving Microneedles

Dissolving microneedles are often constructed from polymers or sugars and contain a drug payload in their matrix. After being inserted into the skin, biodegradable microneedles dissolve, allowing for a controlled release of the drugs for weeks or even months [18, 44]. With this method, the drug is slowly released from the microneedles during the course of treatment. After being applied to the skin, the microneedles must stay in place until the encapsulated drug is delivered [20]. To save production costs and improve product biocompatibility, biopolymers are increasingly employed in dissolving microneedles production [45]. Most microneedles dissolve in the skin by either solubilization or hydrolysis. Microneedles made from biodegradable polymers may provide a more prolonged drug release than those made from sugar [46, 47], which disintegrate quickly and provide a burst drug release [48, 49]. Dissolving microneedles fabricated from various materials, such as maltose, chondroitin sulfate, dextran, dextrin, carboxymethylcellulose, polylactic acid, and others, have been presented in the scientific literature.

According to Lee et al., several criteria should be followed while designing dissolving microneedles [50]:

- Mechanically strong microneedles structure to facilitate effective skin insertion
- Controlled drug release kinetics for rapid or extended drug delivery
- Mild fabrication conditions to avoid drug degradation
- Use of safe, nontoxic, biocompatible, and biodegradable materials

Advantages

- Controlled drug release and delivery
- Biodegradable and biocompatible materials to avoid biosafety issues
- No biohazardous sharp waste
- Precise dosing
- Higher drug-loading capacity than coated microneedles
- No requirement for reconstitution
- Manufactured from safe and inexpensive materials
- Simple, inexpensive, and reproducible fabrication technique (i.e., micromolding)

Disadvantages

- Fabrication at harsh conditions (i.e., high temperature) could compromise drug stability
- Limited drug-loading capacity
- Increased drug loading leads to insufficient mechanical strength
- Requirement of careful material selection for desired dissolution profile.

5.2.11 Swelling Microneedles

Hydrogel-forming swelling microneedles absorb interstitial fluid upon application into the skin, generating continuous, unblockable channels for drug delivery that avoid the obstruction issue of hollow microneedles [51, 52]. In their dry condition, such microneedle arrays are strong and rigid, but once inserted into the skin, they quickly absorb interstitial skin fluid and transform into hydrogel bulbs. The microneedles generally do not carry any drug but are attached to a regular transdermal patch. In this way, the swelling microneedles serve as an unimpeded pathway for the drug to travel from the reservoir to the dermal tissue. Since the quantity of drug that can be applied to the microneedles is no longer a limiting factor, higher doses may be delivered for more extended drug delivery periods [53]. After absorbing skin fluid, these microneedles soften and become unusable for reapplication. Still, they come off the skin without any damage or leaving any polymeric residue in the skin tissue [53, 54]. Even though the generated microchannels are of a tiny size from a clinical perspective, they provide an unobstructed passageway for macromolecules (i.e., proteins and peptides) to move along into the skin. The capability of hydrogel-forming microneedles is particularly relevant for the transdermal delivery of macromolecules. The scientific literature also describes these microneedles as swelling microneedles or phase-transition microneedles [55]. These microneedles are made from hydrogel-forming polymers that expand upon contact with interstitial fluid, which makes them suitable for skin penetration. Hydrogel porosity size may be adjusted to facilitate the diffusion of macromolecules through the channels and into the skin since drug penetration through the swollen hydrogel matrix relies on its hydrodynamic radius and the density of the hydrogel matrix [56]. Since the drug payload is loaded in patches positioned behind the microneedles system, drug diffusion occurs continuously, and the patches can be continually changed to provide the necessary dosage [57]. Drug-loaded patches connected to drug-free hydrogel-forming microneedles have been used effectively to deliver various compounds with different molecular weights [54].

Hydrogel-forming microneedles will allow for the effective transdermal delivery of a broader range of drugs than the roughly 20 that can be delivered transdermally. Regarding the physicochemical characteristics and release patterns of both small molecules and macromolecules, gamma irradiation had no significant effect on hydrogel-forming microneedles [58]. Transdermal delivery of therapeutically effective drug doses through hydrogel-forming microneedles is a promising area of research [59]. There might be drawbacks to using these swelling microneedles if the drug is encapsulated into the hydrogel matrix. In this case, the quantity of drug released is restricted to the drug payload enclosed inside the microneedles [8, 60–63].

5.3 Patents on Microneedles

There has been an increase in the number of published patents relating to the application of microneedles for drugs and vaccine administration. Important microneedles patents holders include Becton Dickinson, Nano Pass Technologies Ltd., Procter & Gamble Company, Life Scan, Inc., Alza Corporation, Massachusetts Institute of Technology, Georgia Tech, Research Corporation, University of California, 3M, Corium International, Inc., Toppan Printing Co., Ltd., Agency for Science, Technology and Research, Pelikan Technologies, Inc., Hisamitsu Pharmaceutical Co., Inc., Industrial Technology Research Institute, Theraject, Inc., All Tranz, Inc., Apogee Technologies, and others. Companies such as Elegaphy, Valeritas, Imtek, Kumetrix, Silex Microsystems, Norwood Abbey, SpectRx, Zeopane, and Zosano Pharma are also developing microneedle products for therapeutic applications [41].

The numbers of patents on microneedles issued in the United States based on patent claims, assignee types, applications of microneedles, and microneedle types were analyzed and presented by Ingrole and colleagues (Fig. 5.1) [1]. Notably, more than 55% of all microneedle patents have been granted in the last five years (2014–2018), compared to 26% in the first decade of research (2001–2010). There has been a significant increase in the number of patents filed for microneedles, with nearly as many filed in the first ten years as in the past two years. Time-series patent analysis also shows variations in microneedle types and applications. The majority of patent assignees were corporations (79%), followed by universities (19%), and, finally, individuals (2%) who submitted the patents themselves. Around 34% of patents dealt with drug applicators, while 31% related to microneedles themselves, and the remaining were split between techniques for making microneedles (20%) and methods of utilizing microneedles (15%) [1]. In the sphere of universities, Georgia Tech Research Corporation ranked first with a 12% share of all patents. After that came the University of California with 10%, followed by the University of Utah Research

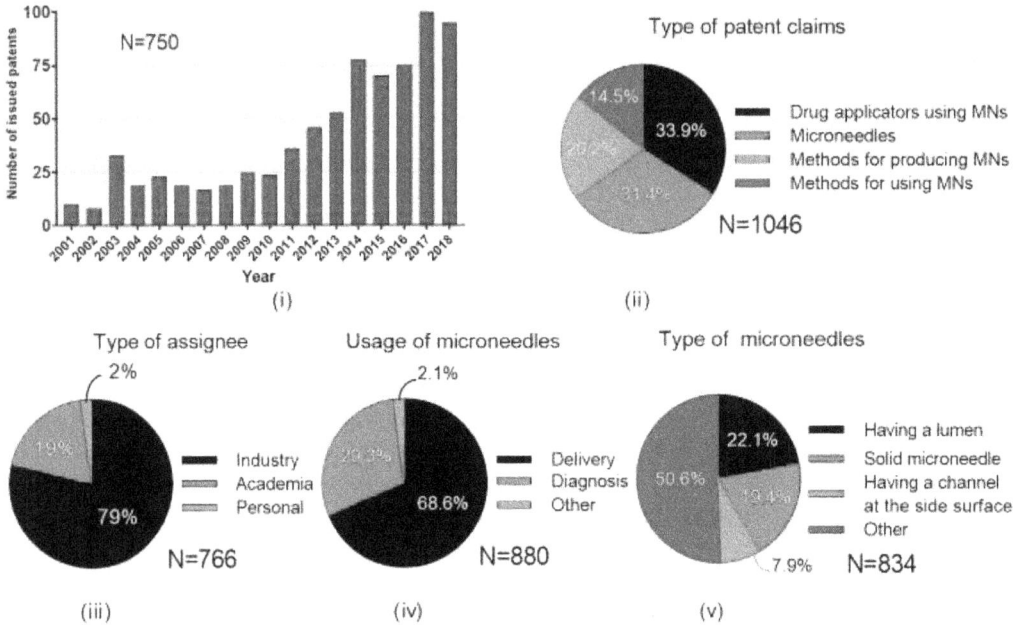

FIGURE 5.1
Number of patents on microneedles issued in the United States. (i) Number of patents per year. (ii) Patent claims. (iii) Assignee types. (iv) Applications of microneedles. (v) Microneedle types. Images reprinted with permission from [1].

Foundation with 4%. To date, 64 academic institutions have been granted patents, with the top 10 colleges receiving roughly half of all patents awarded [1]. BD Technologies has the most patents in the microneedles field (9%). Following a significant distance behind was 3M, with 7%, then came ALZA/Zosano Pharma, with 5%, and Hisamitsu Pharmaceutical, with 4%. To further illustrate how significantly more dynamic the industry has been at patenting than universities, it is noted that the fifth most productive business at patenting (Corium International) holds as many granted patents as the most productive university in the academic area (Georgia Tech Research Corporation). The top 10 patent awardees out of 193 businesses had over 40% of all industry patents combined [1]. As vaccines are a significant field of application for microneedles, researchers also examined relevant patents from academia and industry. The highest number of patents belongs to ALZA/Zosano Pharma (17%) and BD Technologies (14%). Only one academic university made it to the top ten, with Georgia Tech Research Corporation coming in at number four (7%) behind Corium International (9%). There were a total of 1,197 contributors to the microneedle patents, with over 60% of those being sole inventors of a single invention. More than 30% of all microneedle patents came from only ten top innovators. The United States is credited for almost two-thirds of all microneedle patents. Japan produced the second-highest share of microneedles patents in the industry (12%) and total (9%). Israel and Germany were also significant contributors to industry-based innovations, while Taiwan and Korea were major players in the academic sector. There was no difference in the relative prominence of different continents in terms of patent production across either the business sector or academic research. Over 60% of each category came from North America, followed by 20% from Asia, 10% from Europe, and 1% from Australia. This disparity between research articles and patents demonstrates the distinct goals of the academic and business sectors. More research into the delivery of small molecules, macromolecules, and vaccines has been conducted in academic circles, as has an increased focus on solid and dissolving microneedles. Research on hollow and coated microneedles was preferred in the industry, as was a narrower emphasis on macromolecules and vaccines [1].

Increases in microneedle research have coincided with a corresponding increase in patent applications (Fig. 5.2). Most patents were evaluated for their potential use in vaccinations and diabetes monitoring. The most prevalent use of microneedles was for vaccination, whereas the most prominent use of hollow microneedles was for monitoring glucose. Microneedles with a lumen and a side channel were the next most common kind of microneedle after solid microneedles when considering particular applications in vaccination. There was a clear preference for delivery innovations over diagnostic technologies among microneedles patents. Despite the lack of depth in the scholarly literature, patents for drug applicators were common. Vaccination was the most frequent application for delivery patents, while glucose monitoring was the most widely used application for diagnostic patents. Microneedles products have been developed for application in pharmaceuticals and cosmetics fields, and evidence of these functions could be observed in patent literature. A single microneedle (generally hollow microneedles), a collection of microneedles on a substrate (generally solid microneedles), and microneedles integrated

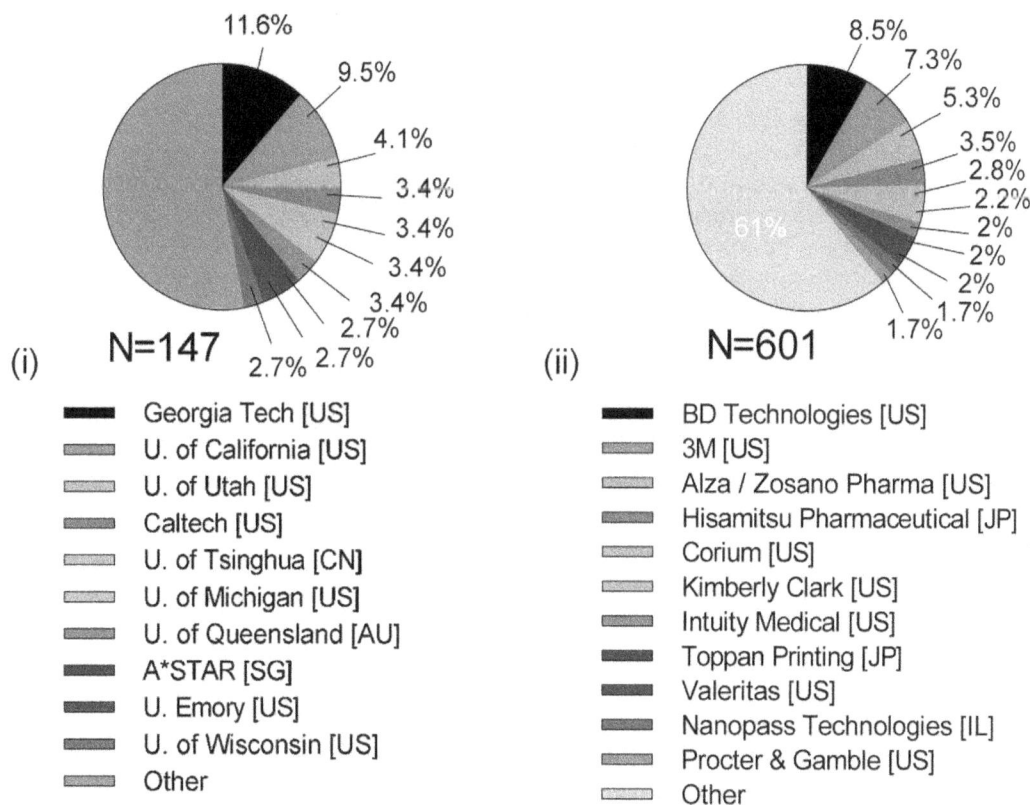

FIGURE 5.2
Patents for microneedles developed in universities and industrial companies. (i) Universities in academia. (ii) Companies in the industry. Images reprinted with permission from [1].

into a finished product are the three most common forms of microneedles. Regarding currently available products, dissolving microneedles have been used popularly in the cosmetics sector. Microneedles made of polymers and metals have been used in collagen induction therapy and other skin treatments. Researchers found that microneedle applicator devices have a significant role in the patent literature. Several microneedle designs require an applicator to ensure consistent pressure is applied rapidly and evenly throughout the microneedle array surface to penetrate skin tissue efficiently. There has been a rise in the number of patents covering the use of solid microneedles in both drug delivery and diagnostics. Reasons for this observation include the less complicated production processes and higher usability of solid microneedles [1]. Microneedles have been widely employed as promising drug carriers in the last several decades. Therefore, the study of microneedles materials and their characteristics receives the researcher's undivided attention. This means it may be employed effectively for administering medications with few adverse effects. The drug delivery system has a number of microneedle-related patents [64]. Researchers have studied microneedles for transdermal and ocular drug delivery and found patents covering the fabrication processes for dissolving, swelling, solid, hollow, and coated microneedles. The investigators also noted patents for emerging microneedle technologies that have shown therapeutic effectiveness across various clinical diseases [65].

5.4 Conclusions

The area of microneedles drug delivery has significantly advanced since the first publication about microneedles applications in drug delivery in 1988. Microneedles substantially improve transdermal drug delivery by physically producing microchannels in the skin. This innovative technology offers several benefits, including painless or minimally invasive application, possible self-administration, and the avoidance of hepatic first-pass metabolism. Clinical studies for various treatments using solid and hollow microneedles have demonstrated success to this point. Coated and dissolving microneedles have been developed recently for use in clinical trials. Despite the widespread consensus that using microneedles is advantageous, specific concerns have been expressed. Microneedle insertion, in particular, has been associated with the creation of microscopic pores in the skin that may serve as entry points for pathogens, including bacteria and fungi. Microneedles have been reported in trials to considerably limit microbial entry through the created pores compared to conventional hypodermic needles [66]. Using a disinfectant at the insertion point prior to microneedles treatment is another way to reduce the likelihood of microbial infection. The entry of allergens may trigger allergic responses in the body. For example, titanium microneedles' corrosion resistance makes them superior to stainless steel alternatives [67]. Polymeric microneedles seldom have this issue since they use superior polymeric materials that are not particularly immunogenic. Thus, the materials used to produce microneedles must be completely risk-free. According to recent research on the safety aspect of microneedles, the microneedles patch is safe to use on human subjects [68–71]. Patients care most about cost and ease of use, although safety is paramount. It is vital to strike a balance between enhanced permeability and noninvasiveness while using microneedles since the depth to which microneedles penetrate is strongly connected with the intensity of any resulting discomfort. Assuming these problems can be resolved, microneedles have the potential to offer a decent alternative to the present technologies.

References

[1] Ingrole RS, Azizoglu E, Dul M, et al. Trends of microneedle technology in the scientific literature, patents, clinical trials and internet activity. Biomaterials. 2021;267:120491.

[2] Kaushik S, Hord AH, Denson DD, et al. Lack of pain associated with microfabricated microneedles. Anesth Analg. 2001;92:502–504.

[3] Davidson A, Al-Qallaf B, Das DB. Transdermal drug delivery by coated microneedles: geometry effects on effective skin thickness and drug permeability. Chem Eng Res Des. 2008;86:1196–1206.

[4] Oh J-H, Park H-H, Do K-Y, et al. Influence of the delivery systems using a microneedle array on the permeation of a hydrophilic molecule, calcein. Eur J Pharm Biopharm. 2008;69:1040–1045.

[5] Jung JH, Jin SG. Microneedle for transdermal drug delivery: current trends and fabrication. J Pharm Investig. 2021;51:503–517.

[6] Kearney M-C, McKenna PE, Quinn HL, et al. Design and development of liquid drug reservoirs for microneedle delivery of poorly soluble drug molecules. Pharmaceutics. 2019;11:605.

[7] Choi I-J, Kang A, Ahn M-H, et al. Insertion-responsive microneedles for rapid intradermal delivery of canine influenza vaccine. J Control Release. 2018;286:460–466.

[8] Chu LY, Prausnitz MR. Separable arrowhead microneedles. J Control Release. 2011;149:242–249.

[9] Li W, Tang J, Terry RN, et al. Long-acting reversible contraception by effervescent microneedle patch. Sci Adv. 2019;5:eaaw8145.

[10] Li W, Terry RN, Tang J, et al. Rapidly separable microneedle patch for the sustained release of a contraceptive. Nat Biomed Eng. 2019;3:220–229.

[11] Banga AK. Microporation applications for enhancing drug delivery. Expert Opin Drug Deliv. 2009;6:343–354.

[12] Prausnitz MR. Microneedles for transdermal drug delivery. Adv Drug Deliv Rev. 2004;56:581–587.

[13] Sivamani RK, Liepmann D, Maibach HI. Microneedles and transdermal applications. Expert Opin Drug Deliv. 2007;4:19–25.

[14] Banks SL, Paudel KS, Brogden NK, et al. Diclofenac enables prolonged delivery of naltrexone through microneedle-treated skin. Pharm Res. 2011;28:1211–1219.

[15] Gupta J, Gill HS, Andrews SN, et al. Kinetics of skin resealing after insertion of microneedles in human subjects. J Control Release. 2011;154:148–155.

[16] Kalluri H, Banga AK. Formation and closure of microchannels in skin following microporation. Pharm Res. 2011;28:82–94.

[17] Kalluri H, Kolli CS, Banga AK. Characterization of microchannels created by metal microneedles: formation and closure. AAPS J. 2011;13:473–481.

[18] Han T, Das DB. Potential of combined ultrasound and microneedles for enhanced transdermal drug permeation: a review. Eur J Pharm Biopharm. 2015;89:312–328.

[19] Sachdeva VK, Banga A. Microneedles and their applications. Recent Pat Drug Deliv Formul. 2011;5:95–132.

[20] van der Maaden K, Jiskoot W, Bouwstra J. Microneedle technologies for (trans)dermal drug and vaccine delivery. J Control Release. 2012;161:645–655.

[21] Bal SM, Ding Z, van Riet E, et al. Advances in transcutaneous vaccine delivery: do all ways lead to Rome? J Control Release. 2010;148:266–282.

[22] Davis SP, Martanto W, Allen MG, et al. Hollow metal microneedles for insulin delivery to diabetic rats. IEEE Trans Biomed Eng. 2005;52:909–915.

[23] Roxhed N, Samel B, Nordquist L, et al. Painless drug delivery through microneedle-based transdermal patches featuring active infusion. IEEE Trans Biomed Eng. 2008;55:1063–1071.

[24] Chandrasekaran S, Frazier AB. Characterization of surface micromachined hollow metallic microneedles. Micro Electro Mech Syst. IEEE; 2003. p. 363–366.

[25] Martanto W, Moore JS, Kashlan O, et al. Microinfusion using hollow microneedles. Pharm Res. 2006;23:104–113.

[26] McAllister DV, Wang PM, Davis SP, et al. Microfabricated needles for transdermal delivery of macromolecules and nanoparticles: fabrication methods and transport studies. Proc Natl Acad Sci. 2003;100:13755–13760.

[27] Wang PM, Cornwell M, Hill J, et al. Precise microinjection into skin using hollow microneedles. J Invest Dermatol. 2006;126:1080–1087.

[28] Paik S-J, Byun S, Lim J-M, et al. In-plane single-crystal-silicon microneedles for minimally invasive microfluid systems. Sens Actuators Phys. 2004;114:276–284.

[29] Cui Q, Liu C, Zha XF. Study on a piezoelectric micropump for the controlled drug delivery system. Microfluid Nanofluidics. 2007;3:377–390.

[30] Reed ML, Lye W-K. Microsystems for drug and gene delivery. Proc IEEE. 2004;92:56–75.

[31] Stoeber B, Liepmann D. Design, fabrication and testing of a MEMS syringe. Proc Solid-State Sens Actuator Workshop. 2002. p. 2–7.

[32] Li GL, Van Steeg TJ, Putter H, et al. Cutaneous side-effects of transdermal iontophoresis with and without surfactant pretreatment: a single-blinded, randomized controlled trial. Br J Dermatol. 2005;153:404–412.

[33] Smart WH, Subramanian K. The use of silicon microfabrication technology in painless blood glucose monitoring. Diabetes Technol Ther. 2000;2:549–559.

[34] Li CG, Lee CY, Lee K, et al. An optimized hollow microneedle for minimally invasive blood extraction. Biomed Microdevices. 2013;15:17–25.

[35] Stoeber B, Liepmann D. Arrays of hollow out-of-plane microneedles for drug delivery. J Microelectromechanical Syst. 2005;14:472–479.

[36] Ashraf MW, Tayyaba S, Nisar A, et al. Design, fabrication and analysis of silicon hollow microneedles for transdermal drug delivery system for treatment of hemodynamic dysfunctions. Cardiovasc Eng. 2010;10:91–108.

[37] Kim Y-C, Park J-H, Prausnitz MR. Microneedles for drug and vaccine delivery. Adv Drug Deliv Rev. 2012;64:1547–1568.

[38] Quinn HL, Kearney M-C, Courtenay AJ, et al. The role of microneedles for drug and vaccine delivery. Expert Opin Drug Deliv. 2014;11:1769–1780.

[39] Watkinson AC, Kearney M-C, Quinn HL, et al. Future of the transdermal drug delivery market-have we barely touched the surface? Expert Opin Drug Deliv. 2016;13:523–532.

[40] Gill HS, Prausnitz MR. Coated microneedles for transdermal delivery. J Control Release. 2007;117:227–237.

[41] Banga AK. Microneedle-mediated transdernal delivery: how to contribute to meaningful research to advance this growing field. Transdermal. 2009;1:8–13.

[42] Daddona P. Macroflux® transdermal technology development for the delivery of therapeutic peptides and proteins. Drug Deliv Technol. 2002;2.

[43] Kim Y-C, Quan F-S, Compans RW, et al. Formulation and coating of microneedles with inactivated influenza virus to improve vaccine stability and immunogenicity. J Control Release. 2010;142:187–195.

[44] Park J-H, Choi S-O, Kamath R, et al. Polymer particle-based micromolding to fabricate novel microstructures. Biomed Microdevices. 2007;9:223–234.

[45] Olatunji O, Igwe CC, Ahmed AS, et al. Microneedles from fish scale biopolymer. J Appl Polym Sci. 2014;131. [Internet] [cited 2016 Aug 13]. Available from: http://onlinelibrary.wiley.com/doi/10.1002/app.40377/full.

[46] Park J-H, Allen MG, Prausnitz MR. Biodegradable polymer microneedles: fabrication, mechanics and transdermal drug delivery. J Control Release. 2005;104:51–66.

[47] Ito Y, Hagiwara E, Saeki A, et al. Sustained-release self-dissolving micropiles for percutaneous absorption of insulin in mice. J Drug Target. 2007;15:323–326.

[48] Migalska K, Morrow DIJ, Garland MJ, et al. Laser-engineered dissolving microneedle arrays for transdermal macromolecular drug delivery. Pharm Res. 2011;28:1919–1930.

[49] Ito Y, Hagiwara E, Saeki A, et al. Feasibility of microneedles for percutaneous absorption of insulin. Eur J Pharm Sci. 2006;29:82–88.

[50] Lee JW, Park J-H, Prausnitz MR. Dissolving microneedles for transdermal drug delivery. Biomaterials. 2008;29:2113–2124.

[51] Donnelly RF, Garland MJ, Morrow DI, et al. Optical coherence tomography is a valuable tool in the study of the effects of microneedle geometry on skin penetration characteristics and in-skin dissolution. J Control Release. 2010;147:333–341.

[52] Mukerjee EV, Collins SD, Isseroff RR, et al. Microneedle array for transdermal biological fluid extraction and in situ analysis. Sens Actuators Phys. 2004;114:267–275.

[53] Donnelly RF, Mooney K, Caffarel-Salvador E, et al. Microneedle-mediated minimally invasive patient monitoring. Ther Drug Monit. 2014;36:10–17.

[54] Donnelly RF, Singh TRR, Garland MJ, et al. Hydrogel-forming microneedle arrays for enhanced transdermal drug delivery. Adv Funct Mater. 2012;22:4879–4890.

[55] Caffarel-Salvador E, Donnelly RF. Transdermal drug delivery mediated by microneedle arrays: innovations and barriers to success. Curr Pharm Des. 2016;22:1105–1117.

[56] Singh TRR, McCarron PA, Woolfson AD, et al. Investigation of swelling and network parameters of poly (ethylene glycol)-crosslinked poly (methyl vinyl ether-co-maleic acid) hydrogels. Eur Polym J. 2009;45:1239–1249.

[57] Donnelly RF, McCrudden MT, Alkilani AZ, et al. Hydrogel-forming microneedles prepared from "super swelling" polymers combined with lyophilised wafers for transdermal drug delivery. PLoS One. 2014;9:e111547.

[58] McCrudden MTC, Alkilani AZ, Courtenay AJ, et al. Considerations in the sterile manufacture of polymeric microneedle arrays. Drug Deliv Transl Res. 2015;5:3–14.

[59] Donnelly RF, Woolfson AD. Patient safety and beyond: what should we expect from microneedle arrays in the transdermal delivery arena? Ther Deliv. 2014;5:653–662.

[60] Jin T. Phase-transition polymeric microneedles. Google Patents; 2016. [Internet] [cited 2016 Aug 16]. Available from: www.google.com/patents/US9320878.

[61] Kim M, Jung B, Park J-H. Hydrogel swelling as a trigger to release biodegradable polymer microneedles in skin. Biomaterials. 2012;33:668–678.

[62] Qiu Y, Qin G, Zhang S, et al. Novel lyophilized hydrogel patches for convenient and effective administration of microneedle-mediated insulin delivery. Int J Pharm. 2012;437:51 56.

[63] Yang S, Feng Y, Zhang L, et al. A scalable fabrication process of polymer microneedles. Int J Nanomedicine. 2012;7:1415–1422.

[64] Ashique S, Khatun T, Upadhyay A, et al. Micro-needles as an effective drug delivery system and associated patents in pharmaceutical field: a review. Biol Sci. 2021;1:53–66.

[65] Queiroz MLB, Shanmugam S, Santos LNS, et al. Microneedles as an alternative technology for transdermal drug delivery systems: a patent review. Expert Opin Ther Pat. 2020;30:433–452.

[66] Donnelly RF, Singh TRR, Tunney MM, et al. Microneedle arrays allow lower microbial penetration than hypodermic needles in vitro. Pharm Res. 2009;26:2513–2522.

[67] Serhan H, Slivka M, Albert T, et al. Is galvanic corrosion between titanium alloy and stainless steel spinal implants a clinical concern? Spine J. 2004;4:379–387.

[68] Hoesly FJ, Borovicka J, Gordon J, et al. Safety of a novel microneedle device applied to facial skin: a subject-and rater-blinded, sham-controlled, randomized trial. Arch Dermatol. 2012;148:711–717.

[69] Kim M, Shin JY, Lee J, et al. Efficacy of fractional microneedle radiofrequency device in the treatment of primary axillary hyperhidrosis: a pilot study. Dermatology. 2013;227:243–249.

[70] Rouphael NG, Paine M, Mosley R, et al. The safety, immunogenicity, and acceptability of inactivated influenza vaccine delivered by microneedle patch (TIV-MNP 2015): a randomised, partly blinded, placebo-controlled, phase 1 trial. The Lancet. 2017;390:649–658.

[71] Zvezdin V, Peno-Mazzarino L, Radionov N, et al. Microneedle patch based on dissolving, detachable microneedle technology for improved skin quality–Part 1: ex vivo safety evaluation. Int J Cosmet Sci. 2020;42:369–376.

6

Microneedle-mediated Delivery of Small Molecules

6.1 Introduction

Approximately 40% of approved molecules have poor water solubility, and almost 90% of products in the development strategies are poorly soluble [1]. The water solubility of molecules approved in 1983 is ten times more than that of those approved in 2012. This fact poses a major challenge for drug development for the oral route of administration regarding drug absorption, bioavailability, and pharmacokinetic profiles. However, several poorly soluble compounds could be excellent candidates for transdermal drug delivery. On a market investigation, the global market of the transdermal delivery system is predicted to reach $81.4 billion by 2024. Most small molecules must be taken at a daily dose below 100 mg via the oral route. Transdermal patches need an estimated size of 10–30 cm^2 to deliver equivalence efficacy. This dimension is well-contained by the marketed patches such as Nicotinell® (nicotine, 30 cm^2, by Novartis, Basel, Switzerland) or Duragesic® CII (fentanyl) patches (32 and 42 cm^2 by Janssen, Beerse, Belgium). However, conventional transdermal drug delivery systems have certain limitations in their pharmacological efficiency: difficulty in precisely controlling the drug delivery due to low skin permeability, poor drug penetration through the stratum corneum, uncontrolled drug diffusion pattern, and nonspecific binding [2]. The stratum corneum layer forms a formidable obstacle to hindering the skin permeability of various molecules. Micrometer-sized needles (microneedles) could completely and effectively bypass this stratum corneum barrier, thus eliminating the dosing variability, creating a path for drug penetration, and facilitating enhanced drug delivery.

6.1.1 Advantages of Microneedles

Microneedles could be incorporated into a self-administrable transdermal patch which provides equivalent bioabsorption and bioavailability as conventional hypodermic needles [3]. Furthermore, microneedles offer several advantages, including, but not limited to, (i) possible delivery of macromolecules, (ii) minimally invasive and painless application, (iii) bypass first-pass metabolism, (iv) enhanced, controlled, and targeted drug delivery, (v) dose reduction, (vi) ease of administration and patient compliance, (vii) rapid healing at the treatment site to avoid infection or irritation, and (viii) low cost of production and distribution. Micrometer-sized needles are designed to be short enough to only penetrate the stratum corneum and part of the viable epidermis layer without deeply entering the dermis layer where the blood capillaries and nerve endings are located, thus avoiding causing pain or bleeding. By bypassing the major skin barrier, microneedles have been found to dramatically enhance the skin delivery of various therapeutic agents, including small

DOI: 10.1201/9780429294433-6

molecules, biotherapeutics, macromolecules, vaccines, micro/nanoparticles, and other materials. The application of microneedles allows a controlled kinetic of drug release. The process of drug release from microneedles consists of two steps: (i) drug transportation from the inner polymeric matrix to the outer surface and (ii) drug release into the surrounding skin tissue [4].

A microneedle array enables rapid bolus drug release and delivery. Also, microneedle formulation could be adjusted to attain sustained-release delivery, where the drug is released slowly from a skin depot formed by the gradual dissolution of the polymeric needles or the coating layer. Interestingly, microneedles could be customized to provide sustained drug delivery where the encapsulated drug is released at a predetermined rate to maintain a steady-state drug level for a certain period and to minimize any potential adverse effects [5] (Table 6.1). Sustainably releasing microneedles helps reduce the frequency of drug administration, decreases product cost, minimizes forgotten or missed doses, reduces the risk of infection (compared to intravenous or intramuscular routes of administration), and improves patient compliance [6, 7]. Altering the polymeric structure, the encapsulation process, or the characteristics of the encapsulated compounds could all affect the release profile of the drug.

When instant or burst drug release is desirable, the needles could penetrate the stratum corneum, dissolve quickly, and immediately release the encapsulated drug load [12]. Rapidly dissolving microneedles could instantly release the drug at the maximum level to the targeted site of action with rapid onset. Burst drug release has proved beneficial in the treatment of various diseases (Table 6.2). This delivery system deems meaningful in analgesia, wound healing, and gene, peptide, and protein delivery in tissue repair [13]. The rapid release allows microneedles to deliver drugs painlessly that are generally administered by intramuscular or intravenous routes. The rapid release could be managed by several factors, such as polymer surface properties, polymer–drug interactions, and the porous structure of the materials [12].

TABLE 6.1

Sustained Drug Release from Polymeric Microneedles

Therapeutics/Drugs	Molecular Weight	Polymer	Release Time	Reference
Levonorgestrel	312.4 Da	PLA/PLGA	30 days	[8]
Etonogestrel	324.5 Da	PVA/HPMC	7 days	[9]
Rhodamine B	479.0 Da	PLGA/poly-*N*-isopropyl acrylamide	3 days	[10]
Doxorubicin	543.5 Da	Gelatin methacryloyl	≤1 day	[11]

TABLE 6.2

Instant Release of Small Molecules from Polymeric Microneedles

Therapeutics/Drugs	Molecular Weight	Polymer	Release Time	Reference
Bleomycin	1415.6 Da	PLA	15 min	[14]
Acyclovir	225.2 Da	Gantrez S-97	15 min	[15]
Artemether	298.4 Da	HA	120 min	[16]
Dihydroergotamine mesylate	679.8 Da	PVP	2 min	[17]
Meloxicam	351.4 Da	PVP	30 min	[18]
Sumatriptan	295.4 Da	Dextran/HA	30 min	[19]

6.1.2 Disadvantages of Microneedles

Most small molecules with a molecular weight of less than 500 Da could permeate into the skin to a certain extent by passive diffusion, depending on their physicochemical properties [20]. However, delivering a sufficiently required dose for therapeutic effects is challenging. Thus, microneedles have been used to enhance the transdermal and intradermal delivery of various small molecules [21–23]. Hydrophilic compounds face a major physical barrier of the stratum corneum layer, while lipophilic compound could diffuse into the stratum corneum and is locked in this layer without further penetrating the hydrophilic epidermis layer. Furthermore, most lipophilic compounds require organic solvents for solubilization, making it more challenging to reach the market [24]. Most small molecules need a high dose for their treatment function. However, microneedles could coat or encapsulate a very limited drug quantity. In specific, a typical needle could contain 0.1–1 µg drug. Thus, only 10–100 µg drug could be delivered with an array consisting of 100 microneedles. If the number of microneedles increases, leading to high needle density, then the "bed of nail" effect will also increase dramatically, resulting in reduced insertion efficiency of microneedles. Among all microneedle types, hollow and solid microneedles (poke and patch method), in which the drug reservoir (i.e., drug concentration and volume) has negligible impact on the properties, design, and performance of microneedles, could allow the large dose of transdermal drug delivery. Due to the excellent diffusion coefficient, these low-molecular-weight molecules could diffuse into skin tissues more easily and rapidly. Besides, there is a risk of skin irritation with microneedle treatment. The needles can break and remain in skin tissue, causing a biosafety concern. Also, the skin's viscoelasticity and hydration level could affect the performance of microneedles.

6.2 Drug Properties for Microneedle Use

To date, more than 20 low-molecular-weight compounds have been approved for transdermal delivery by the US Food and Drug Administration, leading to a \$32 billion global transdermal delivery market [25]. The physicochemical properties of the drug determine its capacity to penetrate the skin. The permeation extent of the drugs is affected by various factors. An ideal candidate for skin delivery possesses (i) low molecular weight (<400 Da), (ii) large diffusion/partition coefficient, (iii) low ionization degree, (iv) low skin binding, (v) suitable solubility in oil and water, (vi) suitable pK, (vii) low melting point, (viii) low dose, and (ix) moderate lipophilicity (hydrophilic molecules with low log P [<1] cannot effectively penetrate the stratum corneum by passive diffusion, while lipophilic molecules with high log P [>3] would be entrapped in the intercellular lipids in the stratum corneum layer without further partitioning into the aqueous environment of the viable epidermis) [26–29].

Microneedles are an effective platform to enhance the delivery of hydrophilic compounds. These molecules could be delivered into and across the skin rapidly and at a large dose. Physical treatment with microneedles disrupts the lipophilic stratum corneum layer—the primary skin barrier, to place the drugs into the hydrophilic viable epidermis, thus, shortening the diffusion pathway. However, the delivery-enhancement efficacy of microneedles for lipophilic compounds is limited. These molecules must be dissolved in organic solvents, thus leading to nonhomogeneity within the needle matrix and aggregation with hydrophilic polymers. Organic solvents also weaken the structure and backbones of microneedles, creating multiple pores in the needles' polymeric matrix [30]. To address this issue, lipophilic drugs in powder form should be encapsulated uniformly in the needle without the use of organic solvents [31]. Besides, particulate systems could be used, or the drug's physicochemical properties could be modified for the effective encapsulation or coating into microneedles.

6.3 Microneedle Design for Delivery of Small Molecules

6.3.1 Solid Microneedles

The majority of low-molecular-weight compounds are delivered into and across the skin using the physical pretreatment of solid microneedles (i.e., silicon, glass, metal, or polymeric microneedles). Microneedle insertion disrupts the skin barrier, thus increasing the skin permeability to various extents, depending on the physicochemical properties of the permeants and the applied formulation. Pretreatment with solid microneedles enables the delivery of a large dose greater than the loading capacity of coated and dissolving microneedles. Furthermore, extended and controlled delivery of drugs through microneedles-created channels could be achieved. The drug could easily diffuse from the formulation into skin tissue as long as the channels remain open. These channels have been reported to reseal after a certain period.

6.3.2 Coated Microneedles

Various therapeutic agents have been successfully coated onto microneedles for enhanced delivery, such as fluorescein [32], sulforhodamine [33], calcein [34], vitamin B [34], pilocarpine [33], and lidocaine [35]. Since the thickness of the coating layer is limited, the quantity of coated drugs is also very limited. Thus, potent compounds with low required doses are preferable. Wearing lidocaine-coated microneedles for 1–5 min was found to provide comparable tissue concentration to EMLA® cream (1 h topical application). Due to its limited surface area, only 225 μg lidocaine could be loaded on coated microneedles array [35].

6.3.3 Hollow Microneedles

Hollow microneedles could be used to deliver a large quantity of drugs in liquid formulations into the skin tissue. For example, a large dose of lidocaine has been successfully administered through hollow microneedles. However, the hollow microneedles system consists of several components, thus being bulky and complicated. It is challenging for patients to use the system by themselves or to use the device for an extended period [36].

6.3.4 Dissolving Microneedles

Even though solid and hollow microneedles enable the administration of a sufficiently large dose, these microneedles could pose a significant biosafety risk of needle fracture in the skin. Dissolving biodegradable polymeric microneedles is a promising, safe, and reliable alternative to address this issue. The quantity of drug encapsulated in dissolving microneedles is markedly greater than the limited amount that could be coated on the surface of solid microneedles. Lee and colleagues first designed the backing layer of the microneedle array as the drug reservoir for a larger drug-loading dose. A maximum quantity of 1–3 mg could be encapsulated in the needles [37]. A simple photolithography technique could be used to fabricate polymeric microneedles, which are capable of loading 3–4 mg of drug [38]. To improve the drug-loading capacity of microneedle arrays, Ito and colleagues revealed the process of attaching drug-loaded chips (produced by depositing a drug-polymer glue inside the molds of tableting equipment) to polymeric microneedle arrays (prepared using the standard micromolding technology) [39]. Consequently, a drug-loading capacity of approximately 12 mg was obtained. Also, this type of microneedles does not require a separate reservoir as the drug source, as in solid and hollow microneedles.

6.3.5 Swelling Microneedles

Swelling microneedles were first fabricated in 2012, thus being the most recent design of microneedles. These needles are produced from a swellable polymer such as cross-linked hydrogels. Swelling microneedles have a different working mechanism from other microneedle types: upon skin insertion, these needles absorb skin interstitial fluid and swell. Drugs could be encapsulated into the polymeric matrix (as in dissolving microneedles) or loaded into a separate reservoir attached on top of the microneedles array (drug releases from the reservoir and diffuses into skin tissue through swelling pores in the hydrogel material). This design of microneedles enables a large drug-loading capacity and controlled drug release kinetics. Hydrogel-forming microneedles could deliver three doses of 60 mg ibuprofen over 160 h [40]. Likewise, reservoir patches of metformin HCl (75 and 50 mg drug) were attached to swelling microneedle to sustainably deliver a high dose of 28 and 23 mg at 24 h, respectively [41]. Hydrogel material is biocompatible, biodegradable, and nontoxic, thus minimizing biosafety issues. Furthermore, the needles could be removed intact after the skin insertion, leaving no polymer in the skin. Swelling microneedles have been reported to enhance the delivery of various small molecules, including donepezil [42], esketamine [43], caffeine, lidocaine hydrochloride [44], ibuprofen [40, 45], and metformin HCl [41].

6.4 Case Studies

Various low-molecular-weight compounds have been delivered into and across the skin using microneedles. A potent molecule to treat warts, bleomycin, is generally administered via intralesional injection. User-friendly PLA microneedles have been reported to enhance the delivery of bleomycin, with more than 80% drug released within 15 min. Thus, microneedles could be a promising technology for wart treatment [14].

Tas et al. fabricated drug-loaded dissolving polyvinylpyrrolidone (PVP) microneedles to enhance transdermal delivery of dihydroergotamine mesylate, an ergot derivative to treat moderate to severe acute migraine. The use of microneedles was revealed to provide painless administration, rapid onset, and enhanced bioavailability. Mechanically strong and uniform PVP microneedles dissolved in skin *ex vivo* within 2 min of insertion. In an *in vivo* pharmacokinetic study on hairless rats, the area under the curve and appreciable plasma levels were comparable to subcutaneous injection [17].

Similarly, microneedles have been employed to enhance transdermal delivery of acyclovir, a small molecule (molecular weight of 225.21 Da) with poor skin permeability (log P = −1.6) used to treat herpes labialis. Pamornpathomkul and coworkers fabricated acyclovir-encapsulated dissolving microneedles from Gantrez S-97. The needles were sharp and strong and could rapidly dissolve within 15 min. The use of microneedles led to a 45-fold enhancement of skin permeability compared to conventional cream products [15]. In another study, Yan and colleagues pretreated skin with solid silicon microneedles with varying needle lengths and density to increase the drug quantity delivered into the skin. The insertion of 600-μm-long microneedles resulted in a 2–8 fold enhancement in the drug delivery, while a 50–100-fold increase could be achieved with longer microneedles. However, increasing the needle density from 2,000 to 5,625 needles/cm² reduced the enhancement magnitude of the delivery flux due to the "bed of nails" effect [46].

A poorly water-soluble model drug, artemether, has been loaded into dissolving oligomeric sodium hyaluronate microneedles in a suspension formulation. The use of microneedles could deliver 72% of the initial drug-loading dose into the skin. In a pharmacokinetic study on rats, a dose-dependent profile of drug plasma level was reported with the area under the curve and bioavailability equivalent to intramuscular injection. In a pharmacodynamic study on collagen-induced arthritis rats, artemether-encapsulated microneedles could reverse paw edema in a similar way as intramuscular injection [16]. Similarly, Hutton and coworkers loaded vitamin K into dissolving microneedles (made from Gantrez® S-97). In an *in vitro* permeation study on neonatal porcine skin, vitamin K-encapsulated microneedles could deliver 1.80 mg drug into the skin after 24 h. Thus, microneedles could replace the painful conventional intramuscular injection to treat vitamin K deficiency bleeding [47].

Naltrexone, a mu-opioid receptor antagonist, is administered orally to treat alcohol and opioid addiction. First-pass metabolism has been a significant hurdle for therapeutic efficacy. Microneedle poration has been reported to enhance skin delivery of naltrexone through guinea pigs and human skin [48–51]. Furthermore, the elevated drug plasma level was maintained for three days [52]. In another study, microneedles pretreatment significantly increases skin delivery of naltrexone [51]. Stainless steel microneedles (650 μm long and 50 needles on an array) porated the skin before the application of a naltrexone-loaded transdermal patch. As a result, the microneedles treatment group achieved the steady-state plasma concentration of naltrexone within 2 h and maintained the level for 48 h, while only a negligible drug plasma concentration was reported in the untreated control group over 72 h. Drug ionization has been employed to alter drug diffusion into and across the skin. Banks and colleagues studied how the ionization of naltrexone affected its permeation across hairless guinea pigs and human skin *in vitro* [48]. The authors revealed that naltrexone base had greater skin permeability than its hydrochloride salt by passive diffusion. However, the opposite was obtained when the skin was treated with an array of 750-μm-long stainless steel microneedles (50 microneedles on the array). In particular, the steady-state flux of the hydrochloride salt was three times higher than that of the base. Interestingly, microneedles treatment caused no improvement in the permeation of the base whose diffusion pathway was not related to the creation of aqueous channels in the skin. Thus, the impact of microneedles pretreatment depends on the physicochemical properties of the compound, especially ionization form and solubility. In another investigation performed by the Prausnitz group, microneedle-mediated delivery of the free base and hydrochloride salt of 6β-naltrexol was studied on hairless guinea pig *in vivo*. The drug-loaded hydroxyethylcellulose-based gel was applied on skin which was previously treated by an array of 50 stainless steel microneedles (750 μm microneedles length).

Consequently, the needles pretreatment resulted in 5- and 20-fold enhancement in the steady-state plasma concentration of the base and salt form, respectively. A follow-up study using naltrexone hydrochloride was carried out on healthy human volunteers [51]. Stainless steel microneedles (50 microneedles of 620 μm length) were used to treat the patients before the application of the drug-loaded patch. No drug was passively delivered into intact, untreated skin after 72 h period, while the needles pretreatment led to a steady-state plasma concentration of 2.5 ng/mL over 48 h. Enhanced delivery of naltrexone was investigated using water-soluble PEGylated naltrexone prodrug [53] and a naltrexone formulation consisting of propylene glycol and water [54] in an *in vitro* permeation study using Yucatan minipig skin. However, the expected enhancement was not obtained due to the nonlinear correlation between the prodrug concentration and the delivery flux and the increase in the formulation viscosity, which negatively affected the drug permeation. PEGylation significantly increases the drug's aqueous solubility; however, it resulted in a negligible enhancement in the skin delivery as compared to the parent molecule.

Microneedle-mediated delivery of lipophilic drugs such as Nile red and capsaicin has been reported by Dangol et al. previously (Fig. 6.1). The authors developed a solvent-free lipophilic system using a mixture of a hydrophilic polymer and a hydrophobic polymer to dissolve the lipophilic drugs and formulate nanoparticles which were then loaded into dissolving microneedles by drawing lithography technique. As a result, microneedles provided a substantially greater quantity and faster onset of *in vitro* and *in vivo* delivery of these compounds than topical formulation [31].

Naloxone (327 Da), a μ-opioid receptor antagonist, has a major issue of high first-pass hepatic metabolism and low bioavailability (about 2%) after oral administration. Thus, the drug is often administered by intravenous, intramuscular, or subcutaneous injection. Burton and coworkers employed microneedles pretreatment to increase the drug's

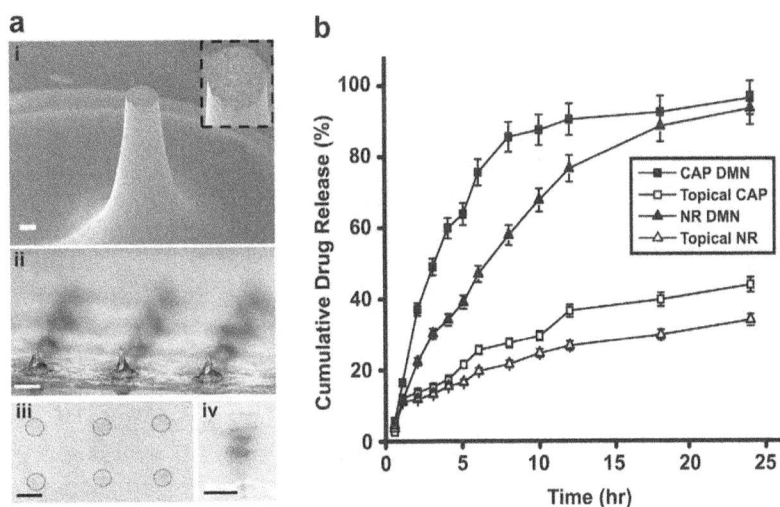

FIGURE 6.1
Schematic representation of Nile red–loaded and capsaicin-loaded dissolving microneedles with an innovative polymeric system (IPS). (a) Nile red–loaded microneedles—(i) scanning electron microscopic image, (ii) bright-field microscopic image, (iii) brightfield microscopic image of porcine skin treated by Nile red–loaded microneedles, and (iv) the histological section of porcine skin treated by Nile red–loaded microneedles. (b) Drug release profiles of Nile red and capsaicin from topical formulations and dissolving microneedles. Images reprinted with permission from [31].

transdermal delivery. In an *in vivo* experiment on domestic swine, the use of solid microneedles resulted in a similar delivery profile compared to subcutaneous injection [55]. Enhanced skin delivery of caffeine and lidocaine HCl was reported with the use of dissolving and hydrogel-forming swelling microneedles. These drug-loaded microneedles resulted in greater drug delivery across dermatomed skin than the respective patch or cream formulation [56]. A 6.1-fold enhancement of caffeine delivery was obtained with swelling microneedles.

Similarly, a large quantity of ibuprofen could be delivered to the skin with the aid of hydrogel-forming swelling microneedles. This needle array could encapsulate 42.5 mg ibuprofen sodium; after 24 h permeation study, about 78% of the loaded quantity was delivered across neonatal porcine skin *in vitro* [57]. Interestingly, hydrogel-forming microneedles provided a burst release at 5 min, followed by the plateau of drug level in the receptor compartment by 4 h. When the drug was loaded into lyophilized wafers, the drug permeation profile *in vitro* was typically the first order, delivering approximately 44 mg (37%) drug across porcine skin in 24 h [45]. Hardy and colleagues fabricated light-responsive materials using a light-responsive ibuprofen conjugate. As a result, the authors could deliver three doses of 60 mg ibuprofen in 160 h [40].

Microneedles have been employed to assist in the delivery of phenylephrine, which is used to treat fecal incontinence. Jun and coworkers injected phenylephrine solution into the anal sphincter of rats via a hollow microneedle, producing local targeted drug delivery in the sphincter muscle. This minimally invasive injection led to a significant increase in resting anal sphincter pressure [58]. In another study, the skin was pretreated with solid microneedles before the topical application of phenylephrine formulation for enhanced local drug delivery. The authors reported an increase in the mean resting anal sphincter pressure in rats in the microneedle treatment group, as compared to the untreated control group [59].

Nicardipine hydrochloride administration with the use of microneedles was investigated in both laboratory and animal setups. Miyano et al. prepared maltose-based dissolving microneedles (500-μm-long pyramidal-shaped microneedles) encapsulated with nicardipine HCl. The needles dissolved within 5 min after the skin insertion. Four times as much flux was observed in the microneedles-treated group compared to the control group. Furthermore, microneedle treatment caused no pain in volunteer subjects [60]. Differently, Kolli and Banga used maltose microneedles (an array of 6×27 microneedles of 500 μm length) to porate hairless rat skin *in vivo* before the application of the drug-loaded formulation. As a result, the microneedle treatment led to significantly higher C_{max} and AUC values than the untreated group. Specifically, C_{max} was 56.45 ng/mL after 7 h in the microneedle treatment group, while passive diffusion of the drug through untreated skin could only result in C_{max} of less than 20 ng/mL after 8 h [61].

Donnelly and colleagues fabricated theophylline-loaded dissolving polymeric microneedles from poly(methyl vinyl ether-*co*-maleic anhydride) using the micromolding technique. Theophylline is a hydrophilic compound with a log P of −0.8 and a molecular weight of 180 Da. The authors revealed that the use of microneedles resulted in a markedly greater drug accumulative delivery across porcine skin [62]. The authors also performed a comparison between drug-loaded microneedles and patches with comparable drug-loading quantities. There was negligible drug permeation after 4 h application of the patch, whereas drug-loaded microneedles could deliver the drug to the skin within only 5 min. The patch delivered 5.5% of the drug load, while the microneedle array could deliver 83% of the drug load across the skin tissue after 24 h [62].

Lidocaine has been efficiently delivered into the skin for local anesthesia after the insertion of coated, hollow, and dissolving microneedles. Ma and Gill fabricated lidocaine-loaded coated microneedles using polyethylene glycol matrix as the coating formulation. The authors reported uniform coating on the needle surface and a significantly higher delivery of lidocaine in 3 min with PEG-lidocaine-coated microneedles compared to 1 h topical delivery of lidocaine from the commercial EMLA® product [63]. Similarly, Zhang et al. coated lidocaine-loaded polymeric formulation on 3M's solid microstructured transdermal system and inserted the needles in domestic swine. As a result, lidocaine is released quickly from the needles and diffused rapidly into skin tissue within 1 min of microneedles-wearing time. The lidocaine level was sufficiently high to cause prolonged local analgesia [35]. In research, lidocaine was administered to human participants using an intradermal hypodermic needle or hollow microneedles. The authors revealed comparable local anesthesia caused by either injection method. The human subjects experienced less pain and a stronger preference for microneedle-based injection [36]. Kwon and coworkers fabricated lidocaine-encapsulated dissolving microneedles from sodium carboxymethyl cellulose by micromolding technique. The results showed that the microneedle insertion led to a threefold enhancement in the flux through human skin compared to the passive diffusion of the drug from a solution [64].

Several groups have used microneedles to increase transdermal delivery of anticancer drugs such as methotrexate, 5-fluorouracil, and doxorubicin. Microneedle insertion increased the transdermal flux of 5-fluorouracil by 4.5-fold and enhanced *in vivo* delivery of the drug to mouse melanoma cells compared to commercially available topical cream [65]. Docetaxel was encapsulated into elastic liposomes for enhanced transdermal delivery through microneedles-porated skin [66]. Luo et al. achieved enhanced and sustained delivery of a chemotherapeutic agent, doxorubicin, using the drug-loaded biodegradable microneedles made from gelatin methacryloyl [13]. Similarly, doxorubicin solution was applied on maltose microneedles-pretreated human skin *in vitro*. The needle insertion led to a marked enhancement in the drug permeability and a reduction in lag time ($p < 0.05$) [67]. In another study, doxorubicin was encapsulated in different locations within the poly(vinyl alcohol) array. The needles were found to be sharp, mechanically robust, and uniform. The *in vitro* drug permeation was significantly enhanced through microneedle-treated skin as compared to the untreated group ($p < 0.01$) [68]. Nguyen et al. fabricated poly(D,L-lactide-*co*-glycolide) acid microneedles by micromolding technique. The microneedles pretreatment substantially increased *in vitro* transdermal delivery of methotrexate across the dermatomed porcine ear and human cadaver skin [69]. Likewise, enhanced delivery of vismodegib was studied on porcine ear skin with regard to needle length (maltose microneedles, Admin Pen™ 1200, and Admin Pen™ 1500), skin equilibration, and microneedle insertion durations. The microneedle treatment resulted in a significant increase in skin permeability. The cumulative amount of drug delivered increased with the needle length. A correlation was reported between the drug permeation and microneedle treatment duration [70].

In vitro transdermal delivery of verapamil hydrochloride and amlodipine besylate has been enhanced using a microneedles roller device (multiple metal microneedles are arranged on a rolling cylinder) and Adminpatch stainless steel microneedle array. The flux of verapamil delivery through porcine skin increased about six times from 8.75 to 49.96 µg/cm²/h after microneedle roller treatment. While the flux of amlodipine besylate increased substantially by 14-fold from 1.57 µg/cm²/h by passive diffusion to 22.39 µg/cm²/h in the microneedles-treated group [71]. Similarly, stainless steel solid microneedles rollers (750 µm long) have been used to facilitate the delivery of captopril and metoprolol tartrate into and across porcine skin *in vitro*. The insertion of microneedles led to a marked increase in the transdermal flux of captopril from 75 µg/cm²/h to 608 µg/cm²/h and the flux of metoprolol tartrate from 62 μg/cm²/h to 291 μg/cm²/h [72]. Likewise, Park and colleagues developed a roller ball device with biodegradable polymeric microneedles (600 μm long) made of polylactic acid and carboxymethylcellulose to improve the delivery of acetylsalicylic acid (a hydrophilic small molecule with a molecular weight of 180 Da). As a result, 21- and 47-fold enhancement of the drug's transdermal delivery was noted when 100 and 200 microchannels were created on the skin by the microneedle device [73]. In another investigation, Wei-Ze and coworkers used super-short microneedles to facilitate the delivery of galantamine across hairless rat skin (a moderately lipophilic small molecule, molecular weight of 287 Da, log P of 1.09) [74]. The authors fabricated two microneedle designs: sharp-tipped (75 μm long) and flat-tipped (80 μm long) solid silicon microneedles. The needles were inserted into the skin by a swaying technique where a finger was rolled on the array substrate, followed by the removal of the microneedle array and the application of galantamine solution (0.5%). The authors reported a significant enhancement in the drug flux when the applied force was more than 5 N. Furthermore, flat-tipped microneedles were superior to sharp-tipped microneedles in enhancing drug delivery. Also, increasing the number on the array resulted in a marked increase in drug delivery [75]. Gardeniers and colleagues used a hollow silicon microneedle array (350 μm long) to enhance skin delivery of diclofenac *in vivo*. A microneedle array attached to a drug-loaded patch was inserted into Sprague-Dawley rats. Microneedle treatment was reported to enhance drug delivery across the skin by several folds [76]. Sivamani and workers injected a liquid formulation of methyl nicotinate (molecular weight of 137 Da) into healthy human volunteers with the use of silicon hollow microneedles (200 μm long). The authors found that the injection through pointed hollow microneedles led to greater drug flux as compared to that through symmetric microneedles [77]. This research group also investigated the delivery of hexyl nicotinate (low molecular weight of 207 Da, a lipophilic vasodilator) in human subjects with the aid of hollow silicon microneedles [78]. Microneedles were found to successfully inject the drug through the stratum corneum, as demonstrated by laser doppler imaging. Hydrogel-forming swelling microneedles have been used to facilitate transdermal and intradermal delivery of various small molecules. Kearney and associates developed hydrogel-forming microneedles to improve the transdermal transport of donepezil hydrochloride for the management of moderate dementia in Alzheimer's disease. The authors could obtain the mean drug release of 855 μg drug in 24 h with an increase in the drug serum level over time. The drug was loaded in a separate reservoir rather than inside the needle matrix. Thus, the loading capacity of swelling microneedles was substantial as compared to dissolving microneedles [42]. Courtenay and coworkers fabricated swelling microneedles to facilitate transdermal delivery of esketamine, a small lipophilic molecule used for treatment-resistant depression (log P = 3.3, molecular weight = 238 Da). The authors reported 24 h drug plasma concentration of 0.26–0.498 μg/mL in rodents [43]. Migdadi et al. could achieve sustained delivery of a large dose of metformin hydrochloride by using hydrogel-forming microneedles [41]. The attached reservoir patch contained 50 and 75 mg drug to deliver 23 and 28 mg drug across the skin over 24 h study, respectively. The enhanced delivery of various small molecules has been reported, such as mannitol [79], cascade blue [80], chondroitin sulfate, dyclonine for topical anesthesia [81], topical photodynamic therapy such as 5-aminolevulinic acid or 5-aminolevulinic acid methyl ester, performed photosensitizer *meso*-tetra(N-methyl-4-pyridyl)porphinetetratosylate [82–84].

Numerous clinical trials have been executed to demonstrate the enhanced transdermal and intradermal delivery of small molecules using microneedles. Gupta et al. performed a randomized, single-blinded clinical study with a minimally invasive injection of lidocaine through hollow borosilicate microneedles (500 μm long). Lidocaine was injected into the forearm of 15 human subjects. The pain and numbness were compared between microneedle treatment and conventional intradermal injection using hypodermic needles. Microneedle therapy was shown to be substantially less intrusive than hypodermic needle injection, as measured by the visual analog (VAS) score. Furthermore, a comparable area or depth of anesthesia was induced by both methods. Even though microneedle injection consumed more time (20–40 s) to deliver a volume of 100–200 μL compared to 3–5 s with hypodermic needle injection, microneedle treatment provided lower pain scores and numbness degree. Moreover, microneedle-based lidocaine injection enabled less pain, rapid onset, and efficacy of local anesthesia as intradermal lidocaine injection [36]. Li and coworkers carried out a randomized, double-blind clinical trial in which microneedle treatment enhanced the effectiveness of topical anesthesia. Dyclonine-loaded cream was applied to 25 healthy human volunteers after microneedle pretreatment. The microneedle group required a markedly shorter time for pain reduction as compared to a sham device [81]. Similar findings were shown in a phase IIb/III clinical trial comparing three different dosages of zolmitriptan-loaded adhesive dermally applied microarray (ADAM) for the management of acute migraine (NCT02745392). As a result, ADAM zolmitriptan 3.8 mg was found well-tolerated and effective in treating migraine headaches [85].

6.5 Conclusions

Microneedles have been found to effectively facilitate the delivery of various small molecules with a wide range of solubility, hydrophilicity, and molecular weight. The enhancing effect was more significant for hydrophilic molecules than lipophilic compounds as microneedles treatment punctured the stratum corneum and allowed the drug to directly reach the aqueous environment of the viable epidermis layer. Various types of microneedles have been used with small molecules, such as solid, coated, dissolving, and swelling microneedles. This chapter also discusses numerous *in vitro*, *in vivo*, and clinical case studies to demonstrate the safety and efficacy of microneedles treatment.

References

[1] Siddalingappa B, Nekkanti V, Betageri GV. Insoluble drug delivery technologies: review of health benefits and business potentials. OA Drug Des Deliv. 2013;1:1.

[2] Langer R. Drug delivery and targeting. Nature. 1998;392:5–10.

[3] Lim D-J, Vines JB, Park H, et al. Microneedles: a versatile strategy for transdermal delivery of biological molecules. Int J Biol Macromol. 2018;110:30–38.

[4] Langer R. New methods of drug delivery. Sci. 1990;249:1527–1533.

[5] Chou S-F, Carson D, Woodrow KA. Current strategies for sustaining drug release from electrospun nanofibers. J Control Release. 2015;220:584–591.

[6] Hong X, Wei L, Wu F, et al. Dissolving and biodegradable microneedle technologies for transdermal sustained delivery of drug and vaccine. Drug Des Devel Ther. 2013;7:945–952.

[7] Natarajan JV, Nugraha C, Ng XW, et al. Sustained-release from nanocarriers: a review. J Control Release. 2014;193:122–138.

[8] Li W, Terry RN, Tang J, et al. Rapidly separable microneedle patch for the sustained release of a contraceptive. Nat Biomed Eng. 2019;3:220–229.

[9] He M, Yang G, Zhang S, et al. Dissolving microneedles loaded with etonogestrel microcrystal particles for intradermal sustained delivery. J Pharm Sci. 2018;107:1037–1045.

[10] Kim M, Jung B, Park J-H. Hydrogel swelling as a trigger to release biodegradable polymer microneedles in skin. Biomaterials. 2012;33:668–678.

[11] Luo Z, Sun W, Fang J, et al. Biodegradable gelatin methacryloyl microneedles for transdermal drug delivery. Adv Healthc Mater. 2019;8:1801054.

[12] Huang X, Brazel CS. On the importance and mechanisms of burst release in matrix-controlled drug delivery systems. J Control Release. 2001;73:121–136.

[13] Parrilla M, Cuartero M, Padrell Sánchez S, et al. Wearable all-solid-state potentiometric microneedle patch for intradermal potassium detection. Anal Chem. 2018;91:1578–1586.

[14] Lee HS, Ryu HR, Roh JY, et al. Bleomycin-coated microneedles for treatment of warts. Pharm Res. 2017;34:101–112.

[15] Pamornpathomkul B, Ngawhirunpat T, Tekko IA, et al. Dissolving polymeric microneedle arrays for enhanced site-specific acyclovir delivery. Eur J Pharm Sci. 2018;121:200–209.

[16] Qiu Y, Li C, Zhang S, et al. Systemic delivery of artemether by dissolving microneedles. Int J Pharm. 2016;508:1–9.

[17] Tas C, Joyce JC, Nguyen HX, et al. Dihydroergotamine mesylate-loaded dissolving microneedle patch made of polyvinylpyrrolidone for management of acute migraine therapy. J Control Release. 2017;268:159–165.

[18] Chen J, Huang W, Huang Z, et al. Fabrication of tip-dissolving microneedles for transdermal drug delivery of meloxicam. AAPS PharmSciTech. 2018;19:1141–1151.

[19] Ito Y, Kashiwara S, Fukushima K, et al. Two-layered dissolving microneedles for percutaneous delivery of sumatriptan in rats. Drug Dev Ind Pharm. 2011;37:1387–1393.

[20] Bos JD, Meinardi MM. The 500 Dalton rule for the skin penetration of chemical compounds and drugs. Exp Dermatol Viewp. 2000;9:165–169.

[21] Dangol M, Kim S, Li CG, et al. Anti-obesity effect of a novel caffeine-loaded dissolving microneedle patch in high-fat diet-induced obese C57BL/6J mice. J Control Release. 2017;265:41–47.

[22] González-Vázquez P, Larrañeta E, McCrudden MT, et al. Transdermal delivery of gentamicin using dissolving microneedle arrays for potential treatment of neonatal sepsis. J Control Release. 2017;265:30–40.

[23] Macedo CG, Jain AK, Franz-Montan M, et al. Microneedles enhance topical delivery of 15-deoxy-Δ12, 14-prostaglandin J2 and reduce nociception in temporomandibular joint of rats. J Control Release. 2017;265:22–29.

[24] Vora LK, Vavia PR, Larrañeta E, et al. Novel nanosuspension-based dissolving microneedle arrays for transdermal delivery of a hydrophobic drug. J Interdiscip Nanomedicine. 2018;3:89–101.

[25] Amjadi M, Sheykhansari S, Nelson BJ, et al. Recent advances in wearable transdermal delivery systems. Adv Mater. 2018;30:1704530.

[26] Hearn EM, Patel DR, Lepore BW, et al. Transmembrane passage of hydrophobic compounds through a protein channel wall. Nature. 2009;458:367–370.

[27] Ita KB. Transdermal drug delivery: progress and challenges. J Drug Deliv Sci Technol. 2014;24:245–250.

[28] Prausnitz MR, Langer R. Transdermal drug delivery. Nat Biotechnol. 2008;26:1261–1268.

[29] Schoellhammer CM, Blankschtein D, Langer R. Skin permeabilization for transdermal drug delivery: recent advances and future prospects. Expert Opin Drug Deliv. 2014;11:393–407.

[30] Santora BP, Gagné MR, Moloy KG, et al. Porogen and cross-linking effects on the surface area, pore volume distribution, and morphology of macroporous polymers obtained by bulk polymerization. Macromolecules. 2001;34:658–661.

[31] Dangol M, Yang H, Li CG, et al. Innovative polymeric system (IPS) for solvent-free lipophilic drug transdermal delivery via dissolving microneedles. J Control Release. 2016;223:118–125.

[32] Gill HS, Prausnitz MR. Pocketed microneedles for drug delivery to the skin. J Phys Chem Solids. 2008;69:1537–1541.

[33] Jiang J, Gill HS, Ghate D, et al. Coated microneedles for drug delivery to the eye. Invest Ophthalmol Vis Sci. 2007;48:4038–4043.

[34] Gill HS, Prausnitz MR. Coated microneedles for transdermal delivery. J Control Release. 2007;117:227–237.

[35] Zhang Y, Brown K, Siebenaler K, et al. Development of lidocaine-coated microneedle product for rapid, safe, and prolonged local analgesic action. Pharm Res. 2012;29:170–177.

[36] Gupta J, Denson DD, Felner EI, et al. Rapid local anesthesia in humans using minimally invasive microneedles. Clin J Pain. 2012;28:129–135.

[37] Lee JW, Park J-H, Prausnitz MR. Dissolving microneedles for transdermal drug delivery. Biomaterials. 2008;29:2113–2124.

[38] Kochhar JS, Goh WJ, Chan SY, et al. A simple method of microneedle array fabrication for transdermal drug delivery. Drug Dev Ind Pharm. 2013;39:299–309.

[39] Ito Y, Hamasaki N, Higashino H, et al. Method to increase the systemically delivered amount of drug from dissolving microneedles. Chem Pharm Bull (Tokyo). 2013;61:8–15.

[40] Hardy JG, Larrañeta E, Donnelly RF, et al. Hydrogel-forming microneedle arrays made from light-responsive materials for on-demand transdermal drug delivery. Mol Pharm. 2016;13:907–914.

[41] Migdadi EM, Courtenay AJ, Tekko IA, et al. Hydrogel-forming microneedles enhance transdermal delivery of metformin hydrochloride. J Control Release. 2018;285:142–151.

[42] Kearney M-C, Caffarel-Salvador E, Fallows SJ, et al. Microneedle-mediated delivery of donepezil: potential for improved treatment options in Alzheimer's disease. Eur J Pharm Biopharm. 2016;103:43–50.

[43] Courtenay AJ, McAlister E, McCrudden MTC, et al. Hydrogel-forming microneedle arrays as a therapeutic option for transdermal esketamine delivery. J Control Release. 2020;322:177–186.

[44] Caffarel-Salvador E, Brady AJ, Eltayib E, et al. Hydrogel-forming microneedle arrays allow detection of drugs and glucose in vivo: potential for use in diagnosis and therapeutic drug monitoring. PLoS One. 2015;10:e0145644.

[45] Donnelly RF, McCrudden MT, Alkilani AZ, et al. Hydrogel-forming microneedles prepared from "super swelling" polymers combined with lyophilised wafers for transdermal drug delivery. PLoS One. 2014;9:e111547.

[46] Yan G, Warner KS, Zhang J, et al. Evaluation needle length and density of microneedle arrays in the pretreatment of skin for transdermal drug delivery. Int J Pharm. 2010;391:7–12.

[47] Aaron RJ H, Helen L. Q, Paul J. M, et al. Transdermal delivery of vitamin K using dissolving microneedles for the prevention of vitamin K deficiency bleeding. Int J Pharm. 2018;541. [Internet] [cited 2022 Jul 12]. Available from: https://pubmed.ncbi.nlm.nih.gov/29471143/.

[48] Banks SL, Pinninti RR, Gill HS, et al. Flux across of microneedle-treated skin is increased by increasing charge of naltrexone and naltrexol in vitro. Pharm Res. 2008;25:1677–1685.

[49] Banks SL, Pinninti RR, Gill HS, et al. Transdermal delivery of naltrexol and skin permeability lifetime after microneedle treatment in hairless guinea pigs. J Pharm Sci. 2010;99:3072–3080.

[50] Banks SL, Paudel KS, Brogden NK, et al. Diclofenac enables prolonged delivery of naltrexone through microneedle-treated skin. Pharm Res. 2011;28:1211–1219.

[51] Wermeling DP, Banks SL, Hudson DA, et al. Microneedles permit transdermal delivery of a skin-impermeant medication to humans. Proc Natl Acad Sci. 2008;105:2058–2063.

[52] Yerramreddy TR, Milewski M, Penthala NR, et al. Novel 3-O-pegylated carboxylate and 3-O-pegylated carbamate prodrugs of naltrexone for microneedle-enhanced transdermal delivery. Bioorg Med Chem Lett. 2010;20:3280–3283.

[53] Milewski M, Yerramreddy TR, Ghosh P, et al. In vitro permeation of a pegylated naltrexone prodrug across microneedle-treated skin. J Control Release. 2010;146:37–44.

[54] Milewski M, Stinchcomb AL. Vehicle composition influence on the microneedle-enhanced transdermal flux of naltrexone hydrochloride. Pharm Res. 2011;28:124–134.

[55] Burton SA, Ng C-Y, Simmers R, et al. Rapid intradermal delivery of liquid formulations using a hollow microstructured array. Pharm Res. 2011;28:31–40.

[56] Caffarel-Salvador E, Tuan-Mahmood T-M, McElnay JC, et al. Potential of hydrogel-forming and dissolving microneedles for use in paediatric populations. Int J Pharm. 2015;489:158–169.

[57] McCrudden MTC, Alkilani AZ, Courtenay AJ, et al. Considerations in the sterile manufacture of polymeric microneedle arrays. Drug Deliv Transl Res. 2015;5:3–14.

[58] Jun H, Han M-R, Kang N-G, et al. Use of hollow microneedles for targeted delivery of phenylephrine to treat fecal incontinence. J Control Release. 2015;207:1–6.

[59] Baek C, Han M, Min J, et al. Local transdermal delivery of phenylephrine to the anal sphincter muscle using microneedles. J Control Release. 2011;154:138–147.

[60] Miyano T, Tobinaga Y, Kanno T, et al. Sugar micro needles as transdermic drug delivery system. Biomed Microdevices. 2005;7:185–188.

[61] Kolli CS, Banga AK. Characterization of solid maltose microneedles and their use for transdermal delivery. Pharm Res. 2008;25:104–113.

[62] Donnelly RF, Majithiya R, Singh TRR, et al. Design, optimization and characterisation of polymeric microneedle arrays prepared by a novel laser-based micromoulding technique. Pharm Res. 2011;28:41–57.

[63] Ma Y, Gill HS. Coating solid dispersions on microneedles via a molten dip-coating method: development and in vitro evaluation for transdermal delivery of a water-insoluble drug. J Pharm Sci. 2014;103:3621–3630.

[64] Kwon S-Y. In vitro evaluation of transdermal drug delivery by a micro-needle patch. Control Release Soc 31st Annu Meet Trans. 2004.

[65] Naguib YW, Kumar A, Cui Z. The effect of microneedles on the skin permeability and antitumor activity of topical 5-fluorouracil. Acta Pharm Sin B. 2014;4:94–99.

[66] Qiu Y, Gao Y, Hu K, et al. Enhancement of skin permeation of docetaxel: a novel approach combining microneedle and elastic liposomes. J Control Release. 2008;129:144–150.

[67] Nguyen HX, Banga AK. Fabrication, characterization and application of sugar microneedles for transdermal drug delivery. Ther Deliv. 2017;8:249–264.

[68] Nguyen HX, Bozorg BD, Kim Y, et al. Poly (vinyl alcohol) microneedles: fabrication, characterization, and application for transdermal drug delivery of doxorubicin. Eur J Pharm Biopharm. 2018;129:88–103.

[69] Nguyen HX, Banga AK. Delivery of methotrexate and characterization of skin treated by fabricated PLGA microneedles and fractional ablative laser. Pharm Res. 2018;35:1–20.

[70] Nguyen HX, Banga AK. Enhanced skin delivery of vismodegib by microneedle treatment. Drug Deliv Transl Res. 2015;5:407–423.

[71] Kaur M, Ita KB, Popova IE, et al. Microneedle-assisted delivery of verapamil hydrochloride and amlodipine besylate. Eur J Pharm Biopharm. 2014;86:284–291.

[72] Nguyen TK, Ita BK, Parikh SJ, et al. Transdermal delivery of captopril and metoprolol tartrate with microneedles. Drug Deliv Lett. 2014;4:236–243.

[73] Park J-H, Choi S-O, Seo S, et al. A microneedle roller for transdermal drug delivery. Eur J Pharm Biopharm. 2010;76:282–289.

[74] Li W-Z, Huo M-R, Zhou J-P, et al. Super-short solid silicon microneedles for transdermal drug delivery applications. Int J Pharm. 2010;389:122–129.

[75] Martanto W, Davis SP, Holiday NR, et al. Transdermal delivery of insulin using microneedles in vivo. Pharm Res. 2004;21:947–952.

[76] Gardeniers HJ, Luttge R, Berenschot EJ, et al. Silicon micromachined hollow microneedles for transdermal liquid transport. J Microelectromechanical Syst. 2003;12:855–862.

[77] Sivamani RK, Stoeber B, Wu GC, et al. Clinical microneedle injection of methyl nicotinate: stratum corneum penetration. Skin Res Technol. 2005;11:152–156.

[78] Sivamani RK, Stoeber B, Liepmann D, et al. Microneedle penetration and injection past the stratum corneum in humans. J Dermatol Treat. 2009;20:156–159.

[79] Badran MM, Kuntsche J, Fahr A. Skin penetration enhancement by a microneedle device (Dermaroller®) in vitro: dependency on needle size and applied formulation. Eur J Pharm Sci. 2009;36:511–523.

[80] Verbaan FJ, Bal SM, van den Berg DJ, et al. Assembled microneedle arrays enhance the transport of compounds varying over a large range of molecular weight across human dermatomed skin. J Control Release. 2007;117:238–245.

[81] Li X, Zhao R, Qin Z, et al. Microneedle pretreatment improves efficacy of cutaneous topical anesthesia. Am J Emerg Med. 2010;28:130–134.

[82] Donnelly RF, Morrow DIJ, McCarron PA, et al. Microneedle-mediated intradermal delivery of 5-aminolevulinic acid: potential for enhanced topical photodynamic therapy. J Control Release. 2008;129:154–162.

[83] Donnelly RF, Morrow DI, McCarron PA, et al. Microneedle arrays permit enhanced intradermal delivery of a preformed photosensitizer. Photochem Photobiol. 2009;85:195–204.

[84] Mikolajewska P, Donnelly RF, Garland MJ, et al. Microneedle pre-treatment of human skin improves 5-aminolevulininc acid (ALA)- and 5-aminolevulinic acid methyl ester (MAL)-induced PpIX production for topical photodynamic therapy without increase in pain or erythema. Pharm Res. 2010;27:2213–2220.

[85] Spierings EL, Brandes JL, Kudrow DB, et al. Randomized, double-blind, placebo-controlled, parallel-group, multi-center study of the safety and efficacy of ADAM zolmitriptan for the acute treatment of migraine. Cephalalgia. 2018;38:215–224.

7

Microneedle-mediated Delivery of Biopharmaceuticals

7.1 Introduction

7.1.1 Introduction of Biopharmaceuticals

Biopharmaceutical products offer substantial potential as safe and effective therapeutic agents [1]. These drugs provide high efficacy and low toxicity. Due to the complex structural arrangement, these biomolecules are highly specific to the treatment target [2, 3]. Furthermore, these highly potent molecules require low doses to provide an effective treatment therapy and favorable safety profile compared to traditional low-molecular-weight drugs [2, 4]. Due to specific functionality and structural hierarchy, biopharmaceuticals have minimal interference in the biological system, thus reducing the risk of adverse effects [5, 6]. Protein drugs can directly substitute the corresponding dysfunctional endogenous proteins in the body. Biomolecules have efficiently treated various diseases, including inflammation, neurodegenerative disorders, genetic disorders, cancer treatment, vaccinations, genetic diseases, hemophilia, infectious diseases, anemia, osteoporosis, lymphoma, leukemia, and diabetes mellitus [7–10]. Among those, immunotherapy is the most employed field for these biopharmaceuticals. These drugs could perform different functions in the body, such as enzymes, immune-stimulators, cellular regulators, molecular transporters, and biological scaffolds [11–14]. Large-scale manufacture of a wide variety of recombinant proteins and biopharmaceutical products has been facilitated by recent developments in biotechnology, particularly recombinant DNA technology. Also, the clinical development of these products is anticipated to grow exponentially [15, 16].

Several limitations have been reported with biomolecules, i.e., proteins, peptides, and biologics. Large molecular weight reduces the drug absorption efficiency and limits its permeability across biological barriers [4]. The drug permeability depends on its physico-chemical properties and the structural difference between the drug and the physiological conditions. Furthermore, biomolecules have poor stability, experiencing significant loss of biological activity due to external environment factors (i.e., moisture and humidity) or endogenous proteolytic enzyme [17]. Metabolic enzymes in the body could easily and rapidly degrade these drugs, thus having short half-lives, requiring repeated and frequency drug administration, and causing poor patient compliance. The poor stability also leads to challenges and difficulties in the development of formulation and delivery technologies for these molecules. Protein denaturation and degradation during drug delivery and storage result in a reduction in the therapeutic efficiency and alteration to regulatory responses [17–19]. Also, hydrolytic attack by proteases leads to poor bioavailability of these drugs [20].

7.1.2 Current Status of Biopharmaceuticals

For 30 years since the first successful launch of Humulin (a recombinant human insulin), the pharmaceutical industry has been tremendously driven by the development of various biopharmaceutical products, including peptides, enzymes, monoclonal antibodies, recombinant proteins, and antibody–drug conjugates [3]. To date, 91 recombinant protein drugs have been approved by the US FDA [21], with 18 approvals for biotech products until 2012 [22], while several other promising candidates are under clinical investigation. Recently, FDA approved semaglutide (a glucagon-like peptide-1 receptor agonist, Rybelsus™) in 2019 as the oral treatment of type 2 diabetes. Proteins and peptides are readily available as the first-line treatment option for various chronic diseases such as diabetes, rheumatoid arthritis, cancers, and hemophilia [23]. By 2024, the global market for biopharmaceutical products is expected to be worth $388 billion. Interestingly, biopharmaceuticals contribute over 50% of the top 20 blockbuster drugs [24]. An exponential growth of the biopharmaceutical market is expected due to substantial potential and interest in this field. The rapid development of biopharmaceutical products is attributed to the improved efficiency of protein expression and synthesis in large-scale manufacturing [9, 25].

7.1.3 Conventional Parenteral Administration

The physicochemical properties of biopharmaceuticals limit the available options for successful drug administration. Different administration methods could be employed, such as intravenous, oral, transdermal, intravesical, nasal, pulmonary, ocular, and rectal routes [26]. In general, biopharmaceuticals (protein and peptide drugs) have been effectively administered via parenteral routes such as intravenous, subcutaneous, and intramuscular injections [2, 27]. Oral administration could easily lead to significant drug degradation in the gastrointestinal tract (by acidic environment or enzymes), first-pass hepatic metabolism, poor absorption (high molecular weight and hydrophilicity of biopharmaceuticals), and compromised molecular stability, thus resulting in low oral bioavailability and limited therapeutic efficiency [28]. Currently, most biotherapeutics are delivered by parenteral injections using a hypodermic needle, which is inexpensive and rapid in drug delivery with 100% bioavailability for intravenous administration [24, 29]. This high bioavailability has benefited proteins and peptides since these drugs could be quickly degraded and cleared from the blood circulation [30, 31].

However, the conventional parenteral injection with hypodermic needles poses several drawbacks and complications. This route generally produces pain, needle phobia, and needlestick injuries, which translate into poor patient compliance, acceptability, and willingness to receive the necessary treatment [24, 32]. Also, patients cannot administer the dose by themselves without trained personnel's assistance [33]. According to a CDC report, annually, around 385,000 caregivers in the United States suffer from needlestick injuries, posing the risk of infectious disease and related health issues. Moreover, biopharmaceuticals have an issue of systemic instability, which is attributed to processes such as proteases, opsonization, rapid metabolism, and agglutination [34, 35]. When biopharmaceutical drugs enter the blood circulation, they can be degraded and eliminated by several environmental factors [36], including sequestration by the reticuloendothelial system, enzymatic degradation, and elimination by the liver [37], thus causing a low efficiency of biological therapies. Furthermore, most proteins and peptides, except for monoclonal antibodies, have short half-lives, have rapid clearance from the body, and require frequent administration. Repeated injections could lead to phlebitis and tissue necrosis, as well as increase the possible risk of adverse reactions [25, 38, 39]. In particular, people with chronic conditions like rheumatoid arthritis and diabetes have found injections unpleasant and inconvenient. Contamination of hypodermic needles during the injections could cause transmission of infectious diseases, including hepatitis B and C [4]. Biomolecules in infusion formulation could induce an immune response if they are recognized as antigens by the body [40, 41]. Hence, parenteral injections could cause inconvenience and complications during the therapy. Several methods, including chemical alteration, colloidal delivery systems, and thermosensitive gels, have been developed to increase the stability of proteins and peptides [42]. Although biopharmaceuticals are generally safer and more effective than chemical compounds, these biomolecules could trigger some side effects in the body, such as autoimmunity or nonspecific inflammatory reactions [43]. Thus, it is crucial to prevent these detrimental effects. Alternative technologies have been developed to stabilize biopharmaceutical drugs and control their adverse effects, such as the development of drug-encapsulated polymeric nanotechnology-based products in which the drugs are protected, transported, and directed to the targeted sites, as well as prevented from causing toxic effects on nonspecific tissues [44]. Extensive investigation has been executed to develop novel delivery technologies that are noninvasive, safe, effective, and user-friendly.

7.1.4 Transdermal Delivery of Biopharmaceuticals

Due to the disadvantages and limitations of injection therapies with biopharmaceutical drugs, an alternative delivery system has to be developed to protect the drug and enhance its treatment efficacy. Recently, transdermal delivery has emerged as a promising platform for the administration of biomolecules (Table 7.1) [2]. The safety and efficacy of transdermal delivery systems for biopharmaceuticals depend on the physicochemical properties of the

TABLE 7.1

Biopharmaceuticals Administered by Transdermal Route

Biopharmaceutical	Product	Indication	Manufacturer
Estradiol/levonorgestrel	Climara Pro®	Menopausal symptoms	Bayer Healthcare Pharmaceuticals
Estradiol	Estraderm®	Menopausal symptoms	Novartis
Estradiol	Estosorb	Female hormone replacement therapy	Exeltis USA, Inc.
Estradiol	Estrogel	Female hormone replacement therapy	Solvay Pharmaceuticals
Estradiol	Elestrin	Female hormone replacement therapy	MEDA Pharmaceuticals, Inc.
Estradiol	Divigel	Female hormone replacement therapy	Upsher-Smith Laboratories
Estradiol	Evamist	Female hormone replacement therapy	Perrigo
Estradiol and norethindrone acetate	Combipatch®	Menopausal symptoms	Novartis
Ethinyl estradiol and gestodene	Apleek™	Contraception	Bayer Healthcare

(Continued)

TABLE 7.1 *(Continued)*

Biopharmaceuticals Administered by Transdermal Route

Biopharmaceutical	Product	Indication	Manufacturer
Ethinyl estradiol and levonorgestrel	Twirla®	Contraception	Agile Therapeutics
Ethinyl estradiol/ norelgestromin	Ortho Evra™	Female contraception	Janssen Pharms
Fertility hormone	Fertility hormone peptide Smart Patch™ transdermal patch	Female infertility	Vyteris/Ferring
Heat-labile enterotoxin of *Escherichia coli*	Drug-loading transdermal patch	Travelers' diarrhea	Iomai
Human growth hormone	Tev-Tropin	Growth hormone deficiency	TransPharma/Teva
Influenza vaccine	Fluzone® Intradermal influenza vaccine	Influenza prophylaxis	Becton Dickinson/ Sanofi-Pasteur
Insulin	Insulin Transdermal AT-1391	Diabetes mellitus	Zealand Pharma/Altea
Parathyroid hormone (1–34)	ZP-PTH	Osteoporosis	Zosano Pharma, Inc.
Testosterone	Testoderm®	Testosterone deficiency (hypogonadism)	Alza Pharmaceuticals
Testosterone	Androgel	Hypogonadism	AbbVie
Testosterone	Testim	Hypogonadism	Auxilium Pharmaceuticals, Inc.
Testosterone	Fortesta	Hypogonadism	Endo Pharmaceuticals, Inc.
Testosterone	Axiron	Hypogonadism	Eli Lilly and Company

drugs and the percutaneous administration system. The drug's physical characteristics, i.e., shape, size, molecular weight, solubility, and amphoteric nature, dictate the appropriate delivery system to be used. The drug's chemical properties should be considered to minimize any reactivity of functional groups of the drug. Also, skin conditions, including age, temperature (hot or freezing), races, abrasion, chemical irritant activity, and skin diseases (i.e., atopic dermatitis and psoriasis), could alter drug permeability.

Transdermal delivery offers several advantages over other routes of administration. Transdermal delivery enables the avoidance of drug degradation in harsh environmental conditions in the gastrointestinal tract and first-pass hepatic metabolism [29, 45]. This noninvasive, convenient, and easy route of administration improves patient compliance and provides a superior safety profile compared to needle-based delivery systems. The transdermal system could provide prolonged, sustained, and continuous drug release to achieve optimal and uniform drug plasma levels, thus reducing the administration frequency [46–48]. This is especially beneficial to drugs with short half-lives or with the frequent-dosing requirement. Drug delivery across the skin offers minimal proteolytic activity, which is significantly lower than that in other routes, such as mucosal, oral, and subcutaneous delivery [2]. This reduction in the enzymatic degradation at the administration site is critical for the therapeutic efficacy of biomolecules. Furthermore, transdermal delivery reduces the risk of adverse effects in the host subjects, enhances the drug's solubility, stability, and pharmacological activity, improves bioavailability and efficacy, and provides rapid drug delivery onset and high drug load and storage. It is feasible that distant immune activation might be triggered via transdermal administration of biomolecules, which shows potential and effectiveness for local skin cancers. Some transdermal systems could deliver ribonucleic acid to regulate localized gene expression or monoclonal antibody for immunotherapy.

Several drawbacks have been reported for transdermally delivered biomolecules. These drugs are hydrophilic and have high molecular weight. These properties are not following the Lipinski rules for effective transdermal drug delivery [27]. Hence, they cannot penetrate the skin by passive diffusion. The transdermal route has been found inappropriate for many macromolecules. Biopharmaceuticals' properties must be thoroughly investigated to ensure minimal impact on drug stability and pharmacokinetic properties [49]. Also, proteolytic enzymes could lead to drug degradation, even though the extent is less severe than other routes [50]. Several instability issues can occur during product development and manufacturing due to the drug's complex structural orientation and potency [27]. Biopharmaceuticals could be easily degraded by environmental insults (i.e., temperature, humidity, oxygen, carbon dioxide, and light) to cause drug decomposition, lead to diminished therapeutic efficacy, or produce harmful by-products [49]. Some biomolecules could have a lower or higher affinity or interaction with lipophilic domains in the stratum corneum layer, thus changing the efficacy of drug permeation across the stratum corneum. Besides, transdermal delivery poses certain risks of skin irritation or local inflammation caused by the delivery system or drug molecules.

Several novel technologies (i.e., methods and devices) have been developed to extend the field of transdermal drug delivery to encompass macromolecules. In particular, the third-generation system directly affects the stratum corneum structure, allowing for the passage of intact biomolecules into and across skin layers. The ideal methods should prevent drug degradation and ensure drug integrity during the fabrication, transportation, and release processes [51]. Among those approaches, thermal ablation and microneedles are the most widely employed techniques to enhance transdermal drug delivery.

7.1.5 Microneedles for Biopharmaceuticals Delivery

Numerous physical enhancement technologies have been developed to effectively enhance the transdermal delivery of various therapeutic agents. Among those, microneedle technology has emerged as a promising platform for the delivery of molecules of any size [52]. Microneedles have been produced to deliver biopharmaceutical drugs into and across the skin (Table 7.2). These micrometer-sized needles breach the skin partially and create channels in the skin. These microneedles-created channels serve as pathways for facilitated drug permeation, allowing the drug to access deeper skin layers. This skin disruption and formation of microchannels effectively facilitate the passage and transport of hydrophilic and macromolecules across the stratum corneum layer to rapidly reach and enter the blood circulation [53]. Certain types of microneedles (coated and dissolving microneedles) could function as a small drug reservoir for a quantity of microliter or microgram drug. Microneedles effectively store, transport, and deliver any molecules into the skin. This capacity depends on the needles' dimensions and drug formulation [49].

Mechanically robust microneedles have been successfully fabricated from various materials such as metal (palladium, stainless steel, nickel, palladium-cobalt titanium [54]), ceramics [55], silicon [56], polymers [14], silica glass [57], and carbohydrates [58]. The most critical characteristics of microneedles are the material of construction and microneedle designs. An attractive feature of microneedles is that the needles can be made from a combination of two or more polymers. This capacity enables the production of microneedles

TABLE 7.2

Currently Active Clinical Trials of Microneedles-assisted Delivery of Biopharmaceuticals

NCT Identifier	Therapeutic Agent	Microneedle Design	Conditions/Diseases
NCT02329457	Zostavax (anti-varicella-zoster antibody)	A novel intradermal microneedle	Varicella-zoster infection
NCT01518478	Fluzone intradermal	An ultrafine microneedle	Atopic dermatitis
NCT01737710	Fluzone intradermal	An ultrafine microneedle	Atopic dermatitis
NCT00602914	Insulin	MicronJet (hollow microneedles)	Intradermal injections
NCT01061216	Insulin	Hollow microneedles BD Research Catheter Set (34G × 1.5 mm needle)	Diabetes mellitus type 1/2
NCT00837512	Insulin	Hollow glass microneedle	Diabetes mellitus type 1
NCT01120444, NCT00553488	Insulin	BD Research Catheter (34G × 1.5 mm needle)	
NCT01557907	Insulin	BD Research Catheter (34G × 1.5 mm needle)	
NCT02837094	C19-A3 GNP peptide	NanoPass microneedles	
NCT01684956	Insulin and glucagon	MicronJet (hollow microneedles)	
NCT02459938	Glucagon	Microneedle patch system	Hypoglycemia
NCT04064411	Abaloparatide	Solid microstructured transdermal system	Postmenopausal osteoporosis
NCT01674621	Abaloparatide	Coated 3M microstructured transdermal system (MTS)	Postmenopausal osteoporosis
NCT02478879	Zosano Pharma parathyroid hormone	ZP-PTH-coated microneedle patch (titanium microneedles)	
NCT03054480	Botulinum toxin type A	Fractional microneedle radiofrequency	Primary axillary hyperhidrosis
NCT01813604	Fractional IPV	MicronJet600 (hollow microneedles)	Poliomyelitis
NCT03607903	Adalimumab	MicronJet600 (hollow microneedles)	Auto-immune/autoinflammatory diseases

with the specifically desired structure to improve penetration efficiency and enhance drug delivery [49]. There are various microneedles systems, namely, hollow, solid [59–61], dissolving [14], coated [62], and swelling microneedles. Microneedles have been found to significantly enhance transdermal and intradermal delivery of various therapeutic agents such as small molecules (hydrophilic or lipophilic compounds), macromolecules (proteins, peptides, vaccines, DNA, etc.), and particulate systems (liposomes, nanoparticle, microparticles, etc.). Examples of microneedles-assisted proteins with enzymatic or regulatory activity include insulin, etanercept, growth hormone, erythropoietin, glucagon, glucagon-like peptide-1, parathyroid hormone, desmopressin, lysozyme [14, 63–65], fluorescein-isothiocyanate labeled bovine serum albumin (BSA) [66], human immunoglobulin A protein [67], oligonucleotides [68], and human IgG [69]. Microneedles have been employed in immunotherapy using monoclonal antibodies to regulate the immune system [67, 70]. Several review articles about microneedles (fabrication, composition, design, and mechanical properties) have been published elsewhere [71].

Microneedle insertion is minimally invasive, thus improving patient compliance and acceptability and being a favorable replacement for conventional injections using hypodermic needles [72]. This is especially beneficial for insulin therapy in which the current hypodermic injection is reported to be inconvenient and painful [73]. Microneedle technology provides various platforms to disrupt the skin barrier and facilitate transdermal delivery of hydrophilic compounds and macromolecules (Fig. 7.1). Furthermore, microneedles minimize the risk of protein denaturation, thereby revolutionizing and expanding the field of transdermal drug delivery to "difficult" molecules such as hydrophilic and macromolecules. Biomolecules could be encapsulated into the polymeric matrix of microneedles at a high loading efficiency. The mild fabrication condition of microneedles production and the dried, solid state of the finished product improve drug stability and maintain the long-term bioactivity of macromolecules. This, in turn, nullifies the requirement for cold-chain storage and transportation, thus reducing the cost and restriction of product transportation [74–77]. Furthermore, certain excipients (i.e., ethylenediaminetetraacetic acid, trehalose, or mannitol) could be included in the formulation to stabilize the drug activity [78]. Drug formulation could be modified and optimized to achieve desired physicochemical properties and spatiotemporal release of the loaded drug [65, 79]. Interestingly, microneedles can provide bolus or sustained drug release to suit the requirement of specific molecules [80]. Coated, dissolving, and swelling microneedles could be fabricated with selected materials to enable a bolus dose or controlled drug release. Extended drug release and permeation could be achieved by skin pretreatment with microneedles followed by a patch application or controlled injection of drug formulation into the skin through hollow microneedles [2]. Besides, microneedles could be used for local drug delivery rather than allowing the drug to enter the blood circulation. This helps reduce the possibilities of immune-related adverse effects by mitigating the overstimulation of self-reactive T cells and preventing immune depletion. This feature is beneficial for therapies using monoclonal antibodies [67].

Even though microneedle technology is a promising and effective tool for enhanced transdermal delivery of macromolecules, this system has several limitations. In particular, the fabrication cost for solid microneedles is expensive, and the two-step application process poses certain risks of inaccurate dosing [81]. Coated microneedles could carry a very limited quantity of drugs on the needles' surface. Hollow microneedles may cause potential toxic effects of uncontrolled drug release and require trained personnel and a complex setup for injection administration [57, 82]. Dissolving microneedles must maintain the needles' sharpness and mechanical strength during production and storage [83]. Furthermore, microneedles penetrate and disrupt the keratinized stratum corneum layer. However, the permeant has to penetrate the epithelium to reach the dermis layer to enter systemic blood circulation or the therapeutic target. Macromolecules are generally less permeable than small molecules and might be degraded by the enzyme present in the epithelium [84]. Therefore, the design and dimensions of microneedles have to be optimized to shorten the pathway from the drug to the targeted skin layers. Moreover, drug loading into the microneedle polymeric matrix is insufficient for some biopharmaceutical drugs to protect its bioactivity and stability. There is still a high risk of the drug undergoing partial or total degradation during microneedle fabrication or drug administration. Thus, sensitive drugs could be encapsulated into specific particulate systems (i.e., nanocapsules or dendrimers) and then loaded into the needle matrix. This way, the drugs cope with negligible risk of structural decomposition and obtain more effective transdermal delivery [85].

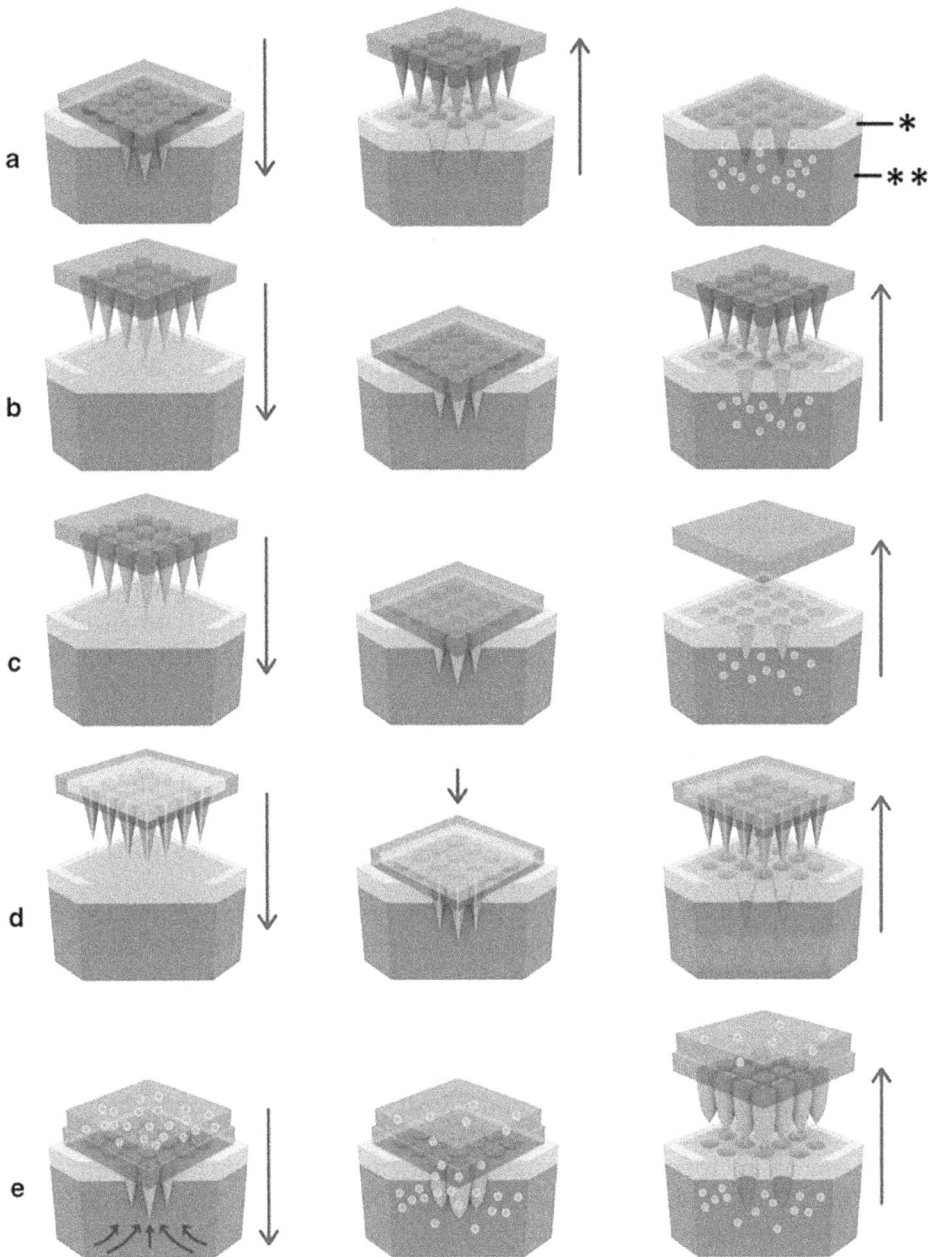

FIGURE 7.1
Mechanism of different microneedle types during skin insertion. * Stratum corneum. ** Epidermis. (a) Solid microneedles produce temporary, micrometer-sized channels in the skin, which are then filled with interstitial skin fluid and covered with topical drug formulation. (b) Solid microneedles may be coated to transport a drug formulation on its surface. Upon microneedle insertion, the coating layer instantly dissolves and releases the drug into the skin tissue. (c) Dissolving microneedles have drug encapsulated in the needles' polymeric matrix. The needles dissolve in the skin upon insertion to release the drug payload. (d) Hollow microneedles porate skin, creating a pathway (the needle bores) through which drug liquid formulation is injected into the skin. (e) Hydrogel-forming swelling microneedles absorb interstitial skin fluid upon skin insertion, creating a swollen porous structure to facilitate drug diffusion into the skin tissue. Images reprinted with permission from [24].

7.2 Physicochemical Stability of Biopharmaceuticals in Microneedles

As opposed to small molecules, biopharmaceutical drugs may be degraded by environmental stimuli such as pH, temperature, and humidity during the production process (Table 7.3) [52]. For instance, proteins, peptides, antibodies, and viruses are more susceptible to breakdown than low-molecular-weight chemical molecules. The degradation of proteins is accelerated in the presence of organic solvents like dichloromethane, ethyl acetate, and dimethyl carbonate. Biomolecules are prone to aggregation, denaturation, and precipitation in aqueous environments [86, 87]. A modification to the structure of biopharmaceuticals not only results in a reduction in treatment effectiveness but may also impair drug safety and produce undesirable immunogenicity. In addition, unwanted immunogenicity may cause the complete loss of a protein's therapeutic effect by neutralizing antibodies and the depletion of endogenous proteins or the destruction of immune tolerance to self-antigens [41, 88–92]. Loss of activity, risks of immunogenicity, and hypersensitivity to immune complexes are all possible risks of antibody delivery that may result from protein deactivation [93–95]. Based on a comprehensive knowledge of the physicochemical and biological properties of biopharmaceuticals and an understanding of the stability concerns of biomolecules, viable and effective formulations of these drugs may be developed. The manufacturing and handling processes must be adjusted and optimized to maintain these drugs' stability, safety, and effectiveness. To protect biopharmaceuticals' integrity, stability, and efficacy, particular materials and formulations must be carefully chosen and developed [14, 96, 97].

TABLE 7.3

Degradation of Biomolecules with Microneedles

Factor Type	Factors	Degradation	Microneedle Types
Induced interface	Microneedle bore, applied pressure, materials/ surface properties, formulation composition	Aggregation, adsorption, unfolding	Hollow microneedle, coated microneedle, and drug patch for "poke and patch" with solid microneedle
High drug concentration	Coating/molding formulation	Aggregation	Coated microneedle, dissolving microneedle
Induced temperature	Microneedle polymerization/transition temperature	Aggregation, unfolding, chemical degradation	Dissolving microneedle
Metal catalysis	Formulation impurities	Aggregation, oxidation	Hollow microneedle, solid metal microneedle
Air exposure	Storage conditions	Aggregation, adsorption, unfolding, oxidation	Coated microneedle, dissolving microneedle, drug patch for "poke and patch" with solid microneedle
Induced pH	pH of coating/molding formulation	Aggregation, unfolding, chemical degradation	Coated microneedle, dissolving microneedle, drug patch for "poke and patch" with solid microneedle

Proteins are complicated molecules with a distinctive three-dimensional structure crucial for their function. The stability of macromolecules in microneedle formulations must be maintained to prevent any adverse effects. As biomolecules diminish their activity and effectiveness in liquid and lyophilized formulations when kept at ambient temperatures, the enhanced thermostability of the pharmaceuticals loaded in microneedles garners considerable interest. Since the skin is a powerful immune organ, undesired protein immunogenicity presents the most significant safety risk. This further emphasizes the need to thoroughly characterize protein aggregates and subvisible particles that may be generated and discharged via transdermal microneedle-based formulations [89, 98, 99]. Protein stability throughout the production process and product storage is a crucial consideration. Conventional production techniques for protein-loaded microneedles entail the use of elevated temperatures, a vacuum, organic solvents, or exposure to UV light, which may be detrimental to protein function and reduce drug stability [100–104]. To preserve the drugs, macromolecules might be encapsulated within micro/nanomaterials utilizing several techniques, including single/double emulsion, microfabrication, and electrospray [105–107]. Then, these particulate systems might be loaded into the microneedles' polymeric matrix. During the microneedle production process, the temperature should be kept at a low level, and the use of organic solvents should be restricted to increase drug stability [101, 102, 108–111]. An excellent review publication by Maaden et al. [112] speculates on the potential sources of protein degradation throughout microneedle manufacturing, storage, application, and delivery.

In research, insulin was encapsulated into dissolving microneedles to deliver insulin percutaneously. This method was able to preserve the insulin's activity after one month of storage at temperatures ranging from −80°C to 40°C [113]. Insulin is more stable when loaded and stored in dissolving microneedles made of a starch/gelatin mixture for at least one month at room temperature or slightly higher [114]. Yang and coworkers [115] employed a photolithography technique for encapsulating BSA in microneedles using modest exposure to UV light. They determined that the protein is completely stable under working conditions by studying the protein's primary, secondary, and tertiary structures. Similarly, encapsulating human growth hormone (HGH) into dissolving microneedles allowed for the preservation of the drug's full activity after encapsulation and the retention of HGH activity after storage at ambient temperature and relative humidity for up to 15 months [65]. Incorporating immunoglobulin G into hyaluronan-based dissolving microneedles led to favorable improvements in drug stability. These needles could penetrate and dissolve quickly in the skin, retaining protein stability throughout the production process. The stability and aggregation of proteins were researched at the molecular, submicrometer, and micrometer levels [116]. Other investigations have examined protein stability in microneedle compositions, highlighting the suitability of this technique for proteins [117–119]. Hiraishi and colleagues [120] revealed that ambient humidity influences the mechanical strength and protein stability in microneedle patches. The mechanical failure force test demonstrated that needle strength declined as the humidity levels increased. In addition, humid environments are unsuitable for preserving the stability of proteins; an uncontrolled atmosphere might result in protein unfolding, aggregation, or chemical decomposition. Park et al. developed dissolving microneedles carrying BSA by casting a drug-containing formulation on a microneedle mold with a molten polymer at 135°C; BSA was preserved in solid form to prevent protein breakdown. They measured protein solubility, dynamic light scattering (DLS), and circular dichroism (CD) to determine the stability of BSA encapsulated in microneedles. After heating BSA in the solid state at 135°C for 10 min, DLS revealed no significant change; however, heating for 20 and 30 min produced aggregates on the order of tens of nanometers. In addition, they detected little or no changes in the secondary structure of the protein following the thermal processing. Nevertheless, 10% BSA was permanently aggregated after 10 min of exposure to the polymer melt, and BSA was totally denatured after 1 h of exposure to 135°C, demonstrating that this method is unsuitable for the delivery of BSA and possibly other macromolecules [104]. Dissolving microneedles containing BSA and lysozyme were produced by Lee et al. at room temperature. Using circular dichroism and enzymatic activity, they examined the structural and functional properties of loaded lysozyme and discovered that, according to both techniques, lysozyme was not significantly damaged after two months of storage at ambient conditions [101]. Migalska et al. developed insulin-loaded dissolving microneedles and observed no chemical changes in denatured insulin and no alteration in the secondary structure of insulin [102]. Fukushima and colleagues enclosed rhGH in dissolving microneedles and revealed that the loaded rhGH was stable for one month, as determined by an enzyme immunoassay and LC/MS/MS [109]. Utilizing rp-HPLC and size exclusion-HPLC methods, Ameri and coworkers investigated the long-term stability of PTH coated on microneedles. Coated PTH was shown to degrade mostly via aggregation and oxidation, and the inclusion of sucrose in the coating formulation reduced PTH aggregation from 7% to 0.5%. The researchers also found that solid-state aggregation accounted for 7% of degradation, while oxidation of PTH contributed to 1% and might be catalyzed by metal elements from excipients or titanium microneedles. When PTH-loaded microneedles were stored at room temperature and 60% humidity, its bioactivity was maintained for up to 18 months [121]. Likewise, Donnelly et al. studied the loaded protein's thermal stability. They reported that during the microneedle production process, the high temperature (160°C) of melted galactose caused a significant loss of 5-aminolevulinic acid and bovine serum albumin [122]. Protein molecules, such as bovine serum albumin and lysozyme [101], have been effectively integrated into carboxymethylcellulose microneedles and remain stable after two months of storage. Microneedles are made from carbohydrates [101]. This method entails pouring the carbohydrate solution into a mold and evaporating it at 37°C. Microneedles patches containing rhGH and insulin were stable for 15 days and 1 month, respectively, when kept at ambient temperature [65, 113]. For antibodies, targeting specificity, molecular structure, and antigen affinity are the qualities that must be evaluated before antibodies may be encapsulated in microneedles [123]. Therefore, research has revealed that after dissolving hyaluronan (HA)-based microneedles [116], more than 80% of monoclonal immunoglobulin G (IgG) was recovered with stable tertiary structure. It was also shown that neither IgG aggregation nor the production of HA/IgG complexes occurred throughout the microneedle production process. Future investigation into drug encapsulation, mechanical integrity, pharmacokinetic, pharmacodynamic, safety, storage, and administration of microneedles will promote the application of microneedles in transdermal delivery of biopharmaceutical drugs.

7.3 Case Studies

7.3.1 Solid Microneedles

Drug administration using solid microneedles is typically a two-step process. In a nutshell, solid microneedles penetrate the skin and then withdraw to create temporary microchannels in the skin. Subsequently, the microchannels are covered with a pharmaceutical dosage form (i.e., gel, cream, ointment, or a transdermal patch) [64]. Applied drugs are passively diffused via the solid microneedles–created microchannels into the skin tissue. Thus, drug delivery into and across the skin will be influenced by the length, sharpness, and density of microneedles employed for skin pretreatment [124, 125]. The efficacy of microneedle-mediated delivery is also affected by the drugs' physicochemical properties and molecular weight [126, 127].

McAllister et al. [128] conducted one of the early tests showing that high-molecular-weight compounds might be administered into and across human skin *in vitro*. Several materials, including metal, glass, and polymers, were used in the researchers' production of solid microneedles. They released an in-depth report showing that solid silicon microneedles were effective in enhancing transdermal delivery of calcein (622 Da) and other large molecules (insulin 58 kDa, bovine serum albumin 67 kDa, and nanoparticles) *in vitro*. Two experiments were conducted. In the first study, drug solutions were applied to the epidermis of human cadaver skin, while microneedle arrays were kept in the skin after the insertion. According to the findings, skin permeation of calcein, insulin, and BSA were all significantly enhanced. In the second study, drug formulations were placed on microneedles-treated skin after the insertion and removal of the microneedle array. Researchers discovered that the removal of microneedles in the second experiment resulted in a higher enhancement of drug delivery compared to the first study.

Solid microneedles have been extensively utilized to enhance the transdermal delivery of insulin. Insulin has been known as an ideal model drug for the transdermal transport of macromolecules facilitated by microneedles. Insulin, with a molecular weight of 5,800 Da, enters intact skin minimally, and its aqueous solubility enables its preparation into conventional liquid and semisolid formulations. Furthermore, its pharmacological effect can be determined by closely monitoring blood glucose levels. By enhancing insulin permeation across the skin, solid microneedles manufactured from various materials, such as silicon [129], metal [130], and polymers [128], have effectively lowered the blood glucose level.

Multiple solid metal microneedles assembled on a Derma Roller device were used to microporate rat skin to enhance insulin delivery and reduce blood glucose levels. Zhou and colleagues studied the effects of various metal microneedle lengths (250, 500, and 1,000 μm) on the enhanced delivery of insulin to diabetic rats' skin. The skin of anesthetized, shaved rats was treated with microneedle rollers ten times in two perpendicular directions. After the application of an insulin-soaked cotton patch, the permeation of insulin increased substantially, and blood glucose levels dropped significantly within 1 h and remained low for 3 h. The drop in blood glucose was more substantial when the insulin dose and the microneedle length were increased. Closing the transient microneedles-created micropores caused a gradual rise in blood glucose levels. Moreover, the rate of increase in blood glucose levels was inversely correlated to the needle length [130]. Similarly, Wu and coworkers [131] examined sustained and controlled intradermal delivery of insulin *in vitro* utilizing solid microneedles 150 μm in length. Microneedles were used to porate the skin before applying an insulin-loaded patch for 3 h. During the patch application, blood glucose levels dropped steadily without apparent peak effects. The drug penetration was greatly improved and remained to rise for many hours after the donor formulation was removed. *In vivo* experiments on diabetic rats indicated that the pharmacodynamic profile of percutaneously delivered insulin was smooth, with an action duration equivalent to that of subcutaneously administered biphasic insulin.

Li et al. [132] have investigated the transdermal delivery of insulin using solid microneedles by analyzing its impact on the blood glucose levels of diabetic mice. At 5 h, the blood glucose level was lowered to 29% of the starting level, demonstrating the enhanced skin penetration of insulin by microneedles treatment. Similarly, Martanto and associates researched the effectiveness of solid microneedles in enhancing the transdermal delivery of insulin. Solid microneedles made of stainless steel were used to puncture the skin, and then a liquid patch was applied. Microneedles enhanced skin permeation of insulin by an amount equivalent to 0.05–0.5 units of subcutaneously administered insulin. In the research, blood glucose concentration decreased by as much as 80% in diabetic rats [133]. Li et al. developed solid microneedles from poly(lactic acid) to capitalize on the advantages of microneedles while also providing the extra benefit of a biodegradable system. The research thoroughly examined how the microneedle dimension, insulin concentration, formulation viscosity, and delivery period affected the transdermal transport of the drug. Increased insulin concentrations enhanced drug permeation quantity *in vitro* but not the delivery rate. The rate of drug permeation was reduced as the formulation's viscosity increased. Then, diabetic mice were treated with solid PLA microneedles of 600 µm in length and 100 microneedles/cm^2 in density in *in vivo* studies. The findings showed that after 5 h, the blood glucose levels were 29%, compared to 19% after 1.5 h of a subcutaneous insulin injection [132]. Another insulin study was conducted by Qiu et al., who used lyophilized hydrogel patches over skin that had been porated with solid silicon microneedles [134]. At least 8 h of continuous insulin release were achieved. Lyophilized hydrogel patches containing insulin were shown to have a longer duration of effect than subcutaneous injection in lowering blood glucose levels. In addition, a stability study revealed that after six months of storage at 4°C, lyophilized hydrogel preserved more than 90% of insulin bioactivity.

In addition to insulin, solid microneedles have been employed to effectively porate skin and enhance transdermal delivery of various biomolecules. A roller-type microneedles (230 µm long) device, designed by Chang and colleagues [135], could generate 267 channels/cm^2 with a single application, yielding a high density of channels. Consequently, the permeation flux of fluorescein isothiocyanate-labeled ovalbumin and insulin was dramatically enhanced after microneedle roller application by 6- and 11-fold, respectively. In another study, pretreatment of skin with Dermaroller^{TM} microneedles (250, 500, and 1,000 µm in length) was assessed for its ability to increase skin penetration of ovalbumin-conjugated nanoparticles *in vitro* and *in vivo*. Microneedle treatment improved ovalbumin absorption in *in vitro* testing considerably higher than the control. In addition, transdermal delivery of ovalbumin from a solution was 28.3% ± 6.5%, whereas the drug delivery from nanoparticles was only 13.6% ± 2.4%. The drug diffusion from nanoparticles was slowed because the ovalbumin nanoparticles were large. The transcutaneous immunization with ovalbumin nanoparticles after microneedle pretreatment was more effective than the subcutaneous immunization using an equivalent dose [136]. Li et al. investigated the skin permeability of human immunoglobulin G (IgG) (RMM ~150 kDa) mediated by sugar (maltose) and metal (stainless steel) microneedles (Dermaroller^{TM}) *in vitro* and *in vivo* in hairless rats. After the microneedle treatment, a liquid reservoir patch loaded with human IgG solution was applied and left on the skin for 24 h. Over the course of 24 h, plasma IgG levels increased steadily. After 24 h, the patch was removed, and transepidermal water loss value and methylene blue staining indicated that microneedles-created channels remained open. The *in vitro* investigation showed that increasing the number of microneedles from 27 to 54 needles and the length of microneedles from 200 to 500 µm each improved IgG flux by roughly ten times and four times, respectively.

The steady-state transdermal flux of IgG was measured to be 45.96 ng/cm^2/h for maltose microneedles and 353.17 ng/cm^2/h for metal microneedles in the subsequent *in vivo* research. C_{max} of maltose and metal microneedles noted at 24 h was 7.27 and 9.33 ng/mL, respectively. Skin treatment with Dermaroller™ resulted in larger microchannels with a mean diameter of 83 μm, as compared to the channel of 58 μm diameter generated by maltose microneedle, which may account for the higher IgG permeation reported by Dermaroller™ [69]. Zhang and collaborators (2014) examined the transdermal permeability of four model peptides through porcine ear skin *in vitro* after a 150-μm solid silicon microneedle insertion. Transdermal delivery of peptides was shown to depend on their molecular weights. Microneedle pretreatment substantially increased the penetration of all peptides; however, an increase in the peptide's molecular weight reduced the quantity of drug delivery [137]. Jae-Ho and colleagues studied the penetration of calcein through excised rat skin using polycarbonate microneedle arrays. The combination of calcein gel and polycarbonate microneedles (500 μm length and 154 needles/cm^2) revealed a 5.46-fold enhancement compared to calcein-loaded gel on its own in the drug permeation after 12-h study. Moreover, increasing microneedle density from 45 microneedles/cm^2 to 154 microneedles/cm^2 enhanced the transdermal flux of calcein from 30.14 ng/cm^2/h to 54.13 ng/cm^2/h [138]. Effective transdermal delivery of fluorescein isothiocyanate–coupled dextran (72 kDa) was achieved using a solid microneedles array [127]. Needles with lengths of 900, 700, and 550 μm were found to efficiently penetrate dermatomed human skin *in vitro*, but shorter needles (300 μm) failed to do so. The permeation of peptides with varying chain lengths (melanostatin, rigin, and palmitoyl-pentapeptide) into human skin was studied by Mohammed et al. They found that lower molecular weight peptides improved local drug delivery [126]. Microneedles could be employed for gene expression and deliver a gene to human skin *ex vivo* [139]. Skin microporation by maltose microneedles substantially increased delivery of Alexa Fluor 555–labeled bovine serum albumin with a rapid onset [140]. Skin pretreatment with solid microneedles has been employed in tandem with iontophoresis to enhance transdermal delivery of human growth hormone [141], Alexa Fluor 555–labeled bovine serum albumin [140], and oligonucleotides [68]. To improve the permeation of bovine serum albumin over porcine ear skin, Han and Das used a combination of low-frequency sonophoresis and solid microneedle treatment. The permeability of BSA was measured to be 0.43 μm/s using microneedles and 0.40 μm/s using sonophoresis individually; however, when these two methods were combined, the drug permeability rose to 1 μm/s. This was estimated to be about ten times more than what could be attained by passive diffusion of BSA [142].

7.3.2 Coated Microneedles

Coating the drug-loaded formulation directly onto the surface of solid microneedles is another method of using microneedles to improve transdermal drug delivery. It is significantly more efficient than solid microneedles, which generally require a two-step application process. To coat therapeutic agents onto the surface of microneedles, various methods, such as dip-coating, casting, and deposition, have been explored [143, 144]. Coated microneedles make transdermal drug delivery more controlled and user-friendly. When drug-coated microneedles penetrate the skin, the coating layer dissolves, allowing the loaded drug to be deposited deeper under the skin [78]. Coated microneedles have been used in most investigations researching *in vivo* delivery of macromolecules employing solid microneedles. Due to the coating layer's weakening effects on the needles' mechanical robustness and sharpness, only a minimal quantity of drug may be deposited onto the needles' surface. Coated microneedles can only be employed in specific scenarios when a relatively small amount is required, such as in the delivery of desmopressin [145], human growth hormone [146], and interferon alpha [147]. The high potency of several macromolecules makes this delivery method a promising platform for drug delivery. The application process also has the additional benefits of only a single-step application. Coated microneedles will be a useful and practical device in clinical settings once the needles can be reliably coated with consistent and reproducible quantities of drugs. Hence, the coating process and formulation compositions must be optimized throughout the development of these coated microneedles systems.

Desmopressin has been used at a dose of 1–20 µg to treat bedwetting in young children, diabetes insipidus, and hemophilia A. This drug is a synthetic peptide of vasopressin with a molecular weight of 1,069 Da. Coated microneedles (microneedles) were evaluated for transdermal delivery of desmopressin, and the findings showed that these needles were safer and more effective than alternative methods [145]. Cormier and colleagues developed coated titanium microneedles loaded with 82 µg desmopressin to treat enuresis. It was estimated that 85% of the drug was administered to hairless guinea pigs, while desmopressin was rapidly released after the disintegration of the coating layer [145]. In another study, Macroflux® microneedle arrays (200-µm-long titanium microneedles) were coated by immersing the solid metal microneedles in 24% or 40% w/w desmopressin formulation to yield coated microneedle array loadings with 56 g and 82 µg drug, respectively. The coated microneedle arrays were inserted into hairless guinea pigs *in vivo* using a spring-loaded, self-activating Macrofux® applicator. Comparing a 5-minute treatment of microneedle arrays containing 82 µg desmopressin to the intravenous injection of 11 µg drug, an equivalent serum drug concentration was observed. This finding indicated that the elimination kinetics of these two delivery methods were comparable [145]. Notably, the system of Macroflux® coated microneedles has also been tested on human subjects. Subjects in a crossover study were administered 30 µg of desmopressin by intravenous infusion in Part 1 and 25 µg of the medication via Macroflux® microneedle patch in Part 2. The microneedles patch was reported to deliver the drug speedily and within the desired therapeutic dose range for its antidiuretic activities. Significantly, both skin inflammation and pain sensation were absent or mild in most subjects [148].

Saurer and coworkers could coat stainless steel microneedles with polyelectrolyte films loaded with DNA and proteins using a layer-by-layer coating technique. Subsequent fluorescence imaging reveals that the coated layer was nearly entirely disintegrated from the solid microneedles, allowing for penetration of the drug payload into the epidermis and dermis layers of the skin tissue [149]. To study antigen-specific immunotherapy for type 1 diabetes, Zhao and associates developed a coating formulation to deliver hydrophobic auto-antigen peptides across the skin. The coating process did not impair the biological activity of the peptides. The capacity of coated microneedles to deliver hydrophobic peptides has been shown in both *in vitro* (human skin) and *in vivo* (mouse skin) experiments [150]. PEG-coated microneedles were employed to deliver BSA transdermally *in vitro* and *in vivo*, as reported by Caudill et al. To prepare for the needles, microneedles were coated with a drug solution in a coating mask equipment, removed once dry, and then inserted into the skin. After 5 min of insertion, 45% of FITC-BSA-loaded microneedles were observed to have penetrated full-thickness pig skin at 24 h. Lesser fluorescence signals were seen in the lower dermis compared to the epidermis, upper dermis, and microneedle insertion areas. The following *in vivo* investigation involved applying BSA-coated microneedles to the backs of BALB/c mice for 2 min. Mice treated with microneedles retained more BSA in the treated area than the control given a subcutaneous injection. Moreover, microneedles treatment resulted in longer-lasting BSA retention than subcutaneous administration [151]. Li and colleagues coated metal solid microneedles with different molecules (immiscible molecules, proteins, and nanoparticles) to provide multiple treatments from a single microneedle patch. The molecules selected were meant to stand in for drugs of varying molecular weights, particle-encapsulated and free drugs. Porcine skin was treated with microneedles for 5 s; the needles were removed after 2 min. All three therapeutic agents were delivered effectively but at varying rates. Sodium fluorescein dye diffused the quickest, followed by fluorescently labeled nanoparticles, and, finally, FITC-BSA. After 4 h, the fluorescence intensity of FITC-BSA had decreased to less than 40%, and after two days, only traces remained [152]. The bioavailability of human growth hormone (hGH)-coated titanium microneedles was reported to be comparable to that of subcutaneous injections [146]. Similarly, equivalent to subcutaneous injections, polymeric solid microneedles coated with interferon-alpha were able to generate anticancer activity in malignant mice [147]. Coated microneedles (microneedles) were also used to deliver parathyroid hormone across the skin. The results were remarkable: a quick peak in the plasma profile even faster than that seen in subcutaneous injections. Furthermore, the drug was stable in the product at a high temperature over more than two years [153]. The coated sMTS used to administer peptide A transdermally was designed by Kapoor and coworkers [154]. A patch with 316 needles was coated with 250 µg peptide A. With microneedle-mediated transdermal delivery, the bioavailability was comparable to that of subcutaneous administration, proving the efficacy of coated microneedle systems. In addition, peptide A's stability was significantly enhanced after being coated on the sMTS [154]. The insulin-loaded polymeric layer was coated onto metal microneedles, as designed by Ross et al. Solid-state insulin administration across the skin using coated microneedles was viable since the thin and homogeneous coating layers were able to preserve insulin's bioactivity, and efficient insulin release was achieved within 20 min [155]. To transdermally administer recombinant human erythropoietin alfa, Peter and coworkers disclosed the development of a sucrose-coated titanium microneedle system. The pharmacokinetic performance of the coated microneedles was assessed in a preclinical study [156]. Using fluorescein isothiocyanate-labeled bovine serum albumin as a model protein, Mutwiri et al. used polyphosphazene polyelectrolyte (PCPP) as the polymeric materials for coated microneedles. The needles' capacity to porate the stratum corneum and the drug release kinetics was studied *in vitro* and *in vivo*. Embedded in the skin of a 4-week-old pig, the polymer dissolved rapidly and released all of the loaded protein within 15 min [157]. Prausnitz and associates devised a method of coating bovine pancreatic ribonuclease A onto metal microneedles using a layer-by-layer deposition of polyelectrolytes. After being inserted into porcine skin, the coating layer was hydrolytically degraded, allowing the loaded protein to be released and driven into skin layers [149].

The solid Microstructured Transdermal System (sMTS), designed by 3M, is a coated microneedle array with a drug-loading capacity of up to 0.3 mg. This system could be used to deliver potent macromolecules transdermally. To facilitate patient self-administration, Zosano Pharma has been developing a coated microneedles device with a reused applicator [153]. Their system employs an array of drug-coated titanium microneedles for transdermal delivery of biomolecules such as biologics, peptides, proteins, and vaccines. Parathyroid hormone (PTH), a medicine for the treatment of osteoporosis, is the company's primary focus. In both phase I and phase II clinical trials, the microneedle patch was shown to effectively and rapidly administer PTH with minimal plasma exposure. Wearing the patch for 0.5–2 h reportedly did not influence the effectiveness of the treatment. Also,

PTH loaded in the microneedle patch is stable at ambient temperature for up to two years, meaning there is no longer a temperature constraint on the product storage [121]. Synthetic strands of nucleic acid called antisense oligonucleotides (ODN) are used to successfully "turn off" certain genes in a process called gene silencing. Lin and coworkers administered these macromolecules transdermally to hairless guinea pigs using the Alza® Macroflux® microneedle patch [68]. At 4 h, the microneedle patches delivered more than 16 µg ODN systemically; however, in the control group, no ODN was absorbed and detected. Similarly, erythropoietin, ovalbumin, and human growth hormone were delivered *in vivo* to hairless guinea pigs using the coated Macroflux® technology [158, 159]. Parathyroid hormone 1–34 (PTH 1–34) loaded on a Macroflux® coated microneedles array has been investigated for its pharmacokinetic (PK) and pharmacodynamic (PD) profile in human subjects [153]. Phase I clinical trials involved the insertion of PTH(1–34)-coated microneedle patches to healthy human participants at various locations (i.e., abdomen, upper forearm, and thigh) for 30 min, followed by a PK assessment. For the control, the marketed product FORTEO® was injected subcutaneously into the subjects. Consequently, it was shown that the insertion of microneedle patches, no matter where they were inserted, caused a sharp increase in plasma PTH(1–34), with a T_{max} three times faster than what was seen after taking FORTEO®. Postmenopausal women with osteoporosis participated in phase II trials to assess the effectiveness of three different patch doses (20, 30, and 40 µg) compared to a placebo patch and an injection of FORTEO®. Dose dependence for PTH(1–34) delivery by microneedle patch was shown by noticing a linear increment in plasma PTH(1–34) AUC with increasing drug dose. Impressively, two years of storage at 25°C showed that 98% of PTH remained stable [121].

7.3.3 Hollow Microneedles

Micrometer-sized hollow needles, which function like small-scale syringes, have been developed to deliver liquid formulation into the epidermis or dermis layers of the skin [160]. The most basic method for drug transport utilizing hollow microneedles is the passive permeation of drugs through the microneedles. Pressure-driven flow has been revealed to be effective in increasing the delivery rate, which is particularly crucial given the slow passive diffusion rate in packed skin tissues [60, 161]. Hence, hollow microneedles may provide a precise drug transport rate while allowing for the delivery of greater drug quantities [60, 162, 163]. During transdermal drug delivery, hollow microneedles should have sufficient mechanical robustness to prevent fracture into the dermis and keep the bores unobstructed. Bypassing the stratum corneum and introducing a drug formulation directly to the epidermis or dermis layers is feasible using hollow microneedles injection. Proteins, oligonucleotides, vaccines, and all of which have relatively high molecular weights benefit significantly from this method of administration. Studies assessing the efficacy of hollow microneedles for the delivery of macromolecules have primarily been conducted *in vivo*. Most experiments using hollow microneedles have used drug infusions via the needles into the skin tissue. One of the primary concerns of using hollow needles is that the needle's bore may become clogged. Microneedles with bores on the side of the tip have been developed and manufactured to address this problem [164, 165]. As an added benefit, positioning the bore off-center minimizes needle blockage and enhances drug exposure to surrounding skin tissue. The integration of hollow microneedles with drug reservoirs is a topic where a significant amount of research has been conducted so far. In the future, the biocompatibility of needles' materials is crucial, and issues like needle clogging and reliability must be resolved.

In many studies, insulin has been widely used as a representative molecule for transdermal delivery via hollow microneedles. Most people with diabetes inject insulin subcutaneously many times daily. Subcutaneous insulin infusions (CSII) may be provided continuously as an alternative option. The CSII system, which contains an insulin pump connected to a subcutaneous needle, could be utilized to simulate basal insulin production and bolus injections along with meals [166]. These insulin infusions may be administered in a painless and noninvasive method with the use of hollow microneedles. Various methods of transdermal drug delivery using microneedles have been investigated for both insulin and BSA, but the "poke and flow" strategy using hollow microneedles has been applied most often in *in vitro* and animal studies [102, 110, 128, 131, 133, 167–171]. Furthermore, in human trials, insulin was administered using hollow microneedles and the "poke and flow" technique [168, 172–174]. Insulin delivery onset is augmented when hollow microneedles are used to administer the drug intradermally, and this effect may be induced by passive diffusion [175], pressure [128], or electricity-driven force [176]. Insulin may be delivered efficiently across the skin using hollow microneedles, such as those manufactured from silicon utilizing MEMS-based etching processes [170]. A preliminary investigation by utilizing insulin highlighted the capability of hollow microneedles to enhance the transdermal delivery of macromolecules was performed by McAllister and colleagues. After 30 min of insertion, a single glass microneedle could inject up to 32 µL insulin solution into hairless rat skin under a pressure of 10 psi. A 70% drop from pre-infusion values in blood glucose level was observed after a 5-h period of injection. A higher pressure was also associated with a speedier reduction in blood glucose levels [128]. Roxhed and coworkers [176] developed a microneedle patch in tandem with an electrically controlled liquid dispenser. At 3 h post-dosing, the plasma insulin level in the electrically powered group was approximately five times greater than in the passive diffusion control [176]. Further research involving human volunteers evaluated insulin lispro infusion through hollow microneedles compared to the subcutaneous injection. It was revealed that insulin injected intradermally via microneedles was absorbed more rapidly. They compared intradermal and subcutaneous injections and found that intradermal delivery resulted in lower values for secondary pharmacodynamic measures (i.e., mean blood glucose, maximum blood glucose, and blood glucose AUC) [177]. Davis and associates also presented a passive delivery device by injecting insulin suspension into diabetic hairless rats using arrays of 16 hollow metal microneedles 500 µm in length. A high-velocity plunger was used to introduce the array into the skin. An insulin-loaded chamber was then positioned on top of the array to function as a reservoir for the drug delivery. As a result, blood glucose levels were observed to decrease gradually over 4 h of insulin delivery period to 47% of baseline values, and to have remained relatively steady for 4 h after the delivery period. The highest level of insulin found in the blood was 0.43 ng/mL [175]. Studies on insulin administration in diabetic hairless rats demonstrated the efficacy of hollow glass microneedles. The glass capillaries were fashioned into needles using the standard micropipette manufacturing processes. Microinfusion was driven at controlled pressures of 5–20 psi for 30 min using microneedle loaded with insulin suspension and attached to compressed CO_2. Reports indicated that the needles penetrated 500–800 µm into the skin and injected around 5 µL during the infusion duration. Significantly lower glucose levels were obtained as compared to the control group. As a result, it was shown that an additional 45% decrease in glucose levels could be achieved by retracting the needles by around 200 µm. A total of about 30 µL might be injected over the course of 30 min after the microneedles were retracted [171]. *In vivo* studies on diabetic rats have also shown that blood glucose levels may be substantially lowered using the Gardeniers microneedle device. Insulin pumps were connected to a patch with arrays of hollow microneedles. A blood glucose profile comparable to that achieved with traditional subcutaneous injection was produced when insulin was injected via the hollow microneedles [178]. The study team led by Dr. Stemme created a patch-like microneedle system in which microneedles were connected to a drug dispenser, and tested its efficacy in diabetic rats. The patch contained an electrical drug dispenser and an array of 21 silicon hollow needles. After the electricity was applied to the heater, the thermally expanding silicone swelled into the reservoir, forcing the housed drug out of the hollow needles. The researchers found that diabetic rats' blood glucose levels dropped after receiving insulin via the patch for 3 h [170]. The same investigators also presented an innovative idea of sealing the hollow needles to prevent the drug contained in the reservoir from degrading, evaporating, or leaking [179]. According to Gupta et al., the use of hollow microneedles to administer insulin to children suffering from type 1 diabetes was associated with a shorter healing time and less discomfort than traditional injection methods [168, 172]. Using a hollow microneedle system, Norman and coworkers showed that insulin could be delivered intradermally to children and adolescents with minimal insertion discomfort and a rapid onset and offset of effect [180]. Significantly, the use of hollow microneedles device for the administration of insulin has already been implemented in humans. Both male and female adult patients with type 1 diabetes were studied to determine if the hollow microneedles were superior than a catheter infusion set at delivering insulin. The insulin infusion rate was modulated by a syringe pump that was coupled to a 3-mL syringe. Microneedles were inserted into the abdomen skin at different depths (1, 3.5, and 5 mm). The findings indicate that the needle penetration depth of 1 mm resulted in fast insulin absorption and decrease in the glucose levels in fasting participants, indicating the efficiency of hollow microneedles in noninvasive transdermal delivery of insulin [168].

In addition to insulin, hollow microneedles have been used to enhance the transdermal delivery of other macromolecules. Conventional administration of botulinum toxin A could be painful; hence Torrisi et al. developed a "pocketed" microneedle device to alleviate these issues while enhancing therapeutic targeting and simplifying the drug administration. Metal microneedles shafts were pocketed, so liquid drug formulation could be loaded into the reservoir. The delivery of β-galactosidase and formaldehyde-inactivated botulinum toxoid across the skin by microneedle showed efficient deposition and diffusion into the dermis layer [181]. Using hollow microneedles, Golombek and colleagues showed that synthetic mRNA could be delivered intradermally *in vitro*. After the injection with hollow microneedles, humanized Guassia luciferase protein levels were found to be high. After 24 and 48 h, the drug concentrations were substantially higher than with the "naked mRNA" control [182]. Transdermal delivery of ovalbumin (OVA)-loaded PLGA nanoparticles through hollow microneedles resulted in greater antibody response and higher levels of interferon-γ than intramuscular injection [183]. Verbaan and associates examined the *in vitro* transdermal delivery of three macromolecules of varying molecular weights through dermatomed human skin: cascade blue (538 Da), dextran-cascade blue (10 kDa), and FITC-dextran (72 kDa). The 30 G hollow needles of 300, 550, 700, and 900 μm height were used to porate the skin. Drug delivery through microneedle-treated skin was observed to be greatly increased as compared to the control group. It was revealed that the flux values dropped drastically as the drug's molecular weight increased. However, compared to untreated skin, the delivery rate of the largest molecule, (FITC-dextran), was significantly improved [166]. Two large molecules, human growth hormone (hGH) and equine tetanus antitoxin (ETAT), were also successfully delivered across skin with the use of the hMTS system. Human growth hormone (hGH) is generally injected subcutaneously to alleviate growth hormone deficiency. Its molecular weight is about 22 kDa. The researchers found that the pharmacokinetic (PK) characteristics of the drug were equivalent whether given to domestic swine through the hMTS or subcutaneously. No significant difference in C_{max} was obtained between the microneedle system and subcutaneous administration; however, the T_{max} reduction was statistically significant in the microneedle group. The authors hypothesized that microneedle-enhanced drug transport to the vascular and lymphatic-rich viable skin tissue could increase systemic absorption. The authors also demonstrated remarkably similar C_{max} and elimination kinetics after hMTS and subcutaneous injection [184]. 3M has designed a hollow microstructured transdermal system (hMTS) to deliver liquid pharmaceutical preparations into the dermis layer. This system is a microneedle-based device that uses a glass cartridge attached to hollow microneedles. This device has been developed to self-administer liquid formulations up to 1.5 mL in volume, with the delivery rate adjusted by a spring. In a specific study, Burton et al. [184] performed pharmacokinetic research on human growth hormones. They reported that the C_{max} was markedly greater, and the T_{max} was shorter for the hMTS system than for subcutaneous injection. Transdermal delivery of large molecules is also investigated by Chen et al., who examine the efficacy of low-frequency ultrasound combined with hollow microneedles. Calcein and bovine serum albumin transdermal delivery was determined using sonophoresis, hollow microneedles, or a combination of both (SEMA). SEMA was found to be superior than sonophoresis alone, hollow microneedles alone, and passive diffusion when it came to efficient transdermal delivery of both molecules [185].

7.3.4 Dissolving Microneedles

Dissolving microneedles are intended to incorporate therapeutic agents inside a water-soluble polymeric matrix and dissolve completely upon skin penetration. Depending on the dissolution rates of the particular polymer and the application time of microneedles, the dissolving and therapeutic duration have been observed to vary substantially from hours to days [186, 187]. It is crucial to consider the polymeric matrix material's physiochemical properties to optimize mechanical attributes and drug release kinetics. To protect the bioactivity of biomolecules, it is required to fabricate the needles under relatively gentle environments [188]. Carboxymethylcellulose [65], maltose [58, 189], chitosan [190], polyvinyl alcohol (PVA) [100], and polyvinylpyrrolidone are noted examples of biodegradable and dissolving polymers often employed in the manufacture of these microneedles.

Researchers have conducted extensive studies in mice, diabetic rats, and dogs using dissolving microneedles to encapsulate insulin, revealing that this technology provides stable drug loading and efficient insulin delivery, leading to lower blood glucose levels [191–193]. In an investigation, the biological activity of the insulin was preserved after the encapsulation and fabrication of insulin-loaded dissolving microneedles [194]. The investigators observed that after 24 h, microneedle insertion and subcutaneous injection both resulted in equivalent plasma insulin levels. Dissolving microneedles also allowed for consistent, reliable, and effective drug delivery. High relative bioavailability and pharmacological availability (90–97%) were achieved due to complete drug release and penetration into the bloodstream from microneedles. Insulin-encapsulated dissolving microneedles were developed by Liu et al. for the treatment of diabetes in rats. Insulin-loaded $CaCO_3$ microparticles and polyvinylpyrrolidone (PVP) were formed into dissolving microneedles using centrifugation and micromolding techniques. As a result, the mechanical strength of the fabricated microneedles was improved, while the solubility was prolonged, resulting in controlled release features, as compared to drug-loaded microneedles made from PVP alone. Due to this, insulin delivery from this microneedle design lagged behind that of a subcutaneous injection [195]. For the treatment of diabetes, Ling and colleagues developed a dissolving microneedle system made from starch and gelatin to rapidly dissolve and efficiently deliver insulin into the skin tissue [114]. Insulin retained more than 90% of its relative bioavailability after being stored for a month at either 25°C or 37°C. Lower blood glucose levels were indicative of stable loading of insulin in dissolving microneedles. Similarly, by blowing controlled air through the pulling polymer droplet to dry and solidify the microneedle structure, Jung and coworkers developed a novel method for fabricating dissolving microneedles, enabling safe and gentle manufacturing conditions for the production of insulin-loaded microneedles. The controlled blood glucose levels in mice with type 1 diabetes verified the remarkable bioavailability result of 96.6% ± 2.4% [196]. Dissolving microneedles for insulin administration was also developed by Migalska et al., who used an aqueous solution of poly(methylvinylether maleic anhydride). This approach significantly decreased the blood glucose levels in diabetic mice [102]. It is important to note that stretchable devices using dissolving and biodegradable microneedles for insulin administration have been produced. The drug was well-protected from enzymatic degradation by encapsulation into the crosslinked hyaluronic acid matrix, and the efficacy of the drug sustained release was maintained after every stretching trigger. Three stretching sessions separated by 4 h showed a pulsatile decrease in blood glucose levels [197]. Yang and associates fabricated phase-transition microneedles that could release insulin by changing the polymeric matrix material from a hard glassy to a hydrogel state after the needle penetration into the skin tissue. After the drug release, the whole PVA needle could be removed from the skin since it had been crosslinked to prevent disintegration in the dermis [198]. The "smart insulin patch" developed by Yu and associates is a transdermal drug delivery device made of crosslinked HA matrix incorporating glucose-responsive vesicles (GRVs). Within 30 min after receiving the GRV-containing microneedles, the blood glucose levels in the chemically induced diabetic mice dropped rapidly to roughly 200 mg/dL. Within 6 h after the treatment, the porated skin returned to normal, showing no signs of irritation and demonstrating the biocompatibility of the insulin-loaded microneedle system [79]. The novel microneedle-based technology disclosed by Ye and colleagues for glucose-responsive control of insulin production from exogenous pancreatic β-cell lines without implantation is particularly interesting. Synthetic glucose-responsive nanovesicles were encased inside the microneedle polymeric matrix, and they were then deployed to enhance glucose signals through a series of enzymatic processes. Pancreatic β-cell capsules housed in the patch's base were activated to secrete insulin in response to the magnified glucose signal inside the microneedle microenvironment. The microneedle patch was reported to rapidly lower blood sugar levels in mice with type 1 diabetes and to keep the levels low for more than 10 h [199]. In addition, insulin was embedded into the needle tip of dissolving microneedles. Results showed that insulin-loaded microneedles had a high relative bioavailability (about 98%) [200]. Insulin was successfully delivered into pig skin using dissolving microneedles manufactured by photopolymerization of vinyl pyrrolidone [102, 111]. In order to make insulin more easily administered transdermally, S. Liu et al. designed an innovative drug-loaded hyaluronic acid (HA) microneedle array. Pharmacokinetic and pharmacodynamic profiles indicated that the insulin released from these dissolving microneedles was almost entirely absorbed into the bloodstream without causing any substantial skin irritation, and that the hypoglycemic activity of insulin-loaded microneedles was mostly equivalent to that of the subcutaneous administration [201].

In addition to insulin, numerous biopharmaceutical drugs have been efficiently delivered across the skin using dissolving microneedles. The use of biodegradable and biocompatible polymers in the fabrication of dissolving microneedles, with the therapeutic agents encapsulated inside the polymer matrix, was reported early by Park et al. For this objective, calcein and bovine serum albumin (BSA) were incorporated into PLGA microneedles as model drugs. In five days, almost 80% of BSA was released. However, this study also revealed several limitations, such as limits on the quantity of the loaded drug, which must be considered to maintain the microneedle's mechanical strength and protein drug stability [104]. Interestingly, polymeric dissolving microneedles have been designed and optimized to effectively and noninvasively deliver a wide range of macromolecules into and across skin tissue. S. Fakhraei Lahiji and coworkers developed a novel hyaluronic acid backbone-based tissue interlocking microneedles array to prevent microneedles from distending from the skin, thus enhancing transdermal delivery of biomolecules (Fig. 7.2) [202].

Microneedles made of hyaluronan that rapidly dissolved in the skin tissue were developed to contain varying amounts of immunoglobulin G (IgG) for efficient *ex vivo* transdermal delivery of IgG [116]. Cyclosporin A is a cyclic peptide with a large molecular weight used to treat a wide variety of skin disorders; however, it is insoluble in water. By using a molding technique, researchers were able to produce cyclosporine A-loaded dissolving microneedles. After 60 min embedded in porcine skin, 65% of the microneedles containing 10% cyclosporine A dissolved, delivering 34 μg drug into skin layers [203]. Hyaluronic acid (HA)-based dissolving microneedles were produced by Liu and coworkers to enhance the transdermal delivery of fluorescein isothiocyanate-labeled dextran (FD4, 4kDa). The scientists demonstrated that after 7 h of insertion of HA microneedles, the quantity of FD4 that penetrated through the skin was substantially more than what was achieved with a drug solution. Drug penetration occurred relatively instantly when microneedles were utilized, as reported by the authors [204]. To facilitate intradermal transport of monoclonal IgG, Mönkäre et al. produced hyaluronan-based dissolving microneedles. With a 10-min insertion into human skin, 65% of the initial tip length was dissolved while IgG and

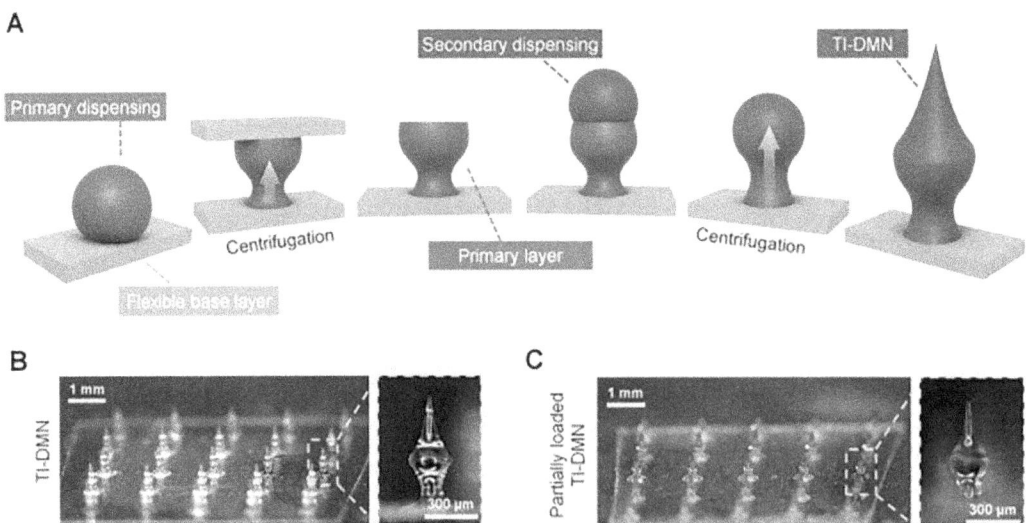

FIGURE 7.2
Schematic representation of tissue interlocking–dissolving microneedles. (A) Manufacturing process. (B) Microscopic images. (C) Partially loaded microneedle array. Images reprinted with permission from [202].

hyaluronan were deposited to a skin depth of 150–200 μm [116]. Dissolving microneedles encapsulating interferon-α-2b were prepared by Chen et al. for enhanced transdermal delivery. As a result, the maximum drug concentration in the blood (C_{max}) was found to be 11.58 ng/mL at 40 min. Interestingly, the drug was found stable in dissolving microneedles for two months. According to the authors, dissolving microneedles were bioequivalent to a control intramuscular injection, indicating that microneedles might substitute intramuscular injections of interferon-α-2b for convenient administration and improved patient compliance [205]. Dillon and associates (2017) developed a dissolving microneedle array made of PVA and trehalose to carry peptides inside the microneedle polymeric matrix. Microneedles loaded with polymyxin B were inserted into pig ear skin. For 4 h after the microneedle treatment, the drug permeation rate and the percentage of drug delivery were greater than those from the drug-loaded disk without microneedles [206]. Several factors, including polymer type, drug concentration, drying conditions, and storage conditions, were studied in relation to lysozyme activity in drug-loaded dissolving microneedles by Lahiji, Jang, Huh, et al. [207] and Lahiji, Jang, Ma, et al. [208]. When lysozyme-encapsulated microneedles were prepared at 4°C, left to dry at room temperature, and manufactured in the presence of stabilizing agents, the drug bioactivity was maintained for up to 99.8% ± 3.8% for 12 weeks [207]. Vora et al. employed a carbohydrate biopolymer (pullulan) to fabricate microneedles to allow efficient transport of FITC-BSA over dermatomed pig skin. Transdermal delivery of FITC-BSA from dissolving microneedles was evaluated by *in vitro* permeation experiments after ensuring the stability of FITC-BSA in the microneedle product was maintained. After 15 min of microneedle insertion, FITC-BSA could be detected, and after 28 h, the dissolving microneedles delivered 1,105 ± 123 μg/cm² across the skin [209]. Thermal-sensitive biomolecules should be cast onto molds and solidified at moderate temperatures that will not disrupt their activity. Microparticles of bovine serum albumin (BSA) and calcein were loaded in poly-lactide-*co*-glycolide (PLGA) microneedles produced by Park and colleagues. They demonstrated the possibility of controlled drug release using polymeric microneedles [104]. However, owing to the usage of increased temperature in manufacturing, protein activity showed a little reduction. To overcome this problem, Lee et al. [101] utilized a gentler preparation procedure to produce dissolving microneedles from ultralow viscosity CMC with complete enzymatic activity. Likewise, using a thread-forming polymer as a basis, researchers were able to manufacture erythropoietin-loaded dissolving microneedles at ambient temperature [110]. Antigen-presenting cells are matured and activated when a model antigen (OVA) and immunostimulatory adjuvant (resiquimod) are delivered to lymph nodes through dissolving microneedles, as shown by Kim and colleagues. When disintegrated in the skin, the amphiphilic triblock copolymer-based dissolving microneedles were able to produce nanomicelles *in situ*, allowing for the more efficient delivery of resiquimod. Tumor-carrying mice were able to produce a remarkable level of antigen-specific cellular and humoral response when treated by microneedles containing OVA and resiquimod [210]. A smart microneedles patch developed by Ghavami Nejad et al. is programmed to generate glucagon only when hypoglycemia is present. Hypoglycemia associated with an excess of insulin was averted using the microneedles patch in an animal model with type 1 diabetes [211]. Dissolving microneedles patches containing human parathyroid hormone were developed by Naito and colleagues to treat osteoporosis. When compared to parathyroid hormone in solution, the drug-loaded microneedles markedly increased the drug stability. According to the *in vivo* testing, the bioavailability of microneedles was determined to be 100% ± 4% when compared to subcutaneous injection. With the intervention of parathyroid hormone-loaded dissolving microneedles, the bone loss was slowed and the bone density was increased in rats with osteoporosis [212]. Chi et al. created chitosan microneedles loaded with vascular endothelial growth factor to aid with wound healing. Drug release might be modulated by a temperature increase caused by the wound's inflammatory reaction. Both the *in vitro* antibacterial experiment and the *in vivo* wound healing investigation showed that the microneedles patch facilitated collagen deposition, inflammatory reduction, and tissue repair in the healing stages of the wound [213]. Martin and coworkers [214] evaluated a moderate-temperature vacuum-forming technique to fabricate dissolving microneedles and showed that microneedles could be made from a dehydrated sugar combination consisting of trehalose anhydrous, trehalose dihydrate, sucrose, and maltose. Studies in rats have tested the viability of dextran microneedles made by spinning polypropylene into thread. After microneedle treatment, rhGH plasma levels in rats peaked and were found to be equivalent to the profile of rhGH solution administered intravenously. The maximal drug concentration in the serum was reached in a dose-dependent fashion, depending on the drug payload in the microneedles [215]. Bouwstra et al. designed hyaluronic acid microneedles for the enhanced transdermal delivery of monoclonal IgG. The micromolding technique was used to successfully fabricate microneedles loaded with either 2% or 10% (w/w) of monoclonal IgG. Dissolving microneedles allowed for the recovery of 80% of the loaded IgG, with negligible disruption to the IgG's tertiary structure. These microneedles were able to penetrate human skin *ex vivo*, dissolve rapidly, and release their drug payload in the epidermis and upper dermis layers of skin [116]. Two-layered dissolving microneedles were fabricated by Takada et al., which were used to deliver rhGH and desmopressin into the abdomen skin of rats. Chondroitin sulfate or dextran, both of which are water-soluble polymers, were used to produce dissolving microneedles containing the proteins [109]. Hammond and colleagues used silk fibroin/poly(acrylic acid) (PAA) composite to fabricate microstructures (microneedles patch) that were biocompatible and biodegradable. The patch included a pedestal base made of polyacrylic acid and a silk needle tip. Therapeutic agents that are sensitive to temperature changes, such as peptides, antibiotics, and vaccines, were able to maintain their therapeutic efficiency owing to the mild micromolding technique, ambient temperature, and atmospheric pressure [216, 217]. Polymeric microneedles have been used to release drugs slowly and selectively by loading them into microparticles. By incorporating CMC and polylactide acid (PLA) microparticles inside PLGA microneedles, it has been demonstrated that the release kinetics of the model protein BSA may be adjusted over a period of hours to months [104]. According to an investigation by Zaric et al., dissolving microneedles arrays effectively delivered PLGA nanoparticles encapsulating chicken OVA into the skin. The antigen-presenting cells in the skin could transfer the nanoparticles through afferent lymphatics to the lymph nodes [218]. To treat melanoma, Wang and collaborators described the application of a biodegradable, dissolving microneedles patch that stimulated the production of acid in the surrounding environment to allow for the prolonged delivery of anti-PD-1 monoclonal antibody. All of the needles consisted of nanoparticles of ethoxypropene-conjugated dextran and hyaluronic acid. By penetrating the epidermis layer, microneedles could deliver the particles to the adjacent lymph and capillaries [219]. Lee and coworkers fabricated dissolving microneedles made of carboxymethylcellulose to carry lysozyme. These microneedles were capable of delivering a bolus dose or controlled drug release by simply modifying the drug payload and microneedle patch design [101]. The same team also produced and evaluated a dissolving microneedle system loaded with hGH. hGH has been observed to retain its functional bioactivity for up to 15 months when stored at ambient conditions. Based on the findings of the *in vivo* experiment on rats, bioavailability was found to be 71% [65]. Microneedles composed of chondroitin sulfate or dextran matrix were employed to deliver hGH in another investigation by Fukushima et al. The acral end of these microneedles was specifically engineered to contain hGH. The bioavailability of these microneedles was estimated to be approximately 70% for the dextran microneedles and 90% for the chondroitin-based microneedles [109]. Likewise, a dissolving microneedle array containing leuprolide acetate was developed employing chondroitin sulfate as the polymeric base. There were reports of poor bioavailability owing to significant drug degradation in the skin [50]. Researchers also developed protein-loaded dissolving microneedles made of carboxymethylcellulose (CMC) and amylopectin that could dissolve in porcine skin within 1 h of insertion [101]. Chen and coworkers also fabricated a microneedle system consisting of chitosan microneedles and a poly(L-lactide-*co*-D,L-lactide) (PLA) supporting base, and employed the needles for transdermal delivery of antigens to skin tissue. The array of chitosan microneedles was affixed to a rigid PLA substrate, which provided the required mechanical robustness for complete skin penetration. Chitosan microneedles effectively detached from their array base and remained in rat skin, allowing for prolonged drug release without the necessity of a transdermal patch [220]. Ito and colleagues developed an innovative thread-forming process for the manufacture of needle-like projections from drug-loaded "dextrin glue" [113]. These systems, named self-dissolving micropiles (SDMP), were fabricated to contain insulin and found to significantly decrease levels of blood glucose *in vivo*. In addition, a hypoglycemic effect was noticed in dogs after the insertion of SDMPs containing chondroitin sulfate and insulin [221]. Likewise, SDMPs composed of dextrin, chondroitin sulfate, and albumin could deliver erythropoietin (EPO, 34 kDa) over the skin of mice *in vivo* [110]. Furthermore, an *in vivo* study on rats demonstrated that the application of drug-loaded SDMPs composed of chondroitin sulfate and dextran enabled the efficient absorption of interferon-alpha (19.5 kDa) into the skin [222]. Human growth hormone (hGH, 22 kDa) was also given *in vivo* through rat skin using dextran SDMPs in another research performed by the same team [215]. This group also developed a self-dissolving micropile array (SDMA) consisting of 100 microneedles arranged in ten rows and ten columns within 1 cm^2 area. *In vivo* evaluation of the effectiveness of a chondroitin sulfate-based SDMA containing EPO was performed on rats and dogs. *In vivo* studies were carried out to investigate the capacity of SDMA to enhance the percutaneous absorption of recombinant human growth hormone and desmopressin in rats [109].

7.3.5 Swelling Microneedles

In most scenarios, the matrix of hydrogel-forming swelling microneedles is made from crosslinked polymeric materials. The needles could penetrate the skin and rapidly absorb interstitial skin fluid. Then, the drug permeation across the swelling structure enables the delivery to deeper skin layers. Hydrogel-forming microneedles may be withdrawn from the skin, with nearly negligible polymeric residue remaining in the skin tissue. Unlike hollow microneedles, drug transport is not impeded by compressed skin tissue when using swelling microneedles [223]. Drugs are often contained within an associated reservoir, while hydrogel-forming microneedles do not carry the drug in their structure [224]. Given that it is not constrained by the needles' dimensions or surface area, a substantially greater quantity of drug can permeate into the skin, and the needles' mechanical robustness is not affected by the drug loading.

First developed in 2012, these swelling microneedles consist of poly(methyl vinyl ether/maleic acid) crosslinked with poly(ethylene glycol) to carry bovine serum albumin (BSA) [66]. Another commonly used polymer that exhibits distinctive phase-transition properties upon temperature alteration is polyvinyl alcohol (PVA) [225]. The swelling mechanism was able to effectively deliver a wide range of pharmaceuticals, including those with high molecular weights [66]. The gap junction blocker, GAP-26, has been incorporated into polyethylene glycol diacrylate microneedles by Liu and coworkers [226] for enhanced transport via the swelling mechanism. The penetration of the loaded peptide was improved significantly in the swelling microneedles. In another study, double-layered microneedle arrays with swelling needles contained within a nonswelling transdermal patch that could interlock upon skin penetration were developed by Seong et al. to enhance skin adhesion. The prolonged release of insulin *in vivo* was demonstrated to be due to this interlocking mechanism. As a result, transdermal delivery efficiency reached 60% over 12 h [227]. A study performed by Courtenay and colleagues (2018) investigated the transdermal delivery of the anticancer drug bevacizumab using dissolving (PVA) and hydrogel-forming microneedles (500 μm in length). Hydrogel-forming microneedles took longer to swell and delivered a lower C_{max} than dissolving microneedles. The pharmacokinetic profile discrepancies were connected to bevacizumab's molecular weight (149 kDa). The delayed C_{max} of swelling microneedles as compared to dissolving microneedles was attributed to the difficulty of large molecules to diffuse through the complicated hydrogel network. Since PVA is hydrophilic, incorporating bevacizumab into PVA microneedles could result in a rapid disintegration and drug release after microneedle application. Dissolving microneedles released the drug as a bolus dose, whereas hydrogel-forming microneedles showed an extended release profile; hence, the microneedle type may be altered to achieve the desired pharmacokinetic profile for the administration of macromolecules [228]. Using polyvinyl alcohol as the microneedle material and a microcrystalline crosslinking technique, Yang et al. developed phase-transition microneedles for the effective transdermal delivery of insulin [198]. In addition, Lutton and colleagues developed a scalable production method for hydrogel-forming microneedles, which included injection molding and roller casting and was performed at room temperature [229]. Interestingly, strong adhesion to skin was achieved by designing bullet-shaped, double-layered microneedle arrays with swelling needle tips. Swelling microneedles loaded with insulin showed extended release, enabling a progressive reduction in blood glucose levels [227]. The super-swelling microneedles delivered about 1.24 mg of the model protein ovalbumin over 24 h for an overall delivery efficiency of about 49% [224]. Transdermal delivery may be further improved by using a combination of iontophoresis and hydrogel-forming microneedles. Donnelly et al. proposed this strategy for addressing "on-demand" needs for post-meal insulin administration and rapid vaccination [164].

7.4 Conclusion

The parenteral injection has been the most efficient method of biopharmaceutical administration. Noninvasive drug delivery methods, such as the transdermal route, will facilitate drug administration and enhance patient compliance. The greatest obstacles in designing a transdermal delivery product for biomolecules are skin barrier function and selective permeability to small, moderately lipophilic compounds. With advancements in physical enhancement technology, the administration of biopharmaceuticals via the skin becomes plausible. Microneedle-enhanced drug delivery appears to be a highly promising method for the delivery of biotherapeutics. Nonetheless, the effectiveness of this sort of delivery system will be contingent on a variety of factors. The microneedle device's performance is crucial since it permits effective penetration into the skin. Several university research groups and pharmaceutical companies are exploring this technique for many biotherapeutics. Extensive academic research in conjunction with the pharmaceutical industry is predicted to speed the clinical translation of microneedles-based products of biopharmaceutical drugs. The delivery of therapeutic biomolecules using polymeric microneedles has garnered substantial interest in various applications. There are about 23 active and 39 completed clinical studies with microneedles at the National Institutes of Health for the treatment of a range of disorders, including type 1 diabetes, psoriatic plaques, and topical anesthesia [230]. A few studies have evaluated the efficacy of polymeric microneedles for biopharmaceutical drug delivery, whereas most investigations use commercially available hollow microneedles devices. Future clinical application success depends heavily on the design of polymeric microneedles with acceptable short-term and long-term biocompatibility. The research findings that have been published so far indicate considerable potential for turning microneedle-based delivery systems into self-use devices that will provide the patient with greater autonomy. Existing limitations might be rectified in the near future, allowing the delivery of biomolecules via the skin practicable.

In addition to drug stability, drug diffusion, manufacturability, and scale-up will impact the timescale for a microneedle product to reach the market. However, these concerns are more particular to the prospective drug in question. Although microneedles have the potential to reduce the stigma related to hypodermic needles, the acceptance of these devices will be impacted by undesirable patient outcomes such as skin irritation, pain, and infection. Future investigations will encompass a comprehensive study of the drug's dermal metabolism, degradation of formulation material, and long-term side effects. In addition, to accelerate the translation process, significant efforts surrounding microneedle production should be considered, covering large-scale manufacturing with fewer errors, simplicity of sterilizing, and increased drug-loading capacity to accommodate diverse applications of microneedles. In the last decade, both developments and translations of microneedles for drug delivery have flourished. With further integration of scientific research and commercialization strategies, an accelerated phase of microneedles products is anticipated to significantly enhance the quality of patients' life, public health, and economic output in developing countries.

References

[1] Han Y, Gao Z, Chen L, et al. Multifunctional oral delivery systems for enhanced bioavailability of therapeutic peptides/proteins. Acta Pharm Sin B. 2019;9:902–922.

[2] Katikaneni S. Transdermal delivery of biopharmaceuticals: dream or reality? Ther Deliv. 2015;6:1109–1116.

[3] Mitragotri S, Burke PA, Langer R. Overcoming the challenges in administering biopharmaceuticals: formulation and delivery strategies. Nat Rev Drug Discov. 2014;13:655–672.

[4] Liu T, Chen M, Fu J, et al. Recent advances in microneedle-mediated transdermal delivery of protein and peptide drugs. Acta Pharm Sin B. 2021;11:2326–2343.

[5] Lu Y, Sun W, Gu Z. Stimuli-responsive nanomaterials for therapeutic protein delivery. J Control Release. 2014;194:1–19.

[6] Ye Y, Yu J, Gu Z. Versatile protein nanogels prepared by in situ polymerization. Macromol Chem Phys. 2016;217:333–343.

[7] Frokjaer S, Otzen DE. Protein drug stability: a formulation challenge. Nat Rev Drug Discov. 2005;4:298–306.

[8] Herwadkar A, Banga AK. Transdermal delivery of peptides and proteins. In: Peptide and protein delivery. Amsterdam, NL: Elsevier; 2011. p. 69–86.

[9] Pavlou AK, Reichert JM. Recombinant protein therapeutics—success rates, market trends and values to 2010. Nat Biotechnol. 2004;22:1513–1519.

[10] Yan M, Du J, Gu Z, et al. A novel intracellular protein delivery platform based on single-protein nanocapsules. Nat Nanotechnol. 2010;5:48–53.

[11] Agyei D, Ahmed I, Akram Z, et al. Protein and peptide biopharmaceuticals: an overview. Protein Pept Lett. 2017;24:94–101.

[12] Jain D, Mahammad SS, Singh PP, et al. A review on parenteral delivery of peptides and proteins. Drug Dev Ind Pharm. 2019;45:1403–1420.

[13] Leader B, Baca QJ, Golan DE. Protein therapeutics: a summary and pharmacological classification. Nat Rev Drug Discov. 2008;7:21–39.

[14] Ye Y, Yu J, Wen D, et al. Polymeric microneedles for transdermal protein delivery. Adv Drug Deliv Rev. 2018;127:106–118.

[15] Hawkins MJ, Soon-Shiong P, Desai N. Protein nanoparticles as drug carriers in clinical medicine. Adv Drug Deliv Rev. 2008;60:876–885.

[16] Reichert JM. Trends in development and approval times for new therapeutics in the United States. Nat Rev Drug Discov. 2003;2:695–702.

[17] Zhu G, Mallery SR, Schwendeman SP. Stabilization of proteins encapsulated in injectable poly (lactide-co-glycolide). Nat Biotechnol. 2000;18:52–57.

[18] Ratanji KD, Derrick JP, Dearman RJ, et al. Immunogenicity of therapeutic proteins: influence of aggregation. J Immunotoxicol. 2014;11:99–109.

[19] Rothe A, Power BE, Hudson PJ. Therapeutic advances in rheumatology with the use of recombinant proteins. Nat Clin Pract Rheumatol. 2008;4:605–614.

[20] Ito Y, Kashiwara S, Fukushima K, et al. Two-layered dissolving microneedles for percutaneous delivery of sumatriptan in rats. Drug Dev Ind Pharm. 2011;37:1387–1393.

[21] Kinch MS. An overview of FDA-approved biologics medicines. Drug Discov Today. 2015;20:393–398.

[22] Rader RA. FDA biopharmaceutical product approvals and trends in 2012. BioProcess Int. 2013;11:18–27.

[23] Tan ML, Choong PF, Dass CR. Recent developments in liposomes, microparticles and nanoparticles for protein and peptide drug delivery. Peptides. 2010;31:184–193.

[24] Kirkby M, Hutton AR, Donnelly RF. Microneedle mediated transdermal delivery of protein, peptide and antibody based therapeutics: current status and future considerations. Pharm Res. 2020;37:1–18.

[25] Morales JO, Fathe KR, Brunaugh A, et al. Challenges and future prospects for the delivery of biologics: oral mucosal, pulmonary, and transdermal routes. AAPS J. 2017;19:652–668.

[26] Ibraheem D, Elaissari A, Fessi H. Administration strategies for proteins and peptides. Int J Pharm. 2014;477:578–589.

[27] Chaulagain B, Jain A, Tiwari A, et al. Passive delivery of protein drugs through transdermal route. Artif Cells Nanomedicine Biotechnol. 2018;46:472–487.

[28] Lundquist P, Artursson P. Oral absorption of peptides and nanoparticles across the human intestine: opportunities, limitations and studies in human tissues. Adv Drug Deliv Rev. 2016;106:256–276.

[29] Asfour MH. Advanced trends in protein and peptide drug delivery: a special emphasis on aquasomes and microneedles techniques. Drug Deliv Transl Res. 2021;11:1–23.

[30] Antosova Z, Mackova M, Kral V, et al. Therapeutic application of peptides and proteins: parenteral forever? Trends Biotechnol. 2009;27:628–635.

[31] Jiskoot W, Randolph TW, Volkin DB, et al. Protein instability and immunogenicity: roadblocks to clinical application of injectable protein delivery systems for sustained release. J Pharm Sci. 2012;101:946–954.

[32] Nir Y, Paz A, Sabo E, et al. Fear of injections in young adults: prevalence and associations. Am J Trop Med Hyg. 2003;68:341–344.

[33] Giudice EL, Campbell JD. Needle-free vaccine delivery. Adv Drug Deliv Rev. 2006;58:68–89.

[34] Bruno BJ, Miller GD, Lim CS. Basics and recent advances in peptide and protein drug delivery. Ther Deliv. 2013;4:1443–1467.

[35] Rawat A, Burgess DJ. Parenteral delivery of peptides and proteins. In: Mariko Morishita, Kinam Park, editors. Biodrug delivery systems. Boca Raton, Florida: CRC Press; 2016. p. 66–84.

[36] Dass CR, Choong PF. Biophysical delivery of peptides: applicability for cancer therapy. Peptides. 2006;27:3479–3488.

[37] Torchilin VP, Lukyanov AN. Peptide and protein drug delivery to and into tumors: challenges and solutions. Drug Discov Today. 2003;8:259–266.

[38] Almeida AJ, Souto E. Solid lipid nanoparticles as a drug delivery system for peptides and proteins. Adv Drug Deliv Rev. 2007;59:478–490.

[39] Ye M, Kim S, Park K. Issues in long-term protein delivery using biodegradable microparticles. J Control Release. 2010;146:241–260.

[40] Jani P, Manseta P, Patel S. Pharmaceutical approaches related to systemic delivery of protein and peptide drugs: an overview. Int J Pharm Sci Rev Res. 2012;12:42–52.

[41] Sauerborn M, Brinks V, Jiskoot W, et al. Immunological mechanism underlying the immune response to recombinant human protein therapeutics. Trends Pharmacol Sci. 2010;31:53–59.

[42] Patel A, Cholkar K, Mitra AK. Recent developments in protein and peptide parenteral delivery approaches. Ther Deliv. 2014;5:337–365.

[43] Riley RS, June CH, Langer R, et al. Delivery technologies for cancer immunotherapy. Nat Rev Drug Discov. 2019;18:175–196.

[44] Lopes AM, Apolinário AC, Valenzuela-Oses JK, et al. Nanostructures for protein drug delivery. Biomater Sci. 2016;4:205–218.

[45] Prausnitz MR, Langer R. Transdermal drug delivery. Nat Biotechnol. 2008;26:1261–1268.

[46] Arora A, Prausnitz MR, Mitragotri S. Micro-scale devices for transdermal drug delivery. Int J Pharm. 2008;364:227–236.

[47] Kalluri H, Banga AK. Transdermal delivery of proteins. AAPS PharmSciTech. 2011;12:431–441.

[48] Teo AL, Shearwood C, Ng KC, et al. Transdermal microneedles for drug delivery applications. Mater Sci Eng B. 2006;132:151–154.

[49] Peña-Juárez M, Guadarrama-Escobar OR, Escobar-Chávez JJ. Transdermal delivery systems for biomolecules. J Pharm Innov. 2021;1–14.

[50] Ito Y, Murano H, Hamasaki N, et al. Incidence of low bioavailability of leuprolide acetate after percutaneous administration to rats by dissolving microneedles. Int J Pharm. 2011;407:126–131.

[51] Blattner CM, Coman G, Blickenstaff NR, et al. Percutaneous absorption of water in skin: a review. Rev Environ Health. 2014;29:175–180.

[52] Jamaledin R, Di Natale C, Onesto V, et al. Progress in microneedle-mediated protein delivery. J Clin Med. 2020;9:542.

[53] Chandrasekhar S, Iyer LK, Panchal JP, et al. Microarrays and microneedle arrays for delivery of peptides, proteins, vaccines and other applications. Expert Opin Drug Deliv. 2013;10:1155–1170.

[54] Donnelly RF, Raj Singh TR, Woolfson AD. Microneedle-based drug delivery systems: microfabrication, drug delivery, and safety. Drug Deliv. 2010;17:187–207.

[55] Ita K. Ceramic microneedles and hollow microneedles for transdermal drug delivery: two decades of research. J Drug Deliv Sci Technol. 2018;44:314–322.

[56] Sharma D. Microneedles: an approach in transdermal drug delivery: a review. PharmaTutor. 2018;6:7–15.

[57] Larrañeta E, Lutton REM, Woolfson AD, et al. Microneedle arrays as transdermal and intradermal drug delivery systems: materials science, manufacture and commercial development. Mater Sci Eng R Rep. 2016;104:1–32.

[58] Miyano T, Tobinaga Y, Kanno T, et al. Sugar micro needles as transdermic drug delivery system. Biomed Microdevices. 2005;7:185–188.

[59] Almazan EA, Castañeda PS, Torres RD, et al. Design and evaluation of losartan transdermal patch by using solid microneedles as a physical permeation enhancer. Iran J Pharm Res IJPR. 2020;19:138.

[60] Prausnitz MR. Microneedles for transdermal drug delivery. Adv Drug Deliv Rev. 2004; 56:581–587.

[61] Serrano Castañeda P, Escobar-Chavez J, Arroyo-Vazquez J, et al. Pravastatin transdermal patch: effect of the formulation and length of microneedles on in-vitro percutaneous absorption studies. Iran J Pharm Res. 2020;19:127–133.

[62] Bhatnagar S, Dave K, Venuganti VVK. Microneedles in the clinic. J Control Release. 2017;260:164–182.

[63] Chen W, Tian R, Xu C, et al. Microneedle-array patches loaded with dual mineralized protein/peptide particles for type 2 diabetes therapy. Nat Commun. 2017;8:1–11.

[64] Kim Y-C, Park J-H, Prausnitz MR. Microneedles for drug and vaccine delivery. Adv Drug Deliv Rev. 2012;64:1547–1568.

[65] Lee JW, Choi S-O, Felner EI, et al. Dissolving microneedle patch for transdermal delivery of human growth hormone. Small. 2011;7:531–539.

[66] Donnelly RF, Singh TRR, Garland MJ, et al. Hydrogel-forming microneedle arrays for enhanced transdermal drug delivery. Adv Funct Mater. 2012;22:4879–4890.

[67] Li G, Badkar A, Nema S, et al. In vitro transdermal delivery of therapeutic antibodies using maltose microneedles. Int J Pharm. 2009;368:109–115.

[68] Lin W, Cormier M, Samiee A, et al. Transdermal delivery of antisense oligonucleotides with microprojection patch (Macroflux®) technology. Pharm Res. 2001;18:1789–1793.

[69] Li G, Badkar A, Kalluri H, et al. Microchannels created by sugar and metal microneedles: characterization by microscopy, macromolecular flux and other techniques. J Pharm Sci. 2010;99:1931–1941.

[70] Reichert JM, Rosensweig CJ, Faden LB, et al. Monoclonal antibody successes in the clinic. Nat Biotechnol. 2005;23:1073–1078.

[71] Escobar-Chávez JJ, Bonilla-Martínez D, Angélica M, et al. Microneedles: a valuable physical enhancer to increase transdermal drug delivery. J Clin Pharmacol. 2011;51:964–977.

[72] Xu B, Jiang G, Yu W, et al. H 2 O 2-responsive mesoporous silica nanoparticles integrated with microneedle patches for the glucose-monitored transdermal delivery of insulin. J Mater Chem B. 2017;5:8200–8208.

[73] Mo R, Jiang T, Di J, et al. Emerging micro-and nanotechnology based synthetic approaches for insulin delivery. Chem Soc Rev. 2014;43:3595–3629.

[74] Cevc G, Vierl U. Nanotechnology and the transdermal route: a state of the art review and critical appraisal. J Control Release. 2010;141:277–299.

[75] Schoellhammer CM, Blankschtein D, Langer R. Skin permeabilization for transdermal drug delivery: recent advances and future prospects. Expert Opin Drug Deliv. 2014;11:393–407.

[76] Shaikh S, Bhan N, Rodrigues FC, et al. Microneedle platform for biomedical applications. In: Kunal Pal, Heinz-Bernhard Kraatz, Anwesha Khasnobish, Sandip Bag, Indranil Banerjee, Usha Kuruganti, editors. Bioelectronics and medical devices. Amsterdam, NL: Elsevier; 2019. p. 421–441.

[77] van der Maaden K, Yu H, Sliedregt K, et al. Nanolayered chemical modification of silicon surfaces with ionizable surface groups for pH-triggered protein adsorption and release: application to microneedles. J Mater Chem B. 2013;1:4466–4477.

[78] Waghule T, Singhvi G, Dubey SK, et al. Microneedles: a smart approach and increasing potential for transdermal drug delivery system. Biomed Pharmacother. 2019;109:1249–1258.

[79] Yu J, Zhang Y, Ye Y, et al. Microneedle-array patches loaded with hypoxia-sensitive vesicles provide fast glucose-responsive insulin delivery. Proc Natl Acad Sci. 2015;112:8260–8265.

[80] Dubin CH. Transdermal, topical and subcutaneous drug delivery: extending pipelines and improving self-administration. Drug Devel Deliv. 2013;13:44–52.

[81] Rejinold NS, Shin J-H, Seok HY, et al. Biomedical applications of microneedles in therapeutics: recent advancements and implications in drug delivery. Expert Opin Drug Deliv. 2016;13:109–131.

[82] He X, Sun J, Zhuang J, et al. Microneedle system for transdermal drug and vaccine delivery: devices, safety, and prospects. Dose-Response. 2019;17:1559325819878585.

[83] Pastor Y, Larrañeta E, Erhard Á, et al. Dissolving microneedles for intradermal vaccination against shigellosis. Vaccines. 2019;7:159.

[84] Cahill EM, O'Cearbhaill ED. Toward biofunctional microneedles for stimulus responsive drug delivery. Bioconjug Chem. 2015;26:1289–1296.

[85] Lim D-J, Vines JB, Park H, et al. Microneedles: a versatile strategy for transdermal delivery of biological molecules. Int J Biol Macromol. 2018;110:30–38.

[86] Di Natale C, La Manna S, Malfitano AM, et al. Structural insights into amyloid structures of the C-terminal region of nucleophosmin 1 in type A mutation of acute myeloid leukemia. Biochim Biophys Acta BBA-Proteins Proteomics. 2019;1867:637–644.

[87] Frieden C. Protein aggregation processes: in search of the mechanism. Protein Sci. 2007;16:2334–2344.

[88] Arakawa T, Philo JS, Ejima D, et al. Aggregation analysis of therapeutic proteins, part 1. Bioprocess Int. 2006;4:32–42.

[89] Hermeling S, Crommelin DJ, Schellekens H, et al. Structure-immunogenicity relationships of therapeutic proteins. Pharm Res. 2004;21:897–903.

[90] Schellekens H. Factors influencing the immunogenicity of therapeutic proteins. Nephrol Dial Transplant. 2005;20:vi3–vi9.

[91] Schellekens H. How to predict and prevent the immunogenicity of therapeutic proteins. Biotechnol Annu Rev. 2008;14:191–202.

[92] Singh SK. Impact of product-related factors on immunogenicity of biotherapeutics. J Pharm Sci. 2011;100:354–387.

[93] Beck A, Wurch T, Bailly C, et al. Strategies and challenges for the next generation of therapeutic antibodies. Nat Rev Immunol. 2010;10:345–352.

[94] Leavy O. Therapeutic antibodies: past, present and future. Nat Rev Immunol. 2010;10:297–297.

[95] Weiner GJ. Building better monoclonal antibody-based therapeutics. Nat Rev Cancer. 2015;15:361–370.

[96] Cobo I, Li M, Sumerlin BS, et al. Smart hybrid materials by conjugation of responsive polymers to biomacromolecules. Nat Mater. 2015;14:143–159.

[97] Karimi M, Sahandi Zangabad P, Baghaee-Ravari S, et al. Smart nanostructures for cargo delivery: uncaging and activating by light. J Am Chem Soc. 2017;139:4584–4610.

[98] Rosenberg AS. Effects of protein aggregates: an immunologic perspective. AAPS J. 2006;8:E501–E507.

[99] Singh SK, Afonina N, Awwad M, et al. An industry perspective on the monitoring of subvisible particles as a quality attribute for protein therapeutics. J Pharm Sci. 2010;99:3302–3321.

[100] Chu LY, Choi S-O, Prausnitz MR. Fabrication of dissolving polymer microneedles for controlled drug encapsulation and delivery: bubble and pedestal microneedle designs. J Pharm Sci. 2010;99:4228–4238.

[101] Lee JW, Park J-H, Prausnitz MR. Dissolving microneedles for transdermal drug delivery. Biomaterials. 2008;29:2113–2124.

[102] Migalska K, Morrow DIJ, Garland MJ, et al. Laser-engineered dissolving microneedle arrays for transdermal macromolecular drug delivery. Pharm Res. 2011;28:1919–1930.

[103] Mistilis MJ, Bommarius AS, Prausnitz MR. Development of a thermostable microneedle patch for influenza vaccination. J Pharm Sci. 2015;104:740–749.

[104] Park J-H, Allen MG, Prausnitz MR. Polymer microneedles for controlled-release drug delivery. Pharm Res. 2006;23:1008–1019.

[105] Pan J, Chan SY, Lee WG, et al. Microfabricated particulate drug-delivery systems. Biotechnol J. 2011;6:1477–1487.

[106] Panyam J, Dali MM, Sahoo SK, et al. Polymer degradation and in vitro release of a model protein from poly (D, L-lactide-co-glycolide) nano-and microparticles. J Control Release. 2003;92:173–187.

[107] Xie J, Wang C-H. Encapsulation of proteins in biodegradable polymeric microparticles using electrospray in the Taylor cone-jet mode. Biotechnol Bioeng. 2007;97:1278–1290.

[108] Donnelly RF, Majithiya R, Singh TRR, et al. Design, optimization and characterisation of polymeric microneedle arrays prepared by a novel laser-based micromoulding technique. Pharm Res. 2011;28:41–57.

[109] Fukushima K, Ise A, Morita H, et al. Two-layered dissolving microneedles for percutaneous delivery of peptide/protein drugs in rats. Pharm Res. 2011;28:7–21.

[110] Ito Y, Yoshimitsu J-I, Shiroyama K, et al. Self-dissolving microneedles for the percutaneous absorption of EPO in mice. J Drug Target. 2006;14:255–261.

[111] Sullivan SP, Koutsonanos DG, Del Pilar Martin M, et al. Dissolving polymer microneedle patches for influenza vaccination. Nat Med. 2010;16:915–920.

[112] van der Maaden K, Jiskoot W, Bouwstra J. Microneedle technologies for (trans)dermal drug and vaccine delivery. J Control Release. 2012;161:645–655.

[113] Ito Y, Hagiwara E, Saeki A, et al. Feasibility of microneedles for percutaneous absorption of insulin. Eur J Pharm Sci. 2006;29:82–88.

[114] Ling M-H, Chen M-C. Dissolving polymer microneedle patches for rapid and efficient transdermal delivery of insulin to diabetic rats. Acta Biomater. 2013;9:8952–8961.

[115] Yang J, Liu X, Fu Y, et al. Recent advances of microneedles for biomedical applications: drug delivery and beyond. Acta Pharm Sin B. 2019;9:469–483.

[116] Mönkäre J, Reza Nejadnik M, Baccouche K, et al. IgG-loaded hyaluronan-based dissolving microneedles for intradermal protein delivery. J Control Release. 2015;218:53–62.

[117] Battisti M, Vecchione R, Casale C, et al. Non-invasive production of multi-compartmental biodegradable polymer microneedles for controlled intradermal drug release of labile molecules. Front Bioeng Biotechnol. 2019;7:296.

[118] Jeon EY, Lee J, Kim BJ, et al. Bio-inspired swellable hydrogel-forming double-layered adhesive microneedle protein patch for regenerative internal/external surgical closure. Biomaterials. 2019;222:119439.

[119] Liu S, Zhang S, Duan Y, et al. Transcutaneous immunization of recombinant Staphylococcal enterotoxin B protein using a dissolving microneedle provides potent protection against lethal enterotoxin challenge. Vaccine. 2019;37:3810–3819.

[120] Hiraishi Y, Nakagawa T, Quan Y-S, et al. Performance and characteristics evaluation of a sodium hyaluronate-based microneedle patch for a transcutaneous drug delivery system. Int J Pharm. 2013;441:570–579.

[121] Ameri M, Daddona PE, Maa Y-F. Demonstrated solid-state stability of parathyroid hormone PTH (1–34) coated on a novel transdermal microprojection delivery system. Pharm Res. 2009;26:2454–2463.

[122] Donnelly RF, Morrow DIJ, Singh TRR, et al. Processing difficulties and instability of carbohydrate microneedle arrays. Drug Dev Ind Pharm. 2009;35:1242–1254.

[123] Chennamsetty N, Voynov V, Kayser V, et al. Design of therapeutic proteins with enhanced stability. Proc Natl Acad Sci. 2009;106:11937–11942.

[124] Cheung K, Han T, Das DB. Effect of force of microneedle insertion on the permeability of insulin in skin. J Diabetes Sci Technol. 2014;8:444–452.

[125] Yan G, Warner KS, Zhang J, et al. Evaluation needle length and density of microneedle arrays in the pretreatment of skin for transdermal drug delivery. Int J Pharm. 2010;391:7–12.

[126] Mohammed YH, Yamada M, Lin LL, et al. Microneedle enhanced delivery of cosmeceutically relevant peptides in human skin. PLoS One. 2014;9:e101956.

[127] Verbaan FJ, Bal SM, van den Berg DJ, et al. Assembled microneedle arrays enhance the transport of compounds varying over a large range of molecular weight across human dermatomed skin. J Control Release. 2007;117:238–245.

[128] McAllister DV, Wang PM, Davis SP, et al. Microfabricated needles for transdermal delivery of macromolecules and nanoparticles: fabrication methods and transport studies. Proc Natl Acad Sci. 2003;100:13755–13760.

[129] Xie Y, Xu B, Gao Y. Controlled transdermal delivery of model drug compounds by MEMS microneedle array. Nanomedicine Nanotechnol Biol Med. 2005;1:184–190.

[130] Zhou C-P, Liu Y-L, Wang H-L, et al. Transdermal delivery of insulin using microneedle rollers in vivo. Int J Pharm. 2010;392:127–133.

[131] Wu Y, Gao Y, Qin G, et al. Sustained release of insulin through skin by intradermal microdelivery system. Biomed Microdevices. 2010;12:665–671.

[132] Li QY, Zhang JN, Chen BZ, et al. A solid polymer microneedle patch pretreatment enhances the permeation of drug molecules into the skin. Rsc Adv. 2017;7:15408–15415.

[133] Martanto W, Davis SP, Holiday NR, et al. Transdermal delivery of insulin using microneedles in vivo. Pharm Res. 2004;21:947–952.

[134] Qiu Y, Qin G, Zhang S, et al. Novel lyophilized hydrogel patches for convenient and effective administration of microneedle-mediated insulin delivery. Int J Pharm. 2012;437:51–56.

[135] Lee CR, Kim MS, Lee HB, et al. The effect of molecular weight of drugs on transdermal delivery system using microneedle device. Key Eng Mater. Trans Tech Publ; 2007;342–343:945–948.

[136] Kumar A, Li X, Sandoval MA, et al. Permeation of antigen protein-conjugated nanoparticles and live bacteria through microneedle-treated mouse skin. Int J Nanomedicine. 2011;6:1253–1264.

[137] Zhang S, Qiu Y, Gao Y. Enhanced delivery of hydrophilic peptides in vitro by transdermal microneedle pretreatment. Acta Pharm Sin B. 2014;4:100–104.

[138] Oh J-H, Park H-H, Do K-Y, et al. Influence of the delivery systems using a microneedle array on the permeation of a hydrophilic molecule, calcein. Eur J Pharm Biopharm. 2008;69:1040–1045.

[139] Pearton M, Allender C, Brain K, et al. Gene delivery to the epidermal cells of human skin explants using microfabricated microneedles and hydrogel formulations. Pharm Res. 2008;25:407–416.

[140] Bai Y, Sachdeva V, Kim H, et al. Transdermal delivery of proteins using a combination of iontophoresis and microporation. Ther Deliv. 2014;5:525–536.

[141] Cormier M, Daddona PE. Macroflux technology for transdermal delivery of therapeutic proteins and vaccines. In: Michael Rathbone, Jonathan Hadgraft, editors. Modified-release drug delivery technololgy. Boca Raton, Florida: CRC Press; 2002. p. 613–622.

[142] Han T, Das DB. Permeability enhancement for transdermal delivery of large molecule using low-frequency sonophoresis combined with microneedles. J Pharm Sci. 2013;102:3614–3622.

[143] Chen X, Kask AS, Crichton ML, et al. Improved DNA vaccination by skin-targeted delivery using dry-coated densely-packed microprojection arrays. J Control Release. 2010;148:327–333.

[144] Ma Y, Gill HS. Coating solid dispersions on microneedles via a molten dip-coating method: development and in vitro evaluation for transdermal delivery of a water-insoluble drug. J Pharm Sci. 2014;103:3621–3630.

[145] Cormier M, Johnson B, Ameri M, et al. Transdermal delivery of desmopressin using a coated microneedle array patch system. J Control Release. 2004;97:503–511.

[146] Ameri M, Kadkhodayan M, Nguyen J, et al. Human growth hormone delivery with a microneedle transdermal system: preclinical formulation, stability, delivery and PK of therapeutically relevant doses. Pharmaceutics. 2014;6:220–234.

[147] Kusamori K, Katsumi H, Sakai R, et al. Development of a drug-coated microneedle array and its application for transdermal delivery of interferon alpha. Biofabrication. 2016;8:015006.

[148] Sathyan G, Sun YN, Weyers R, et al. Macroflux® desmopressin transdermal delivery system: pharmacokinetics and pharmacodynamic evaluation in healthy volunteers. AAPS J. 2004;6:665.

[149] Saurer EM, Flessner RM, Sullivan SP, et al. Layer-by-layer assembly of DNA-and protein-containing films on microneedles for drug delivery to the skin. Biomacromolecules. 2010;11:3136–3143.

[150] Zhao X, Coulman SA, Hanna SJ, et al. Formulation of hydrophobic peptides for skin delivery via coated microneedles. J Control Release. 2017;265:2–13.

[151] Caudill CL, Perry JL, Tian S, et al. Spatially controlled coating of continuous liquid interface production microneedles for transdermal protein delivery. J Control Release. 2018;284:122–132.

[152] Li S, Li W, Prausnitz M. Individually coated microneedles for co-delivery of multiple compounds with different properties. Drug Deliv Transl Res. 2018;8:1043–1052.

[153] Daddona PE, Matriano JA, Mandema J, et al. Parathyroid hormone (1–34)-coated microneedle patch system: clinical pharmacokinetics and pharmacodynamics for treatment of osteoporosis. Pharm Res. 2011;28:159–165.

[154] Kapoor Y, Milewski M, Dick L, et al. Coated microneedles for transdermal delivery of a potent pharmaceutical peptide. Biomed Microdevices. 2020;22:1–10.

[155] Ross S, Scoutaris N, Lamprou D, et al. Inkjet printing of insulin microneedles for transdermal delivery. Drug Deliv Transl Res. 2015;5:451–461.

[156] Peters EE, Ameri M, Wang X, et al. Erythropoietin-coated ZP-microneedle transdermal system: preclinical formulation, stability, and delivery. Pharm Res. 2012;29:1618–1626.

[157] Andrianov AK, DeCollibus DP, Gillis HA, et al. Poly[di(carboxylatophenoxy)phosphazene] is a potent adjuvant for intradermal immunization. Proc Natl Acad Sci U S A. 2009;106:18936–18941.

[158] Ameri M, Peters EE, Wang X, et al. Erythropoietin (EPO) coated microprojection transdermal system: pre-clinical formulation, stability and delivery. AAPS J. 2009;11:T2245.

[159] Daddona P. Macroflux® transdermal technology development for the delivery of therapeutic peptides and proteins. Drug Deliv Technol. 2002;2.

[160] Shrestha P, Stoeber B. Fluid absorption by skin tissue during intradermal injections through hollow microneedles. Sci Rep. 2018;8:1–13.

[161] Donnelly RF, Singh TRR, Larrañeta E, et al. Microneedles for drug and vaccine delivery and patient monitoring. New Jersey: John Wiley & Sons; 2018.

[162] Terashima S, Tatsukawa C, Takahashi T, et al. Fabrication of hyaluronic acid hollow microneedle array. Jpn J Appl Phys. 2020;59:SIIJ03.

[163] Zaid Alkilani A, McCrudden MT, Donnelly RF. Transdermal drug delivery: innovative pharmaceutical developments based on disruption of the barrier properties of the stratum corneum. Pharmaceutics. 2015;7:438–470.

[164] Griss P, Stemme G. Side-opened out-of-plane microneedles for microfluidic transdermal liquid transfer. J Microelectromechanical Syst. 2003;12:296–301.

[165] Stoeber B, Liepmann D. Two-dimensional arrays of out-of-plane needles. ASME international mechanical engineering congress and exposition. Orlando, Florida: American Society of Mechanical Engineers; 2000. p. 355–359.

[166] Valla V. Therapeutics of diabetes mellitus: focus on insulin analogues and insulin pumps. Exp Diabetes Res. 2010;2010.

[167] Gill HS, Prausnitz MR. Coating formulations for microneedles. Pharm Res. 2007;24:1369–1380.

[168] Gupta J, Felner EI, Prausnitz MR. Minimally invasive insulin delivery in subjects with type 1 diabetes using hollow microneedles. Diabetes Technol Ther. 2009;11:329–337.

[169] Harvey AJ, Kaestner SA, Sutter DE, et al. Microneedle-based intradermal delivery enables rapid lymphatic uptake and distribution of protein drugs. Pharm Res. 2011;28:107–116.

[170] Nordquist L, Roxhed N, Griss P, et al. Novel microneedle patches for active insulin delivery are efficient in maintaining glycaemic control: an initial comparison with subcutaneous administration. Pharm Res. 2007;24:1381–1388.

[171] Wang PM, Cornwell M, Hill J, et al. Precise microinjection into skin using hollow microneedles. J Invest Dermatol. 2006;126:1080–1087.

[172] Gupta J, Felner EI, Prausnitz MR. Rapid pharmacokinetics of intradermal insulin administered using microneedles in type 1 diabetes subjects. Diabetes Technol Ther. 2011;13:451–456.

[173] Pettis RJ, Ginsberg B, Hirsch L, et al. Intradermal microneedle delivery of insulin lispro achieves faster insulin absorption and insulin action than subcutaneous injection. Diabetes Technol Ther. 2011;13:435–442.

[174] Pettis RJ, Hirsch L, Kapitza C, et al. Microneedle-based intradermal versus subcutaneous administration of regular human insulin or insulin lispro: pharmacokinetics and postprandial glycemic excursions in patients with type 1 diabetes. Diabetes Technol Ther. 2011;13:443–450.

[175] Davis SP, Martanto W, Allen MG, et al. Hollow metal microneedles for insulin delivery to diabetic rats. IEEE Trans Biomed Eng. 2005;52:909–915.

[176] Roxhed N, Samel B, Nordquist L, et al. Painless drug delivery through microneedle-based transdermal patches featuring active infusion. IEEE Trans Biomed Eng. 2008;55:1063–1071.

[177] McVey E, Hirsch L, Sutter DE, et al. Pharmacokinetics and postprandial glycemic excursions following insulin lispro delivered by intradermal microneedle or subcutaneous infusion. J Diabetes Sci Technol. 2012;6:743–754.

[178] Gardeniers HJ, Luttge R, Berenschot EJ, et al. Silicon micromachined hollow microneedles for transdermal liquid transport. J Microelectromechanical Syst. 2003;12:855–862.

[179] Roxhed N, Griss P, Stemme G. Membrane-sealed hollow microneedles and related administration schemes for transdermal drug delivery. Biomed Microdevices. 2008;10:271–279.

[180] Norman JJ, Brown MR, Raviele NA, et al. Faster pharmacokinetics and increased patient acceptance of intradermal insulin delivery using a single hollow microneedle in children and adolescents with type 1 diabetes. Pediatr Diabetes. 2013;14:459–465.

[181] Torrisi BM, Zarnitsyn V, Prausnitz MR, et al. Pocketed microneedles for rapid delivery of a liquid-state botulinum toxin a formulation into human skin. J Control Release. 2013;165:146–152.

[182] Golombek S, Pilz M, Steinle H, et al. Intradermal delivery of synthetic mRNA using hollow microneedles for efficient and rapid production of exogenous proteins in skin. Mol Ther-Nucleic Acids. 2018;11:382–392.

[183] Niu L, Chu LY, Burton SA, et al. Intradermal delivery of vaccine nanoparticles using hollow microneedle array generates enhanced and balanced immune response. J Control Release. 2019;294:268–278.

[184] Burton SA, Ng C-Y, Simmers R, et al. Rapid intradermal delivery of liquid formulations using a hollow microstructured array. Pharm Res. 2011;28:31–40.

[185] Chen B, Wei J, Iliescu C. Sonophoretic enhanced microneedles array (SEMA)—Improving the efficiency of transdermal drug delivery. Sens Actuators B Chem. 2010;145:54–60.

[186] An M, Liu H. Dissolving microneedle arrays for transdermal delivery of amphiphilic vaccines. Small. 2017;13:1700164.

[187] Hong X, Wei L, Wu F, et al. Dissolving and biodegradable microneedle technologies for transdermal sustained delivery of drug and vaccine. Drug Des Devel Ther. 2013;7:945–952.

[188] Moga KA, Bickford LR, Geil RD, et al. Rapidly-dissolvable microneedle patches via a highly scalable and reproducible soft lithography approach. Adv Mater. 2013;25:5060 5066.

[189] Lee K, Lee CY, Jung H. Dissolving microneedles for transdermal drug administration prepared by stepwise controlled drawing of maltose. Biomaterials. 2011;32:3134–3140.

[190] Chen M-C, Ling M-H, Lai K-Y, et al. Chitosan microneedle patches for sustained transdermal delivery of macromolecules. Biomacromolecules. 2012;13:4022–4031.

[191] Fukushima K, Yamazaki T, Hasegawa R, et al. Pharmacokinetic and pharmacodynamic evaluation of insulin dissolving microneedles in dogs. Diabetes Technol Ther. 2010;12:465–474.

[192] Ito Y, Hagiwara E, Saeki A, et al. Sustained-release self-dissolving micropiles for percutaneous absorption of insulin in mice. J Drug Target. 2007;15:323–326.

[193] Ito Y, Yamazaki T, Sugioka N, et al. Self-dissolving micropile array tips for percutaneous administration of insulin. J Mater Sci Mater Med. 2010;21:835–841.

[194] Chen M-C, Ling M-H, Kusuma SJ. Poly-γ-glutamic acid microneedles with a supporting structure design as a potential tool for transdermal delivery of insulin. Acta Biomater. 2015;24:106–116.

[195] Liu D, Yu B, Jiang G, et al. Fabrication of composite microneedles integrated with insulin-loaded $CaCO_3$ microparticles and PVP for transdermal delivery in diabetic rats. Mater Sci Eng C. 2018;90:180–188.

[196] Kim JD, Kim M, Yang H, et al. Droplet-born air blowing: novel dissolving microneedle fabrication. J Control Release. 2013;170:430–436.

[197] Di J, Yao S, Ye Y, et al. Stretch-triggered drug delivery from wearable elastomer films containing therapeutic depots. ACS Nano. 2015;9:9407–9415.

[198] Yang S, Wu F, Liu J, et al. Phase-transition microneedle patches for efficient and accurate transdermal delivery of insulin. Adv Funct Mater. 2015;25:4633–4641.

[199] Ye Y, Yu J, Wang C, et al. Microneedles integrated with pancreatic cells and synthetic glucose-signal amplifiers for smart insulin delivery. Adv Mater. 2016;28:3115–3121.

[200] Ito Y, Nakahigashi T, Yoshimoto N, et al. Transdermal insulin application system with dissolving microneedles. Diabetes Technol Ther. 2012;14:891–899.
[201] Alexander A, Dwivedi S, Giri TK, et al. Approaches for breaking the barriers of drug permeation through transdermal drug delivery. J Control Release. 2012;164:26–40.
[202] Fakhraei Lahiji S, Kim Y, Kang G, et al. Tissue interlocking dissolving microneedles for accurate and efficient transdermal delivery of biomolecules. Sci Rep. 2019;9:7886.
[203] Jeong H-R, Kim J-Y, Kim S-N, et al. Local dermal delivery of cyclosporin A, a hydrophobic and high molecular weight drug, using dissolving microneedles. Eur J Pharm Biopharm. 2018;127:237–243.
[204] Liu S, Jin M, Quan Y, et al. Transdermal delivery of relatively high molecular weight drugs using novel self-dissolving microneedle arrays fabricated from hyaluronic acid and their characteristics and safety after application to the skin. Eur J Pharm Biopharm. 2014;86:267–276.
[205] Chen J, Qiu Y, Zhang S, et al. Dissolving microneedle-based intradermal delivery of interferon-α-2b. Drug Dev Ind Pharm. 2016;42:890–896.
[206] Dillon C, Hughes H, O'Reilly NJ, et al. Formulation and characterisation of dissolving microneedles for the transdermal delivery of therapeutic peptides. Int J Pharm. 2017;526:125–136.
[207] Fakhraei Lahiji S, Jang Y, Huh I, et al. Exendin-4–encapsulated dissolving microneedle arrays for efficient treatment of type 2 diabetes. Sci Rep. 2018;8:1–9.
[208] Lahiji SF, Jang Y, Ma Y, et al. Effects of dissolving microneedle fabrication parameters on the activity of encapsulated lysozyme. Eur J Pharm Sci. 2018;117:290–296.
[209] Vora LK, Courtenay AJ, Tekko IA, et al. Pullulan-based dissolving microneedle arrays for enhanced transdermal delivery of small and large biomolecules. Int J Biol Macromol. 2020;146:290–298.
[210] Kim NW, Kim S-Y, Lee JE, et al. Enhanced cancer vaccination by in situ nanomicelle-generating dissolving microneedles. ACS Nano. 2018;12:9702–9713.
[211] GhavamiNejad A, Li J, Lu B, et al. Glucose-responsive composite microneedle patch for hypoglycemia-triggered delivery of native glucagon. Adv Mater. 2019;31:1901051.
[212] Naito C, Katsumi H, Suzuki T, et al. Self-dissolving microneedle arrays for transdermal absorption enhancement of human parathyroid hormone (1–34). Pharmaceutics. 2018;10:215.
[213] Chi J, Zhang X, Chen C, et al. Antibacterial and angiogenic chitosan microneedle array patch for promoting wound healing. Bioact Mater. 2020;5:253–259.
[214] Martin CJ, Allender CJ, Brain KR, et al. Low temperature fabrication of biodegradable sugar glass microneedles for transdermal drug delivery applications. J Control Release. 2012;158:93–101.
[215] Ito Y, Ohashi Y, Shiroyama K, et al. Self-dissolving micropiles for the percutaneous absorption of recombinant human growth hormone in rats. Biol Pharm Bull. 2008;31:1631–1633.
[216] DeMuth PC, Min Y, Irvine DJ, et al. Implantable silk composite microneedles for programmable vaccine release kinetics and enhanced immunogenicity in transcutaneous immunization. Adv Healthc Mater. 2014;3:47–58.
[217] Tsioris K, Raja WK, Pritchard EM, et al. Fabrication of silk microneedles for controlled-release drug delivery. Adv Funct Mater. 2012;22:330–335.
[218] Zaric M, Lyubomska O, Touzelet O, et al. Skin dendritic cell targeting via microneedle arrays laden with antigen-encapsulated poly-D,L-lactide-co-glycolide nanoparticles induces efficient antitumor and antiviral immune responses. ACS Nano. 2013;7:2042–2055.
[219] Wang C, Ye Y, Hochu GM, et al. Enhanced cancer immunotherapy by microneedle patch-assisted delivery of anti-PD1 antibody. Nano Lett. 2016;16:2334–2340.
[220] Chen M-C, Huang S-F, Lai K-Y, et al. Fully embeddable chitosan microneedles as a sustained release depot for intradermal vaccination. Biomaterials. 2013;34:3077–3086.
[221] Ito Y, Ohashi Y, Saeki A, et al. Antihyperglycemic effect of insulin from self-dissolving micropiles in dogs. Chem Pharm Bull (Tokyo). 2008;56:243–246.
[222] Ito Y, Saeki A, Shiroyama K, et al. Percutaneous absorption of interferon-α by self-dissolving micropiles. J Drug Target. 2008;16:243–249.
[223] Tuan-Mahmood T-M, McCrudden MT, Torrisi BM, et al. Microneedles for intradermal and transdermal drug delivery. Eur J Pharm Sci. 2013;50:623–637.

[224] Donnelly RF, McCrudden MT, Alkilani AZ, et al. Hydrogel-forming microneedles prepared from "super swelling" polymers combined with lyophilised wafers for transdermal drug delivery. PLoS One. 2014;9:e111547.

[225] Jiang S, Liu S, Feng W. PVA hydrogel properties for biomedical application. J Mech Behav Biomed Mater. 2011;4:1228–1233.

[226] Liu S, Yeo DC, Wiraja C, et al. Peptide delivery with poly (ethylene glycol) diacrylate microneedles through swelling effect. Bioeng Transl Med. 2017;2:258–267.

[227] Seong K-Y, Seo M-S, Hwang DY, et al. A self-adherent, bullet-shaped microneedle patch for controlled transdermal delivery of insulin. J Control Release. 2017;265:48–56.

[228] Courtenay AJ, McCrudden MT, McAvoy KJ, et al. Microneedle-mediated transdermal delivery of bevacizumab. Mol Pharm. 2018;15:3545–3556.

[229] Lutton REM, Larrañeta E, Kearney M-C, et al. A novel scalable manufacturing process for the production of hydrogel-forming microneedle arrays. Int J Pharm. 2015;494:417–429.

[230] Rouphael NG, Paine M, Mosley R, et al. The safety, immunogenicity, and acceptability of inactivated influenza vaccine delivered by microneedle patch (TIV-MNP 2015): a randomised, partly blinded, placebo-controlled, phase 1 trial. The Lancet. 2017;390:649–658.

8

Microneedle-mediated Delivery of Vaccines

8.1 Introduction

8.1.1 Introduction of Vaccination

Vaccination is widely recognized among the most effective therapeutic strategies ever developed and one of the most critical innovations in the battle against infectious diseases in contemporary preventive medicine. Vaccines have always been essential in lowering the global incidence of infectious diseases. Vaccination considerably decreases infectious disease-related morbidity and mortality [1, 2]. Vaccination not only protects people directly but also promotes herd immunity in a particular region, delaying the spread of infectious illnesses and lowering the risk of infection among vulnerable groups [3].

The World Health Organization (WHO) claims that vaccination saves between 2 and 3 million deaths annually and is the most effective technique for protecting individuals against infectious diseases. Globally, such illnesses claimed around 15 million lives in 2010. From 2011 and 2020, vaccination campaigns in 94 poor and middle-income nations cost approximately $62 billion. The delivery cost was $34 billion, and the supply chain cost was $4 billion, or 54% and 6%, respectively, of the overall vaccination cost [4]. According to a survey in 2015, barely 60% of qualifying children in these areas have received adequate vaccination [5]. According to research by the WHO, at least 50% of children immunizations were deemed unsafe in 14 countries spread across five distinct developing world regions [6, 7]. Between 1994 and 2013, immunizations prevented approximately 732,000 premature deaths and 320 million cases of the disease, as reported by the Centers for Disease Control and Prevention [8]. Vaccines have been employed to protect from over 25 life-threatening illnesses, averting around 2.5 million fatalities each year from influenza, diphtheria, measles, polio, typhoid, meningitis, tetanus, and cervical cancer. As stated by the WHO, vaccination expenditure amounts for just around 2–3% of the whole pharmaceutical industry. The Health Service Executive (HSE) of Ireland suggests 15 immunizations (16 for females) to be taken from birth to about 14 years of age. Vaccination rates continue to fall short of the European Centre for Disease Prevention and Control's expected coverage rate of 75% [9]. WHO's primary objectives include vaccine development, coverage, and mass immunization, particularly for certain diseases such as influenza, HIV/AIDS, TB, hepatitis B, Ebola, and Zika [10]. The emergence of "blockbuster vaccines," classified as those generating at least $1 billion in annual sales in the United States, has been documented [11], such as Pfizer's Prevnar 7 and Prevnar 13, GSK's Rotarix, and MSD's Rotateq. Indeed, among more than 5 billion vaccination doses administered annually to humans, 3 billion are provided through needles [6, 7].

DOI: 10.1201/9780429294433-8

Many individuals continue to reject or postpone immunizations. Around 10% of the population suffers from unpleasant vaccination-related experiences, such as painful injections and needle phobia [12, 13]. Other vaccination-related challenges include an increase in the risk of needle-caused injury issues, needle reuse, poor vaccine stability, the requirement of skilled practitioners for administration, low patient compliance, high cost of transportation and storage due to the use of cold-chain systems, the likelihood of mishandling and risk during clinical procedures [14, 15], low-risk perception, lack of reliable information about vaccination, and a fear of adverse effects, cost factors, availability, and convenience [9]. Capital expenditures related to vaccination services include cold-chain equipment and vehicles [9], while recurring costs comprise vaccines and training activities. The cold-chain system is projected to cost vaccination programs globally $200–300 million yearly due to the cost of maintaining cold storage facilities, cold transportation, and cold containers that keep vaccines at the appropriate temperatures. The United States and Canada have the lowest rate of sharp (needlestick) injuries at work (0.18 per healthcare professional per year). In contrast, Egypt and Pakistan have the highest rate (4.7 per care provider annually). Each year, an estimated 3 million healthcare workers are injured by a sharp item associated with hepatitis C, hepatitis B, or human immunodeficiency virus [6, 7]. Pain and trauma related to needle-based vaccination might act as obstacles to vaccine uptake, especially for needle-phobic individuals, who account for at least 10% of the population [16].

Vaccines resemble infections and stimulate the immune system to generate antibodies against the invading pathogen without resorting to the disease's pathogenesis. Vaccines are biological compositions that include a live or attenuated antigen that induce an immune response when administered to a healthy human subject. The vaccination aids the immune system in producing a long-lasting immunological memory, enabling it to detect and attack disease-causing microorganisms such as viruses and bacteria [17, 18]. Vaccines often include an agent that mimics the pathogenic microbe and are frequently derived from weakened or dead forms of the pathogen or its toxins. The agent induces the body's immune system to detect it as foreign, eliminate it, and "memorize" it so that the immune system may more quickly recognize and remove subsequent contacts with these microorganisms.

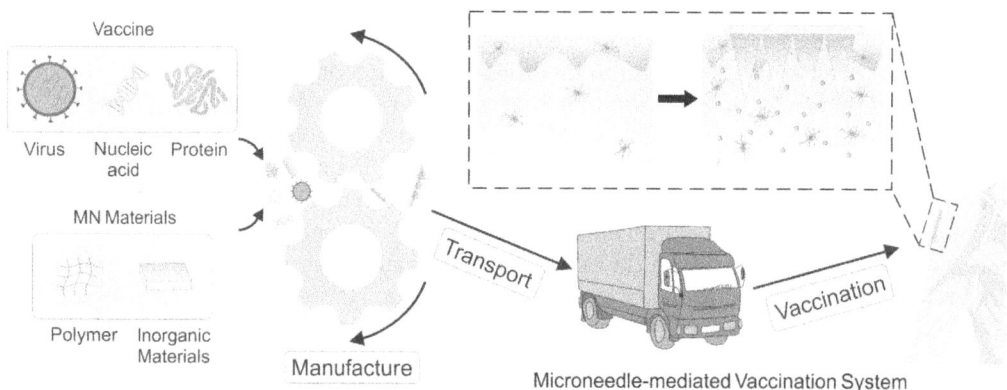

FIGURE 8.1

Diagram depicting microneedles' manufacturing, shipping, and vaccination for immunization applications. Images reprinted with permission from [19].

To contribute to public health sustainably via vaccination, vaccine delivery methods must enable effective delivery without jeopardizing product stability during storage and shipping or adversely affecting patient perception [6]. The novel vaccine should be needle-free or have a retractable or self-disabling needle to avoid reuse and minimize the danger of needlestick injuries. It should alleviate or completely remove pain, require minimal healthcare expertise, and permit mass immunization during a natural pandemic or bio-terrorism incident. New vaccine products should not be more expensive to manufacture, ship, store, or administer than existing vaccines and should eliminate the need for a cold chain (Fig. 8.1). Once administered, the vaccine must reach the immune system and generate a protective response, indicating that it is at least as immunogenic and protective as parenteral vaccination.

8.1.2 Route of Vaccine Delivery

Vaccines are currently given through one of five routes: intramuscular, subcutaneous, intra-dermal, intranasal, and oral administration [6, 16]. Prophylactic immunizations are often regarded as the most efficient method of controlling infectious diseases [20]. With a few exceptions, most vaccinations are delivered intramuscularly and subcutaneously by needles and syringes, with certain rotavirus, adenovirus, cholera, and typhoid vaccines provided orally [21]. The only vaccinations available for mucosal administration are live attenuated versions for poliomyelitis [6, 22], typhoid fever, rotavirus, and influenza. Vaccination via the mucosa removes the possibility of blood-borne illness transmission and needlestick injuries. Workers may provide it with minimal medical training, which has significant practical and financial advantages, particularly in large-scale vaccination programs in developing countries. Furthermore, this approach has the potential to provoke mucosal and humoral immunity. A disadvantage of this approach is that the live attenuated viruses in the oral poliomyelitis vaccine (OPV) might return to virulence, resulting in vaccine-associated para-lytic poliomyelitis (VAPP) in the vaccinated children or their close contacts, especially immu-nocompromised individuals. Oral immunizations must overcome barriers to absorption and destruction in the gastrointestinal tract. Intradermal immunization has several poten-tial disadvantages, including needlestick injuries, low thermostability, disease transmission via reused needles, the requirement for administration by a trained health professional, a lack of reaching to antigen-presenting cells (APCs) in the body, and the necessity for vaccine shipping and storage (cold-chain system) in remote and underdeveloped areas around the world [14, 23]. Transdermal drug delivery system (TDDS) may resolve some significant issues associated with oral and hypodermic routes, including rapid pass metabolism, decreased dose frequency, and degradation in the gastrointestinal tract [24]. The administration of drugs and vaccines through the skin is minimally invasive, painless, affordable, and conve-nient [25, 26]. On the other hand, the stratum corneum layer of the skin significantly limits the effective transport of drugs, particularly high-molecular-weight proteins, peptides, and live or attenuated organisms for immunization applications [27–29].

8.2 Roles of Skin in Vaccination

The skin serves as a protective barrier and an immunocompetent organ. The skin's stra-tum corneum is the body's outermost and most protective layer. It is composed of a lipid-rich network of corneocytes and simulates a physical barrier constructed of "bricks and mortar." Keratinocytes, Langerhans cells (LCs), dermal dendritic cells, macrophages, and mast cells in the epidermis and dermis layers, as well as T and B lymphocytes in the lymph nodes, contribute to immune protection for the skin and form the skin immune system, which are critical elements in the vaccine-elicited specific immune reaction [30, 31]. The Langerhans cells function as antigen-presenting cells (APCs), delivering antigens or vaccines to T cells to stimulate the immune system [32, 33]. APCs are abundant in the dermis and epidermis layers of the skin. The dermis is highly vascularized and contains glands, nerve fibers, and hair follicles. Dermal dendritic cells are also located in the dermis and capable of activating antigen-specific immune reactions. Even though intramuscular and subcutaneous injection is by far the most common route of administration for vaccines, only a small number of circulating dendritic cells may be able to take the antigen and travel to draining lymph nodes or spleens for antigen presentation [34]. Transdermal vaccination, as compared to intramuscular injection, has the potential to reduce vaccine doses and further enhance immunogenicity, while also likely cutting immunization costs [35–37]. When the vaccine is administered to the skin's surface, it is discharged from the formulation and picked up by APCs, effectively delivering the antigen to T cells for priming [38]. Then, the T cells trigger the B cells to release the antibodies. The B cells internalize the vaccine complex, change into plasmocytes, proliferate by cloning, and generate immense quantities of antibodies. At this stage, B cells also develop some memory B cells, which are later triggered in response to repeated exposure to target antigens or pathogens and generate antibodies to attack the pathogens [39–41].

8.3 Skin Vaccination Strategies

8.3.1 Conventional Intradermal Vaccination

Until now, the most frequently used vaccine delivery method has been traditional intradermal immunization. Since its creation in 1853, the hypodermic needle has grown to be the most commonly utilized medical device, with approximately 16 billion injections given globally [42]. Disposable needles and syringes may now be manufactured in large quantities for as low as $0.03–0.04. By circumventing first-pass hepatic metabolism and the harsh conditions of the gastrointestinal system, this method of administration enables quick attainment of desired plasma levels, appropriate titration of medicines with a narrow therapeutic index, and delivery of drugs with low oral bioavailability. It has been extensively documented that vaccines delivered intradermally often generate more robust immune responses than those given intramuscularly or subcutaneously. This observation has been linked to the skin's greater capacity for accumulating immune components compared to the subcutaneous or intramuscular routes [43, 44]. Notably for massive vaccination in the event of a pandemic or bioterrorism, as well as cost savings in resource-limited countries, intradermal immunization seems to be dose-efficient, with comparable immune responses frequently obtained with lesser vaccine doses than those given by the traditional routes [22, 43, 44]. The typical intradermal injection method, devised by Mantoux, is linked to a lack of consistency in the injection volume, primarily due to the complex technique and inevitable vaccine leakage from the area of injection, vaccine wastage when filling syringes and removing the needle of air, and the significant dead volume of the needle and syringe.

Nevertheless, the use of hypodermic needles involves significant drawbacks [16, 24, 45]:

- Anxiety before the procedure.
- If reused, the risk of disease transmission increases and dosing requires a skilled professional.
- Unpredictable delivery, speedy degradation, and inadequate absorption result in low bioavailability, necessitating a greater drug dose to attain the therapeutic level.
- Challenge in adjusting the depth of needle insertion and dose leaking from the injection area after the needle is removed from the skin.
- The risk of experiencing a needlestick injury.
- Hazardous biological waste and sharps disposal.
- Possibility of developing a hematoma or bleeding.
- A lack of belief in healthcare practitioners and a desire to avoid healthcare.
- Side effects, including inflammatory responses and abscess formation.

Contemporary vaccination procedures for the pediatric population often include the simultaneous delivery of two or three shots during a single visit, resulting in significant pain and suffering [46]. Indeed, vaccination is among children's most prevalent causes of iatrogenic discomfort [47].

8.3.2 Noninvasive Skin Vaccination

Several noninvasive and minimally invasive methods are available for skin vaccination. Because minimally invasive treatments are intrusive, they raise more safety and sterility issues than noninvasive procedures [48]. Not only would an ideal skin vaccination technique be reliable, but it would also alleviate the risks and discomfort linked to the use of hypodermic needles. Noninvasive skin vaccination techniques strive to accomplish this by negating the needle and substituting it with noninvasive ways, increasing skin permeability and avoiding sharps waste [49]. These technologies alleviate patient discomfort and apprehension associated with hypodermic injections, minimize or lessen the possibility of needlestick injuries and reuse of needle and syringe, and could be performed by modestly trained professionals or perhaps even by patients themselves, thus facilitating expanded immunization coverage. This is particularly critical during mass vaccination against a potential pandemic since the injection with hypodermic needles is relatively slow, and congregating persons at centralized vaccination locations increase the danger of cross-contamination and pathogen spreading [48].

Skin vaccination techniques that are minimally invasive, most prominently via the use of different microneedle types, provide advantages over noninvasive alternatives by effectively delivering vaccines into the skin in a timely, consistent, and effective way. Furthermore, they have many benefits beyond hypodermic needles, including the elimination or reduction of pain or irritation, hazardous sharps waste, and the requirement for professionally trained health workers. Becton Dickinson's microneedle-based prefilled injectable system (BD Soluvia™ with microneedles connected to a glass syringe) for influenza vaccination was authorized for practical use in Europe in 2009 under the brand name Intanza (Sanofi-Pasteur). BD devised Onvax™ (a skin microabrader composed of an array of plastic microneedles) to rupture the stratum corneum and pass vaccine antigen toward APCs in the epidermis layer [50, 51]. Utilizing a variety of microneedle designs, antigens, adjuvants, inactivated and attenuated pathogens, and genes encoding antigen production have been researched *in vitro* and *in vivo*. Coated microneedles, the poke-and-patch method, and, most interestingly, dissolving biodegradable microneedles have been the most frequently used methods for microneedle-assisted transdermal delivery.

Tattooing is a long-established technique of depositing materials into the skin for decorative reasons. This method has been employed to deliver DNA vaccines into the skin. Tattoo needles with high-frequency oscillations may puncture the skin and carry vaccine formulation to the dermis. DNA tattooing generated a superior humoral and cellular immune response in animal experiments than intramuscular vaccination [52].

The most well-known needle-free vaccination technique is the *liquid jet injection*, which involves driving a pressurized liquid formulation into the skin and delivering the vaccine intradermally. This procedure was widely used for intramuscular and subcutaneous immunization in the mid-20th century and has also been developed for intradermal injections. The intradermal jet injection is capturing renewed attention as a method of administering inactivated poliovirus vaccine and is now undergoing clinical trials [53].

Epidermal powder immunization (EPI) is essentially similar to liquid jet injection; however, it uses supersonic-speed flow to drive dried-powder vaccine particles into the skin instead of liquid. Vaccination utilizing this strategy has been demonstrated in human studies to provide comparable immune responses to intramuscular immunization [54]. *Particle-mediated epidermal delivery* (PMED) is another variant of this technique in which DNA vaccines are coated on gold microparticles and injected into the skin. Clinical trials of PMED vaccination revealed excellent outcomes, although with weaker immunogenic responses than traditional vaccine delivery techniques [55]. Abrasion of the skin with a razor and a toothbrush provided favorable therapeutic benefits in humans [56]. Recent research revealed immunization in animals using this technique [57].

Thermal ablation creates micrometer-sized pores in the stratum corneum by vaporizing the tissue with heat energy [58]. In animal research, electrical energy or radiofrequency-based resistive heating has been devised and found to induce protective immune responses to vaccine antigens [59, 60].

Furthermore, *ultrasound* has been demonstrated to enhance skin permeability and may be utilized to administer vaccines to the skin. Ultrasound not only improved vaccine transport but also promoted antigen-presenting cells stimulation in the epidermis layer of animal skin [61].

Electroporation has been employed to increase transdermal drug delivery by improving skin permeability. One research used electroporation to increase the permeation of a peptide vaccine [62]. Generally, electroporation has been employed to enhance the permeability of skin cells to facilitate the intracellular transport of DNA vaccines, thus increasing cell transfection and resulting in efficient antigen protein production [63]. Electroporation has been applied successfully in animal studies and, notably, human clinical investigations for DNA vaccination targeting prostate cancer to induce efficient immune responses. Possible usage of a combination of chemical penetration enhancers for vaccination purposes, when tailored by high-throughput screening, may improve skin permeation to vaccine antigen and serve as a novel adjuvant [64]. The needle-free, high-velocity injection devices are typically capable of rapidly and effectively injecting vaccines into the skin while eliminating the risks associated with hypodermic needles. However, these techniques often need cumbersome apparatus, may induce discomfort comparable to hypodermic needles, and can fail to provide consistent injections [65, 66]. The other noninvasive strategies enhance skin permeability to varying degrees and then need a slow and sometimes ineffective process of vaccine antigen permeation into the skin, which generally results in a significant amount of vaccine remaining on the surface of the skin [24].

8.4 Microneedle-mediated Vaccination Strategies

8.4.1 Introduction of Different Microneedle Types for Vaccination

Microneedles are classified as solid, hollow, coated, and dissolving microneedles (Table 8.1). The schematic representation of different microneedle types is displayed in Fig. 8.2 As the drug is not preloaded or deposited onto solid microneedles, the production procedure is less expensive than coated or dissolving microneedles. However, since solid microneedles must penetrate the skin to release the drug load, the dose administered is modest and

TABLE 8.1

Comparison between Different Types of Microneedles

Criteria	Solid Microneedles	Hollow Microneedles	Coated Microneedles	Dissolving Microneedles
Low manufacturing cost	+++	++	++	+
Ease of large-scale manufacturing	+++	++	++	+
Potential for self-administration	+	++	+++	+++
Short wearing time	+++	+	+	+
Biocompatibility of microneedles material	+++	+++	++	+
Safety of microneedle insertion	+	++	++	+++
Controlled delivery of the right dose	+	++	+++	+++
Ease of sterilization/aseptic compounding	+++	+++	++	+
Physical stability against humidity	+++	+++	+++	+
Minimal waste	+	+	+	+++

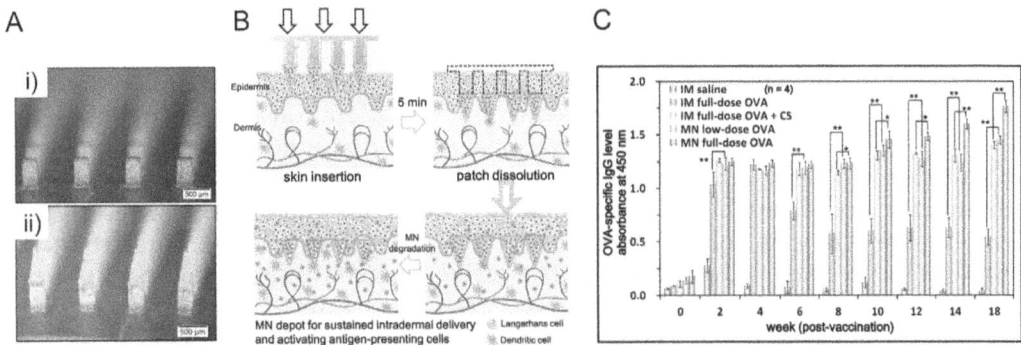

FIGURE 8.2
(A) Microscopic images of the PVA/PVP supporting array patch (i) and chitosan (CS) microneedles combined with the patch (ii). (B) Schematic illustrations of transdermal delivery of vaccine using a chitosan microneedles patch. (C) OVA-specific IgG level of rats after a single administration of OVA on day 0. Images reprinted with permission from [67].

unpredictable. As for coated and dissolving microneedles, the wearing time (the duration supposed to hold the microneedles on the skin) is significantly longer, as adequate adhesion duration is required to deliver the entire quantity of drug contained in the coated microneedles or dissolving microneedles matrix. As the dissolving microneedles matrix dissolves in the skin, the mechanical properties and biocompatibility of the microneedles component are crucial [68]. Compared to solid microneedles or coated microneedles, most dissolving microneedles are composed of soluble polymers, which may make them more prone to degrade when exposed to humidity [10, 69, 70]. Since hollow microneedles are downsized from hypodermic needles, their production and sterilizing processes are identical to those of hypodermic needles. This needle type is sturdy and physically stable at high temperatures and humidity. However, sharp waste management continues to be a challenge.

8.4.1.1 Solid Microneedles

Solid microneedles form micrometer-sized pores in the stratum corneum layer, enhancing skin permeability. A vaccine placed on the microneedle-treated site effectively diffuses into the skin through the channels generated by microneedle pretreatment (via a drug-loaded patch or semi-solid topical formulation) [72]. Solid microneedles have been employed to deliver diphtheria [73], influenza [74], hepatitis B [75], and malaria vaccines to mice [76]. Solid microneedles in a Nanopatch™ array with 10,000 micro projections/cm^2 and each 250 µm in length increased the antigenicity of the HPV vaccination. This strategy permits the HPV vaccine to be administered without adjuvant with a transfer efficiency of approximately 20% [77]. Ding and colleagues reported that pretreatment with solid microneedles raised serum IgG levels specific for diphtheria toxoids in mice [74, 78]. *In vivo* studies revealed that compared to mice treated with transcutaneous vaccination, those treated with solid microneedles demonstrated a nearly 1,000-fold increase in diphtheria toxoid-specific serum IgG levels, indicating that the microneedle-created channels effectively enhanced the vaccine's transdermal delivery.

For transdermal immunization, a hydrogel patch has been combined with solid microneedles treatment. Guo et al. [75] used a combination of hydrogel patches and solid microneedles for enhanced delivery of hepatitis B. The microneedles array consisted of solid silicon microneedles positioned on a polymer supporting plate. The hydrogel patch was composed of carbomer polymer and was loaded with hepatitis B surface antigen (HBsAg) and cholera toxin B adjuvant. Consequently, even after three weeks of storage at 45°C, HBsAg in the hydrogel formulation retained immunogenicity, but HBsAg in the liquid form was much less immunogenic. Compared to standard percutaneous immunization, hydrogel-based vaccination considerably reduced the necessity for HBsAg. Moreover, passive vaccine permeation across the transitory microchannels formed by microneedles might be improved further with the use of external stimuli such as electrical current (iontophoresis) and ultrasound (sonophoresis) [79, 80]. Scraping the skin with solid microneedle, comparable to noninvasive abrasive procedures, was also employed to deliver DNA vaccines, which resulted in markedly stronger humoral and cellular immune responses against hepatitis B than intramuscular or intradermal vaccination via injection [50]. However, solid microneedles have lost favor in recent years, perhaps owing to the necessity for a multistep application procedure, an absence of consistency, and an expanding number of benefits offered by alternative microneedles systems [72].

8.4.1.2 Hollow Microneedles

This microneedle design contains the vaccine antigens, which are contained within the hollow needles. When administered, the vaccine antigens are injected and delivered to the skin. In general, hollow microneedles function as micrometer-scale needles and syringes, requiring external pressures (e.g., syringe thrust, pressure difference, spring elasticity) to assist the transportation of drug formulation via the hollow microneedle' channels to the intended region in the skin [81]. An external liquid pumping device may construct a measurable, accurate, and speed-controllable drug delivery system. Currently, two types of hollow microneedles are available: a single microneedle or mini-needle that resembles a standard hypodermic needle [82] and an array of several hollow microneedles [83]. The latter enables simultaneous delivery of a vaccine formulation across a larger skin region, thereby enhancing bioavailability and increasing the possibility of delivered antigens being taken up by the lymphatic system [84]. The vaccine might well be administered passively via microneedles [72]. On the other hand, a syringe may be affixed to the microneedle, allowing for active vaccine administration. There are multiple commercially marketed hollow microneedles systems; Soluvia® is licensed for human use [85], and MicronJet® is currently undergoing clinical trials [86]. Soluvia® is a prefilled microneedles system with a single 1,500-μm-long hollow silicon microneedle, while MicronJet® is an array of four 600 μm hollow silicon microneedles assembled on a plastic adapter for connection to a conventional syringe barrel [87]. Hollow microneedles have been effectively used to immunize humans against polio, influenza, and plague and to deliver the polio vaccine to rats. Medical professionals may provide intradermal injections using hollow microneedles easily with minimal training. Moreover, human studies using hollow microneedles show considerable dose reduction compared to intramuscular vaccination [86]. Furthermore, hollow microneedles have been utilized to deliver DNA vaccines that have been encapsulated in nanoparticles. Compared to conventional intradermal injection, a therapeutic cancer vaccine delivered using a digitally controllable hollow microneedles device requires substantially less antigen. Van der Maaden and coworkers fabricated hollow microneedles for the enhanced delivery of inactivated polio vaccine (IPV) [88]. They tested the efficiency of hollow microneedles to traditional hypodermic needles in inoculating rats with IPV. The findings indicate that the immunological response caused by IPV intradermal injection through hollow microneedles was comparable to that elicited by standard subcutaneous injection.

8.4.1.3 Coated Microneedles

Coated microneedles are typically manufactured by coating solid microneedles with a vaccination solution or dispersion. Following the insertion of the microneedles into the skin, the loaded vaccine is gradually released from the needles' surface and permeates into the dermis layer. Following that, the delivered vaccine is captured by Langerhans cells or dermal dendritic cells, triggering immune responses and attaining vaccination. The coating thickness and the size of the solid microneedles influence the total amount of coated drugs. Coated microneedles have been employed to deliver various vaccines, including influenza, human papillomavirus, chikungunya virus, West Nile virus, rotavirus, herpes simplex virus and hepatitis C, Bacillus Calmette–Guerin, hepatitis B virus, measles, and polio vaccines. Also, microneedles have been coated with a variety of influenza vaccines, namely, inactivated viruses [89] and virus-like particles [90]. Kines et al. revealed that when mice were immunized with microneedles or intramuscular injections, comparable levels of neutralizing antibodies were produced, demonstrating that the neutralizing antibody caused by the HPV vaccine was remarkably efficient and comparable *in vivo* irrespective of the path of vaccination, and implying the suitability of using coated microneedles for vaccine delivery. Moreover, the HPV pseudovirus loaded on the surface of solid microneedles could remain antigenically stable at ambient conditions, obviating the necessity for cold-chain distribution and storage of vaccines [91]. Zhang et al. found that DNA vaccines delivered using coated microneedles outperformed traditional syringe injections in respect of antigen expression and immunogenicity [92]. Microneedles covered with several layers of charge reversal pH-sensitive copolymers improved DNA vaccine delivery to antigen-presenting cells, resulting in an increased immune response [93]. Numerous ways might considerably enhance the stability of vaccination coated on solid microneedles. Polymers, e.g., polyvinyl alcohol (PVA) and trehalose added to the coating formulation may improve vaccine stability throughout the fabrication and storage. Turvey et al. similarly coated PLA microneedles with live-attenuated dengue vaccine [94]. With the addition of controlled saccharide formulations into the coating mixture (i.e., 0.5% carboxymethylcellulose, 7.5% trehalose, and 2.5% maltodextrin), the vaccine-coated microneedles can be stored at room temperature for three weeks and yet still produce substantial protective immunity. As per Kaplan and colleagues, when microneedles were coated with a 1% silk fibroin vaccine formulation, the antigen was less vulnerable to environmental and temperature fluctuations throughout the drying and storage periods [95].

8.4.1.4 Dissolving Microneedles

Polymeric dissolving microneedles contain vaccines inside their matrix [96]. These microneedles are made of FDA-approved polymeric materials and may encapsulate vaccine antigens or antigen-loaded nanoparticles. Microneedle insertion into the skin causes the breakdown of the polymeric component, therefore discharging the vaccine [68]. Dissolving microneedles are biocompatible and produce no biohazardous waste, which is a significant benefit [24, 97]. Furthermore, robustness and scalability are advantageous features of dissolving microneedles [98]. In contrast to hollow microneedles, however, a restriction is imposed on the quantity of vaccine that may be integrated into the microneedles matrix [99], and vaccines may be required to undergo a lengthy releasing period to allow full microneedles disintegration [97]. Numerous dissolving microneedles prepared with water-soluble polymers have been researched due to their remarkable biocompatibility, mechanical strength, and excellent water solubility (e.g., sucrose, maltose, hyaluronic acid, CMC, polyvinylpyrrolidone [PVP], and polyvinyl alcohol). Chitosan and PVA/PVP dissolving microneedles are presented in Fig. 8.3. Thermostable microneedles have been fabricated to include vaccines against influenza virus, hepatitis B, tetanus, diphtheria, malaria, and HIV in mice, as well as measles and polio in rhesus macaques. Dissolving microneedles combine the simplicity and efficacy of coated microneedles with the elimination of sharp and biohazardous waste. Dissolving microneedles are composed of water-soluble polymers and sugars that fully dissolve in the skin interstitial fluid. Besides, dissolving microneedles preloaded with microparticles offer the benefit of gradual and prolonged antigen release, which promotes the development of a strong adaptive immune response.

The first dissolving microneedles used for vaccination was to administer the influenza vaccine. The microneedles product was made of polyvinylpyrrolidone and could deliver the lyophilized antigen in 5 min [100]. Numerous dissolving microneedles for

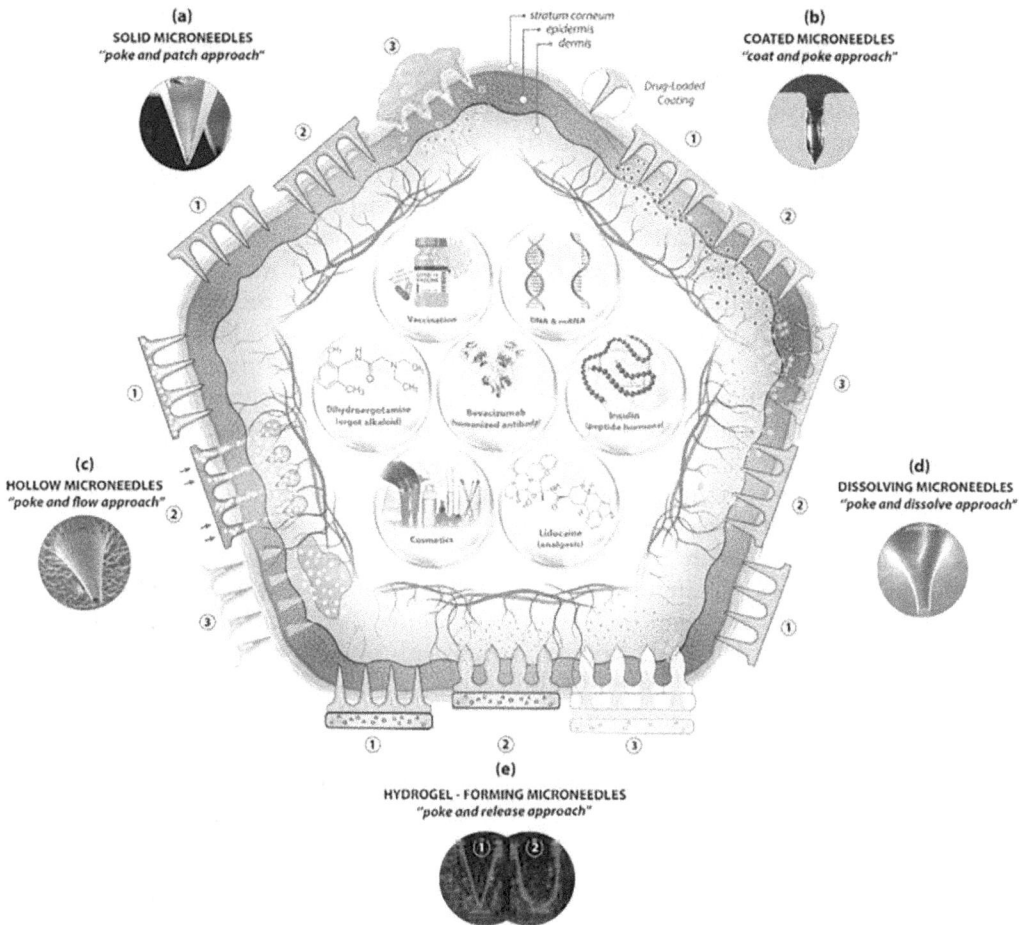

FIGURE 8.3
Schematic representation of microneedles drug delivery systems. (a) Solid microneedles. (b) Coated microneedles. (c) Hollow microneedles. (d) Dissolving microneedles. (e) Hydrogel-forming microneedles. Images reprinted with permission from [71].

immunizations have been developed using various polymers and sugars [101]. Moreover, it has been shown that dissolving microneedles could preserve the antigen's stability at ambient conditions (25°C) for more than a year. Influenza vaccine encapsulated in dissolving microneedles comprised of polyvinyl alcohol (PVA) and sucrose which were stable for up to 24 and 4 months at 25°C and 60°C, respectively [102]. Likewise, a malaria antigen was more stable in a dissolving sugar microneedles array than in the liquid formulation of the vaccine [103]. Also, dissolving PVA microneedles have been extensively researched and have been shown to generate incredibly strong immune responses. Moreover, they have proved an effective platform for administering preventive DNA vaccines against cervical cancer [104, 105]. Dissolving microneedles have generated a superior antibody response to the adenovirus-based *Plasmodium falciparum* malaria vaccine AdHu5–PfRH5 [103]. Similarly, microneedles made of PVA and sugars also boosted the immune response to the *Neisseria gonorrhoeae* challenge [106]. Vaccines for hepatitis B might be encapsulated into microneedles composed of polylactic acid and carboxymethylcellulose, resulting in a dual-release profile and allowing the microneedles to perform the functions of both a prime and booster immunization. Consequently, the microneedle-assisted vaccination could elicit an immunological response comparable to or greater than that produced by two doses via standard administration [107]. Moreover, a phase I clinical trial revealed that the influenza vaccine-loaded dissolving microneedles had superior patient compliance than the traditional intramuscular method [18]. Prausnitz and colleagues demonstrated the efficacy of dissolving polymeric microneedles for influenza vaccine delivery [108]. The comparison between dissolving and solid metal microneedles for transdermal vaccination indicated that dissolving needles produced a more efficient cellular immune response, as indicated by increased IL-4 and IFN-c release from lymphoid cells. Kim et al. attempted to produce microneedles by simply casting anhydrous organic solvent (chloroform) containing lyophilized vaccine and PVP polymer onto the molds [109]. Without the use of additional stabilizers or adjuvants, the resulting microneedles carrying influenza vaccine could be preserved at 40°C for 12 weeks and still elicit a robust immunological response in mice. Tran et al. fabricated a transdermal microneedles patch with customizable burst release of vaccine antigen loads at various controllable time points spanning from days to months, permitting several immunizations with a single microneedles patch with a single application [110]. During the worldwide SARS-CoV-2 outbreak, researchers have been devoted to integrating the COVID-19 vaccine into dissolving microneedles to facilitate self-vaccination, minimize interpersonal contact, and potentially increase COVID-19 immunization rates, thus possibly saving more lives [111]. The researchers discovered that microneedles loaded with the SARS-CoV-2-S1 protein and manufactured with CMC generated high levels of antigen-specific antibodies [112]. SARS-CoV-2 S1 subunit vaccine administered through dissolving CMC microneedles significantly increased efficient antigen-specific antibodies in mice two weeks after the vaccine administration [18].

8.4.2 Advantages of Microneedles-based Vaccination

Microneedles provide the following advantages:

- Microneedles products contain a low bioburden.
- Microneedles provide a more convenient, painless, and less invasive delivery method owing to their capacity to reduce nerve stimulation, hence avoiding the formation of the pain perception.
- Absence of bleeding or pathogen introduction associated with microneedles application.
- Suitability and relative simplicity of microneedles application or convenient usage for nonskilled and self-administration abolish the requirement for trained healthcare professionals. This advantage allows for widespread vaccination in poor and developing countries. Microneedles enhance patient acceptability and compliance by enabling self-vaccination to comply with the vaccination program (particularly when multiple booster doses have to be given).
- A reduction in the possibility of needlestick injury and cross-contamination, as well as greater disposal simplicity.
- Microneedle-assisted vaccination may reduce capital and recurrent costs related to standard immunization programs: their thermostability negates the need for

cold-chain storage and distribution [113, 114], and their self-administration feature may eliminate the necessity for trained caregivers to deliver the vaccine [9].

- Compared to traditional intramuscular and subcutaneous vaccination, microneedle-assisted administration of vaccines may result in dose-sparing, longer-lasting, and more robust antibody responses [115]. Microneedles stimulate the immune system more effectively at a relatively low dosage.

- Microneedles are compatible with live, inactivated, and subunit vaccines [108, 116] to elicit equivalent and, in some instances, enhanced immunogenicity compared to standard vaccination [86, 117].

- Reduce the package size of the product in comparison to a set of a hypodermic needle, syringe, and vaccine vial, which then simplifies storage, transportation, and disposal. This lowers expense and infrastructure requirements, as well as the space needed in the cold chain for vaccines that require refrigeration [48].

- Lower vaccination costs result from these logistical benefits, potential dosage reduction, superior vaccine immunogenicity, and enhanced vaccination efficiency and coverage [48].

- Without the addition of adjuvants, vaccination with microneedles was shown to be still efficient [118].

- Microneedles coated or loaded with vaccines are formulated in the finished dry form. This promotes vaccine stability in the dry state, potentially without refrigeration, and eliminates the requirement for vaccine reconstitution by health professionals, which is labor-intensive and time-consuming, may result in vaccine waste, and cause medical errors.

- Acceptability by patients: when provided this product, 30% of formerly unvaccinated subjects changed their minds and agreed to get vaccinated [119].

- Microneedles significantly enhance vaccine permeability, allowing for accurate and effective delivery of the vaccine into the skin's vascular dermis and epidermis layers, stimulating antigen-presenting cells and producing antigen-specific antibodies [32].

8.4.3 Barrier to Microneedles-based Vaccination

If a microneedle product encapsulating a vaccine is sterilized with radiation, the vaccine's immunogenicity may be compromised. As a consequence, microneedles may require aseptic manufacturing to preserve sterility. This could impose a further obstacle to the mass production of vaccine-loaded microneedles to battle pandemics that need widespread immunization. The potential for skin irritation exists upon microneedle insertion and the risk of microneedles breaking off and remaining underneath the skin [120]. Since microneedles are so minute, they may go undetected, resulting in unanticipated adverse effects. Concerns about microneedles centered on their convenience, the expense of developing them, and their safety and effectiveness. Moreover, it is critical to construct microneedles in such a way that variation in application pressure across persons has no effect on the dosage form's efficacy. Clinical translation of microneedle-based vaccinations is also challenging. The scarcity of clinical evidence also shows that scaling up microneedles production is another impediment to the clinical translation of this technology. Consequently, industrial-scale manufacturing of microneedles will necessitate numerous in-depth considerations. Conforming to WHO guidelines, vaccination products employing microneedles must give stability records for vaccine vial monitor (VVM) type 7 or higher. A higher VVM category, e.g., VVM 14 or VVM 30, would be excellent for vaccines stored at room temperature. Vaccines for human use must be sterile and devoid of pyrogens other than the vaccine antigens. If microneedles are regarded as medical devices, regulatory requirements will involve needle length, sharpness, capacity to penetrate the skin, and level of control over the application. Regulatory registrations for vaccine-loaded microneedles will be required for both the vaccine and the microneedles, as well as the combination product.

8.5 Studies of Microneedle-mediated Vaccination

8.5.1 Clinical Studies of Microneedle-mediated Vaccination

Numerous preclinical research investigations using microneedles for immunization have been conducted; the target animal subjects ranged from mice to monkeys. Most challenge testing was conducted on mice, while one trial involving a measles vaccination was conducted on infant rhesus macaques. The findings indicated that the microneedles group obtained complete protection compared to the subcutaneous injection group [121]. Microneedle-based vaccination produced a robust immune response to particular antigens and provided protective activity immediately after the vaccine delivery and over an extended period.

8.5.2 Safety, Efficacy, and Stability of Microneedles

In clinical studies, the principal outcome measures for microneedle-mediated vaccines were safety, efficacy, and stability. Carter and colleagues confirmed the safety and efficacy of a MicronJet 600™-mediated vaccine in combination with a TLR4 agonist-based adjuvant, presenting a novel system for dose-sparing and self-administrable vaccine delivery design [122]. Van Damme and associates studied and analyzed the safety and immunogenicity of three virosomal vaccines delivered by MicronJet 600™ to healthy volunteers aged 65. Furthermore, this research indicated that MicronJet 600™ is not inferior to Soluvia™ and intramuscular delivery of conventional and high doses of influenza vaccine. MicronJet 600™ treatment resulted in a greater frequency of local adverse effects, primarily erythema and induration, compared to intramuscular injection. However, there were no systemic adverse events. Moreover, immunogenicity evaluations revealed that intradermal transmission through microneedles enhanced the immunogenicity of at least two of the three experimental virosomal vaccine strains compared to Inflexal intramuscular injection [123]. Besides, a safe and efficient microneedle product is BD Soluvia™ hollow microneedle, a novel prefilled intradermal delivery device approved for distribution in the Europe market in 2009 as Intanza (Sanofi-Pasteur) seasonal flu vaccination [85]. BD Soluvia™ has been studied in humans for influenza and rabies vaccine administration [124, 125]. Furthermore, the DebioJect™ device was shown to be capable of safely and well-tolerated delivering at least 100 µL of vaccine into the dermis, thus optimizing its advantages, such as dose-sparing effects [126]. Along with immunological benefits and a low incidence of adverse effects, both dissolving and coated microneedles demonstrated a prolonged storage duration at room temperature or even high temperatures. Microneedles were developed and mainly employed to provide vaccines in a dry solid form and preserve the vaccine's thermal stability while kept at room temperature [37, 127, 128]. In contrast to microneedle-based drug-device combinations, hollow microneedles enable the administration of larger drug doses, exhibiting a safe vaccine delivery method that also ensures a higher degree of immunogenicity in clinical testing [129]. Nevertheless, obstacles such as the absence of a guarantee for the long-term stability of liquid vaccine formulation, the demand for skilled healthcare personnel, and unanticipated mishaps continue to hinder the widespread use of microneedle-based skin vaccination.

8.5.3 Acceptability of Microneedles

The factors determining the acceptance of microneedle-assisted immunization have been identified to emerge predominantly inside microneedles products and may be further classified as follows: (1) individual opinions regarding microneedle; (2) physician, family, and friend recommendations for microneedles products; (3) endorsement of the microneedle' convenience and effectiveness; (4) evaluation of physical adverse effects associated with microneedles and injectables; and (5) challenges in validating proper microneedles administration. The Prausnitz group assessed the acceptance of their polymeric microneedles and reported that, albeit individual experience and awareness of microneedles influenza vaccine impacted the acceptability of the product, the majority of subjects favored influenza microneedles vaccination over traditional injections [130]. In a notable survey of 10,740 adults from different European countries and Australia, 96.6% asserted that they were "satisfied" or "very satisfied" taking the microneedles vaccination, and 93.7% stated that they would favor microneedles in the future if offered the option [9]. According to a study conducted on physicians in France and Germany, the choice of microneedles devices may motivate healthcare professionals to advocate the influenza vaccine and encourage the general population to receive the vaccine [131]. However, unfamiliarity, doubts regarding practicality and application in pediatrics, the risk of allergy, and the difficulty in validating immunization effectiveness are all obstacles to microneedles acceptance among parents.

8.5.4 Cost-effectiveness of Microneedles

Vaccine administration through hypodermic injection has historically been deemed costly for various reasons. These include the requirement for cleanrooms, autoclaving, freeze-drying, sophisticated distribution systems, cold-chain supply, needles, syringes, and water for injection to reconstitute the lyophilized powder, as well as the requirement for trained healthcare professionals to provide the injection [132]. Conversely, with numerous significant benefits, microneedle-mediated vaccination delivery has evolved as a more cost-effective approach than traditional hypodermic injections. Microneedles patches are provided without the need for clean-room facilities, cold-chain supply, or trained caregivers. Furthermore, they utilize less costly polymers, plastics, metals, and other materials and have a lower dosing frequency and dose-sparing potential. The cost-effectiveness of microneedle patches depends on several parameters, including vaccination acceptance rates, vaccine efficacy, and manufacturing and storage expenses. However, most of the expenditures were not spent on vaccine production but on vaccine administration [133]. Moreover, microneedles may help boost voluntary vaccination compliance, vaccination coverage, and reduced incidence of infectious diseases, all of which benefit the entire population. The intramuscular and microneedles vaccination program successfully reduced influenza infection rates, hospitalization rates, and influenza-associated mortality, increasing economic efficiency and lowering general health care costs [134, 135]. Also, microneedle-assisted vaccination can decrease secondary influenza transmission and influenza-related medical usage in both public and private settings. Bishwa and colleagues examined the cost-effectiveness of measles vaccine administration using microneedles to traditional vaccine delivery via a hypodermic needle. Microneedle-aided vaccine administration was predicted to cost $1.66 per case at 95% immunization coverage, compared to $2.64 per case with traditional subcutaneous injection, a cost savings of around 40% [132]. Microneedles are expected to save third-party payers $950 million and society $2.6 billion during a flu season [136]. Meltzer and his team created a simple spreadsheet model. The findings indicated that the use of microneedles products in pediatric measles vaccination programs in low- and middle-income countries might decrease vaccination costs and improve vaccination coverage, particularly among hard-to-reach communities in developing countries [132].

8.5.5 Clinical Studies of Microneedles-based Vaccination

Numerous clinical studies have been conducted to investigate the safety and efficacy of microneedles technology for the skin delivery of various vaccines (Table 8.2).

8.6 Future of Microneedle-mediated Vaccination

8.6.1 Commercialization of Microneedles-based Vaccines

Multiple microneedle products are available on the market, and several manufacturers have attempted to commercialize microneedle-based products (Table 8.3). Despite widespread interest in microneedle-enhanced vaccine delivery within the scientific world, only a few microneedle systems are commercially accessible for immunization, and an even smaller number is on the verge of commercialization [10]. Numerous elements contribute to the effectiveness of this delivery system. Most fabrication processes need a complex cleanroom facility, costly equipment, and a long production time, all of which reduce the commercial appeal of these systems [137, 138]. Funding and investment are always critical components of research [139]. Fewer than 20% of microneedles candidates may reach clinical trials directly from the preclinical stage. Onvax™ (a BD business) comprises an array of 200-μm-long plastic microprojections. Rubbing such devices over the skin surface disrupted the skin and delivered the vaccine into the epidermal layer [51, 140]. Vaxxas developed a Nanopatch™, a coated microneedles array containing an influenza vaccine formulation. The needle length of a Nanopatch™ is 250 μm, which is applied with a spring-loaded applicator [141]. Zosano Pharma's ZP microneedles system comprises 1,300 microneedles spread throughout a 2 cm^2 array. The drug formulation is coated on a 190-μm-long microneedles array and delivered using a handheld applicator. This device delivers the drug to the upper layers of the skin and achieves the desired result [142]. In the near future, cleanroom-free manufacturing techniques, the employment of Nanopatch® and micro-additives, or 3D printing, will redefine the success of this technology [38].

TABLE 8.2

List of Clinical Trials for Microneedle-mediated Vaccine Delivery

NCT Number	Phase	Study Title	Interventions	Microneedles System	Conditions	Sponsor/ Collaborators
NCT00703651	2	Study of Inactivated, Split-Virion Influenza Vaccine Administered by Intradermal Route versus Vaxigrip® in Adults	Biological: inactivated, split-virion influenza vaccine Trivalent influenza vaccine (inactivated, split-virion vaccine)	Microprojection system	Influenza Orthomyxoviridae infection Myxovirus infection	Sanofi Pasteur, a Sanofi Company
NCT04064554	NA	Clinical Study to Evaluate Safety and Immunogenicity of Bacillus Calmette–Guerin (BCG) Delivery via Novel Micronjet600 Device Compared to Those via Conventional Needle	Device: Bacillus Calmette–Guerin vaccination with MicronJet600 Device: BCG vaccination with conventional needle	MicronJet 600®	Tuberculosis BCG vaccination	Yonsei University
NCT01049490	NA	Dose Sparing Intradermal S-OIV H1N1 Influenza Vaccination Device	Biological: S-CIV H1N1 vaccine	Micron Jet 600®	Influenza infection	The University of Hong Kong Hospital Authority, Hong Kong
NCT01304563	NA	2010/2011 Trivalent Influenza Vaccination	Biological: TIV 2010/2011 influenza vaccine Biological: INT	Micron Jet	Influenza	The University of Hong Kong Hospital Authority, Hong Kong
NCT01686503	2	Intradermal versus Intramuscular Polio Vaccine Booster in HIV-infected Subjects	Drug: IPOL (Sanofi Pasteur) inacivated polio vaccine booster dose	NanoPass MicronJet 600® microneedles device	Polio immunity	Eastern Virginia Medical School NanoPass Technologies Ltd.

(Continued)

TABLE 8.2 (*Continued*)

List of Clinical Trials for Microneedle-mediated Vaccine Delivery

NCT Number	Phase	Study Title	Interventions	Microneedles System	Conditions	Sponsor/ Collaborators
NCT04394689	1 and 2	Measles and Rubella Vaccine Microneedles Patch Phase I–II Age De-escalation Trial	Biological: measles rubella vaccine (MRV-SC) Biological: MRV-MNP	Dissolving microneedles patch	Measles rubella vaccination healthy	Micron Biomedical, Inc. Medical Research Council Centers for Disease Control and Prevention
NCT02438423	1	Inactivated Influenza Vaccine Delivered by Microneedles Patch or by Hypodermic Needle	Biological: inactivated influenza vaccine	Dissolvable microneedles patch	Influenza	Mark Prausnitz Emory University Georgia Institute of Technology
NCT02621112	2 and 3	HBV Vaccine in Renal Failure Patients	Biological: intradermal HBVv with imiquimod Biological: intradermal HBVv with aqueous cream Biological: intramuscular HBVv with aqueous cream	Microneedles	Renal failure	The University of Hong Kong
NCT02329457	2 and 3	VZV Vaccine for Hematopoietic Stem Cell Transplantation	Biological: Zostavax	Microneedles	Varicella-zoster Infection	The University of Hong Kong
NCT01707602	1 and 2	Routes of Immunization and Flu Immune Responses	Biological: INTANZA® 15 Biological: Vaxigrip® Biological: INTANZ® 15 T	Microneedles	Influenza	Assistance Publique— Hôpitaux de Paris Institut National de la Santé Et de la Recherche Médicale, France

NCT Number	Phase	Title	Intervention	Device	Condition	Sponsor
NCT03207763	NA	Microneedles Patch Study in Healthy Infants/Young Children	Device: Microneedles Formulation 1; Device: Microneedles Formulation 2	Microneedles	Vaccination; Skin absorption	Emory University; Micron Biomedical, Inc.
NCT05315362	2	Establishing Immunogenicity and Safety of Needle-free Intradermal Delivery of mRNA COVID-19 Vaccine	Device: solid microneedles skin patch	Solid microneedles patch	Vaccination; infection COVID-19	Leiden University Medical Center
NCT00558649	NA	A Pilot Study to Evaluate the Safety and Immunogenicity of Low-Dose Flu Vaccines	Biological: flu vaccine (FLUARIX®)	Microneedles injectors	Influenza, human	NanoPass Technologies Ltd.
NCT01767324	NA	Site Selection for Intracutaneous Saline Delivery	Device: injection to deltoid; Device: injection to the forearm; Device: injection to thigh	FLUGEN 101.2 microneedle-based device	Intracutaneous drug delivery	FluGen, Inc. Accelovance
NCT01039623	NA	Assessment of Safety and Immunogenicity of Intradermal Unadjuvanted Portion of Pandemrix® via a Microneedles Device with Intramuscular Adjuvanted Pandemrix® as Reference	Biological: Pandemrix® (H1N1 pandemic influenza)	Microneedles	Healthy	Hadassah Medical Organization

TABLE 8.3

Companies Developing Microneedles Products for Vaccination

Company	Type of Microneedle	Vaccine
Micron Biomedical	Dissolving microneedle	IRV-IPV Measles
Vaxxas (Nanopatch™)	Coated microneedle	Influenza, COVID-19
QuadMedicine	Coated microneedle	Influenza, hepatitis B, canine influenza
Vaxess	Dissolving microneedle	Influenza, COVID-19, skin cancer
Raphas	Dissolving microneedle	HPV, polio, Tdap, HBV, IPV, hepatitis B
3M	Coated microneedle	Influenza
	Hollow microneedle	Cancer vaccines
JUVIC	Dissolving microneedle	Scrub typhus
BD Technologies (BS Soluvia)	Stainless steel microneedle	Influenza
Flugen	Metal microneedle	Influenza
Debiotech	Hollow microneedle	COVID-19
Verndari (Vaxipatch)	Stainless steel microneedle	Influenza, COVID-19
NanoPass (MicroJet™)	Silicon microneedle	Influenza, polio, varicella-zoster, cancers, hepatitis B, COVID-19
BioSerenTach, Inc.	Dissolving microneedle	Vaccine
Sorrento therapeutics (Sofusa®)	Nanotopographical imprinted microneedle (coated)	Immuno-oncology

There are several requirements of microneedles for commercialization:

- *Environment:* Under biosafety level 3 for specific pathogens.
- *Quality attributes:* Physicochemical stability without cold-chain storage, minimal adverse effects, self-administration, desired immunogenicity, and dose-sparing effects.
- *Manufacturing:* Simple manufacture process, large-scale production possibility, scalability and repeatability, minimum waste, low cost of manufacturing.
- *Pre-market management:* Standardization of GMP laboratory, product safety, and efficacy demonstrated by FDA approval.
- *Post-marketing management:* Management of feedback and pharmacovigilance supervision, fail-free on microneedles application, confirm the dose of adminis-tered vaccine.

8.6.2 Manufacturing Issues

Multiple pharmaceutical companies have sought to mass-produce vaccine-loaded microneedles. Specifically, HBsAg dissolving microneedles were manufactured in a GMP pilot facility using an aseptic Grade A isolator [143], while influenza-coated microneedles were constructed using 3M's solid microstructured transdermal system using a GMP-scalable procedure [144]. The 3M's patented GMP manufacturing and aseptic coating technique offers a daily production capacity of up to 10,000 microneedles patches [145]. Lohmann Therapie-Systeme AG (LTS) and Corium, Inc., hold manufacturing licenses for microneedle patches used as drug delivery systems [133]. In terms of cost and scalability, microneedle-based products necessitate the establishment of large-scale production machinery and procedures [119]. Significant expenditure is required for machining, casting, and fabricating microneedles at the earliest phases of large-scale production. However, if these early phases are established successfully, the cost of production is expected to be lower than that of injectables [36]. The polymer-based microneedles casting method may be cost-effective due to the cheap cost of certain polymers such as cellulose derivatives, engineering plastics, and sugars. Yet, owing to the dependency on master molds and the inherent multistep filling process, scaling up the handling systems may be challenging. Moreover, the temperature may rise due to the drying process used to fabricate vaccine-loaded microneedles. As a result, a low-temperature technique may be necessary to generate thermosensitive antigens. While special packaging or desiccants may be critical to enhance storage stability, the inclusion of moisture-resistant material may drive up the price of packing. Also, sterilization is required for vaccine microneedle. Even though microneedles have a negligible bioburden, it is crucial to evaluate the expense of the aseptic procedure. Furthermore, the cost of validation of vaccine microneedles products should be evaluated. It is also critical to standardize microneedles for quality control purposes throughout production and marketing. Manufacturers must construct an efficient pharmaceutical quality assurance system that is well-designed and properly executed in accordance with a Pharmaceutical Quality System that incorporates Good Manufacturing Practices and Quality Risk Management. The effective fabrication of vaccine microneedles is contingent upon adhering to both existing rules for conventional pharmaceuticals and specialized requirements for each form of microneedles [146].

8.6.3 Regulatory Issues

According to the current FDA guideline, a vaccine microneedle product is a combination of a biopharmaceutical and a device. A prefilled syringe, an autoinjector, or a microneedles array patch loaded with a biological formulation are all examples of this sort of drug-device combined product (21 CFR 3.2e) [147]. Regulation of vaccine-loaded microneedles should consider the safety and efficacy of each component and the whole product (21 CFR Part 4 Subpart A: Sec. 4.4 (b)). Self-administration of microneedles products will require regulatory guidance on the validity and appropriate usage of self-vaccination [119].

8.7 Future Perspectives of Microneedles-based Vaccines

Extensive studies into preferred materials for microneedles are critical to enhancing the performance and biosafety of vaccine products. The mechanical qualities of materials should be deliberately constructed to provide effective transdermal vaccine delivery with a low risk of fracture inside the skin tissue. Furthermore, further research comprising a comprehensive assessment of microneedles' biocompatibility *in vitro* and *in vivo* are necessary. How to scale up production successfully remains a roadblock in the development and commercialization of microneedle-based vaccine products. Future research is required to ensure the uniformity of microneedles parameters and vaccine dose levels during large-scale manufacturing. Successful vaccination, in conjunction with proper recordkeeping, is also critical for enhancing immunization coverage.

Formulation, manufacturing, and production will all be essential determinants in the future and will demand special attention. The suitability of industrial production of this microneedle-based system in developing countries should be considered and supported critically [38]. The majority of clinical studies have been on different types of influenza vaccines. Other, more deadly infectious illnesses, such as whooping cough, measles, tuberculosis, rubella, and chickenpox, kill many people globally, particularly in resource-limited areas. These locations require substantial attention and may also be the focus of future investigations to save more lives. Regulatory considerations, such as the toxicity of the different polymers and metals used to fabricate microneedle systems, should be prioritized to influence the registration of this novel delivery technology.

8.8 Conclusions

Numerous vaccines, including emerging global pandemic vaccines, have been evaluated utilizing the microneedles technology, with equivalent or greater antibody response compared to intramuscular and other routes of immunization [10]. Besides being patient-friendly, microneedles have been shown to be very effective in enhancing a strong immune response against a range of viral and bacterial infections and cancer immunotherapy. Clinical trials have also demonstrated the vaccine microneedle's stability, safety, and immunological efficiency. Nevertheless, questions concerning mass manufacturing, cost-effectiveness, aseptic processing, and consistent quality continue to exist. Multiple microneedles manufacturers with mass-production capacity have previously developed vaccine microneedles in collaboration with vaccine makers, with documented improvements in immunological outcomes. The capacity to produce vaccines in the dry state represents a substantial advantage in efforts to bypass the cold chain, while the absence of medical skills necessary for microneedles administration should prove to be a benefit in impoverished nations. Owing to the lack of discomfort during administration, the absence of noticeable needles is expected to be beneficial in the vaccination of a considerable number of needle-phobic individuals and young children. Microneedles cannot be reused after they have been removed from a patient and do not need complicated disposal. The successful commercialization of this innovative vaccine delivery technology will be revolutionary and will likely save countless lives globally, particularly in resource-constrained areas with unacceptably high mortality rates from numerous infectious diseases [38]. Despite a few impediments, microneedles vaccinations have a promising future and will fundamentally alter how the world is immunized.

References

[1] Ehreth J. The global value of vaccination. Vaccine. 2003;21:596–600.
[2] Finco O, Rappuoli R. Designing vaccines for the twenty-first century society. Front Immunol. 2014;5:12.
[3] Fine P, Eames K, Heymann DL. "Herd immunity": a rough guide. Clin Infect Dis. 2011;52:911–916.

[4] Portnoy A, Ozawa S, Grewal S, et al. Costs of vaccine programs across 94 low-and middle-income countries. Vaccine. 2015;33:A99–A108.

[5] Restrepo-Méndez MC, Barros AJ, Wong KL, et al. Inequalities in full immunization coverage: trends in low-and middle-income countries. Bulletin of the World Health Organization. 2016;94:794.

[6] Kersten G, Hirschberg H. Needle-free vaccine delivery. Expert opinion on drug delivery. 2007;4:459–474.

[7] Simonsen L, Kane A, Lloyd J, et al. Unsafe injections in the developing world and transmission of bloodborne pathogens: a review. Bulletin of the World Health Organization. 1999;77:789.

[8] Rappuoli R. Vaccines: science, health, longevity, and wealth. Proc Natl Acad Sci. 2014;111:12282–12282.

[9] Marshall S, Sahm LJ, Moore AC. Microneedle technology for immunisation: perception, acceptability and suitability for paediatric use. Vaccine. 2016;34:723–734.

[10] Nguyen TT, Oh Y, Kim Y, et al. Progress in microneedle array patch (MAP) for vaccine delivery. Human Vaccines & Immunotherapeutics. 2021;17:316–327.

[11] Aggarwal SR. What's fueling the biotech engine—2012 to 2013. Nat Biotechnol. 2014;32:32–39.

[12] Clark SJ, Cowan AE, Wells K. Improving childhood vaccination coverage rates: the case of fourth dose of DTaP. Human Vaccines & Immunotherapeutics. 2020;16:1884–1887.

[13] Diekema DS. Improving childhood vaccination rates. N Engl J Med. 2012;366:391–393.

[14] Songane M. Challenges for nationwide vaccine delivery in African countries. Int J Health Econ Manag. 2018;18:197–219.

[15] Wouters OJ, Shadlen KC, Salcher-Konrad M, et al. Challenges in ensuring global access to COVID-19 vaccines: production, affordability, allocation, and deployment. The Lancet. 2021;397:1023–1034.

[16] Giudice EL, Campbell JD. Needle-free vaccine delivery. Adv Drug Deliv Rev. 2006;58:68–89.

[17] Griffin P, Elliott S, Krauer K, et al. Safety, acceptability and tolerability of uncoated and excipient-coated high density silicon micro-projection array patches in human subjects. Vaccine. 2017;35:6676–6684.

[18] Kim E, Erdos G, Huang S, et al. Microneedle array delivered recombinant coronavirus vaccines: immunogenicity and rapid translational development. EBioMedicine. 2020;55:102743.

[19] Sheng T, Luo B, Zhang W, et al. Microneedle-mediated vaccination: innovation and translation. Adv Drug Deliv Rev. 2021;179:113919.

[20] Gamazo C, Pastor Y, Larrañeta E, et al. Understanding the basis of transcutaneous vaccine delivery. Ther Deliv. 2019;10:63–80.

[21] Ramirez JEV, Sharpe LA, Peppas NA. Current state and challenges in developing oral vaccines. Adv Drug Deliv Rev. 2017;114:116–131.

[22] Kendall M. Engineering of needle-free physical methods to target epidermal cells for DNA vaccination. Vaccine. 2006;24:4651–4656.

[23] Kaufmann JR, Miller R, Cheyne J. Vaccine supply chains need to be better funded and strengthened, or lives will be at risk. Health Affairs. 2011;30:1113–1121.

[24] Prausnitz MR, Langer R. Transdermal drug delivery. Nat Biotechnol. 2008;26:1261–1268.

[25] Haj-Ahmad R, Khan H, Arshad MS, et al. Microneedle coating techniques for transdermal drug delivery. Pharmaceutics. 2015;7:486–502.

[26] Ma G, Wu C. Microneedle, bio-microneedle and bio-inspired microneedle: a review. J Control Release. 2017;251:11–23.

[27] Bediz B, Korkmaz E, Khilwani R, et al. Dissolvable microneedle arrays for intradermal delivery of biologics: fabrication and application. Pharm Res. 2014;31:117–135.

[28] van der Maaden K, Jiskoot W, Bouwstra J. Microneedle technologies for (trans)dermal drug and vaccine delivery. J Control Release. 2012;161:645–655.

[29] Zhang Y, Yu J, Kahkoska AR, et al. Advances in transdermal insulin delivery. Adv Drug Deliv Rev. 2019;139:51–70.

[30] Combadiere B, Liard C. Transcutaneous and intradermal vaccination. Human Vaccines. 2011;7:811–827.

[31] Korkmaz E, Balmert SC, Sumpter TL, et al. Microarray patches enable the development of skin-targeted vaccines against COVID-19. Adv Drug Deliv Rev. 2021;171:164–186.

[32] Rodgers AM, Cordeiro AS, Kissenpfennig A, et al. Microneedle arrays for vaccine delivery: the possibilities, challenges and use of nanoparticles as a combinatorial approach for enhanced vaccine immunogenicity. Expert Opin Drug Deliv. 2018;15:851–867.

[33] Suh H, Shin J, Kim Y-C. Microneedle patches for vaccine delivery. Clin Exp Vaccine Res. 2014;3:42–49.

[34] Nicolas J-F, Guy B. Intradermal, epidermal and transcutaneous vaccination: from immunology to clinical practice. Expert Rev Vaccines. 2008;7:1201–1214.

[35] Choi YH, Perez-Cuevas MB, Kodani M, et al. Feasibility of Hepatitis B vaccination by microneedle patch: cellular and humoral immunity studies in rhesus macaques. J Infect Dis. 2019;220:1926–1934.

[36] Prausnitz MR. Engineering microneedle patches for vaccination and drug delivery to skin. Ann Rev Chem Biomol Eng. 2017;8:177–200.

[37] Rouphael NG, Paine M, Mosley R, et al. The safety, immunogenicity, and acceptability of inactivated influenza vaccine delivered by microneedle patch (TIV-MNP 2015): a randomised, partly blinded, placebo-controlled, phase 1 trial. The Lancet. 2017;390:649–658.

[38] Hossain MK, Ahmed T, Bhusal P, et al. Microneedle systems for vaccine delivery: the story so far. Expert Rev Vaccines. 2020;19:1153–1166.

[39] Chaplin DD. Overview of the immune response. J Allergy Clin Immunol. 2010;125:S3–S23.

[40] Corrie SR, Depelsenaire ACI, Kendall MAF. Introducing the nanopatch: a skin-based, needle-free vaccine delivery system. Australian Biochemist. 2012;43:17–20.

[41] He X, Sun J, Zhuang J, et al. Microneedle system for transdermal drug and vaccine delivery: devices, safety, and prospects. Dose-Response. 2019;17:1559325819878585.

[42] Hauri AM, Armstrong GL, Hutin YJ. The global burden of disease attributable to contaminated injections given in health care settings. Int J STD & AIDS. 2004;15:7–16.

[43] Lambert PH, Laurent PE. Intradermal vaccine delivery: will new delivery systems transform vaccine administration? Vaccine. 2008;26:3197–3208.

[44] Laurent A, Mistretta F, Bottigioli D, et al. Echographic measurement of skin thickness in adults by high frequency ultrasound to assess the appropriate microneedle length for intradermal delivery of vaccines. Vaccine. 2007;25:6423–6430.

[45] Birchall JC. Microneedle array technology: the time is right but is the science ready? Expert Rev Med Devices. 2006;3:1–4.

[46] Bakhache P, Rodrigo C, Davie S, et al. Health care providers' and parents' attitudes toward administration of new infant vaccines—a multinational survey. Eur J Pediatr. 2013;172:485–492.

[47] Shah V, Taddio A, Rieder MJ, et al. Effectiveness and tolerability of pharmacologic and combined interventions for reducing injection pain during routine childhood immunizations: systematic review and meta-analyses. Clin Ther. 2009;31:S104–S151.

[48] Kim Y-C, Prausnitz MR. Enabling skin vaccination using new delivery technologies. Drug Deliv Transl Res. 2011;1:7–12.

[49] Mitragotri S. Immunization without needles. Nat Rev Immunol. 2005;5:905–916.

[50] Mikszta JA, Alarcon JB, Brittingham JM, et al. Improved genetic immunization via micro-mechanical disruption of skin-barrier function and targeted epidermal delivery. Nat Med. 2002;8:415–419.

[51] Mikszta JA, Sullivan VJ, Dean C, et al. Protective immunization against inhalational anthrax: a comparison of minimally invasive delivery platforms. J Infect Dis. 2005;191:278–288.

[52] Bins AD, Jorritsma A, Wolkers MC, et al. A rapid and potent DNA vaccination strategy defined by in vivo monitoring of antigen expression. Nat Med. 2005;11:899–904.

[53] Mohammed AJ, AlAwaidy S, Bawikar S, et al. Fractional doses of inactivated poliovirus vaccine in Oman. N Eng J Med. 2010;362:2351–2359.

[54] Dean HJ, Chen D. Epidermal powder immunization against influenza. Vaccine. 2004;23:681–686.

[55] Jones S, Evans K, McElwaine-Johnn H, et al. DNA vaccination protects against an influenza challenge in a double-blind randomised placebo-controlled phase 1b clinical trial. Vaccine. 2009;27:2506–2512.

[56] Van Kampen KR, Shi Z, Gao P, et al. Safety and immunogenicity of adenovirus-vectored nasal and epicutaneous influenza vaccines in humans. Vaccine. 2005;23:1029–1036.

[57] Gill HS, Andrews SN, Sakthivel SK, et al. Selective removal of stratum corneum by microdermabrasion to increase skin permeability. Eur J Pharm Sci. 2009;38:95–103.

[58] Park J-H, Lee J-W, Kim Y-C, et al. The effect of heat on skin permeability. Int J Pharm. 2008;359:94–103.

[59] Bramson J, Dayball K, Evelegh C, et al. Enabling topical immunization via microporation: a novel method for pain-free and needle-free delivery of adenovirus-based vaccines. Gene Therapy. 2003;10:251–260.

[60] Fagnoni FF, Zerbini A, Pelosi G, et al. Combination of radiofrequency ablation and immunotherapy. Front Biosci. 2008;13:369–381.

[61] Dahlan A, Alpar HO, Stickings P, et al. Transcutaneous immunisation assisted by low-frequency ultrasound. Int J Pharm. 2009;368:123–128.

[62] Zhao YL, Murthy SN, Manjili MH, et al. Induction of cytotoxic T-lymphocytes by electroporation-enhanced needle-free skin immunization. Vaccine. 2006;24:1282–1290.

[63] Drabick JJ, Glasspool-Malone J, Somiari S, et al. Cutaneous transfection and immune responses to intradermal nucleic acid vaccination are significantly enhanced by in vivo electropermeabilization. Mol Ther. 2001;3:249–255.

[64] Karande P, Arora A, Pham TK, et al. Transcutaneous immunization using common chemicals. J Control Release. 2009;138:134–140.

[65] Baxter J, Mitragotri S. Needle-free liquid jet injections: mechanisms and applications. Exp Rev Med Dev. 2006;3:565–574.

[66] Hogan M-E, Kikuta A, Taddio A. A systematic review of measures for reducing injection pain during adult immunization. Vaccine. 2010;28:1514–1521.

[67] Chen M-C, Lai K-Y, Ling M-H, et al. Enhancing immunogenicity of antigens through sustained intradermal delivery using chitosan microneedles with a patch-dissolvable design. Acta Biomaterialia. 2018;65:66–75.

[68] Lee JW, Park J-H, Prausnitz MR. Dissolving microneedles for transdermal drug delivery. Biomaterials. 2008;29:2113–2124.

[69] Lee JW, Choi S-O, Felner EI, et al. Dissolving microneedle patch for transdermal delivery of human growth hormone. Small. 2011;7:531–539.

[70] Shim DH, Nguyen TT, Park P, et al. Development of botulinum toxin A-coated microneedles for treating palmar hyperhidrosis. Mol Pharm. 2019;16:4913–4919.

[71] Avcil M, Çelik A. Microneedles in drug delivery: progress and challenges. Micromachines (Basel). 2021;12:1321.

[72] Marshall S, Sahm LJ, Moore AC. The success of microneedle-mediated vaccine delivery into skin. Human Vaccines & Immunotherapeutics. 2016;12:2975–2983.

[73] Bal SM, Ding Z, Kersten GFA, et al. Microneedle-based transcutaneous immunisation in mice with N-trimethyl chitosan adjuvanted diphtheria toxoid formulations. Pharm Res. 2010;27:1837–1847.

[74] Ding Z, Verbaan FJ, Bivas-Benita M, et al. Microneedle arrays for the transcutaneous immunization of diphtheria and influenza in BALB/c mice. J Control Release. 2009;136:71–78.

[75] Guo L, Qiu Y, Chen J, et al. Effective transcutaneous immunization against hepatitis B virus by a combined approach of hydrogel patch formulation and microneedle arrays. Biomed Microdevices. 2013;15:1077–1085.

[76] Carey JB, Vrdoljak A, O'Mahony C, et al. Microneedle-mediated immunization of an adenovirus-based malaria vaccine enhances antigen-specific antibody immunity and reduces antivector responses compared to the intradermal route. Sci Rep. 2014;4:6154.

[77] Fernando GJ, Hickling J, Flores CMJ, et al. Safety, tolerability, acceptability and immunogenicity of an influenza vaccine delivered to human skin by a novel high-density microprojection array patch (Nanopatch™). Vaccine. 2018;36:3779–3788.

[78] Ding Z, Van Riet E, Romeijn S, et al. Immune modulation by adjuvants combined with diphtheria toxoid administered topically in BALB/c mice after microneedle array pretreatment. Pharm Res. 2009;26:1635–1643.

[79] Ma S, Liu C, Li B, et al. Sonophoresis enhanced transdermal delivery of cisplatin in the xeno-grafted tumor model of cervical cancer. OTT. 2020;13:889–902.

[80] Toyoda M, Hama S, Ikeda Y, et al. Anti-cancer vaccination by transdermal delivery of antigen peptide-loaded nanogels via iontophoresis. Int J Pharm. 2015;483:110–114.

[81] Waghule T, Singhvi G, Dubey SK, et al. Microneedles: a smart approach and increasing potential for transdermal drug delivery system. Biomed Pharm. 2019;109:1249–1258.

[82] Wonglertnirant N, Todo H, Opanasopit P, et al. Macromolecular delivery into skin using a hollow microneedle. Biol Pharm Bull. 2010;33:1988–1993.

[83] Davis SP, Martanto W, Allen MG, et al. Hollow metal microneedles for insulin delivery to diabetic rats. IEEE Trans Biomed Eng. 2005;52:909–915.

[84] Harvey AJ, Kaestner SA, Sutter DE, et al. Microneedle-based intradermal delivery enables rapid lymphatic uptake and distribution of protein drugs. Pharm Res. 2011;28:107–116.

[85] Laurent PE, Bonnet S, Alchas P, et al. Evaluation of the clinical performance of a new intradermal vaccine administration technique and associated delivery system. Vaccine. 2007;25:8833–8842.

[86] Van Damme P, Oosterhuis-Kafeja F, Van der Wielen M, et al. Safety and efficacy of a novel microneedle device for dose sparing intradermal influenza vaccination in healthy adults. Vaccine. 2009;27:454–459.

[87] Donnelly RF, Singh TRR. Novel delivery systems for transdermal and intradermal drug delivery. New Jersey: John Wiley & Sons; 2015.

[88] van der Maaden K, Trietsch SJ, Kraan H, et al. Novel hollow microneedle technology for depth-controlled microinjection-mediated dermal vaccination: a study with polio vaccine in rats. Pharm Res. 2014;31:1846–1854.

[89] Kim Y-C, Quan F-S, Compans RW, et al. Formulation and coating of microneedles with inactivated influenza virus to improve vaccine stability and immunogenicity. J Control Release. 2010;142:187–195.

[90] Fernando GJ, Chen X, Prow TW, et al. Potent immunity to low doses of influenza vaccine by probabilistic guided micro-targeted skin delivery in a mouse model. PLoS One. 2010;5:e10266.

[91] Kines RC, Zarnitsyn V, Johnson TR, et al. Vaccination with human papillomavirus pseudovirus-encapsidated plasmids targeted to skin using microneedles. PLoS One. 2015;10:e0120797.

[92] Zhang S, Zhao S, Jin X, et al. Microneedles improve the immunogenicity of DNA vaccines. Human Gene Therapy. 2018;29:1004–1010.

[93] Meyer BK, Kendall MA, Williams DM, et al. Immune response and reactogenicity of an unadjuvanted intradermally delivered human papillomavirus vaccine using a first generation Nanopatch™ in rhesus macaques: an exploratory, pre-clinical feasibility assessment. Vaccine: X. 2019;2:100030.

[94] Turvey ME, Uppu DS, Mohamed Sharif AR, et al. Microneedle-based intradermal delivery of stabilized dengue virus. Bioeng Transl Med. 2019;4:e10127.

[95] Stinson JA, Raja WK, Lee S, et al. Silk fibroin microneedles for transdermal vaccine delivery. ACS Biomat Sci Eng. 2017;3:360–369.

[96] Sullivan SP, Murthy N, Prausnitz MR. Minimally invasive protein delivery with rapidly dissolving polymer microneedles. Adv Mat. 2008;20:933–938.

[97] Lahiji SF, Dangol M, Jung H. A patchless dissolving microneedle delivery system enabling rapid and efficient transdermal drug delivery. Sci Rep. 2015;5:7914.

[98] Donnelly RF, Raj Singh TR, Woolfson AD. Microneedle-based drug delivery systems: microfabrication, drug delivery, and safety. Drug Deliv. 2010;17:187–207.

[99] Chu LY, Choi S-O, Prausnitz MR. Fabrication of dissolving polymer microneedles for controlled drug encapsulation and delivery: bubble and pedestal microneedle designs. J Pharm Sci. 2010;99:4228–4238.

[100] Arya JM, Dewitt K, Scott-Garrard M, et al. Rabies vaccination in dogs using a dissolving microneedle patch. J Control Release. 2016;239:19–26.

[101] Mistilis MJ, Joyce JC, Esser ES, et al. Long-term stability of influenza vaccine in a dissolving microneedle patch. Drug Deliv Transl Res. 2017;7:195–205.

[102] Flynn O, Dillane K, Lanza JS, et al. Low adenovirus vaccine doses administered to skin using microneedle patches induce better functional antibody immunogenicity as compared to systemic injection. Vaccines. 2021;9:299.

[103] Ali AA, McCrudden CM, McCaffrey J, et al. DNA vaccination for cervical cancer; a novel technology platform of RALA mediated gene delivery via polymeric microneedles. Nanomed Nanotechnol Biol Med. 2017;13:921–932.

[104] Duong HTT, Yin Y, Thambi T, et al. Highly potent intradermal vaccination by an array of dissolving microneedle polypeptide cocktails for cancer immunotherapy. J Mat Chem B. 2020;8:1171–1181.

[105] Esser ES, Romanyuk Andrey A, Vassilieva EV, et al. Tetanus vaccination with a dissolving microneedle patch confers protective immune responses in pregnancy. J Control Release. 2016;236:47–56.

[106] Gala RP, Zaman RU, D'Souza MJ, et al. Novel whole-cell inactivated Neisseria gonorrhoeae microparticles as vaccine formulation in microneedle-based transdermal immunization. Vaccines. 2018;6:60.

[107] Li Z, He Y, Deng L, et al. A fast-dissolving microneedle array loaded with chitosan nanoparticles to evoke systemic immune responses in mice. J Mat Chem B. 2020;8:216–225.

[108] Sullivan SP, Koutsonanos DG, Del Pilar Martin M, et al. Dissolving polymer microneedle patches for influenza vaccination. Nat Med. 2010;16:915–920.

[109] Kim YC, Lee JW, Esser ES, et al. Fabrication of microneedle patches with lyophilized influenza vaccine suspended in organic solvent. Drug Deliv and Transl Res. 2021;11:692–701.

[110] Tran K, Gavitt TD, Farrell NJ, et al. Transdermal microneedles for the programmable burst release of multiple vaccine payloads. Nat Biomed Eng. 2021;5:998–1007.

[111] O'Shea J, Prausnitz MR, Rouphael N. Dissolvable microneedle patches to enable increased access to vaccines against SARS-CoV-2 and future pandemic outbreaks. Vaccines. 2021;9:320.

[112] Ingrole RS, Azizoglu E, Dul M, et al. Trends of microneedle technology in the scientific literature, patents, clinical trials and internet activity. Biomaterials. 2021;267:120491.

[113] Chen X, Fernando GJ, Crichton ML, et al. Improving the reach of vaccines to low-resource regions, with a needle-free vaccine delivery device and long-term thermostabilization. J Control Release. 2011;152:349–355.

[114] Choi H-J, Yoo D-G, Bondy BJ, et al. Stability of influenza vaccine coated onto microneedles. Biomaterials. 2012;33:3756–3769.

[115] Jacoby E, Jarrahian C, Hull HF, et al. Opportunities and challenges in delivering influenza vaccine by microneedle patch. Vaccine. 2015;33:4699–4704.

[116] Kommareddy S, Baudner BC, Oh S, et al. Dissolvable microneedle patches for the delivery of cell-culture-derived influenza vaccine antigens. J Pharm Sci. 2012;101:1021–1027.

[117] Arnou R, Eavis P, De Juanes Pardo J-R, et al. Immunogenicity, large scale safety and lot consistency of an intradermal influenza vaccine in adults aged 18–60 years: randomized, controlled, phase III trial. Human Vaccines. 2010;6:346–354.

[118] Shakya AK, Gill HS. A comparative study of microneedle-based cutaneous immunization with other conventional routes to assess feasibility of microneedles for allergy immunotherapy. Vaccine. 2015;33:4060–4064.

[119] Norman JJ, Arya JM, McClain MA, et al. Microneedle patches: usability and acceptability for self-vaccination against influenza. Vaccine. 2014;32:1856–1862.

[120] Indermun S, Luttge R, Choonara YE, et al. Current advances in the fabrication of microneedles for transdermal delivery. J Control Release. 2014;185:130–138.

[121] Joyce JC, Carroll TD, Collins ML, et al. A microneedle patch for measles and rubella vaccination is immunogenic and protective in infant rhesus macaques. J Infect Dis. 2018;218:124–132.

[122] Carter D, van Hoeven N, Baldwin S, et al. The adjuvant GLA-AF enhances human intradermal vaccine responses. Sci Adv. 2018;4:eaas9930.

[123] Levin Y, Kochba E, Shukarev G, et al. A phase 1, open-label, randomized study to compare the immunogenicity and safety of different administration routes and doses of virosomal influenza vaccine in elderly. Vaccine. 2016;34:5262–5272.

[124] Holland D, Booy R, De Looze F, et al. Intradermal influenza vaccine administered using a new microinjection system produces superior immunogenicity in elderly adults: a randomized controlled trial. J Infect Dis. 2008;198:650–658.

[125] Leroux-Roels I, Vets E, Freese R, et al. Seasonal influenza vaccine delivered by intradermal microinjection: a randomised controlled safety and immunogenicity trial in adults. Vaccine. 2008;26:6614–6619.

[126] Vescovo P, Rettby N, Ramaniraka N, et al. Safety, tolerability and efficacy of intradermal rabies immunization with DebioJect™. Vaccine. 2017;35:1782–1788.

[127] Arya J, Henry S, Kalluri H, et al. Tolerability, usability and acceptability of dissolving microneedle patch administration in human subjects. Biomaterials. 2017;128:1–7.

[128] Hirobe S, Azukizawa H, Hanafusa T, et al. Clinical study and stability assessment of a novel transcutaneous influenza vaccination using a dissolving microneedle patch. Biomaterials. 2015;57:50–58.

[129] Bhatnagar S, Gadeela PR, Thathireddy P, et al. Microneedle-based drug delivery: materials of construction. J Chem Sci. 2019;131:1–28.

[130] Frew PM, Paine MB, Rouphael N, et al. Acceptability of an inactivated influenza vaccine delivered by microneedle patch: results from a phase I clinical trial of safety, reactogenicity, and immunogenicity. Vaccine. 2020;38:7175–7181.

[131] Arnou R, Frank M, Hagel T, et al. Willingness to vaccinate or get vaccinated with an intradermal seasonal influenza vaccine: a survey of general practitioners and the general public in France and Germany. Adv Ther. 2011;28:555–565.

[132] Adhikari BB, Goodson JL, Chu SY, et al. Assessing the potential cost-effectiveness of microneedle patches in childhood measles vaccination programs: the case for further research and development. Drugs in R&D. 2016;16:327–338.

[133] Richter-Johnson J, Kumar P, Choonara YE, et al. Therapeutic applications and pharmacoeconomics of microneedle technology. Exp Rev of Pharmacoecon Outcomes Res. 2018;18:359–369.

[134] Leung M-K, You JH. Cost-effectiveness of an influenza vaccination program offering intramuscular and intradermal vaccines versus intramuscular vaccine alone for elderly. Vaccine. 2016;34:2469–2476.

[135] Wong C, Jiang M, You JH. Potential cost-effectiveness of an influenza vaccination program offering microneedle patch for vaccine delivery in children. PLoS One. 2016;11:e0169030.

[136] Lee BY, Bartsch SM, Mvundura M, et al. An economic model assessing the value of microneedle patch delivery of the seasonal influenza vaccine. Vaccine. 2015;33:4727–4736.

[137] Balmert SC, Carey CD, Falo GD, et al. Dissolving undercut microneedle arrays for multicomponent cutaneous vaccination. J Control Release. 2020;317:336–346.

[138] Krieger KJ, Bertollo N, Dangol M, et al. Simple and customizable method for fabrication of high-aspect ratio microneedle molds using low-cost 3D printing. Microsyst Nanoeng. 2019;5:1–14.

[139] Fogel DB. Factors associated with clinical trials that fail and opportunities for improving the likelihood of success: a review. Contemp Clin Trials Commun. 2018;11:156–164.

[140] Laurent PE, Bourhy H, Fantino M, et al. Safety and efficacy of novel dermal and epidermal microneedle delivery systems for rabies vaccination in healthy adults. Vaccine. 2010;28:5850–5856.

[141] Carey JB, Pearson FE, Vrdoljak A, et al. Microneedle array design determines the induction of protective memory CD8+ T cell responses induced by a recombinant live malaria vaccine in mice. PLoS One. 2011;6:e22442.

[142] Daddona PE, Matriano JA, Mandema J, et al. Parathyroid hormone (1–34)-coated microneedle patch system: clinical pharmacokinetics and pharmacodynamics for treatment of osteoporosis. Pharm Res. 2011;28:159–165.

[143] Poirier D, Renaud F, Dewar V, et al. Hepatitis B surface antigen incorporated in dissolvable microneedle array patch is antigenic and thermostable. Biomaterials. 2017;145:256–265.

[144] Kommareddy S, Baudner BC, Bonificio A, et al. Influenza subunit vaccine coated microneedle patches elicit comparable immune responses to intramuscular injection in guinea pigs. Vaccine. 2013;31:3435–3441.

[145] Zhang Y, Brown K, Siebenaler K, et al. Development of lidocaine-coated microneedle product for rapid, safe, and prolonged local analgesic action. Pharm Res. 2012;29:170–177.

[146] Lutton REM, Moore J, Larrañeta E, et al. Microneedle characterisation: the need for universal acceptance criteria and GMP specifications when moving towards commercialisation. Drug Deliv Transl Res. 2015;5:313–331.

[147] Bayarri L. Drug-device combination products: regulatory landscape and market growth. Drugs of Today. 2015;51:505–513.

9

Microneedles for Cosmetic Applications

9.1 Introduction

Numerous variables affect skin health, including lifestyle, environmental factors (exposure to sunlight and ultraviolet radiation), genetics, hormones, and diet [1]. Several biological processes contribute to skin aging. Both intrinsic aging (the destruction of elastin fibers and a significant decrease in collagen that causes wrinkles) and extrinsic aging (photoaging) ensue from years of exposure to harmful conditions, particularly ultraviolet radiation. Many individuals also have to cope with the unpleasant phenomena of facial scarring [2, 3], which may be brought on by various causes such as depigmentation, acne scars, burn scars, and the development of enlarged pores. Research into novel strategies for preventing the formation of stretch marks is ongoing [4]. Acne vulgaris, which may be psychologically disturbing, is one of the most prevalent skin illnesses that causes scarring. Its pathophysiology is based on active inflammation leading to the destruction to the elastic support structures underneath the skin's surface [5, 6].

The primary goal of the cosmetics field is to restore the skin's natural beauty by treating a variety of skin disorders (such as acne, psoriasis, and hyperpigmentation) and mending the skin's general structure (such as treatment of scar, cellulite reduction, skin tightening, and wrinkles). It is important to emphasize that cosmetic products are not designed to be administered systemically to obtain these benefits. Because the stratum corneum, viable epidermis, and dermis layer are often the targeted site for cosmeceuticals, it is more accurate to refer to the delivery of cosmeceuticals as topical "dermal delivery" [7]. Typically, cosmeceuticals are topical products (i.e., creams, gels, lotions, and serums), meaning they are applied to the skin, and then the active components are absorbed into the skin [8]. Nevertheless, the stratum corneum, the uppermost skin layer, functions as a protective barrier to external elements; thus, only compounds with suitable physicochemical qualities, including low molecular weight, moderate lipophilicity, and low melting point, may permeate this layer [9]. Because of this, even if the products are targeted to have a localized action in the skin, a considerable portion of them are lost from the skin's surface and have limited diffusion into the skin.

The cosmetic sector places a strong emphasis on the viable epidermis and dermis layers of skin since they are responsible for the skin's texture, moisture levels, and pigmentation [10]. The stratum corneum, the protein- and lipid-rich topmost layer of the epidermis, inhibits water evaporation from the skin and is the principal barrier to the transport of all reagents into and across the skin [11]. The cosmetic industry aims to temporarily remove this layer. Besides, damage to or loss of collagen, the main structural protein in the dermis layer, may lead to skin distortion, such as wrinkles and scars [12].

DOI: 10.1201/9780429294433-9

Over the years, several novel technologies have been developed to tackle the issue of limited skin permeability [13]. Physical enhancement technologies employ a device to either noninvasively puncture the protective stratum corneum barrier or provide a physical force to drive the compounds into the skin (Table 9.1). These technologies facilitate the movement of cosmeceuticals across the skin's cellular layers and to the targeted site in the skin. Iontophoresis, microdermabrasion, sonophoresis, and microporation (microneedles or laser ablation) are only a few physical enhancement techniques used in the cosmetic field [11]. When it comes to skin penetration, the effectiveness of various physical enhancement technologies is limited by the molecular size and mass of cosmeceutical compounds. Since molecules used in the cosmetic field may differ widely in terms of size and lipophilicity, the delivery method must be tailored to the specific molecule. Moreover, identifying the location of action in the skin is essential for the effective delivery of cosmeceuticals.

More invasive methods may be preferred over aesthetic technologies that use minimally or noninvasive procedures, according to the extent of the skin issues to be remedied and the targeted site of delivery. Exfoliating dry skin and removing mild hyperpigmentation after acne scars are two examples of common uses for minimally invasive methods. For significantly damaged skin (i.e., wrinkles or atrophic acne scars), more invasive techniques, such as ablative and nonablative laser therapy, are employed to produce more extensive skin structural disruption and repair [14]. Scarred and aged skin may be treated using

TABLE 9.1

Physical Enhancement Technologies in the Cosmetic Field [14]

Technology	Mechanism of Action	Devices
Microneedles	Physical microporation of skin layers	DermaRoller® (DermaRoller), Dermapen® (EquipMED™), Revive™ HAP (AMIEA MED), Beauty Mouse (derma roller), Derma stamp (derma roller), Skinpen® (Bellus Medical), Exceed Microneedling device (AMIEA MED)
Iontophoresis	Electrical current-based mechanisms: electro-repulsion and electroosmosis	WrinkleMD™ (WrinkleMD), BioBliss™ (Iontera, Inc.), NuFace® Trinity (NuFace)
Sonophoresis	Ultrasound-induced disruption of the stratum corneum lipids	Clarisonic® Opal Sonic Infusion (Clarisonic)
Laser	For nonablative laser resurfacing, an intense laser beam targets and heats the dermis layer to promote collagen production. The ablative laser disrupts and removes the epidermis layer	Quasar® MD Plus (Quasar Bio-Tech, Inc.), QS ND: YAG; Er: YAG, CO_2, Er: glass, Titan™ (Cutera), Triactive™ (Cynosure), SmoothShapes™ (Cynosure)
Microdermabrasion	Abrasive crystals are propelled against the skin, causing mechanical abrasion to the skin and disrupting the stratum corneum layer	PMD® (Personal Microderm) (Age Sciences, Inc.), MegaPeel™ (DermaMed Solutions, LLC), Pristine™ (Viora)
Combination of microneedles and radiofrequency	Physical microporation combined with low-energy radiation (heat the dermis layer to stimulate cutaneous collagen, elastin, and hyaluronic acid production)	IntraCel™ (JEISYS Medical, Inc.), Vivace Microneedling RF (Aesthetics Biomedical, Inc.)

ablative techniques such as laser resurfacing and dermabrasion. A comprehensive report in 2014 describes the many skin laser resurfacing procedures presently accessible to doctors and those in the development pipeline [15]. Some invasive procedures carry high risks of undesirable effects, such as discomfort, erythema, pruritus, and severe edema, among others, to the users [16]. Injections of botulinum toxin and other cosmetic products are painful and require trained professionals to administer, although they provide desirable aesthetic outcomes [13]. Many aesthetic devices and treatments that use physical technologies are only offered by dermatologists; however, at-home cosmetic gadgets are becoming increasingly accessible to the public [14].

9.1.1 Microneedles for Cosmetics

9.1.1.1 History of Microneedle Use in Cosmetics

Skin needling technique had been used in dermatology before microneedles were widely utilized. Subcision, sometimes called dermal needling, was first proposed by Orentreich and Orentreich in 1995 [17]. This method requires making minor puncture wounds in the skin and then drawing the needle into the dermis to scarify this layer to produce connective tissue underneath the scars. However, owing to bleeding and excessive bruising, this method was not feasible for application over vast skin regions. In 1997, Camirand and Doucet "needle abraded" scars using a tattoo gun [18]. This method is widely believed to be very time-consuming since the epidermal pores are too shallow and closely spaced [19]. Later, microneedling was devised by Fernandes (a drum-shaped gadget with numerous tiny protruding needles) to stimulate the body's post-traumatic inflammatory response [20]. This method relies on the controlled penetration of very fine needles into the skin to produce microscopic tears in the collagen fibers that anchor the scar to the dermis. This triggers the body's wound-healing cascade, leading to the formation of new blood vessels and collagen. Microneedling, also widely recognized as percutaneous collagen induction, collagen induction therapy, dry tattooing, and intra-dermabrasion, is a relatively new method that has shown promise as a noninvasive approach to reducing the presence of scars (i.e., acne scars, surgical scars, fine lines, wrinkles, stretch marks, cellulite, and more) and enhancing skin texture, firmness, and hydration [19, 20]. The application of microneedling fractional radiofrequency in acne treatments is a novel strategy; this method has been demonstrated to be clinically effective in the management of acne scars without generating direct harm to the epidermis layer.

9.1.1.2 Introduction of Microneedles

Microneedle technology has been the subject of extensive research worldwide since its potential as a drug delivery platform was proposed in 1976. Micrometer-sized needles (microneedles) have been thoroughly studied for use in various pharmaceutical and cosmetic applications; they may target either the epidermis or the dermis layer, depending on the needle's length and design. Cosmetic microneedles devices have been devised to disturb the stratum corneum's barrier function, allowing skin rejuvenation and enhanced skin texture through induced collagen production and deposition. In addition, they are being employed in conjunction with topical treatments or light sources and as carriers to transport cosmeceuticals into the skin. Producers of cosmetic microneedle devices for aesthetic applications have produced some remarkable proof, giving hope to individuals with unpleasant burns and scars and anybody who wants to look youthful. Microneedles have a promising future in this cosmetic field, and it is not difficult to envision a new generation of microneedles devices carrying various active molecules to enhance the skin's beauty. In contrast, this could necessitate a higher standard of regulatory approval than is often expected for cosmetic products, which would jack up the industry costs.

The following benefits of microneedles have contributed to their increase in popularity in the cosmetics industry over the last several decades.

- Acceptability and convenience of self-administration.
- Minimal to no pain during microneedle treatment.
- No size restriction on the delivered molecules, including antioxidants, vitamins, peptides, and potent molecules of low lipophilicity or larger molecular size.
- Minimal undesired postoperative epidermal injury, thus requiring short healing or recovery times.
- Low risk of hyperpigmentation and scarring, excellent for individuals with thin, sensitive, or ethnic skin types.
- Significant enhancement of skin permeability.
- Relatively cheap in comparison to alternative treatments. Dermatologists' services and other cosmetic surgeries may be highly pricey.
- Use in areas where invasive methods are not an option, such as in the eye's surrounding region.
- Scars may be reduced with collagen deposition from microneedling more so than with intense pulsed light therapy [21].

Microneedle use in the cosmetic field is based on two primary principles: increasing skin permeability of cosmeceutical molecules and promoting skin healing from microinjuries caused by microneedles treatment [8]. Microneedles are used for skin microporation, a process that allows macromolecules or hydrophilic molecules to enter the skin by creating micrometer-sized channels in the skin [11]. Cosmetic devices are utilized not only for the dermal transport of cosmeceutical compounds but also for the significant benefit of the physical technology on the skin's structure. The epidermal barrier may be disrupted using microneedling to increase the skin's capacity to absorb topical compounds. As cosmeceuticals diffuse into the skin, they penetrate directly to the site of skin damage and assist in accelerating the skin's natural healing process. Nonactive-encapsulated microneedles are licensed in several countries for collagen induction therapy, scar and hyperpigmentation treatment, and wrinkle prevention and reduction. Multiple micrometer-sized needles penetrating the skin generate minuscule controlled injuries that disrupt collagen strands tethering the scar to the dermis. This procedure yields angiogenesis and collagenesis via post-traumatic inflammation response and natural wound-healing cascade [22]. Microneedling stimulates wound healing in three stages: (i) initiation/inflammatory, (ii) proliferation, and (iii) remodeling. Microneedle insertion to the stratum corneum triggers the release of growth factors that stimulate neocollagenesis and neovascularization, which are central to the microneedling mechanism. Researchers indicate that the procedure's efficacy in reducing scarring and restoring the effects of sunlight exposure is due to the release of growth factors [23]. An endogenous biochemical mechanism causes "enhanced keratinocyte proliferation and differentiation, improved generation of corneocytes, and formation, processing, and secretion of barrier lipids" in the epidermis layer during the healing process [24]. Microneedling is a minimally invasive technique that stimulates the skin's natural healing mechanisms in a way similar to that observed in response to an injury. The electrical signals sent by the stimulated nerves set off a chain reaction that ultimately leads to the healing of the injury [25]. This triggers the proliferation of undifferentiated skin cells and the transformation of fibroblasts into collagen and elastin fibers in the skin. These latter cells then function to thicken the skin and fill in scars by merging with the surrounding collagen layer. A distinct layer of collagen forms when the insertion of numerous microneedles triggers this mechanism. When collagen is produced, the skin revives its flexibility and hydration, while wrinkles disappear [25]. Moreover, the signals mentioned earlier promote the growth of endothelia cells in dermal capillaries, resulting in the branching or formation of capillaries and an improved blood flow to the dermis layer [25]. Consequently, the epidermis and dermis are remodeled, which is an effective treatment for skin-related issues. Percutaneous collagen induction (PCI) is a process in which dermal collagen is induced to repair itself by means of an immune response triggered inside the skin upon piercing by microneedles [15].

Despite the apparent therapeutic advantages of microneedles devices and their growing availability and use, questions have been raised about the patient acceptability of such products, as well as possible erythema, discomfort, and patient safety in administration and sterilization [26]. In the grand scheme, using microneedles in cosmetics is safe and effective. Crusting, swelling (edema), redness (erythema), and minor pain are all possible mild to moderate adverse effects of microneedles [27]. When microneedles are tested on humans, most participants reported little or minor skin irritation and adverse effects, which often subsided on their own and were well-tolerated [28, 29]. Concerns about local skin irritation or erythema after the application of microneedles device are warranted due to the skin's robust immune-stimulatory property [30], although studies have shown that the skin's barrier function recovers rapidly within a few hours [3, 31]. One research demonstrated that erythema was resolved within 24–48 h, with no notable difference seen in erythema index ratios between the varied needle lengths used in the study [3]. The ability of microneedles to stimulate collagen restoration has been extensively utilized in the field of percutaneous collagen induction technology. Slight bleeding from contact with cutaneous blood capillaries is possible during the collagen induction process with a needle length of 1.5 mm [32]. A microneedle of this length causes far less discomfort than the standard hypodermic needle. Typically, the length of cosmetic microneedles is less than 620 μm so as not to cause any painful sensation. Depending on the kind of aesthetic procedure, microneedles may be as short as 200 μm [11].

In addition to performing as intended, the future commercial and therapeutic success of microneedle devices will be determined by how positively they are received by patients and healthcare providers [33]. For this reason, the Birchall team [34] and the Donnelly group [35] reported their perspectives on how users regard microneedles. Eighty percent of participants in both studies reported feeling "strongly positive" about the microneedle devices employed in the research, indicating that they were aware of the potential advantages of the microneedle system. It is still unclear what, if any, long-term impacts microneedles application, or repeated microneedles exposure, may have on the skin. Researchers should pay attention to the necessity for vigilance in the use of topical drugs in conjunction with physical enhancement technologies. Only properly approved and tested cosmeceutical products developed for this purpose should be combined with microneedles treatment. Early research on an animal model reveals that repeated application of polymeric microneedle arrays did not result in any unfavorable local or systemic adverse effects [36]. Regardless of the fact that many microneedle devices are classified as either "home use" or "medical use" in the product's documentation, anyone may buy them online from a wide variety of retailers. There is an obvious possibility for misuse and exploitation of these devices, and this is further exacerbated by the lack of restrictions on acquiring them.

The issue of whether or not microneedles devices used for cosmetic purposes need terminal sterilization has also been discussed. This issue has to be answered in a way that is consistent with the guidelines set out by regulatory agencies since improper use of microneedling devices might result in their early, unjustified rejection. Microneedles devices are not comparable to traditional transdermal patches since they do not just stick to the skin [33]. This is true regardless of how the pharmaceutical and cosmetics industry classifies microneedles. Since they are more similar to a typical hypodermic injection, they may need to be sterilized. For example, derma roller and Dermapen products come sterilized and may be easily re-sterilized due to their metal material [33]. The majority of the cosmetic devices sold in the United States are either class I devices (which do not require FDA pre-market approval) or class II devices (which require clearance via the 510(k) application), in which the safety and efficacy of the device are compared to that of a "substantially equivalent" commercial cosmetic device [24, 37].

Several researchers have examined to see if microneedle technology is safe to use. Skin barrier recovery after microneedling was a crucial factor. Studies have shown that pore closure on human forearm skin occurs within 2 h when the treated area is not occluded [38] but may take up to 48–72 h when the site is occluded [39]. After the occlusion is lifted, the skin's natural barrier function is restored rapidly without causing any harm to the skin, and pore closure often occurs within a few hours. Most cosmeceuticals are used on the face; thus, it is significant that this skin area's protective barrier is restored. Facial barrier healing was also observed within a short duration, suggesting that microneedles may be used for optimal aesthetic purposes without risk [3]. It has also been demonstrated that the skin barrier function may be recovered safely and efficiently in various Fitzpatrick skin types (I–VI) after microneedle application [32]. Several factors, including age, skin elasticity, application location, and insertion pressure, influence how long it takes for the skin to heal after microneedles treatment [3, 31]. The application of cosmetic gadgets has usually been linked to certain skin irritation. Using a cosmetic device with a topical product containing skin sensitizer excipients is indeed common. The integration of physical treatment may enhance the penetration of these sensitizers, thus elevating the skin irritation potential [7].

9.2 Types of Microneedles in Cosmetics

Different types and designs of microneedles have been used in the cosmetic field. The most common types of microneedles for cosmetic application are solid microneedles (especially metal microneedles) (Fig. 9.1) and dissolving microneedles (Fig. 9.2). It has been shown that using a solid metal microneedle to create micrometer-sized channels in the skin may increase collagen production and speed up the body's natural healing process, as shown in several studies [40–42]. Furthermore, microneedles are used prior to the application of cosmeceutical preparations to increase the skin's capacity to absorb the active ingredients [43–45]. As a result of the two-step procedure, more of the active substance will be delivered into the skin, but not all of it [46]. Solid microneedles raised safety issues due to the sharp residues/waste left after usage.

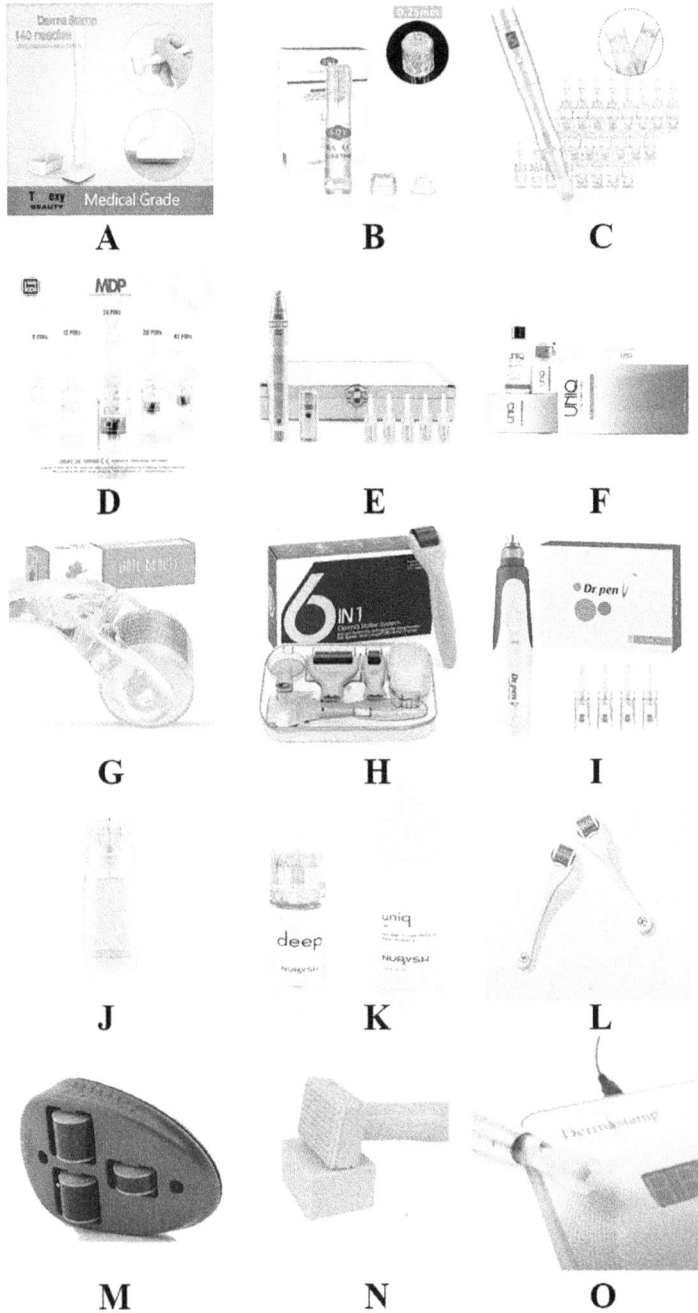

FIGURE 9.1

Solid microneedles for cosmetic applications. (A) Microneedles Derma Stamp. (B) Automatic Gold Derma Stamp. (C) Beautlinks Electric Microneedling Pen. (D) Auto Stamp Pen. (E) Angel Kiss Derma Auto Pen. (F) Titanium Microneedle Facial Roller. (G) Titanium Microneedle derma roller. (H) 6 in 1 Derma Roller (Microneedle Kit for Face and Body). (I) Shake Beauty Derma Auto Pen (Wireless Electric Microneedle Microneedling Pen). (J) Hydra Needle Microneedle Tool and Serum Applicator. (K) DEEP + UNIQ Titanium Microneedle/Dermapen Kit. (L) Titanium Microneedle Derma Roller. (M) Beauty Mouse®. (N) White Lotus Dermastamp™. (O) eDermastamp®. Images reprinted with permission from respective sources.

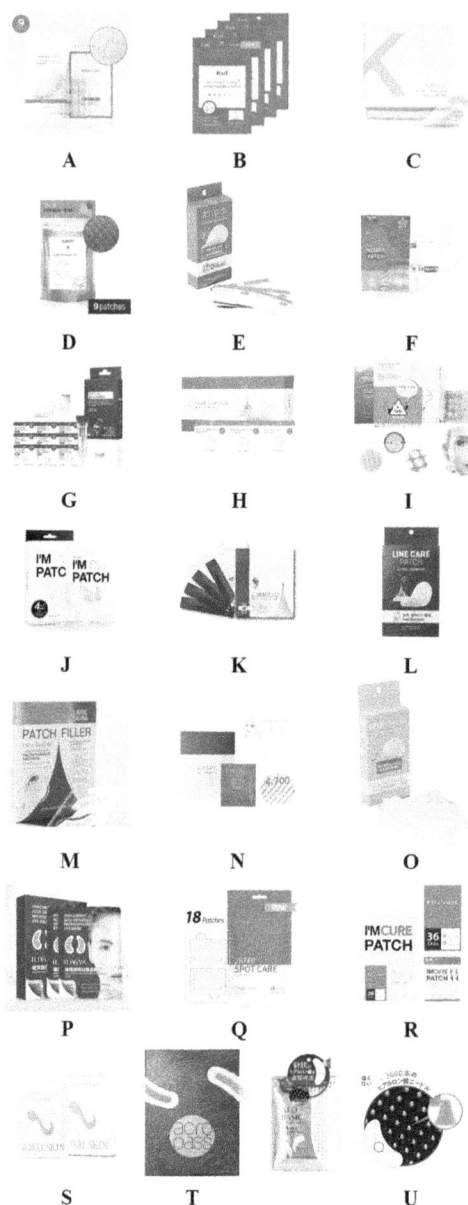

FIGURE 9.2
Dissolving microneedles for cosmetic applications. (A) Pimtox microneedle patch for acne, pimple, and skin trouble. (B) Rael microneedle acne healing patch. (C) Pimple patch for spot treatment. (D) Microneedle for healing acne, pimple, and blemish. (E) Acne care treatment (Acropass). (F) Patch Pro microneedle patch for eye mask antiaging and anti-wrinkle. (G) Anti-trouble microneedle patch for acne and blemish care. (H) Acropass trouble cure plus, instant acne pimple patch. (I) Microneedle solution patch for acnes, skin calming, and sebum control. (J) Karatica I'm fill patch. (K) Spa treatment HAS iMicro microneedle patch. (L) Acropass facial wrinkles care microneedle patch. (M) Librederm Patch-Filler with microneedles for antiaging. (N) Artpe smile care solution multi-spot patch for eye and smile wrinkles. (O) Acropass age spot/dark spot eraser. (P) Rouse microneedle patch for wrinkles and fine lines. (Q) Derma microneedle two-step acne treatment. (R) Karatica hydrocolloid I'm cure patch for acne care. (S) Royal skin hyaluronic acid micro-patch (Junmok International Co., Ltd.), (T) Acropass (RAPHAS Co., Ltd.). (U) Neo basic HA fill micro patch (Nissha Co., Ltd.). Images reprinted with permission from respective sources.

Microneedles made of biodegradable polymers have also been developed to deliver cosmeceutical ingredients into skin tissue, which may exert a profound effect [13]. Dissolving microneedles could penetrate and disrupt the skin barrier and release cosmetic agents into the skin by dissolution in skin interstitial fluid. Dissolving microneedle arrays improve the efficacy of aesthetic treatments over metal microneedles since more cosmeceutical is absorbed into the skin in a shorter period with minimal drug loss [47]. In addition, the polymeric matrix of microneedles is biocompatible and biodegradable; thus, it does not cause any biohazardous effects [48, 49]. Dissolving microneedles leave no sharp or hazardous waste, and the reuse of needles is prohibited, so enhancing safety and convenience. Microneedles with adequate mechanical robustness to pierce the skin may be fabricated from materials with a high molecular weight of >10,000 Da [50]. However, materials with such a molecular weight tend to dissolve more slowly. Recently, issues with the commercial viability of dissolving microneedles products—specifically, the limited amounts of encapsulated active agents and the drug delivery efficiency—have been brought to light [51].

An antiaging or skin-moisturizing microneedle patch has recently achieved significant popularity in the cosmetic industry. Most commercially available microneedle patches are made of hyaluronic acid, which dissolves in the skin's interstitial fluid after skin insertion. Hyaluronic acid–based microneedles can release cosmeceutical agents for skin improvement while moisturizing skin tissue. Karatica Co., Ltd. produced the cosmetic microneedle array for use on the skin around the lips and eyes. The I'm Fill Needle Patch comprises 400 hyaluronic acid dissolving microneedles loaded with acetyl hexapeptide-8. Junmok International Co., Ltd. provides the Royal Skin Hyaluronic Acid Micro Patch, a hyaluronic acid–based microneedle array that enables the active agent to permeate the stratum corneum layer. Moisturizing and erasing fine lines and wrinkles, I'm Fill Needle Patch and Royal Skin Hyaluronic Acid Micro Patch both gain over-the-counter (OTC) drug approval from the Food and Drug Administration (FDA). The Acropass dissolving microneedle patch was manufactured by RAPHAS Co., Ltd. and is composed of hyaluronic acid. The swelling polymeric matrix that encapsulates the epidermal growth factor for antiaging serves as the skeleton component of the microneedles patch. RAPHAS Co., Ltd. holds worldwide patents for a droplet-born air blowing process to manufacture Acropass microneedles. Clinical investigations using hyaluronic acid microneedle arrays successfully improved the skin's flexibility and general health. Acropass is a human over-the-counter product that was approved by the FDA. The Nissaha Co., Ltd. developed the MicroCure® dissolving microneedle technology upon which the Neo Basic HA Fill Micro Patch is built. Flat-ended microneedles were designed by Cosmetex Roland Co., Ltd. using the MicroCure® technology, which increased patient safety.

SkinPen microneedling device from Bellus Medical (Addison, Texas) is the first and only microneedles-based system to be granted FDA De Novo clearance as a class II medical device (Fig. 9.3). This certification offers the clearance and marketing license for a device designed to improve facial acne scars in individuals aged 22 and above. SkinPen has created new technical and safety benchmarks for microneedling by providing minimally invasive skin rejuvenation solutions. Using straight and sharp needles that enter the skin at a 90° angle, SkinPen generates thousands of tiny channels in the dermis to stimulate skin remodeling without inducing scar tissue development. It just takes about 30 min to complete this comfortable procedure. It triggers the body's natural tissue regeneration mechanism while minimizing cell injury via the induction of controlled microdamage. The outcome is the successful remodeling of scar tissue while maintaining the integrity of the skin's general structure. Most patients experience the sensation of just a minor vibration

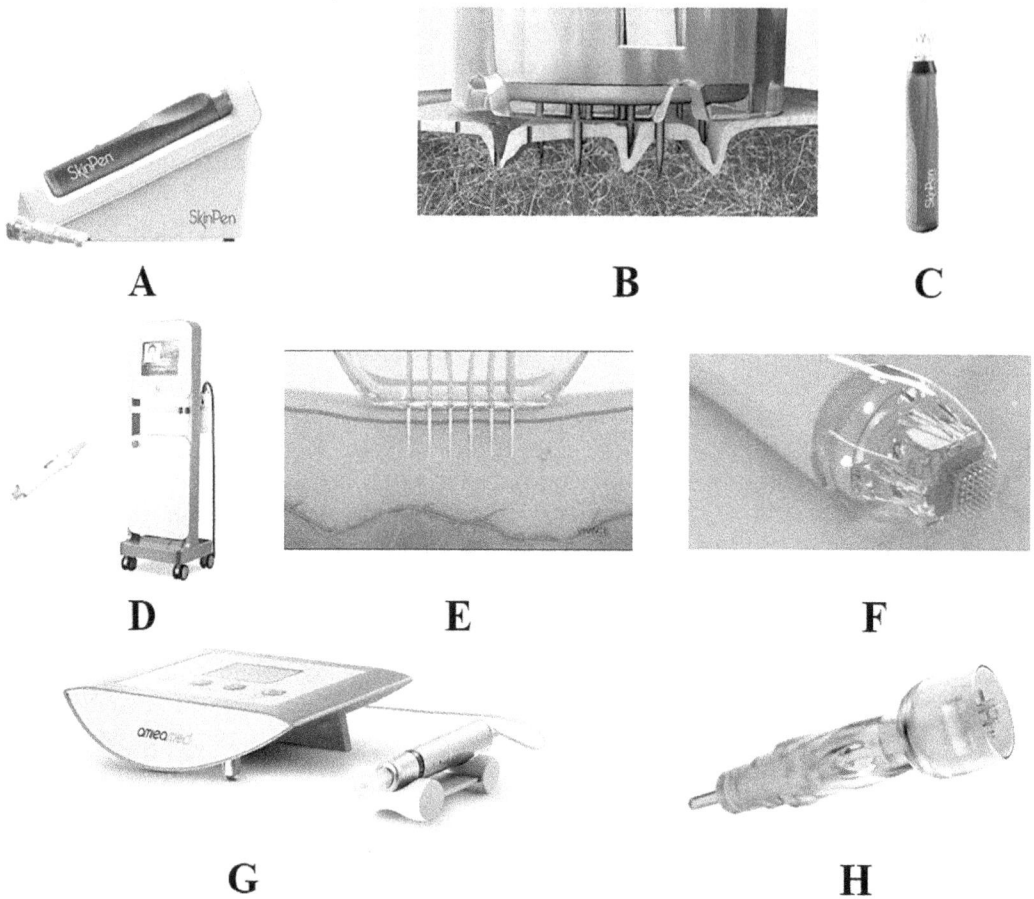

FIGURE 9.3
(A–C) SkinPen® microneedling device by Bellus Medical. (D–F) Vivace™ fractional radiofrequency microneedling system. (F and H) AMIEA MED EXCEED microneedling device by MT.DERM GmbH. Images reprinted with permission from respective sources.

during the treatment. Immediately after the treatment, the skin will seem somewhat pink to red, akin to a mild to moderate sunburn. This condition disappeared rapidly without further complications.

Vivace's microneedling device using the combination of microneedles and radiofrequency was granted FDA approval in January 2016 (Fig. 9.3). This noninvasive procedure has been demonstrated to reduce the appearance of fine lines and wrinkles and tighten and tone the skin on the face, neck, hands, and body by stimulating the body's natural synthesis of collagen. As opposed to other products, Vivace is the only one to have a precise robotic motor that effectively eliminates pain. With Vivace, users may stimulate and tighten their skin down to its innermost layers with the use of microneedling and radiofrequency. Radiofrequency treatment is utilized to warm skin tissue and promote collagen formation in deep skin layers. The device also depends on the process of producing numerous microchannels in the face tissues to stimulate collagen and cellular regeneration. Vivace microneedling device is effective for minimizing the appearance of acne scars on any skin type, and it may be applied on almost any part of the face or body. Vivace works by applying the portable device over the target region of the skin, which then releases the radiofrequency energy. The handpiece has a multi-needles head that may be adjusted to a specific depth for optimal results with the individual user. These microneedles cause microscopic "injuries" to the skin, which in turn trigger the body's natural synthesis of skin-tightening hyaluronic acid and elastin. The ultimate outcome is healthier, more flexible, and more youthful skin.

The FDA approved the first automated microneedling medical device (Exceed, made by MT.DERM GmbH in Berlin, Germany) to treat facial wrinkles and reduce acne scars. Minimally invasive percutaneous collagen induction (PCI) is achieved by microneedling with the AMIEA MED EXCEED to treat face wrinkles and acne scars (Fig. 9.3). In clinical research, the Exceed microneedling device was utilized to rejuvenate the face skin of 48 individuals showing symptoms of facial skin aging, and its effectiveness and safety were assessed. Participants were evaluated for changes in wrinkle extent, skin laxity, and texture after four microneedling treatments spaced 30 days apart. Individuals in the research showed statistically and clinically significant improvements in face wrinkles, skin texture, and laxity 60 days after the completion of the treatment sequence (day 90) [52]. The EXCEED premium needle cartridge provides superior safety and aesthetic outcomes owing to its innovative safety membrane and six-needle tilting plate for robust and accurate skin treatment at 900 perforations per second. Because of the needle plate's ability to tilt, it may be positioned at any angle on the skin's surface, allowing for perpendicular needle insertion, circular therapy for speedier, more efficient treatment, and no drooping of the skin's surface. The presence of the safety membrane dramatically reduces the possibility of liquid contamination in the handpiece. In addition to its scientifically verified efficiency and minimal risk of post-inflammatory hyperpigmentation, this device also boasts excellent accuracy and penetration force, a short recovery period, scarless healing, reduced pain for the users, and no ablation of the epidermis.

One of the most widely utilized solid metal microneedles in the cosmeceutical industry is the DermaRoller® (Dermaroller®, Deutsch-land GmbH, Wolfenbuttel, Germany), a device that has been approved by the FDA and has been on the field for many years. The early concept layout for microneedling was devised by Fernandes and is now commercially available under the trademark Dermaroller®. The Dermaroller® and MTS Roller™ [53] are the two most popular microneedling devices on the market for cosmetic applications. Microneedles are arranged on a rotating concentric head of this gadget. The FDA-approved derma roller is a handheld device with a cylindrical roller and medical-grade, solid stainless steel microneedles that protrude from the roller [54]. This device is used by rolling it directly over the skin in vertical, horizontal, and diagonal directions. Dermarollers® may be used in both at-home care and in-office clinical treatments.

Currently, the FDA has approved five different types of Dermarollers®, each with a different needle length: Dermaroller C-8, Dermaroller C-8HE, Dermaroller CIT 8, Dermaroller MF-8, and Dermaroller MS-4 [55]. Dermarollers® for at-home use comprise the C-8 and C-8HE models. The needle lengths of C-8 and C-8HE devices range from 130 μm to 200 μm, and their penetration diameter is about 70 μm [55]. DermaRoller® C8, a reusable home care product, has 192 microneedles measuring 0.2 mm in length on a cylindrical roller to aid skin rejuvenation. The C-8HE model, with its 0.2 mm needle length, is excellent for use on hairy areas like the scalp [55]. Because of its shorter needles, the home device is more convenient and favorable and provides a pleasant experience without the need for local anesthesia [44]. A medical type of DermaRoller® with microneedles of 0.3–1.5 mm in length is presently available for collagen induction therapy in clinical settings. To ensure proper operation, the CIT-8, MF-8, and MS-4 medical devices are restricted to qualified medical personnel only. The MF-8 model has needle lengths up to 1,500 μm [30], while the derma roller CIT 8 has 192 microneedles that are 0.5 mm in length and 0.2 mm in diameter [44]. With its compact cylinder, four circular arrays of 24 needles (for a total of 96 needles), and the ability to use needles up to 1,500 μm in length, the MS-4 model is the only Dermaroller® of its kind. Acne scars on the face are an excellent example of a location where its usage is warranted [55]. The deeper skin penetration of Dermaroller MF-8 and MS-4 models made it possible to treat deep scars, wrinkles, and lines [55]. The length of the needles used in any given treatment modality is determined by the requirement of that treatment [56]. Needle lengths of 1,500–2,000 μm are often used, for instance, for addressing acne and other types of scarring. Needles with a length of 500–1,000 μm are often suggested for use in microneedling procedures intended to address wrinkled and aged skin [55]. Acne scars, burns, cellulite, lost hair, hyperpigmentation, melasma, and aging skin may all be treated using Dermaroller® microneedling for cosmetic applications [6].

Microneedling is a rapidly expanding industry. Over the last 15 years, several improvements have been made to the original Dermaroller® that Fernandes invented. Since the first Dermaroller® was released, several upgrades and changes have been developed as the therapeutic application of microneedling has expanded beyond scar therapy. The present Dermaroller® market is increasing rapidly, with many manufacturers releasing a wide range of Dermaroller® models with varying needle lengths and drum dimensions. Companies like Hansderma, White Lotus, Royal Derma Roller, bioGenesis London, and MTS Roller are just a few examples. Microneedles on Hansderma's Genosys® rollers are 25% smaller in diameter than those of competing manufacturers, and there are 450 of them on each device. In addition, the heads of their Dermarollers® are designed to be removable so that the device handles may be reused several times. End users with metal allergies may now use the Dermaroller® (or Lotus Roller), manufactured by White Lotus, since it is built from a biocompatible polymer. Titanium alloy microneedles are used in the production of Royal Derma Rollers' Dermaroller® products. BioGenesis London manufactures the DNS® Classic 3- and 8-Line Roller. Numerous Dermaroller® models, such as Dr. Roller, MT Roller, MRS Roller, Body Roller, Elimiscar Roller, and ZGTS Titanium Derma Roller, are produced by MTS Roller. Designs for the handles and rollers of these models vary significantly. For instance, the Body Roller's larger roller head (total of 1,080 titanium needles) is designed to treat broader skin regions, such as the chest, back, buttocks, thighs, and arms.

There are some drawbacks to using a derma roller, even though they are simple to operate and can even be used at home. For example, mastering the level of pressure required to roll the device effectively takes time and practice; furthermore, treating small skin regions or localized scars is challenging because the roller also damages adjacent skin [57]. Cosmetic derma rollers create numerous microchannels in the skin after being rolled over, which increases the permeation of active compounds [58]. This procedure is two-step since the cosmetic cream is used after the microneedle treatment. Furthermore, the majority of the active cosmeceuticals are still retained on the skin surface. There is still a demand for innovative technologies to enhance the permeability of active agents further while minimizing loss, although this microneedling method improves the treatment efficacy of conventional topical products [13].

The "Beauty Mouse®" is a cosmetic roller device similar to the Derma roller. It was designed to guarantee the covering of wider skin areas at various body locations, such as the arms, legs, and buttocks, for treating stomach or thigh stretch marks and cellulite [59, 60]. This gadget is constructed like a computer mouse and has three distinct Dermaroller® heads, each containing 480 microneedles of 200 μm length. When increased collagen fiber production, microcirculation, or improved delivery of active molecules into deeper skin layers is expected, the device is preferred since it covers a wider skin area and short-ens treatment duration. The Beauty Mouse® is a medically approved microneedling device designed for use in the convenience of one's own home, just like the Dermaroller® device. Furthermore, it is included in the Australian Register of Therapeutic Products. Scalproller®, a commercially available alternative to the Derma roller, is indicated for increasing the effectiveness of topical therapies for baldness (i.e., minoxidil) and stimulating new hair growth by increasing blood flow to the scalp.

A miniaturized version of derma roller, known as Dermastamps™, represents a sig-nificant advancement in percutaneous collagen induction technology. These are portable medical needles with a 5-mm diameter circular arrangement and a needle length of 200 µm [55]. They are designed to fit in confined, congested spaces that a regular derma roller would have difficulty reaching. This device that employs "vertical penetration to form infusion channels" in the skin is suitable for usage on isolated scars and wrinkles. The very same company that brought customers the Dermaroller® has also produced a newer, more effective device termed the eDermastamp®. These needles are of medical grade stainless steel and measure a maximum of 1,500 µm in length; the device is an electroni-cally driven stamping mechanism with a circular arrangement of the needles. Because of its complexity, the developers of this product insist that it be used only by licensed medical professionals at clinical facilities.

The Dermapen®, a state-of-the-art microneedling device, was released to address the problems caused by the disparity between the pressure applied by healthcare providers or users and the resulting microneedle penetration depth. The Dermapen's stainless steel microneedles may be set between 0.25 and 2.5 mm in length by simply rotating an adjust-ment ring and stamped into the skin through a spring-loaded mechanism. According to the manufacturer, the device performs the function of "fractional mechanical resurfacing." Ergonomically speaking, this gadget is a spring-loaded, oscillating microneedling device made of an electric hand piece and a sterile, single-use needle cartridge. A vibrating stamp-resembling, vertical movement is applied to the skin using an electrically driven, automated pen to create numerous microchannels [61]. It has been reported that its "auto-matic stamping" skin microneedling function may be used at either fast or low speeds (Arora & Gupta, 2012). The Dermapen, with its sleek, user-friendly design, has penetrated the cosmetics industry. The manufacturers are looking into using this device as a treat-ment for acne scars, burn scars, and the effects of photoaging on the skin. Using Dermapen microneedling device, the skin is subjected to a more uniform level of pressure, and the chance of the needles tips' fracturing in the skin is reduced compared to when using a derma roller [46, 55]. The Dermapen is currently utilized only in medical settings and is not available for retail purchase for home use [14].

There has been a lot of interest in these microneedling devices; thus, additional commer-cial products based on the same ideas are being developed presently [56, 59]. The newest and most sophisticated model of the Dermapen® series, Dermapen 3™, was released by AOVNTM technologies. Its major improvement over previous versions of the Dermapen® is its ability to quickly puncture the skin, producing more than 1,300 microchannels per second. According to the company behind the Dermapen®, this version is superior to its predecessors because it is stronger, easier to use, and more capable of meeting the demands of clinical usage. The Dermapen 3™ gadget comes in two different versions: the Dermapen 3MD™ and the Dermapen 3PRO™. The Dermapen 3MD™ and Dermapen 3PRO™ are only meant for usage in medical clinics and by trained professionals. The Dermapen 3MD™ model (with a penetration depth of up to 2,500 µm) is best suited for more intensive skin remodeling therapies like scars, while the Dermapen 3PRO™ (with a penetration depth of up to 1,000 μm) may be used to treat superficial skin issues like fine lines, pigmentation, and enlarged pores [62]. MDerma™ FDS is an upgraded version of the original Dermapen® that incorporates the proprietary microneedles tip technology, SurSpace™. With its innovative 12-needle tip configuration, it generates a powerful pressure effect. The scalloped edge and two opposing vents on the needle cartridge work together to avoid suction and contamination. Furthermore, a modified elastomeric spring and an upgraded motor enhance the needles' oscillating performance, allowing for greater power and efficiency. Based on Clinical Resolution Lab, Inc.'s proprietary INNO™ Technology, the INNOPen™ is designed as a Dermapen®-alternative microneedling device with a detachable needle cartridge (the INNOTip™). As opposed to single-walled open-tip cartridges used by competing microneedle devices, the INNOTip™ has a patented double-protective, sealed tip system constructed of sterile, medical-grade polycarbonate resin. The first protective wall of the INNOTip™, which consists of 13 stainless steel microneedles, stabilizes the device at any speed, preventing the needle housing from swaying and going off-center owing to vibrations from the device's motor. Moreover, it provides better safety by guaranteeing a uniformly vertical arrangement of needles, which eliminates the risk of needle trauma and damage due to slanted needle application. The system is completely enclosed, with just the 13 apertures visible through the second exterior protective covering. Therefore, all 13 needles must fit through these minuscule openings prior to penetrating the skin. Precise needle penetration and patient safety are guaranteed by its outer safety covering's ability to identify needle deformation or misalignment. The dual-spring design is an additional innovation of the INNOTip™ that puts the users in control of the needle's movement. Both the INNOPen MD™ and INNOPen PRO™ models are commercially available for purchase. The INNOPen MD is designed for doctors, while the INNOPen PRO™ is intended for clinic usage. The INNOPen MD™, like the Dermapen 3™ versions, can penetrate as deeply as 2,500 μm, making it suitable for treating deep wrinkles and atrophic scars. The INNOPen PRO™ may be used to treat aging skin, hyperpigmentation, and other skin disorders, owing to its maximum needle length of 1,000 μm [62].

For scar-free postoperative healing, physicians employ the Revive™ HAP clinical microneedling device from AMIEA MED (Berlin, Germany). The Revive HAP's microneedles are battery-powered and can be adjusted in length from 0 mm to 2 mm; they can penetrate the skin at a rate of "50–150 hits/s," comparable to that of the Dermapen. The Revive HAP topical serum works best on the skin post-treatment since it contains skin-repairing cosmeceuticals such as hyaluronic acid, peptides, amino acids, minerals, and vitamins. Postoperative restorative dermatological operations are the primary use for Revive HAP, which is not sold commercially.

9.3 Applications of Microneedles in Skin Care

Microneedling has gained popularity in the cosmetics industry as a means of treating a wide range of skin issues, including seborrheic keratosis [63], scars [64], striae, acne, depigmentation [6], hyperpigmentation (melasma, post-acne scarring), collagen induction therapy, and photodamaged skin (wrinkles, age spots, and sun damage). Microneedling devices for cosmetic use often combine the administration of cosmeceuticals with the stimulation of the skin's underlying structural layers to promote healing. Skin-tightening (required after weight loss or aging), skin resurfacing, and scar therapy are some methods that do not require cosmeceutical administration [14].

Wrinkles are an inevitable consequence of getting aged with time. Wrinkles are exacerbated by several other conditions, such as stress, pollution, cigarette use, and extended exposure to sunlight (ultraviolet light) [65]. Skin microneedling is a painless and effective alternative to ablative or surgical facial rejuvenation treatments. Wrinkles around the eyes, mouth, cheeks, neck, and chest may all be smoothed out with skin needling. The backs of the hands and arms, among other places, are amenable to this kind of treatment [66]. Ascorbic acid, an antioxidant often used as an antiaging and anti-wrinkle agent in cosmetics, may be effectively administered using microneedles since they can penetrate the skin's barrier while entering deeper dermis layers with the aid of microneedles treatment. It has been observed that derma roller microneedle mesotherapy may increase L-ascorbic acid delivery, resulting in improved skin hydration, tone, and elasticity [67]. Dissolving microneedles encapsulated with ascorbic acid and composed of a biodegradable polymer may be applied in a single-step procedure and dissolve in the skin's interstitial fluid to release the active ingredient. The effects of ascorbic acid-loaded dissolving microneedle arrays on wrinkles around the eyes were studied by Lee C. and colleagues in research with 23 participants. After 12 weeks, the Global Photodamage Score and visiometer R-values improved in the microneedles intervention group, suggesting a lower wrinkle severity score [68]. It has been demonstrated that adenosine inhibits calcium-induced cellular contractions and helps reduce wrinkles around the eyes [69]. Kang and associates conducted a study to determine whether dissolving microneedle arrays with 49 adenosine microneedles per patch is more effective than topical cream administration [28]. With a lower dose of adenosine and less frequent application, the microneedle group showed a comparable but longer-lasting wrinkle reduction effect, increased hydration effect, enhanced dermal density, and improved skin elasticity on periorbital wrinkles. Microneedles have been shown to increase the absorption of cosmeceutical compounds, as shown by research using botulinum toxin type A [70]. An innovative pocketed stainless steel microneedles device has been revealed to expedite the delivery of botulinum toxin A (BoTox®), used in the treatment of wrinkles. Compared with the number of intradermal injections that would have been needed when using a standard hypodermic needle, the number of treatments required when using the microneedle device was markedly lower [70]. The application of microneedles in antiaging skin treatments is also a growing trend. An innovative antiaging therapy is the use of growth factors. Stem cells contain a wide variety of growth factors and cytokines. Seo et al. investigated the efficacy and safety of the noninvasive technique of microneedle fractional radiofrequency for skin rejuvenation. Microneedle fractional radiofrequency, as they observed, is safe and effective for skin rejuvenation, and it yields even greater outcomes when used in tandem with stem cells [71]. There is no concern for depigmentation with percutaneous collagen treatments, which allow for the rejuvenation and restoration of the skin's appearance. Moreover, several active antiaging compounds might be incorporated into dissolving microneedle patches. Due to their ease of use, safety, and success in reducing wrinkles, these microneedle patches have found widespread use in the cosmetics industry [13].

Melanin prevents sunlight-exposed damage by acting as an antioxidant, free radical scavenger, and broadband UV absorber. Nevertheless, melasma, lentigines, and freckles all are forms of skin hyperpigmentation issues caused by the overproduction of melanin, and they may lead to aesthetic issues that, in turn, lead to poor self-esteem and psychological frustration [72]. Melasma is a prevalent form of acquired symmetrical hypermelanosis, manifesting as macules and patches ranging in color from light to dark brown and appearing almost exclusively in parts of the skin that are often exposed to sunlight. When tranexamic acid is injected intradermally or used topically, the severity of melasma is reduced. Machekposhti and colleagues developed dissolving microneedles made of polyvinylpyrrolidone (PVP) and methacrylic acid to deliver tranexamic acid. These microneedles possessed the proper attributes to penetrate the skin and to release in the encapsulated tranexamic acid, suggesting they may be used as an alternative method of treating melasma [73]. Seborrheic keratosis and senile lentigo are prominent forms of pigmentation that are frequently observed in adults over the age of 50 and respond well to treatment with all-trans retinoic acid (ATRA). To improve the skin permeability of ATRA, Sachiko and coworkers created a dissolving microneedle patch filled with the drug. ATRA-loaded microneedles were used to treat the lesion areas of all subjects. There were no notable adverse effects, either locally or systemically, associated with the use of microneedles. Microneedle therapy shows excellent potential as a safe and effective treatment for seborrheic keratosis and senile lentigo [74]. The skin depigmentation-treated substances such as hydroquinone, arbutin, kojic acid, and 4-n-butyl resorcinol may be delivered directly to the melanocytes, where the enzyme tyrosinase is housed, by incorporating them into dissolving microneedles. In particular, significant depigmentation effectiveness was observed in an eight-week randomized, double-blind, placebo-controlled investigation using 4-n-butyl resorcinol-loaded dissolving microneedles [75]. It was shown that the patch containing the active ingredient was twice as effective as the placebo patch. In sensitization testing, the dissolving microneedle patch only caused minor skin irritation and no allergic responses. Since this is such a novel method of skin depigmentation treatment, it stands to reason those studies examining the efficiency of various skin-lightening agents administered using dissolving microneedle patches will proliferate in the not-too-distant future.

Furthermore, it has been found that hypertrophic scars might be less noticeable after treatment with microneedling. Scar tissue has a reorganized network of collagen fibers that may be prompted by microneedles [64]. The lower cost of microneedles is a significant benefit compared to laser therapy. In addition, microneedling is a safe and effective treatment that may be employed in skin areas where a laser simply cannot [76]. Scarring from acne occurs when the dermal follicular wall is damaged due to inflammation. There are three primary forms of acne scars: atrophic, hypertrophic, and keloidal [77]. Chemical peels, dermabrasion/microdermabrasion, laser therapy, punch methods, dermal grafting, silicone gels, cryotherapy, and surgery are some of the current therapies for acne scars [77]. Acne scars are also treatable with a microneedle derma roller [78, 79]. The microinjuries induced by the microneedles promote the production of new collagen and elastin in the dermis and the destruction of damaged collagen in the scars [78, 80]. Acne scarring has been addressed with skin microneedling since it is a simple and inexpensive method [54, 64]. Acne scars may also be treated with microneedle radiofrequency. Mechanical disruption of the dermal fibrotic strands (the cause of skin retraction in an atrophic scar) is generated by microneedles treatment [81]. This is followed by the delivery of radiofrequency energy to stimulate collagen remodeling, which ultimately leads to the synthesis of new collagen fibers to replace the damaged fibrous tissue. Acne scarring is not the only skin issue that may receive benefits from this treatment; patients could also see reductions in roughness, dermal density, wrinkles, skin laxity, and pigmentation [82]. Alopecia areata, a chronic autoimmune disorder damaging hair follicles, has been treated using microneedles. Delivering corticosteroids with microneedles is a noninvasive alternative for treating significant areas of hair loss. In addition, they enhance microcirculation to the scalp, which supports hair follicles. Furthermore, it has been hypothesized that the microinjury produced by microneedles aids in recruiting and activating growth factors [83].

Excessive hair growth in a masculine pattern in women is known as hirsutism [84]. Lifestyle changes like dieting and exercise, hair removal techniques like shaving, waxing, electrolysis, laser, and photoepilation, and medications like topical eflornithine cream, oral contraceptive pills, spironolactone, cyproterone acetate, and finasteride are the standard methods of treating hirsutism [84, 85]. The FDA has approved eflornithine, a topical therapy for hirsutism, as safe and effective [86]. Eflornithine is only recommended as a monotherapy for moderate conditions; however, in severe cases, the drug is frequently used as an auxiliary to other treatments [87]. According to a 2014 research on a mouse model, using a microneedle roller in combination with applying eflornithine cream topically to prevent hair growth was more effective than using only eflornithine cream [86]. The *in vivo* efficiency of eflornithine cream at suppressing hair growth after skin pretreatment with microneedles was examined in a mouse study [86]. The researchers concluded that this strategy provides a potentially effective way to improve eflornithine's capacity to control hair growth in patients with face hirsutism. On the other hand, microneedles have also been combined with topically applied drugs, like minoxidil, to promote hair growth. Research in 2013 assessed the effects of topical minoxidil therapy and physical microneedling on human volunteers with androgenetic alopecia. The derma roller and the minoxidil-applied group was shown to have substantially greater hair growth than minoxidil alone, as demonstrated by three key efficacy outcomes of hair count and patient/investigator evaluation [43].

9.4 Case Studies

Recent years have seen a plethora of promising research published on the topic of using microneedle technology to improve the efficiency with which cosmeceuticals can be administered into the skin. Minimally invasive microneedles treatment can enhance the permeation of topically applied products containing the cosmeceutical active(s) and stimulate percutaneous collagen induction for dermal rejuvenation. In a research performed by Sharad et al., the authors found that using the derma roller MF8 to treat atrophic box and rolling acne scars with post-inflammatory hyperpigmentation was successful when combined with a glycolic acid peel [88].

Related to this field is current research on microneedles-based intradermal delivery of cosmetic peptides. The skin does not readily absorb protein-based molecules because of their high molecular weights and hydrophilicity [89]. It is potential that microneedles, which have been found to improve skin permeability significantly, might be an efficient method for increasing peptide delivery. Melanostatin, rigin, and pal-KTTKS are three examples of cosmetic peptides. Specifically, pal-KTTKS has been reported to enhance collagen formation when injected into the skin dermis. Recently, the efficiency of microneedles on the skin permeation of these peptides was compared to the passive diffusion of the same peptides. After being pretreated with solid stainless steel microneedles, the skin was applied with the peptides; the smallest peptide, melanostatin, could penetrate more effectively into the skin. Nevertheless, this tendency did not hold true for peptides with larger molecular weights [90].

Park and colleagues evaluate the effectiveness and safety of a novel hyaluronic acid microneedle patch for skin whitening. Thirty-four Korean women participated in a split-face trial to assess the product's efficacy on one cheek while the other cheeks received a control whitening essence. Consequently, after eight-week therapy, there were noticeable changes between the whitening microneedles patch and whitening essence groups. Compared to the topically applied formulation, the microneedles patch performed better in brightness enhancement. It is reported that the microneedle patch with whitening ingredients enhanced skin tone and pigmentation more efficiently than a topical formulation with the same active components. Subjects' evaluations of the aesthetic effects of the whitening patches and essence revealed moderate improvement. There were no reports of side effects or skin irritation (such as itching, stinging, erythema, or edema) [91].

Dermapen was utilized by Amer et al. to alleviate face wrinkles caused by smoking and skin aging. Dermapen has the benefit of being a low-cost, in-office therapy that carries a low risk of major depigmentation or complications. All individuals in the aging group exhibited statistically marked improvements in skin texture and firmness. All patients presented improvement, and the only adverse effects were temporary redness and swelling that went away after two to three days [66]. To further clarify, consider what happens when a needle punctures the skin: small blood vessels are ruptured, resulting in localized microinjuries and perhaps moderate bleeding. Needling treatment stimulates keratinocyte proliferation and growth factor release, which activates fibroblasts to deposit collagen. A number of genes involved in extracellular matrix remodeling (including vascular endothelial growth factor, fibroblast growth factor, epidermal growth factor, and collagen types I and III) are altered in expression after microneedling treatment. [6]. Microneedling also causes fibroblast development, enhanced collagen arrangement, increased deposition of fibronectin and extracellular matrix, epithelium regrowth, and angiogenesis. The skin tightens and regains its elasticity as collagen grows and repairs. Since the skin's structure is being repaired, the skin will look more attractive. Six months following a microneedling treatment, there is conclusive evidence of an increase in collagen and elastin fibers [92].

To reduce the appearance of fine lines and wrinkles, Kim and colleagues designed two innovative cosmetic dissolving microneedle patches: one containing retinyl retinoate and the other containing ascorbic acid. Clinical trials using these cosmetic microneedle patches demonstrated that the skin effectively absorbed retinyl retinoate and ascorbic acid. These microneedle patches were shown to be efficient in reducing wrinkles and were found to be safe in the research. After 6 h, all of the microneedles had dissolved. Considerable differences were reported in all visiometer R-values for retinyl retinoate and ascorbic acid–loaded microneedle patches. Notably, there were substantial differences in skin roughness (R1) and arithmetic average roughness (R5). These patches were considered safe for cosmetic use since they did not cause severe adverse reactions. No allergic or irritating contact dermatitis cases were seen in any individuals. Because of their convenience, safety, and efficacy in reducing wrinkles for patients, these novel microneedles patches have a promising future in the cosmetics industry [13].

Kang and colleagues employed an adenosine-loaded dissolving microneedle patch in conjunction with an adenosine-loaded topical cream to increase the penetration of the encapsulated active agent into the dermal layer. Channels in the skin were generated by the insertion of microneedles, allowing the encapsulated agent to be administered from the microneedles and the cream. Applying the cream formulation shortly after removing the microneedles patch would enable efficient transport of adenosine in the cream formulation through microneedles-created channels. A randomized clinical experiment on humans found that after eight weeks of use, the wrinkles, dermal density, elasticity, and moisture in the crow's feet area were significantly better with the combination treatment than with the cream alone. The longer duration of action seen with the combination suggests a higher concentration of adenosine penetrated the skin and was maintained under the skin, even after treatment was completed and left alone for two weeks. Wrinkle and dermal density photographs showed that a higher quantity of adenosine, responsible for the rapid disappearance of wrinkles and the enhancement in dermal density, could be delivered by the combinatorial application. Furthermore, no major subjective or objective adverse effects, such as irritation or allergic response, were detected; hence this combinatorial application is believed to be safe for human usage [51]. In another study by Kim et al., to circumvent the limited quantity of drugs loaded in dissolving microneedles, a skin-depigmenting agent (4-*n*-butyl resorcinol) was given topically in the form of a serum, followed by the insertion of a dissolving microneedles patch, in a stepwise order. Since the liquid formulation of topical serum dissolved these microneedles before penetrating the skin, the best interval to avoid microneedles dissolution was examined to ensure efficient drug delivery. The application of topical formulation combined with dissolving microneedles was more effective than either serum or microneedles alone [93].

One intriguing *in vitro* research investigated the intradermal delivery of epigallocatechin-3-gallate (EGCG) using maltose microneedles to improve skin texture. Compared to untreated skin, skin that had been pierced by microneedles demonstrated significantly improved transport of EGCG from both aqueous solution and hydrogel to the epidermis and dermis layers. Because of its lipophilicity offered by the gallate group and strong binding affinity to skin tissues, especially the collagen network, EGCG was observed to accumulate in the dermis, despite its high aqueous solubility and, therefore, capacity to diffuse through the aqueous microchannels. Accordingly, this investigation proved that solid maltose microneedles assisted EGCG in penetrating the skin's stratum corneum and into the dermis [94].

Fifty-five women with facial hyperpigmentation participated in research examining microneedles-based therapy for skin depigmentation. In this trial, individuals' faces were treated with dissolving microneedles made of hyaluronic acid and carrying the depigmentation chemical 4-*n*-butyl resorcinol either every four days or every three days for eight weeks. On the opposite side of the face, both groups of subjects wore an unloaded microneedles patch (4-*n*-butyl resorcinol-free, control). In this experiment, the innovative dissolving microneedles patch was twice as effective as the control patch in administering 4-*n*-butyl resorcinol, with no serious adverse events and minimal skin irritation. Due to its practicality, safety, and effectiveness, the researchers determined that this unique dissolving microneedle patch may be manufactured by integrating various depigmentation and antiaging chemicals [75].

9.5 Conclusion

Since the first discussion on microneedles appeared in the literature in 1998, there has been extensive study into their potential applications. The field is still expanding and improving as better materials, production techniques, and needle designs become available [95]. The use of microneedles to deliver cosmeceutical compounds is one area where steady study and progress have been made. Multiple microneedle technologies have found use in the field of cosmetics, such as the Dermaroller®, Beauty Mouse®, Dermastamp™, and Dermapen®, with more on the horizon. However, as the field moves toward further commercialization of microneedle devices, it is clear that involvement with regulatory agencies is critical to identify concerns about the microneedles aseptic manufacturing process and prevent misuse of such devices, as highlighted in the safety and public perception studies. All those experiencing unattractive burns and scars and the majority of the public who seek to retain a youthful look should take heart from the findings offered by producers of microneedle devices for cosmetic applications. Microneedles have a promising future in this field, and it is reasonable to imagine a new generation of these devices containing various active chemicals designed to enhance the skin's appearance. Nevertheless, this may call for a higher standard of regulatory approval, not often expected for skincare products, driving up the associated costs.

References

[1] Schagen SK, Zampeli VA, Makrantonaki E, et al. Discovering the link between nutrition and skin aging. Dermatoendocrinol. 2012;4:298–307.

[2] El-Domyati M, Medhat W. Minimally invasive facial rejuvenation: current concepts and future expectations. Expert Rev Dermatol. 2013;8:565–580.

[3] Han TY, Park KY, Ahn JY, et al. Facial skin barrier function recovery after microneedle transdermal delivery treatment. Dermatol Surg. 2012;38:1816–1822.

[4] Liu L, Ma H, Li Y. Interventions for the treatment of stretch marks: a systematic review. Cutis. 2014;94:66–72.

[5] Harvey A, Huynh TT. Inflammation and acne: putting the pieces together. J Drugs Dermatol JDD. 2014;13:459–463.

[6] Majid I. Microneedling therapy in atrophic facial scars: an objective assessment. J Cutan Aesthetic Surg. 2009;2:26.

[7] Wiechers JW. Skin barrier: chemistry of skin delivery systems. Carol Stream, Illinois: Allured Publishing Corporation; 2008.

[8] Bhatnagar S, Dave K, Venuganti VVK. Microneedles in the clinic. J Control Release. 2017;260:164–182.

[9] Donnelly RF, Raj Singh TR, Woolfson AD. Microneedle-based drug delivery systems: microfabrication, drug delivery, and safety. Drug Deliv. 2010;17:187–207.

[10] Baumann LS, Baumann L. Cosmetic dermatology. New York: McGraw-Hill Professional Publishing; 2009.

[11] Banga AK. Transdermal and intradermal delivery of therapeutic agents: application of physical technologies. Florida: CRC Press; 2011.

[12] Humbert P, Viennet C, Legagneux K, et al. In the shadow of the wrinkle: theories. J Cosmet Dermatol. 2012;11:72–78.

[13] Kim M, Yang H, Kim H, et al. Novel cosmetic patches for wrinkle improvement: retinyl retinoate- and ascorbic acid-loaded dissolving microneedles. Int J Cosmet Sci. 2014;36:207–212.

[14] Scott JA, Banga AK. Cosmetic devices based on active transdermal technologies. Ther Deliv. 2015;6:1089–1099.

[15] Loesch MM, Somani A-K, Kingsley MM, et al. Skin resurfacing procedures: new and emerging options. Clin Cosmet Investig Dermatol. 2014;7:231.

[16] Alster TS, Lupton JR. Prevention and treatment of side effects and complications of cutaneous laser resurfacing. Plast Reconstr Surg. 2002;109:308–316.

[17] Orentreich DS, Orentreich N. Subcutaneous incisionless (subcision) surgery for the correction of depressed scars and wrinkles. Dermatol Surg. 1995;21:543–549.

[18] Camirand A, Doucet J. Needle dermabrasion. Aesthetic Plast Surg. 1997;21:48–51.

[19] Fernandes D. Minimally invasive percutaneous collagen induction. Oral Maxillofac Surg Clin N Am. 2005;17:51–63, vi.

[20] Fernandes D. Percutaneous collagen induction: an alternative to laser resurfacing. Aesthet Surg J. 2002;22:307–309.

[21] Kim S-E, Lee J-H, Kwon HB, et al. Greater collagen deposition with the microneedle therapy system than with intense pulsed light. Dermatol Surg. 2011;37:336–341.

[22] Fernandes D, Signorini M. Combating photoaging with percutaneous collagen induction. Clin Dermatol. 2008;26:192–199.

[23] Majid I, Sheikh G, September PI. Microneedling and its applications in dermatology. Prime Int J Aesthetic Anti-Ageing Med Healthc. 2014;4:44–49.

[24] Draelos ZD. Cosmetic dermatology: products and procedures. Hoboken, New Jersey: John Wiley & Sons; 2022.

[25] Sachdeva VK, Banga A. Microneedles and their applications. Recent Pat Drug Deliv Formul. 2011;5:95–132.

[26] Soltani-Arabshahi R, Wong JW, Duffy KL, et al. Facial allergic granulomatous reaction and systemic hypersensitivity associated with microneedle therapy for skin rejuvenation. JAMA Dermatol. 2014;150:68–72.

[27] Lu W, Wu P, Zhang Z, et al. Curative effects of microneedle fractional radiofrequency system on skin laxity in Asian patients: a prospective, double-blind, randomized, controlled face-split study. J Cosmet Laser Ther. 2017;19:83–88.

[28] Kang G, Tu TNT, Kim S, et al. Adenosine-loaded dissolving microneedle patches to improve skin wrinkles, dermal density, elasticity and hydration. Int J Cosmet Sci. 2018;40:199–206.

[29] Tanaka Y. Long-term three-dimensional volumetric assessment of skin tightening using a sharply tapered non-insulated microneedle radiofrequency applicator with novel fractionated pulse mode in Asians. Lasers Surg Med. 2015;47:626–633.

[30] Badran MM, Kuntsche J, Fahr A. Skin penetration enhancement by a microneedle device (Dermaroller®) in vitro: dependency on needle size and applied formulation. Eur J Pharm Sci. 2009;36:511–523.

[31] Kalluri H, Kolli CS, Banga AK. Characterization of microchannels created by metal microneedles: formation and closure. AAPS J. 2011;13:473–481.

[32] Fabbrocini G, De Vita V, Monfrecola A, et al. Percutaneous collagen induction: an effective and safe treatment for post-acne scarring in different skin phototypes. J Dermatol Treat. 2014;25:147–152.

[33] Donnelly RF, Woolfson AD. Patient safety and beyond: what should we expect from microneedle arrays in the transdermal delivery arena? Ther Deliv. 2014;5:653–662.

[34] Birchall JC, Clemo R, Anstey A, et al. Microneedles in clinical practice–an exploratory study into the opinions of healthcare professionals and the public. Pharm Res. 2011;28:95–106.

[35] Donnelly RF, Moffatt K, Alkilani AZ, et al. Hydrogel-forming microneedle arrays can be effectively inserted in skin by self-application: a pilot study centred on pharmacist intervention and a patient information leaflet. Pharm Res. 2014;31:1989–1999.

[36] Vicente-Perez EM, Larrañeta E, McCrudden MT, et al. Repeat application of microneedles does not alter skin appearance or barrier function and causes no measurable disturbance of serum biomarkers of infection, inflammation or immunity in mice in vivo. Eur J Pharm Biopharm. 2017;117:400–407.

[37] Newburger AE. Cosmetic medical devices and their FDA regulation. Arch Dermatol. 2006;142:225–228.

[38] Gupta J, Park SS, Bondy B, et al. Infusion pressure and pain during microneedle injection into skin of human subjects. Biomaterials. 2011;32:6823–6831.

[39] Brogden NK, Milewski M, Ghosh P, et al. Diclofenac delays micropore closure following microneedle treatment in human subjects. J Control Release. 2012;163:220–229.

[40] Cachafeiro T, Escobar G, Maldonado G, et al. Comparison of nonablative fractional erbium laser 1,340 nm and microneedling for the treatment of atrophic acne scars: a randomized clinical trial. Dermatol Surg. 2016;42:232–241.

[41] Kim ST, Lee KH, Sim HJ, et al. Treatment of acne vulgaris with fractional radiofrequency microneedling. J Dermatol. 2014;41:586–591.

[42] Park JY, Lee EG, Yoon MS, et al. The efficacy and safety of combined microneedle fractional radiofrequency and sublative fractional radiofrequency for acne scars in Asian skin. J Cosmet Dermatol. 2016;15:102–107.

[43] Dhurat R, Sukesh M, Avhad G, et al. A randomized evaluator blinded study of effect of microneedling in androgenetic alopecia: a pilot study. Int J Trichology. 2013;5:6–11.

[44] Fabbrocini G, De Vita V, Fardella N, et al. Skin needling to enhance depigmenting serum penetration in the treatment of melasma. Plast Surg Int. 2011;2011:158241.

[45] Fabbrocini G, Marasca C, Ammad S, et al. Assessment of the combined efficacy of needling and the use of silicone gel in the treatment of C-section and other surgical hypertrophic scars and keloids. Adv Skin Wound Care. 2016;29:408–411.

[46] Park Y, Park J, Chu GS, et al. Transdermal delivery of cosmetic ingredients using dissolving polymer microneedle arrays. Biotechnol Bioprocess Eng. 2015;20:543–549.

[47] Oh J-H, Park H-H, Do K-Y, et al. Influence of the delivery systems using a microneedle array on the permeation of a hydrophilic molecule, calcein. Eur J Pharm Biopharm. 2008;69:1040–1045.

[48] Lee K, Lee CY, Jung H. Dissolving microneedles for transdermal drug administration prepared by stepwise controlled drawing of maltose. Biomaterials. 2011;32:3134–3140.

[49] Park J-H, Allen MG, Prausnitz MR. Biodegradable polymer microneedles: fabrication, mechanics and transdermal drug delivery. J Control Release. 2005;104:51–66.

[50] Shim WS, Hwang YM, Park SG, et al. Role of polyvinylpyrrolidone in dissolving microneedle for efficient transdermal drug delivery: in vitro and clinical studies. Bull Korean Chem Soc. 2018;39:789–793.

[51] Kang G, Kim S, Yang H, et al. Combinatorial application of dissolving microneedle patch and cream for improvement of skin wrinkles, dermal density, elasticity, and hydration. J Cosmet Dermatol. 2019;18:1083–1091.

[52] Ablon G. Safety and effectiveness of an automated microneedling device in improving the signs of aging skin. J Clin Aesthetic Dermatol. 2018;11:29.

[53] Baran R, Maibach H. Textbook of cosmetic dermatology. Florida: CRC Press; 2010.

[54] Harris AG, Naidoo C, Murrell DF. Skin needling as a treatment for acne scarring: an up-to-date review of the literature. Int J Womens Dermatol. 2015;1:77–81.

[55] Singh A, Yadav S. Microneedling: advances and widening horizons. Indian Dermatol Online J. 2016;7:244.

[56] Kim Y-C, Park J-H, Prausnitz MR. Microneedles for drug and vaccine delivery. Adv Drug Deliv Rev. 2012;64:1547–1568.

[57] Arora S, Gupta PB. Automated microneedling device-a new tool in dermatologist's kit-a review. J Pak Assoc Dermatol. 2012;22.

[58] Park J-H, Choi S-O, Seo S, et al. A microneedle roller for transdermal drug delivery. Eur J Pharm Biopharm. 2010;76:282–289.

[59] Donnelly RF, Singh TRR, Morrow DI, et al. Microneedle-mediated transdermal and intradermal drug delivery. New Jersey: John Wiley & Sons; 2012.

[60] McCrudden MTC, McAlister E, Courtenay AJ, et al. Microneedle applications in improving skin appearance. Exp Dermatol. 2015;24:561–566.

[61] Clementoni MT, B-Roscher M, Munavalli GS. Photodynamic photorejuvenation of the face with a combination of microneedling, red light, and broadband pulsed light. Lasers Surg Med. 2010;42:150–159.

[62] McAlister E, McCrudden MT, Donnelly RF. Microneedles in improving skin appearance and enhanced delivery of cosmeceuticals. Microneedles Drug Vaccine Deliv Patient Monit. 2018;1.

[63] Hiraishi Y, Hirobe S, Iioka H, et al. Development of a novel therapeutic approach using a retinoic acid-loaded microneedle patch for seborrheic keratosis treatment and safety study in humans. J Control Release. 2013;171:93–103.

[64] Kim SK, Park JM, Jang YH, et al. Management of hypertrophic scar after burn wound using microneedling procedure (dermastamp). Burns. 2009;S37.

[65] Chauhan P, Shakya M. Modeling signaling pathways leading to wrinkle formation: identification of the skin aging target. Indian J Dermatol Venereol Leprol. 2009;75.

[66] Amer M, Farag F, Amer A, et al. Dermapen in the treatment of wrinkles in cigarette smokers and skin aging effectively. J Cosmet Dermatol. 2018;17:1200–1204.

[67] Zasada M, Markiewicz A, Drożdż Z, et al. Preliminary randomized controlled trial of antiaging effects of l-ascorbic acid applied in combination with no-needle and microneedle mesotherapy. J Cosmet Dermatol. 2019;18:843–849.

[68] Lee C, Yang H, Kim S, et al. Evaluation of the anti-wrinkle effect of an ascorbic acid-loaded dissolving microneedle patch via a double-blind, placebo-controlled clinical study. Int J Cosmet Sci. 2016;38:375–381.

[69] Park J-H, Allen MG, Prausnitz MR. Polymer microneedles for controlled-release drug delivery. Pharm Res. 2006;23:1008–1019.

[70] Torrisi BM, Zarnitsyn V, Prausnitz MR, et al. Pocketed microneedles for rapid delivery of a liquid-state botulinum toxin A formulation into human skin. J Control Release. 2013;165:146–152.

[71] Seo KY, Yoon MS, Kim DH, et al. Skin rejuvenation by microneedle fractional radiofrequency treatment in Asian skin; Clinical and histological analysis. Lasers Surg Med. 2012;44:631–636.

[72] Brenner M, Hearing VJ. The protective role of melanin against UV damage in human skin. Photochem Photobiol. 2008;84:539–549.

[73] Machekposhti SA, Soltani M, Najafizadeh P, et al. Biocompatible polymer microneedle for topical/dermal delivery of tranexamic acid. J Control Release. 2017;261:87–92.

[74] Hirobe S, Otsuka R, Iioka H, et al. Clinical study of a retinoic acid-loaded microneedle patch for seborrheic keratosis or senile lentigo. Life Sci. [Internet] [cited 2016 Aug 13]. Available from: www.sciencedirect.com/science/article/pii/S0024320515301442.

[75] Kim S, Yang H, Kim M, et al. 4-n-butylresorcinol dissolving microneedle patch for skin depigmentation: a randomized, double-blind, placebo-controlled trial. J Cosmet Dermatol. 2016;15:16–23.

[76] Aust MC, Knobloch K, Reimers K, et al. Percutaneous collagen induction therapy: an alternative treatment for burn scars. Burns. 2010;36:836–843.

[77] Simmons BJ, Griffith RD, Falto-Aizpurua LA, et al. Use of radiofrequency in cosmetic dermatology: focus on nonablative treatment of acne scars. Clin Cosmet Investig Dermatol. 2014;7:335.

[78] Doddaballapur S, others. Microneedling with dermaroller. J Cutan Aesthetic Surg. 2009;2:110.

[79] Sunil D, Savita Y, Rishu S. Microneedling for acne scars in Asian skin type: an effective low cost treatment modality. J Cosmet Dermatol. 2014;13. [Internet] [cited 2022 Oct 11] Available from: https://pubmed.ncbi.nlm.nih.gov/25196684/.

[80] Chen M-C, Ling M-H, Kusuma SJ. Poly-γ-glutamic acid microneedles with a supporting structure design as a potential tool for transdermal delivery of insulin. Acta Biomater. 2015;24:106–116.

[81] Pudukadan D. Treatment of acne scars on darker skin types using a noninsulated smooth motion, electronically controlled radiofrequency microneedles treatment system. Dermatol Surg. 2017;43:S64–S69.

[82] Cho SI, Chung BY, Choi MG, et al. Evaluation of the clinical efficacy of fractional radiofrequency microneedle treatment in acne scars and large facial pores. Dermatol Surg. 2012;38:1017–1024.

[83] Chandrashekar BS, Yepuri V, Mysore V. Alopecia areata-successful outcome with microneedling and triamcinolone acetonide. J Cutan Aesthetic Surg. 2014;7:63.

[84] Kini S, Mahmood T. Hirsutism and virilism. EBCOG Postgrad Textb Obstet Gynaecol. Cambridge: Cambridge University Press; 2021.

[85] com AMW dtp@ adis. Identify underlying cause of hirsutism and individualize treatment as required. Drugs Ther Perspect. 2014;30:417–421.

[86] Kumar A, Naguib YW, Shi Y-C, et al. A method to improve the efficacy of topical eflornithine hydrochloride cream. Drug Deliv. 2016;23:1495–1501.

[87] Somani N, Turvy D. Hirsutism: an evidence-based treatment update. Am J Clin Dermatol. 2014;15:247–266.

[88] Sharad J. Combination of microneedling and glycolic acid peels for the treatment of acne scars in dark skin. J Cosmet Dermatol. 2011;10:317–323.

[89] Park B-S, Jang KA, Sung J-H, et al. Adipose-derived stem cells and their secretory factors as a promising therapy for skin aging. Dermatol Surg. 2008;34:1323–1326.

[90] Mohammed YH, Yamada M, Lin LL, et al. Microneedle enhanced delivery of cosmeceutically relevant peptides in human skin. PloS One. 2014;9:e101956.

[91] Park KY, Kwon HJ, Lee C, et al. Efficacy and safety of a new microneedle patch for skin brightening: a randomized, split-face, single-blind study. J Cosmet Dermatol. 2017;16:382–387.

[92] Zencker S. Skin rejuvenation with microneedling. Prime J. 2013;3:62–68.

[93] Kim S, Dangol M, Kang G, et al. Enhanced transdermal delivery by combined application of dissolving microneedle patch on serum-treated skin. Mol Pharm. 2017;14:2024–2031.

[94] Puri A, Nguyen HX, Banga AK. Microneedle-mediated intradermal delivery of epigallocatechin-3-gallate. Int J Cosmet Sci. 2016;38:512–523.

[95] Henry S, McAllister DV, Allen MG, et al. Microfabricated microneedles: a novel approach to transdermal drug delivery. J Pharm Sci. 1998;87:922–925.

10

Laboratory Techniques for Microneedle Research

10.1 Introduction

Microneedles have been extensively recognized as a preferable delivery method for the transdermal administration of a broad range of therapeutic agents. Given its versatility and wide range of applications, microneedles technology has recently attracted a lot of attention in biomedical research and drug delivery worldwide. Micrometer-sized needles could easily, noninvasively, and painlessly bypass the skin's primary barrier, the stratum corneum, and transport a variety of small and large molecules into the epidermis, dermis, and, eventually, into the systemic circulation. The majority of investigations into microneedles have been carried out in laboratories. These studies include *in vitro* experiments on various skin models and *in vivo* studies on animal subjects. The relevance of microneedles research is affected by several factors, such as different microneedle materials, varying designs and geometries, different therapeutic agents to be delivered, experimental protocols, and various skin models [1].

10.2 Selection of Skin or Membranes

10.2.1 Introduction of Skin Models

Microneedle characterization using various human or animal skin models is crucial due to its clinical relevance. The microneedles must be effective for use on persons of varying ages, skin types, and ethnicities [2]. Microneedle performance has been investigated using a variety of skin models and membranes. Human cadaver skin, epidermal membrane from human breast skin, synthetic membranes, heat-separated epidermis, hairless rat skin, and dermatomed or full-thickness porcine skin are all employed as models for human skin [3–8]. For the *in vitro* assessment of microneedle-mediated transdermal drug delivery, there has been no widespread agreement on the preference for the skin model. Unfortunately, the mechanics of fresh skin in its natural conditions and microneedles-to-tissue interactions during microneedle insertions are poorly understood. Despite the many studies defining microneedle insertions into different kinds of skin [9–13], the difficulties of a wide variety in penetration pressures, efficient drug delivery, and nonreproducible results remain unaddressed.

Human skin is best suited for testing transdermal drug delivery, but its usage has been restricted by regulatory and ethical concerns [14]. Therefore, to simulate *in vivo*

DOI: 10.1201/9780429294433-10

studies on human skin, scientists often use skin samples taken from pigs and mice [15–17]. Research into transdermal drug delivery has often used pig skin as a surrogate for human skin due to its comparable histological and physiological attributes [18, 19]. The stratum corneum of a pig's back skin is 26 μm thick, but that of an ear skin is just 10 μm thick [20]. Epidermis thickness, dermal:epidermal layer ratio, hair follicle density, blood vessel density, and dermal collagen:elastin ratio is very similar between human and pig skins [14]. Microneedles are considered to be capable of entering into human skin if they can be effectively inserted into the skin of a pig's flank. However, if insertion studies are conducted on pig ear skin, which is substantially thinner than human skin, the equivalency is absent [21]. Similar problems arise when conducting insertion experiments on mouse skin with a thin stratum corneum layer of just 5 μm thickness [21].

Skin tissues with consistent mechanical characteristics for mechano-analysis are typically challenging to acquire. Therefore, artificial skin models are useful for addressing the difficulties and limitations of investigations using biological skins. Specifically, nonbiological polymeric membranes that can replicate the mechanical qualities of human skin are beneficial [22]. Many laboratories use artificial membranes in their hypodermic needle evaluation, and standardized bench tests have been created for this application [23]. Unfortunately, there is a lack of research on artificial membranes for the mechanical assessment of microneedle insertion [24]. In previously reported studies, several synthetic membranes and artificial films have been developed and used as an alternative skin model to evaluate the performance of microneedles (uniformity, penetration depth, and penetration efficiency) and study drug delivery from microneedles [24–28]. Various artificial skin models have been developed in recent years using soft materials such as polydimethylsiloxane, polyurethane, and hydrogels [24, 26, 28, 29]. It is critical to choose a skin model membrane that is representative of the skin barrier and can reproduce the *in vivo* results for drug release, microneedle penetration depth, microneedles adherence to the skin, and microneedles dissolution [26]. Compared to using animal or human skin, synthetic membranes have been shown to be advantageous owing to their wide availability and low cost, as well as the fact that they do not need sophisticated pretreatment or cumbersome transportation or storage conditions [30].

As a potential alternative to biological tissues, commercial polymeric films may be used as a model membrane to test microneedle insertion [29]. One such film is Parafilm® M, a combination of hydrocarbon wax and polyolefin. Compared to the artificial skin model, biological skin has several drawbacks, such as an expensive cost, a shortage of readily available fresh human skin tissues, a challenge in complying with its *in vivo* setup, and issues with handling safety [14]. Eight layers of parafilm have been employed in recent experiments to simulate skin and test the insertion capabilities of microneedles [31, 32]. Prior to testing on humans [17], mice [15, 16], or pig skin *ex vivo* [33], skin penetration tests using polymeric films are generally conducted. Paraffin wax and agarose gel are viable substitutes for animal skin models. Agarose gel, a carbohydrate polymer, is often used as a skin model because its mechanical characteristics may be tailored to mimic human skin. Also, since the material is transparent, the depth of microneedle penetration may be observed over time [34, 35]. Furthermore, gelatin gels and other polysaccharide-based gels are used to simulate human skin. Collagen extracted from animals is the typical source of gelatin [36]. Gelatin is employed as a substrate for a layer of PDMS (~10 μm thick) that mimics the stratum corneum layer of human skin. This method may be used to study drug release kinetics and needle penetration.

10.2.2 Case Studies of Skin Models

Topical and transdermal drug delivery has been studied *in vitro* and *in vivo* using a number of skin models (Fig. 10.1). To investigate how fluorescent nanoparticles pass through a synthetic membrane, Coulman and colleagues employed Isopore® polycarbonate track-etched membranes. The microchannels in these membranes are

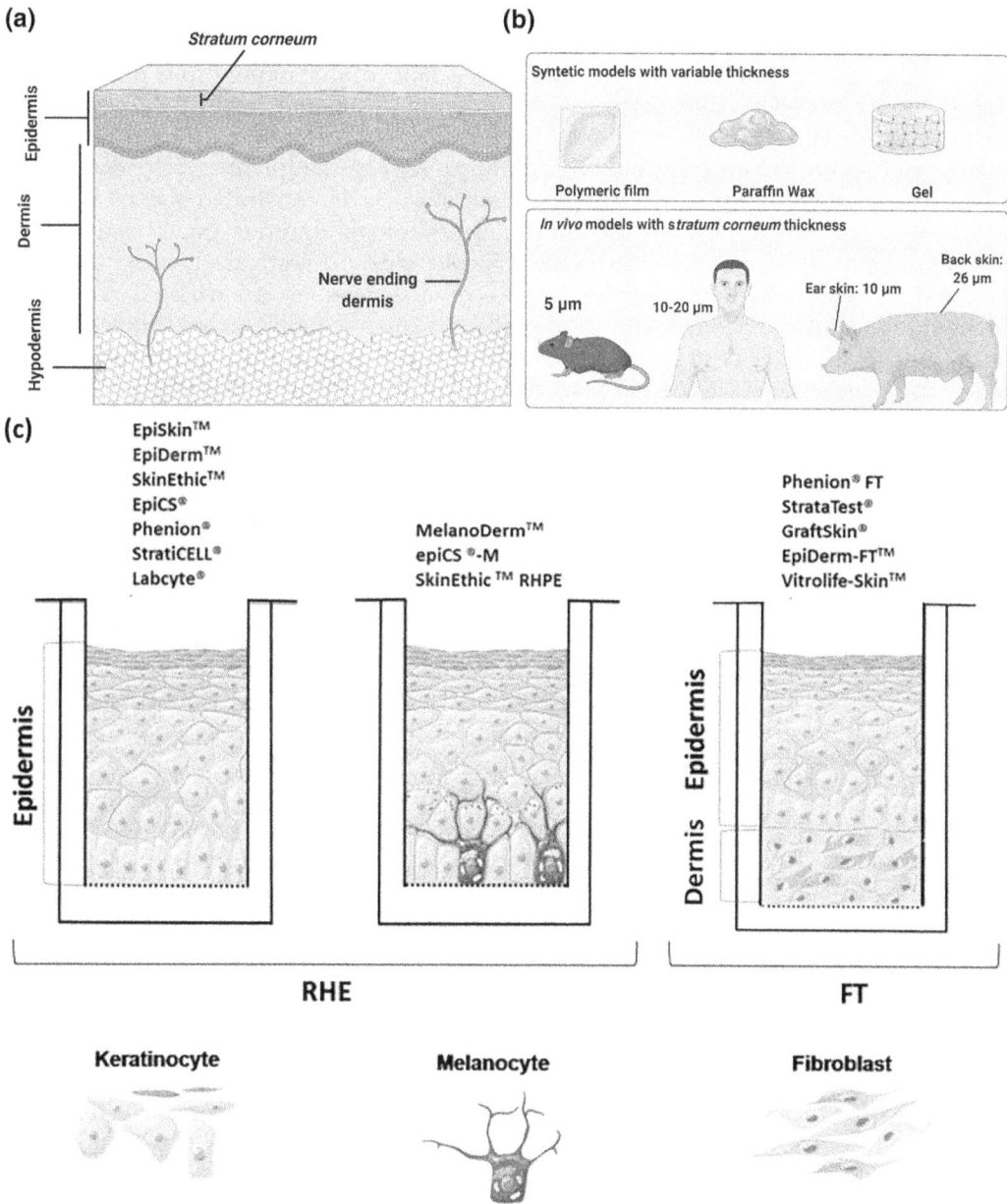

FIGURE 10.1

(a) Representation of human skin. (b) Synthetic membranes and *in vivo* skin models with varying thickness. (c) 3D skin models. Images reprinted with permission from [37, 38].

homogeneous and well-characterized; their diameter and length have been precisely determined [39]. Examining how nanoparticles diffuse via microchannels was made possible with the help of these membranes. The membrane's negative surface potential is also comparable to the features of the skin surface. The skin barrier and the Isopore® membrane both have their inherent hydrophobic properties. Isopore® membranes were considered an approximate analogue of microchannel-containing human skin, which was treated by microneedles [3]. Verhoeven et al. conducted an experiment using eggplants to mimic human skin to evaluate the efficacy of ceramic nanoporous microneedles for skin extraction and drug delivery. A purple eggplant (*Solanum melongena*) was employed as a simple skin model to evaluate the concept that nanoporous microneedle arrays could be used to collect interstitial skin fluids. Transdermal drug delivery capabilities of microneedles were evaluated by inserting an array of microneedles loaded with toluidine blue O onto the skin of a light green Thai eggplant and observing the skin sample using a stereomicroscope. These studies demonstrated the viability of using eggplant skin to investigate the efficiency of nanoporous microneedles [40]. Another group of researchers, Garland and colleagues, investigate how to choose a model skin membrane to test the effectiveness of microneedles. An artificial hydrophobic membrane (Silescol® 7–4107 silicone membrane) and neonatal porcine skin were used as the models for the *in vitro* permeation study. Microneedles made of poly(methyl vinyl ether-*co*-maleic acid) were loaded with drugs and inserted into these skin models. It was determined that after applying the dissolving microneedles, only around 3.7% of the methylene blue quantity loaded into the microneedle device was permeated when Silescol® was utilized as the model membrane. Meanwhile, when microneedle arrays were inserted into skin models of dermatomed and full-thickness neonatal pig skin, roughly 67.4% and 47.5% of the loaded amount of methylene blue was transported across the skin. The penetration and adhesion of microneedles *in vivo* did not correspond to those seen when using a Silescol® membrane. The level of microneedle-mediated transdermal delivery in an *in vivo* rat model was comparable to that obtained from *in vitro* experiments using dermatomed neonatal pig skin. Based on the results of this research, the rate and extent of transdermal delivery of small hydrophilic molecules from dissolving microneedles varied dramatically among skin models [26]. Koelmans and coworkers studied the mechanical interaction between silicon solid microneedles and the skin model. The microneedle design was optimized by using a double-layer skin simulant (comprised of an agarose gel layer and a layer of needle-testing foil). The researchers discovered that microneedle shape affects the force curve and that increasing the insertion speed of microneedles from 100 µm/s to 500 µm/s resulted in a 14% increase in the insertion force [24]. The penetration of pulsed microjets has been studied in agarose gel, a skin model used by Arora and colleagues [34]. As an artificial model, agarose gel has been utilized to successfully simulate the viscoelasticity of pig skin. To accurately measure the depth of microneedle penetration, the gel can be made into a homogeneous and transparent medium whose properties can be controlled and reproduced. Different microneedle insertions into the gel have been analyzed, and the results show that as agarose concentration increased, so did the depth of the holes created by the insertions [28]. This study suggests that agarose gel (0.0265 g/mL) is equivalent to the structure of pig skin. The findings indicated that the dynamic viscoelastic characteristics of porcine skin might be mimicked by utilizing an agarose gel as a model. The holes in agarose gel made by the microneedles were smaller than the needles themselves; the depth of the hole was shallower than the length of the microneedles. After the removal of microneedles, the holes quickly returned to their original dimensions, indicating that the material had a fast elastic response. The concentration of agarose was positively correlated with the depth of the pores. Experiments on skin-mimicking agarose and actual skin show a strong correlation regarding hole shrinkage [28]. Larrañeta and colleagues used a commercial polymeric film (Parafilm M®) for microneedle insertion experiments as a model membrane. Microneedles penetrated a stack of multiple layers of parafilm that approximately imitate skin tissue. Needle insertion depth was measured by optical coherence tomography and light microscopy. Comparing the penetration depth of microneedles in the parafilm layer and neonatal pig skin, the researchers noted that the penetration depth of microneedles in parafilm layers was less than that of the skin tissue. They stated that this parafilm model might be a simple, fast, and reliable method for evaluating microneedles and comparing various microneedle designs and formulations [29]. Similarly, Nguyen et al. used Parafilm M® film as a skin model to evaluate the uniformity of length and mechanical properties of maltose microneedles. After the insertion and removal of the microneedles, parafilm layers were separated and viewed under a light microscope. The researchers revealed that maltose microneedles of similar length had equivalent mechanical characteristics. In addition, an indentation region around each pore was noticed, as has often been described for microneedle insertion into the skin tissue. Importantly, microneedle penetration was deeper in parafilm layers than in the skin [41]. Moronkeji et al. designed a skin model consisting of subcutaneous and muscular mimics to assess microneedle performance. Neonatal pig skin was employed as the uppermost layer, followed by gelatin gels of varying water content to simulate subcutaneous tissue and Perma-Gel®, ballistic gelatin, to imitate muscular tissue. Each of these layers' mechanical characteristics was tested. Microneedles made of polymethylmethacrylate were inserted into the model with a specified force and velocity. According to the authors, the skin model matched the predicted values for subcutaneous and muscular tissue. Moreover, bigger and deeper microneedle-created channels were observed in skin models with a higher water content [42]. Ranamukhaarachchi and colleagues used a comprehensive mechanical analysis of fresh human and pig skin samples to guide the development of an artificial mechanical skin model (AMSM). The mechanical properties of the AMSM are compared to those of fresh human skin, and the AMSM's interaction with microneedles is evaluated in the same fashion. Mechanical interactions between microneedles and skin can be studied using the artificial mechanical skin model, but the diffusion of molecules through skin tissue cannot. The AMSM is a viable mechanical model that represents the properties of human skin, as shown by the mechanical measures (out-of-plane and in-plane Young's modulus, ultimate tensile strength, insertion force, displacement, and stiffness) [22]. In a subsequent investigation, the same team utilized the same validated artificial mechanical human skin model to determine what aspects of microneedle insertion dynamics were most important. Successful insertion of microneedle devices with varying geometric characteristics and array size was shown to be largely dependent on the insertion velocity of the microneedles [43]. In another study, Jing and colleagues developed a novel epidermal cells (HaCaT cells) membrane which was coated with pH-sensitive micelles. This membrane facilitated therapeutic active targeting of epidermal disease, thus improving the treatment efficacy. The authors loaded shikonin in biomimetic nanocarriers and reported that the nanocarriers were mostly delivered to the target of the active epidermis by dissolving microneedles [44].

10.3 Computational Modeling of Microneedles

10.3.1 Introduction of Computational Modeling

Recently, computational modeling has received much attention to improve technologies and enhance drug delivery efficiency. Moss et al. summarized the most current findings in simulating and predicting drug absorption into and across the skin. In addition, suggestions for future model building, improvement, and validation are discussed [45]. Also, Chen and colleagues published modeling research predicting the transdermal delivery of hydrophobic and hydrophilic permeants [46]. There has been a lot of research on the physical mechanism of microneedle insertion to optimize the system variables and enhance the efficacy of microneedle-mediated transdermal delivery. Computational models have lately been noticeable and may become more so in the future to predict the ideal microneedle design for the transdermal delivery of a particular therapeutic agent [47, 48]. Given that computational models can be verified, this would eliminate the requirement to obtain *ex vivo* skin tissues, which is beneficial since microneedles need to be approved by regulatory authorities to become a therapeutic success. The elimination of the need for *ex vivo* skin tissue for mechanical testing increases the likelihood that microneedles will be accepted [37]. Sanders and colleagues constructed models that characterize the skin's reaction to a force of stretching [49]. Kong and Wu investigated the insertion of a sharp tip into human skin [50]. By measuring transepidermal water loss, Gomaa et al. examined the impact of microneedle length, density, and insertion duration on improving drug permeation [51]. The majority of existing theoretical models for solid microneedles concentrate on the insertion procedure [9]. Shergold and Fleck designed a micromechanical model for the perforation of a soft solid by microneedles [52]. The researchers have developed an analytical model based on liquid expansion in a soft material to compute a solution's initial infusion through a micropump-powered microneedle array [53].

10.3.2 Case Studies of Computational Modeling

The finite element method (FEM) has lately emerged as a preferred simulation technique for engineering and mathematics models. For instance, the analytical model of skin with viscoelastic properties [12] includes differential terms with such a complex analytical solution [54]. FEM software employs a specific numerical approach to assist the solution of the partial differential equations that dictate physical modeling. This instrument enables engineers to study physical simulations without the necessity for experimental studies and hence anticipates the behavior of actual systems. ANSYS [55, 56], ABAQUS [57, 58], COMSOL [11, 59–61], and AutoFEM Lite [62] are critical software in this field. Simulation software is employed to anticipate the results of drug delivery investigations, skin penetration research, and structural evaluations [37]. Microneedle geometry, material characteristics, and insertion force are all examples of data needed for the simulation to accurately simulate a drug permeation study using microneedles. The skin's mechanical attributes provide a considerable challenge for simulation programs. The behavior of the skin may be simulated in many models. It is possible to replicate skin behavior using hyperelastic models such as the Neo Hookian model [57, 58] or the linear elastic model [60, 63]. Another approach is to model skin as a monolayer [58] or, more realistically, a multilayer [56, 57, 60, 63] in computer simulations. The multilayer skin model allows for the simulation of layers with varying parameters within the same model. Mostly all simulations involving microneedles have used the linear elastic model [55, 56, 59, 60, 62]. The load is often modeled as a force exerted on the needle array. Displacement is another kind of presentation for this load. The rate of needle penetration is constant and, within a short range, quasi-static [56, 57]. Notably, in most cases, the substrate (i.e., skin) breaks, allowing the needles to penetrate. An element deletion algorithm will often display this failure. As a result, the element will be eliminated once a prerequisite is met [57]. FEM modeling is frequently employed to study how microneedles material affects its efficiency, manufacturability, and mechanical properties. Accordingly, Parker and colleagues used a two-dimensional FEM simulation to study the buckling load as the mechanical behavior of titanium micromachining for the production of microneedles [61]. Another research used 3D FEM simulations to compare the strength of microneedles made from PMVE/MA to microneedles made from fish scales, determining which kind of material could better withstand the force required to penetrate the skin without breaking [62]. The FEM modeling is also useful for studying the microneedles' geometry and dimensions. Using this technique, researchers could determine the areas and magnitudes of stress concentrations in various needle geometries, including those with straight, jagged, and harpoon shapes [55]. Kong and coworkers examined how the tip area, wall angle, and wall thickness influenced skin deformation, failure, and insertion force [57]. Using FEM modeling, they revealed the force–displacement curve of microneedle penetration in skin tissue. The point at which the needle enters the skin causes a sharp drop in applied pressure. Specifically, the researchers examined the relationships between insertion force and the thickness of the stratum corneum, the dermis, the hypodermis, the area of the microneedle tip, and the angle and thickness of hollow microneedle wall. These studies found that the characteristics of the stratum corneum, the size of the needle tip, and the angle of the needle wall all contribute to the optimal insertion depth of tapered microneedles. Furthermore, increasing the wall thickness of hollow microneedles with a large tip diameter increases the insertion force, whereas increasing the wall thickness of hollow microneedles with a small tip has no influence on the insertion force. Mechanical evaluation metrics such as Von Mises stress and critical load factor were derived from FEM simulations of microneedles with triangular, square, and hexagonal base geometries [60]. The calculations showed that microneedles could tolerate more compressive stresses if the polygon structure had more vertices. Compressive loads were shown to be less of an issue for hexagonal microneedles than for triangular microneedles.

According to Olatunji and workers, microneedle insertion force may be roughly described as in Eq. (10.1) [11]:

$$F_{\text{Insertion}} = F_{\text{Bending}} + F_{\text{Indentation}} + F_{\text{Cutting}} + F_{\text{Buckling}} + F_{\text{Friction}} \qquad \text{(Eq. 10.1)}$$

Here, F_{Bending} bends the skin, $F_{\text{Indentation}}$ disrupts the stratum corneum layer, F_{Cutting} punctures the skin, F_{Buckling} deforms the skin, and F_{Friction} applies frictional force on the skin. Researchers have built several analytical relations for each of these forces. A further 2D finite element simulation is performed and compared to the results produced from such analytical relations. The authors suggested that the force components are impacted by the skin's mechanical characteristics as well as by the geometry and alignment of microneedles on the array [37].

Using computational models, in which various conditions may be modeled, is one way to circumvent the difficulties in experimentation [1]. Without the high costs of manufacturing and experimentation, software models allow researchers to explore a wide variety of variables and factors. Using the dynamic finite element program ANSYS/LS-DYNA, Chiu and colleagues simulated the penetration of PLA microneedles into the skin to determine the ideal design for polymeric microneedles patches. According to the findings, the stress distribution of the microneedle increases by a factor of 3 as its base size decreases [64].

Furthermore, Chen et al. simulated a microneedle insertion into the skin using a nonlinear finite element model supported by the skin's biomechanical characteristics [65]. To achieve optimal microneedle design [1], this research simulated the effects of various geometries on microneedles fracture. A study on mouse skin was used as experimental validation. The model found that the buckling force for a microneedle of 1,000 µm length and 100 µm width would increase with the needle angle but remained unaffected by the change in tip width. Contrastingly, a smaller tip would require significantly less force to penetrate the skin. The model overestimated the microneedle insertion force, but the findings were similar to their experimental observations. While it is not a drawback to overestimate the insertion force since doing so gives a safety margin, doing so by as much as 40% in this situation is not optimal when trying to optimize the needle's geometry. Since skin is a nonlinear material, it does not display the ideal elastic behavior; some models dismiss the skin deformation prior to puncturing; boundary patterns alter as the contact between the microneedle and skin evolves over time; the impact of underlying tissues, i.e., muscle and bone, is neglected; and the thickness of skin layers is assumed to be the same for all subjects [65, 66]. As a consequence of these assumptions and challenges, predictions may be too conservative and unreliable. Groves and colleagues conducted computational modeling to reduce errors as much as feasible and subsequently refined the computer algorithms using experimental data [66]. To anticipate skin deformation and allow the rational design of optimal microneedles, they carried out research similar to Chen et al., employing the same prediction model [65]. Groves and coworkers [66] optimized the material coefficients using an algorithm for extracting material parameters based on *in vivo* indentation studies. Subsequently, the Ogden material characteristics derived from the indentation tests were compared to the experimental values. Despite the known constraints, there was 95.1–99% agreement between the simulated curves and the *in vivo* results. This research emphasizes the role of computational simulations in applied research by demonstrating the value of modeling while also demonstrating the continued requirement for experimental evidence.

Since current detection methods are inadequate, a thorough understanding of how a microneedle dissolves in the skin is a significant challenge. Hence, Kim K.S. and collaborators created a mathematical model to estimate the quantity of drug delivered across the skin from dissolving microneedles. The drug permeation and microchannels' depth in the skin were estimated using dimensionless governing equations [67]. The research showed that the amount of fentanyl given by a microneedle was directly related to its mass fraction, with smaller-pitch needles being more effective than larger-pitch microneedles. A moderately nonlinear model was built to account for the influence of the pitch on drug permeation. There was also no change in the elimination rate constant due to the needle dissolution. The optimization algorithm was also utilized to evaluate the validity of the experimental findings [67]. Enhancing skin permeability using conical solid or hollow microneedles has previously been demonstrated with the use of an algorithm. Increases in drug delivery occur with larger needle radii, whereas decreases happen at larger patch sizes [68]. Other research has established algorithm models for both square and nonsquare microneedle distribution on arrays [69, 70]. As liquid drugs are injected into the skin using hollow microneedles, it is crucial to construct a proper numerical model for these microneedles with fluid flow features and account for "lumen dimensions." As a result, mathematical models are created and documented in the literature to assess and understand the theoretical performance of microneedles [71]. Microelectromechanical system (MEMS)– based silicon hollow out-of-plane microneedle arrays were modeled, designed, and simulated by Amin et al. Bernoulli equation–based numerical simulations have been used to compare how fluid flows through these microneedles with and without the presence of gravitational forces. Microneedle geometry was modeled to examine the effects of flow rate, needle diameter, and pressure drop on drug delivery. The Bernoulli equation was shown to be a reasonable approximation for fluid flow through microneedle lumens when MEMS PRO was employed. Furthermore, physical process simulations on TCAD SILVACO have been used to fine-tune the design of these microneedles in accordance with the conventional Si-fabrication lines [72]. A computational model has been developed to predict the ideal microneedle geometry for skin penetration, especially dermal vaccination [47]. This research examined how the needle penetration depth and immune response changed depending on needle-to-needle distance, needle length, and the diameter of the array base. It was hypothesized that the optimal distance between microneedles was associated with the immunological response caused by the antigen-presenting cells, and the findings showed that this distance was affected by both the number of active antigen-presenting cells and the target location (epidermis or dermis layer). The greatest number of antigen-presenting cells were achieved when microneedles were spaced 1 mm apart when aiming toward the epidermis and 1.5 mm apart when aiming for the dermis layer. Antigen-presenting cell activation was also shown to be dependent on microneedle length, with longer microneedles being more suited to dermal antigen-presenting cell activation. There was hardly any correlation between the array base diameter and the number of responding immune cells [47]. In another investigation, structural properties of sugar microneedles were studied [59]. The findings showed that the mechanical strength of carboxymethylcellulose/maltose microneedles was higher than that of carboxymethylcellulose/trehalose and carboxymethylcellulose/sucrose microneedles. Most microneedles failed by buckling, and the Young's modulus of the sugar ingredients of each microneedle correlated positively with the order of buckling [59].

Lv and colleagues presented the first quantitative modeling of fluid injection kinetics across the skin using a microneedle array. The injection flow and drug delivery were quantitatively modeled at the same time. Dispersed drug injection kinetics using a microneedle array were also predicted using numerical solutions. The authors also looked at how factors including microneedle tip dimension, the velocity with which solutions were injected at the needle's tip, tissue porosity, and blood perfusion rate affected transdermal drug delivery. Improved transdermal drug delivery was calculated to result from increasing the initial injection velocity and enhancing blood circulation in highly porous skin [73]. In another study, Chen and collaborators proposed a quantitative, analytical model to simulate the infusion flow of a micropump-driven array of hollow microneedles. They hypothesized that each microneedle's initial injection would expand and diffuse in a spherical pattern. The model can predict the diffusion boundary and the time-dependent expansion radius. The results of the calculations demonstrate that without an increase in the pressure from the micro-pump, the expansion generated by the infusion of microneedles ceases quickly, and the flow rate goes to zero in a brief duration. Nevertheless, if the surroundings are highly absorbent, the diffusion boundary is markedly greater than the expansion, and the infusion persists. The qualitative agreement between the calculated findings and the actual results of jet infusion with a single needle in silicon rubber and polyacrylamide gel is remarkable [74]. To estimate the systemic pharmacokinetics of microneedle arrays containing cabotegravir and rilpivirine, Rajoli and coworkers created a unique intradermal pharmacokinetic model. This model predicted the optimum dosage and release rates for microneedle arrays to keep the drug plasma levels above specified antiretroviral goals throughout treatment durations

[75]. Microneedle shape, the material of construction, needle length, needle-to-needle distance, and diameter all play a role in the fracture force and the capacity of the microneedles to puncture human skin. In 2008, Al-Qallaf et al. presented a mathematical algorithm to anticipate how changing these variables would affect macromolecules' absorption through the skin using solid and hollow microneedles. Collectively, their findings revealed the model's significance in determining the patch size for maximum skin permeability and blood concentration [68]. Ever since, numerous diffusion models have been created to estimate drug delivery with the use of solid, hollow, or swelling microneedles [76–78]. However, in the case of dissolving microneedles, where dissolution and penetration processes predominate, these models are inapplicable. Mathematical modeling by Ronnander and coworkers allowed researchers to anticipate how much sumatriptan would be absorbed into the skin from drug-loaded dissolving polyvinylpyrrolidone-based microneedles. Mass balance equations were created to model the drug's dissolution and delivery. The researchers utilized a theoretical method to evaluate and predict how altering critical design variables would affect the drug release kinetics. Therefore, the loading quantity and the microneedle length contributed to an increase in the drug level in the skin. The quantity of drug delivered to the dermal layer was shown to be inversely related to the pitch width. The maximum amount of drug in the skin was shown to increase with an increase in the drug load in microneedles. An increase in drug concentration was observed after a marginal increase in the needle length [79]. To precisely identify the "ideal" design of microneedles, it is necessary to examine the influence of multiple factors (i.e., microneedle length, patch surface area) and varied drug transport aspects with microneedles. For transdermal delivery of a macromolecule through microneedles, a parametric study was provided by Al-Qallaf and colleagues. Computational simulations have allowed the researchers to determine the role of different variables (i.e., microneedle length, application time, patch size) in determining the efficacy of microneedle array designs. Moreover, a scaling analysis was carried out, which demonstrated the drug concentration's functional dependency on skin and microneedle array variables [80]. Olatunji and coworkers provided a framework for quantifying the impact of design factors of microneedles on transdermal delivery of drugs. Effects of compressive strain on skin during microneedle insertion were also investigated. When the impact of microneedles strain on the diffusion coefficient was modeled, the model discovered that the steady-state flux was lower than expected for all examined cases. The findings suggest that decreasing drug permeability may be achieved by increasing the size and density of microneedle on an array due to the increased compressive force [77]. Similarly, a framework was presented by Davidson and coworkers to determine which types of drug-coated microneedles are most effective for transdermal drug delivery by enhancing skin permeability. For various microneedle designs, the effective skin thickness and permeability were computed. The hypothesized correlation between effective skin permeability and skin thickness enables the prediction of permeation through the skin and the correlation of microneedle geometries for small/large molecule drug delivery utilizing microneedles [81].

10.4 Microneedles-assisted Drug Permeation

Solid microneedles are generally inserted into the skin using a thumb or an applicator. A manual insertion using a thumb is the most convenient method; however, it cannot control the desired pressure and uniformity of force received by individual microneedles on the array. This issue becomes more serious when the microneedle array has a flat substrate and the skin surface is nonuniform. This can cause incomplete penetration of some needles on the array. Furthermore, there is no controlled application velocity for thumb insertion. The insertion velocity of microneedles has been found to play an essential role in effective microneedle penetration. Besides, several types of applicators have been developed to aid microneedle insertion [82–84]. The designs of applicators are discussed in another chapter. After microneedle insertion, the needles are then removed intact from the skin, leaving no or negligible traces of microneedle materials remaining in skin tissue. This is essential for the safety of microneedles. Following microneedle removal, a drug-loaded formulation (solution, topical gel, cream, or transdermal patch) is applied to the microneedle-treated skin area for the permeation study [41, 85]. For *in vitro* studies, dermatomed or full-thickness cadaver skin tissue is placed flat on a supporting material (i.e., parafilm layers). Microneedles are inserted into the skin for a certain period before the needle removal. After that, the skin sample is assembled into permeation cells (i.e., Franz vertical or horizontal cells. Franz cells are widely used to evaluate microneedle-mediated transdermal drug delivery *in vitro* since they are an established method for assessing pharmaceutical semisolid dosage forms [86]) with the stratum corneum facing the donor compartment. The formulation is then added to the donor chamber to initiate *in vitro* permeation study. The cumulative quantity of drugs that permeated through a particular skin area is estimated and presented. For *in vivo* experiments, the method of microneedle insertion and formulation application is different from those in *in vitro* studies. Initially, animal subjects (i.e., mice and rats) are lightly anesthetized before shaving hairs on a particular skin area. Then, microneedles are inserted into the shaved area using a thumb or an applicator. A plastic ring or a liquid reservoir patch is employed to keep the drug formulation on the skin and prevent drug leakage. The reservoir ring adheres to the skin after microneedles treatment and removal. Drug formulation is then applied on the treated skin area inside the reservoir ring before this reservoir is tightly sealed with a film. At predetermined intervals, the blood samples were collected, processed, and analyzed [87]. Interestingly, Derma Roller microneedles are applied without the use of an applicator. The treatment is performed by rolling the Derma Roller on the skin surface at a movement pattern and the number of rolling times [88]. Thus, this microneedle design enables the generation of numerous microchannels at various channel-to-channel distances.

Coated microneedles carry the drug payload in the coating layer. Thus, the application of coated microneedles is a simple single-step process. Microneedle array is inserted into the skin using a thumb or an applicator for a certain period, as in solid microneedles. The use of an applicator is typically preferable since a controlled, consistent, and uniform force can be applied on a microneedle array. The needles are then kept in skin tissue for the disintegration of the coating layer to release the coated drug into skin layers. After that, microneedles are removed intact from the skin with a negligible amount of drug on the needles' surface. The majority of the coated drug is placed deeply in skin layers, thus preventing any significant drug loss. The needles must remain firmly inserted in the skin (i.e., using a self-adhesive bandage) for a predetermined period required to dissolve the coated layer without any needle breakage in the skin. Coated microneedles have a lot in common across the *in vitro* and *in vivo* study designs. For *in vitro* studies, skin pieces are laid flat on a surface. Coated microneedles are then inserted into the skin tissue. Skin and microneedles are positioned between the donor and receptor chambers. The permeation study is initiated as soon as the skin is in touch with the receptor solution [89]. For *in vivo* studies, hairs on a selected skin area of an animal subject are shaved before the application of coated microneedles. The needles are then kept in the skin for a predetermined period before microneedle removal. Blood samples are then collected and analyzed [90, 91]. In general, the quantity of drug adhered on coated microneedles after the skin insertion and the amount remaining on the skin surface are captured and analyzed to evaluate the drug delivery efficiency of coated microneedles.

Hollow microneedles are micrometer-sized hypodermic needles with a bore inside the needles, which serve as a channel for drug diffusion into the skin tissue. Sharp microneedles penetrate the skin, and then the drug solution is driven through the needles into the skin by passive diffusion or pressure-based micropump. The application of hollow microneedles includes two steps: (i) microneedle insertion and (ii) drug injection. After microneedle insertion, the needle has to be kept in place to avoid the "pushing out" effect, which can cause incomplete needle penetration and drug leakage. The drug solution is injected continuously into the skin using a micropump at a predefined infusion flow rate, injection depth, and injection volume [93–95]. For *in vitro* experiments, hollow microneedles are inserted into cadaver skin tissue before the drug solution is injected directly into the skin. The drug-contained skin sample is then mounted on diffusion cells for *in vitro* permeation study [96]. *In vitro* permeation studies are not as popular and practical as *in vivo* studies. The thickness of the skin has to be appropriately selected to ensure that hollow microneedles do not pierce through the skin. For *in vivo* studies, hollow microneedles are inserted into an anesthetized animal whose hairs of a selected area have been shaved. A drug reservoir or chamber is located on top of the needle array in which the drug formulation is not in direct contact with the skin. This setup allows the drug to enter the skin only via the hollow bore of the needle. The drug solution is injected into the skin at a specific flow rate using a controlled application pressure [97, 98]. Interestingly, extraction of skin interstitial fluid using hollow microneedles has also been reported. Microneedles equipped with pipet capillary tubes have been used to extract fluid from the skin [99]. Blood was also extracted *in vivo* by connecting a microneedle with an elastic self-recovery actuator, which converted the pressure from the researcher's finger into elastic energy for sample extraction. When the pressure was released, the resulting vacuum caused blood to be drawn into the chamber [100]. Similarly, pressure-driven force is generated inside a vacuum chamber to draw blood from the skin using hollow microneedles [101].

Dissolving microneedles contain drug load inside the polymeric matrix of microneedles. Upon skin insertion, these polymeric microneedles dissolve and release the loaded drug into skin layers. The application of dissolving microneedles is a single-step procedure, which is similar to that of coated microneedles. After skin insertion, the needles are kept in skin tissue for a certain period to completely dissolve [102]. Thus, microneedles are usually attached to the skin using adhesive tape. The encapsulated drug is first released from disintegrated microneedles and then delivered into skin layers. After microneedles dissolution and removal from the skin, only the array substrate remained, producing no sharp waste and minimal drug loss. Dissolving microneedles could be arranged on a rigid or flexible array substrate. Chen and coworkers fabricated chitosan microneedles on a poly(L-lactide-*co*-D,L-lactide) rigid supporting array for sustained transdermal delivery of ovalbumin as a model molecule for vaccines (Fig. 10.2) [92]. Microneedle application can be performed with the aid of a thumb or an applicator. A similar insertion technique is employed for both *in vitro* and *in vivo* studies [103, 104]. Swelling microneedles are known as the latest design of microneedles which offer several advantages over other microneedle types. Upon skin insertion, microneedles swell and create a porous structure in the polymeric microneedles. These porous structures facilitate drug diffusion into skin layers. The application procedure for swelling microneedles is similar to dissolving and coated microneedles [105, 106].

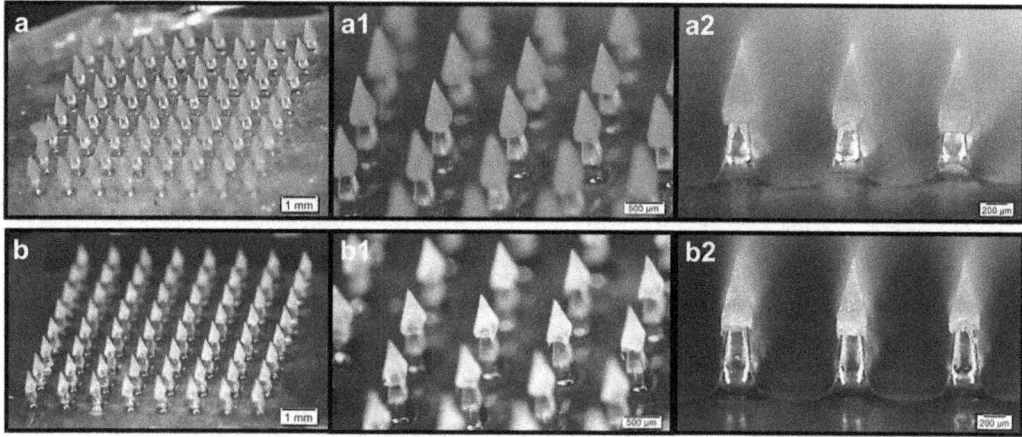

FIGURE 10.2
Microscopic images of rhodamine B-dextran-loaded (a–a2) and ovalbumin-loaded (b–b2) chitosan poly(L-lactide-*co*-D,L-lactide) microneedle arrays. Images reprinted with permission from [92].

10.5 Conclusions

Microneedle technology is a promising platform for the transdermal delivery of various therapeutic agents. Numerous variables of microneedles (i.e., shape, design, type, length, tip dimension, needle density, and array size) have been found to significantly affect the efficiency of microneedle treatment. A thorough evaluation of the effects of these variables on microneedle-mediated drug delivery is required to propose an ideal microneedle design. Researchers have developed multiple synthetic skin models to examine microneedles' mechanical properties and observe the skin penetration process. These models provide a rapid, effective, and reliable tool to characterize microneedle products. Besides, computational modeling is a practical and cost-effective approach to evaluating microneedles' performance. The development and optimization of skin models and mathematical simulation will significantly advance the field of microneedles.

References

[1] Lutton REM, Moore J, Larrañeta E, et al. Microneedle characterisation: the need for universal acceptance criteria and GMP specifications when moving towards commercialisation. Drug Deliv Transl Res. 2015;5:313–331.

[2] Matsuo K, Yokota Y, Zhai Y, et al. A low-invasive and effective transcutaneous immunization system using a novel dissolving microneedle array for soluble and particulate antigens. J Control Release. 2012;161:10–17.

[3] Coulman SA, Anstey A, Gateley C, et al. Microneedle mediated delivery of nanoparticles into human skin. Int J Pharm. 2009;366:190–200.

[4] Lee JW, Park J-H, Prausnitz MR. Dissolving microneedles for transdermal drug delivery. Biomaterials. 2008;29:2113–2124.

[5] Li G, Badkar A, Nema S, et al. In vitro transdermal delivery of therapeutic antibodies using maltose microneedles. Int J Pharm. 2009;368:109–115.

[6] Verbaan FJ, Bal SM, van den Berg DJ, et al. Assembled microneedle arrays enhance the transport of compounds varying over a large range of molecular weight across human dermatomed skin. J Control Release. 2007;117:238–245.

[7] Wang P, Prausnitz M. Drilling microneedle device. Google Patents; 2007. [Internet] [cited 2016 Aug 23]. Available from: www.google.com/patents/US20080027384.

[8] Yoon J, Son T, Choi E, et al. Enhancement of optical skin clearing efficacy using a microneedle roller. J Biomed Opt. 2008;13:021103–021103.

[9] Davis SP, Landis BJ, Adams ZH, et al. Insertion of microneedles into skin: measurement and prediction of insertion force and needle fracture force. J Biomech. 2004;37:1155–1163.

[10] Khanna P, Luongo K, Strom JA, et al. Sharpening of hollow silicon microneedles to reduce skin penetration force. J Micromechanics Microengineering. 2010;20:045011.

[11] Olatunji O, Das DB, Garland MJ, et al. Influence of array interspacing on the force required for successful microneedle skin penetration: theoretical and practical approaches. J Pharm Sci. 2013;102:1209–1221.

[12] Park J-H, Allen MG, Prausnitz MR. Biodegradable polymer microneedles: fabrication, mechanics and transdermal drug delivery. J Control Release. 2005;104:51–66.

[13] Yang M, Zahn JD. Microneedle insertion force reduction using vibratory actuation. Biomed Microdevices. 2004;6:177–182.

[14] Flaten GE, Palac Z, Engesland A, et al. In vitro skin models as a tool in optimization of drug formulation. Eur J Pharm Sci. 2015;75:10–24.

[15] Dong L, Li Y, Li Z, et al. Au nanocage-strengthened dissolving microneedles for chemo-photothermal combined therapy of superficial skin tumors. ACS Appl Mater Interfaces. 2018;10:9247–9256.

[16] Lee H, Choi TK, Lee YB, et al. A graphene-based electrochemical device with thermoresponsive microneedles for diabetes monitoring and therapy. Nat Nanotechnol. 2016;11:566–572.

[17] Li W, Terry RN, Tang J, et al. Rapidly separable microneedle patch for the sustained release of a contraceptive. Nat Biomed Eng. 2019;3:220–229.

[18] Lermen D, Gorjup E, Dyce PW, et al. Neuro-muscular differentiation of adult porcine skin derived stem cell-like cells. PLoS One. 2010;5:e8968.

[19] Shergold OA, Fleck NA, Radford D. The uniaxial stress versus strain response of pig skin and silicone rubber at low and high strain rates. Int J Impact Eng. 2006;32:1384–1402.

[20] Todo H. Transdermal permeation of drugs in various animal species. Pharmaceutics. 2017;9:33.

[21] Wei JC, Edwards GA, Martin DJ, et al. Allometric scaling of skin thickness, elasticity, viscoelasticity to mass for micro-medical device translation: from mice, rats, rabbits, pigs to humans. Sci Rep. 2017;7:1–16.

[22] Ranamukhaarachchi SA, Schneider T, Lehnert S, et al. Development and validation of an artificial mechanical skin model for the study of interactions between skin and microneedles. Macromol Mater Eng. 2016;301:306–314.

[23] Vedrine L, Prais W, Laurent PE, et al. Improving needle-point sharpness in prefillable syringes. Med Device Technol. 2003;14:32–35.

[24] Koelmans WW, Krishnamoorthy G, Heskamp A, et al. Microneedle characterization using a double-layer skin simulant. Mech Eng Res. 2013;3:51.

[25] Donnelly RF, Singh TRR, Tunney MM, et al. Microneedle arrays allow lower microbial penetration than hypodermic needles in vitro. Pharm Res. 2009;26:2513–2522.

[26] Garland MJ, Migalska K, Tuan-Mahmood T-M, et al. Influence of skin model on in vitro performance of drug-loaded soluble microneedle arrays. Int J Pharm. 2012;434:80–89.

[27] Ng S-F, Rouse JJ, Sanderson FD, et al. The relevance of polymeric synthetic membranes in topical formulation assessment and drug diffusion study. Arch Pharm Res. 2012;35:579–593.

[28] Zhang D, Das DB, Rielly CD. Microneedle assisted micro-particle delivery from gene guns: experiments using skin-mimicking agarose gel. J Pharm Sci. 2014;103:613–627.

[29] Larrañeta E, Moore J, Vicente-Pérez EM, et al. A proposed model membrane and test method for microneedle insertion studies. Int J Pharm. 2014;472:65–73.

[30] Huong SP, Bun H, Fourneron J-D, et al. Use of various models for in vitro percutaneous absorption studies of ultraviolet filters. Skin Res Technol. 2009;15:253–261.

[31] Permana AD, Mir M, Utomo E, et al. Bacterially sensitive nanoparticle-based dissolving microneedles of doxycycline for enhanced treatment of bacterial biofilm skin infection: a proof of concept study. Int J Pharm X. 2020;2:100047.

[32] Permana AD, Paredes AJ, Volpe-Zanutto F, et al. Dissolving microneedle-mediated dermal delivery of itraconazole nanocrystals for improved treatment of cutaneous candidiasis. Eur J Pharm Biopharm. 2020;154:50–61.

[33] Chen M-C, Ling M-H, Wang K-W, et al. Near-infrared light-responsive composite microneedles for on-demand transdermal drug delivery. Biomacromolecules. 2015;16:1598–1607.

[34] Arora A, Hakim I, Baxter J, et al. Needle-free delivery of macromolecules across the skin by nanoliter-volume pulsed microjets. Proc Natl Acad Sci. 2007;104:4255–4260.

[35] Fonseca DF, Costa PC, Almeida IF, et al. Swellable gelatin methacryloyl microneedles for extraction of interstitial skin fluid toward minimally invasive monitoring of urea. Macromol Biosci. 2020;20:2000195.

[36] Padil VVT, Cheong JY, Kp A, et al. Electrospun fibers based on carbohydrate gum polymers and their multifaceted applications. Carbohydr Polym. 2020;247:116705.

[37] Makvandi P, Kirkby M, Hutton AR, et al. Engineering microneedle patches for improved penetration: analysis, skin models and factors affecting needle insertion. Nano-Micro Lett. 2021;13:1–41.

[38] Sanches PL, Geaquinto LR de O, Cruz R, et al. Toxicity evaluation of TiO_2 nanoparticles on the 3D skin model: a systematic review. Front Bioeng Biotechnol. 2020;8:575.

[39] Apel P. Track etching technique in membrane technology. Radiat Meas. 2001;34:559–566.

[40] Verhoeven M, Bystrova S, Winnubst L, et al. Applying ceramic nanoporous microneedle arrays as a transport interface in egg plants and an ex-vivo human skin model. Microelectron Eng. 2012;98:659–662.

[41] Nguyen HX, Banga AK. Fabrication, characterization and application of sugar microneedles for transdermal drug delivery. Ther Deliv. 2017;8:249–264.

[42] Moronkeji K, Todd S, Dawidowska I, et al. The role of subcutaneous tissue stiffness on microneedle performance in a representative in vitro model of skin. J Control Release. 2017;265:102–112.

[43] Ranamukhaarachchi SA, Stoeber B. Determining the factors affecting dynamic insertion of microneedles into skin. Biomed Microdevices. 2019;21:1–8.

[44] Jing Q, Ruan H, Li J, et al. Keratinocyte membrane-mediated nanodelivery system with dissolving microneedles for targeted therapy of skin diseases. Biomaterials. 2021;278:121142.

[45] Moss GP, Wilkinson SC, Sun Y. Mathematical modelling of percutaneous absorption. Curr Opin Colloid Interface Sci. 2012;17:166–172.

[46] Chen L, Lian G, Han L. Modeling transdermal permeation. Part I. Predicting skin permeability of both hydrophobic and hydrophilic solutes. AIChE J. 2010;56:1136–1146.

[47] Römgens AM, Bader DL, Bouwstra JA, et al. Predicting the optimal geometry of microneedles and their array for dermal vaccination using a computational model. Comput Methods Biomech Biomed Engin. 2016;19:1599–1609.

[48] Zoudani EL, Soltani M. A new computational method of modeling and evaluation of dissolving microneedle for drug delivery applications: extension to theoretical modeling of a novel design of microneedle (array in array) for efficient drug delivery. Eur J Pharm Sci. 2020;150:105339.

[49] Sanders JE, Goldstein BS, Leotta DF. Skin response to mechanical stress: adaptation rather than breakdown-a review of the literature. J Rehabil Res Dev. 1995;32:214–214.

[50] Kong X, Wu C. Measurement and prediction of insertion force for the mosquito fascicle penetrating into human skin. J Bionic Eng. 2009;6:143–152.

[51] Gomaa YA, Morrow DI, Garland MJ, et al. Effects of microneedle length, density, insertion time and multiple applications on human skin barrier function: assessments by transepidermal water loss. Toxicol In Vitro. 2010;24:1971–1978.

[52] Shergold OA, Fleck NA. Mechanisms of deep penetration of soft solids, with application to the injection and wounding of skin. Proc R Soc Lond Ser Math Phys Eng Sci. 2004;460:3037–3058.

[53] Yang F, Chen K, Feng Z-G. Analytical model of initial fluid infusion by a microneedle drug delivery system. 2011 4th Int Conf Biomed Eng Inform BMEI. IEEE; 2011. p. 913–917.

[54] Shabani M, Jahani K, Di Paola M, et al. Frequency domain identification of the fractional Kelvin-Voigt's parameters for viscoelastic materials. Mech Mater. 2019;137:103099.

[55] Aoyagi S, Izumi H, Fukuda M. Biodegradable polymer needle with various tip angles and consideration on insertion mechanism of mosquito's proboscis. Sens Actuators Phys. 2008;143:20–28.

[56] Xenikakis I, Tzimtzimis M, Tsongas K, et al. Fabrication and finite element analysis of stereolithographic 3D printed microneedles for transdermal delivery of model dyes across human skin in vitro. Eur J Pharm Sci. 2019;137:104976.

[57] Kong XQ, Zhou P, Wu CW. Numerical simulation of microneedles' insertion into skin. Comput Methods Biomech Biomed Engin. 2011;14:827–835.

[58] Leyva-Mendivil MF, Lengiewicz J, Page A, et al. Skin Microstructure is a Key Contributor to Its Friction Behaviour. Tribol Lett. 2016;65:12.

[59] Loizidou EZ, Williams NA, Barrow DA, et al. Structural characterisation and transdermal delivery studies on sugar microneedles: experimental and finite element modelling analyses. Eur J Pharm Biopharm. 2015;89:224–231.

[60] Loizidou EZ, Inoue NT, Ashton-Barnett J, et al. Evaluation of geometrical effects of microneedles on skin penetration by CT scan and finite element analysis. Eur J Pharm Biopharm. 2016;107:1–6.

[61] Parker ER, Rao MP, Turner KL, et al. Bulk micromachined titanium microneedles. J Microelectromechanical Syst. 2007;16:289–295.

[62] Olatunji O, Igwe CC, Ahmed AS, et al. Microneedles from fish scale biopolymer. J Appl Polym Sci. 2014;131. [Internet] [cited 2016 Aug 13]. Available from: http://onlinelibrary.wiley.com/doi/10.1002/app.40377/full.

[63] Boonma A, Narayan RJ, Lee Y-S. Analytical modeling and evaluation of microneedles apparatus with deformable soft tissues for biomedical applications. Comput-Aided Des Appl. 2013;10:139–157.

[64] Chiu CY, Kuo HC, Lin Y, et al. Optimal design of microneedles inserts into skin by numerical simulation. Key Eng Mater. 2012;516:624–628.

[65] Chen S, Li N, Chen J. Finite element analysis of microneedle insertion into skin. Micro Nano Lett. 2012;7:1206–1209.

[66] Groves RB, Coulman SA, Birchall JC, et al. Quantifying the mechanical properties of human skin to optimise future microneedle device design. Comput Methods Biomech Biomed Engin. 2012;15:73–82.

[67] Kim KS, Ita K, Simon L. Modelling of dissolving microneedles for transdermal drug delivery: theoretical and experimental aspects. Eur J Pharm Sci. 2015;68:137–143.

[68] Al-Qallaf B, Das DB. Optimization of square microneedle arrays for increasing drug permeability in skin. Chem Eng Sci. 2008;63:2523–2535.

[69] Al-Qallaf B, Das DB. Optimizing microneedle arrays for transdermal drug delivery: extension to non-square distribution of microneedles. J Drug Target. 2009;17:108–122.

[70] Al-Qallaf B, Das DB. Optimizing microneedle arrays to increase skin permeability for transdermal drug delivery. Ann N Y Acad Sci. 2009;1161:83–94.

[71] Stoeber B, Liepmann D. Arrays of hollow out-of-plane microneedles for drug delivery. J Microelectromechanical Syst. 2005;14:472–479.

[72] Amin F, Ahmed S. Design, modeling and simulation of MEMS-based silicon Microneedles. J Phys Conf Ser. IOP Publishing; 2013. p. 012049. [Internet] [cited 2016 Aug 16]. Available from: http://iopscience.iop.org/article/10.1088/1742-6596/439/1/012049/meta.

[73] Lv YG, Liu J, Gao YH, et al. Modeling of transdermal drug delivery with a microneedle array. J Micromechanics Microengineering. 2006;16:2492.

[74] Chen K, Pan M, Feng Z-G. Modeling of drug delivery by a pump driven micro-needle array system. Open Biomed Eng J. 2016;10:19.

[75] Rajoli RK, Flexner C, Chiong J, et al. Modelling the intradermal delivery of microneedle array patches for long-acting antiretrovirals using PBPK. Eur J Pharm Biopharm. 2019;144:101–109.

[76] Mansoor I, Lai J, Ranamukhaarachchi S, et al. A microneedle-based method for the characterization of diffusion in skin tissue using doxorubicin as a model drug. Biomed Microdevices. 2015;17:9967.

[77] Olatunji O, Das DB, Nassehi V. Modelling transdermal drug delivery using microneedles: effect of geometry on drug transport behaviour. J Pharm Sci. 2012;101:164–175.

[78] Zhang R, Zhang P, Dalton C, et al. Modeling of drug delivery into tissues with a microneedle array using mixture theory. Biomech Model Mechanobiol. 2010;9:77–86.

[79] Ronnander P, Simon L, Spilgies H, et al. Modelling the in-vitro dissolution and release of sumatriptan succinate from polyvinylpyrrolidone-based microneedles. Eur J Pharm Sci. 2018;125:54–63.

[80] Al-Qallaf B, Das DB, Mori D, et al. Modelling transdermal delivery of high molecular weight drugs from microneedle systems. Philos Transact A Math Phys Eng Sci. 2007;365:2951–2967.

[81] Davidson A, Al-Qallaf B, Das DB. Transdermal drug delivery by coated microneedles: geometry effects on effective skin thickness and drug permeability. Chem Eng Res Des. 2008;86:1196–1206.

[82] Hartmann XHM, van der Linde P, Homburg EFGA, et al. Insertion process of ceramic nanoporous microneedles by means of a novel mechanical applicator design. Pharmaceutics. 2015;7:503–522.

[83] Leone M, Van Oorschot BH, Nejadnik MR, et al. Universal applicator for digitally-controlled pressing force and impact velocity insertion of microneedles into skin. Pharmaceutics. 2018;10:211.

[84] van der Maaden K, Sekerdag E, Jiskoot W, et al. Impact-insertion applicator improves reliability of skin penetration by solid microneedle arrays. AAPS J. 2014;16:681.

[85] Nguyen HX, Banga AK. Microneedle-mediated delivery of vismodegib across skin. J Invest Dermatol. 2015;135:S58–S58.

[86] Ross S, Scoutaris N, Lamprou D, et al. Inkjet printing of insulin microneedles for transdermal delivery. Drug Deliv Transl Res. 2015;5:451–461.

[87] Ilić T, Savić S, Batinić B, et al. Combined use of biocompatible nanoemulsions and solid microneedles to improve transport of a model NSAID across the skin: in vitro and in vivo studies. Eur J Pharm Sci. 2018;125:110–119.

[88] Kalluri H, Kolli CS, Banga AK. Characterization of microchannels created by metal microneedles: formation and closure. AAPS J. 2011;13:473–481.

[89] Lee HS, Ryu HR, Roh JY, et al. Bleomycin-coated microneedles for treatment of warts. Pharm Res. 2017;34:101–112.

[90] Pawley DC, Goncalves S, Bas E, et al. Dexamethasone (DXM)-coated poly (lactic-co-glycolic acid)(PLGA) microneedles as an improved drug delivery system for intracochlear biodegradable devices. Adv Ther. 2021;4:2100155.

[91] Tort S, Mutlu Agardan NB, Han D, et al. In vitro and in vivo evaluation of microneedles coated with electrosprayed micro/nanoparticles for medical skin treatments. J Microencapsul. 2020;37:517–527.

[92] Chen M-C, Huang S-F, Lai K-Y, et al. Fully embeddable chitosan microneedles as a sustained release depot for intradermal vaccination. Biomaterials. 2013;34:3077–3086.

[93] Mönkäre J, Pontier M, van Kampen EEM, et al. Development of PLGA nanoparticle loaded dissolving microneedles and comparison with hollow microneedles in intradermal vaccine delivery. Eur J Pharm Biopharm. 2018;129:111–121.

[94] Resnik D, Možek M, Pečar B, et al. In vivo experimental study of noninvasive insulin microinjection through hollow Si microneedle array. Micromachines. 2018;9:40.

[95] Vinayakumar KB, Kulkarni PG, Nayak MM, et al. A hollow stainless steel microneedle array to deliver insulin to a diabetic rat. J Micromechanics Microengineering. 2016;26:065013.

[96] Pamornpathomkul B, Wongkajornsilp A, Laiwattanapaisal W, et al. A combined approach of hollow microneedles and nanocarriers for skin immunization with plasmid DNA encoding ovalbumin. Int J Nanomedicine. 2017;12:885.

[97] Davis SP, Martanto W, Allen MG, et al. Hollow metal microneedles for insulin delivery to diabetic rats. IEEE Trans Biomed Eng. 2005;52:909–915.

[98] Wang PM, Cornwell M, Hill J, et al. Precise microinjection into skin using hollow microneedles. J Invest Dermatol. 2006;126:1080–1087.

[99] Miller PR, Taylor RM, Tran BQ, et al. Extraction and biomolecular analysis of dermal interstitial fluid collected with hollow microneedles. Commun Biol. 2018;1:1–11.

[100] Li CG, Lee CY, Lee K, et al. An optimized hollow microneedle for minimally invasive blood extraction. Biomed Microdevices. 2013;15:17–25.

[101] Li CG, Dangol M, Lee CY, et al. A self-powered one-touch blood extraction system: a novel polymer-capped hollow microneedle integrated with a pre-vacuum actuator. Lab Chip. 2015;15:382–390.

[102] Lee B-M, Lee C, Lahiji SF, et al. Dissolving microneedles for rapid and painless local anesthesia. Pharmaceutics. 2020;12:366.

[103] Ronnander P, Simon L, Spilgies H, et al. Dissolving polyvinylpyrrolidone-based microneedle systems for in-vitro delivery of sumatriptan succinate. Eur J Pharm Sci. 2018;114:84–92.

[104] Yao G, Quan G, Lin S, et al. Novel dissolving microneedles for enhanced transdermal delivery of levonorgestrel: in vitro and in vivo characterization. Int J Pharm. 2017;534:378–386.

[105] Donnelly RF, McCrudden MT, Alkilani AZ, et al. Hydrogel-forming microneedles prepared from "super swelling" polymers combined with lyophilised wafers for transdermal drug delivery. PLoS One. 2014;9:e111547.

[106] Turner JG, White LR, Estrela P, et al. Hydrogel-forming microneedles: current advancements and future trends. Macromol Biosci. 2021;21:2000307.

11

Combination of Microneedles with Other Enhancement Techniques

11.1 Introduction

The promising platform given by skin microporation by microneedle devices has allowed researchers to investigate the skin as a viable path for drug delivery. According to the scientific literature, these micrometer-sized devices have been demonstrated to be remarkably successful in delivering a diverse range of drugs into and across the skin. There is no limit to how microneedles might be employed for drug delivery. Microneedles may be made in various shapes, sizes, and materials. Microneedles are available in various delivery techniques, allowing individualized treatment programs based on the patient's condition. Coated or dissolving microneedles that discharge the drug payload immediately upon application into the skin may be used to provide a bolus dose. Hollow microneedles can be employed for more than only taking blood samples for glucose testing; they can also be utilized to inject drug solutions into a certain skin depth. Modifying the needle's length allows for precise drug deposition into the desired skin depth. There is also the option of a controlled drug release and delivery. It is possible to alter the release profile of drugs delivered by microneedles by encapsulating them in polymeric materials having controlled release capabilities [1].

When microneedles are used in conjunction with other physical enhancement technologies, it could pave the way for a new avenue in drug delivery. Two complementary and synergistic methods, each with a unique mechanism of action, might enhance drug delivery and provide superior results to each technique alone. Microneedles have been studied in conjunction with a variety of delivery methods for molecules of varying molecular weight, including iontophoresis, ultrasound, and electroporation. The combined strategy has been successful in most previously reported investigations. Most of these studies, nevertheless, are in their infancy stages. At this moment, combining multiple physical enhancement methods seems feasible on a small laboratory scale. The continued endeavors to advance the development of a therapeutic product will be supported by the results of more research in the future. Prototype construction and preclinical findings collection should drive future research. The introduction of a microneedle product that has been authorized by the Food and Drug Administration (FDA) will encourage researchers to explore this topic further. Some preclinical research is essential to build credibility in these combinatorial strategies, and further consideration has to be given to product design, production processes, product safety, and regulatory requirements [1].

DOI: 10.1201/9780429294433-11

11.2 Combination of Microneedles with Physical Enhancement Technologies

11.2.1 Microneedles and Iontophoresis

For iontophoresis-mediated transdermal drug delivery, a physiologically tolerable electrical current (<0.5 mA/cm^2) is applied to the skin to facilitate the transport of charged and polar compounds through the skin barrier. Electromigration and electroosmosis are recognized as the primary drug delivery processes in iontophoresis. The electromigration of charged molecules in the presence of an electrical current is the essential mechanism for iontophoretic drug delivery. When the charged ions move, aqueous flow ensues, transporting the dissolved drugs over the skin through a process called electroosmosis. This noninvasive method has been applied in drug administration and clinical diagnostics [2]. It has been reported that the drug delivery rate through iontophoresis is directly correlated to the applied electrical current [3]. Bok et al. employed the combination of hyaluronic acid dissolving microneedles with sonophoresis and iontophoresis to enhance the efficiency of microneedles (Fig. 11.1) [4]. The risk of burns, irritation and local skin

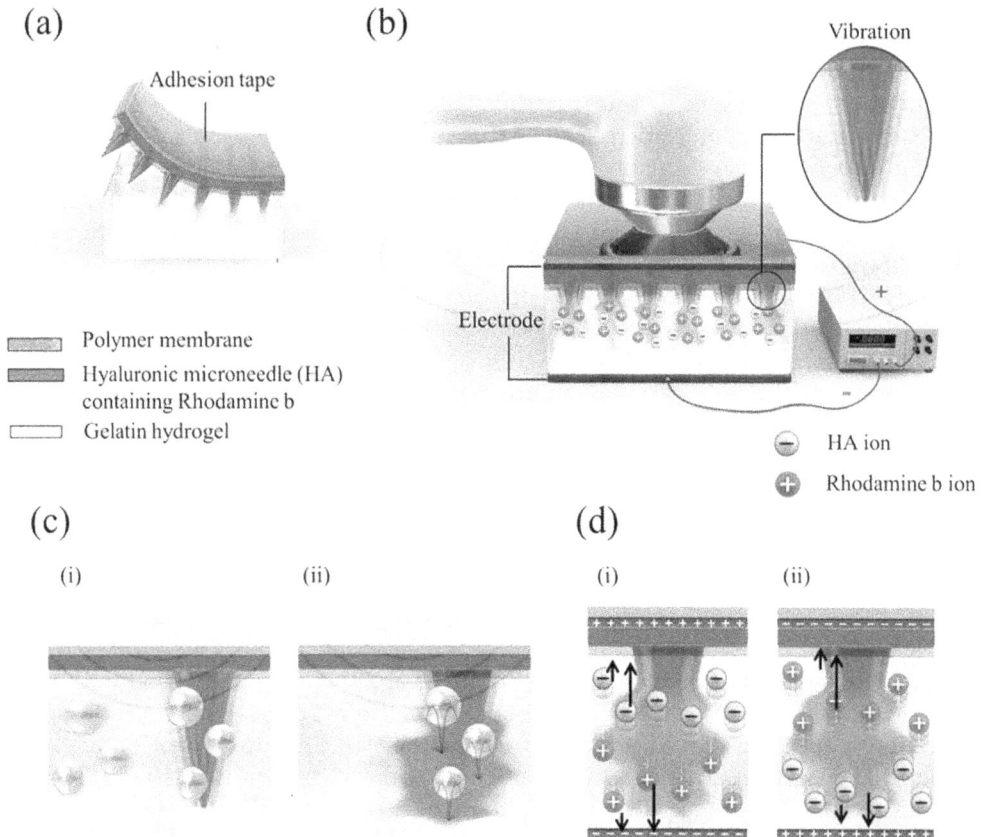

FIGURE 11.1
Schematic representation of (a) insertion of microneedles into gelatin hydrogel, (b) combination of microneedles and the ultrasonic and electric field in gelatin hydrogel, (c) microneedles dissolution under the ultrasonic field, and (d) microneedles dissolution and ion movement under the electric field. Images reprinted with permission from [4].

responses observed at high currents limits the applied current intensity to below 0.5mA/cm^2 [3, 5, 6]. Iontophoresis has several drawbacks, the most notable being that it can only transport molecules up to around 15 kDa in molecular weight [7–11].

Many researchers have studied how transdermal drug delivery is enhanced when iontophoresis is used in conjunction with microneedles. The combination of microneedles and iontophoresis has been noticed and shown to improve drug delivery [8, 9, 11–13]. This is because the former allows transporting a wider variety of molecules through the skin, while the latter increases drug delivery efficiency. Using an electrical driving force provided by iontophoresis, drug molecules could be pushed through the skin and into the microneedles-created channels in the skin. When iontophoresis is paired with the "poke and patch" method of solid microneedles, charged molecules are delivered at a substantially higher rate than they would be with either iontophoresis or microneedles alone [8, 11, 12, 14, 15]. Iontophoresis combined with microneedles causes a disturbance in the skin barrier, expanding the range of therapeutic agents that might be delivered to the skin. Also, by adjusting the intensity of the electric current, customized and precise drug delivery may be attained [16]. Due to this synergistic effect of iontophoresis and microneedles, undesired side effects, including tingling, burns, erythema, irritation, or discomfort caused by excessive electric exposure, will be minimized during drug delivery. The combination of microneedles and iontophoresis has been used to effectively and successfully enhance the transdermal delivery of various compounds such as insulin [12], fluorescein isothiocyanate-labeled bovine serum albumin [17], antisense oligonucleotide [15], high-molecular-weight fluorescent tagged dextran molecules [11], low-molecular-weight heparin [13], methotrexate [9], daniplestim [18], interferon α-2b [14], calcein, human growth hormone [19], salmon calcitonin [10], oligodeoxynucleotide ISIS 2302 [15], and others.

11.2.2 Microneedles and Sonophoresis

Sonophoresis, also known as phonophoresis, employs ultrasound energy to deliver therapeutic agents into the skin. Two methods have been suggested for delivering ultrasonic waves to the skin: (i) a skin pretreatment strategy, in which ultrasound is applied to the skin before the drug formulation application, and (ii) a simultaneous strategy, in which ultrasound is delivered to the skin via the drug-loaded coupling medium. Since concurrent administration of ultrasound and drug formulation may lead to drug degradation or induce other side effects, strategy (i) is more often adopted. Treatment duration, duty cycle, ultrasound transducer-to-skin distance, and coupling medium formulation are some variables that affect ultrasound-assisted drug delivery. This sonophoresis method utilizes ultrasound waves to generate temporary channels in the skin for drug administration [20]. It is hypothesized that the enhanced delivery is the result of temperature effects on the skin and mechanical impacts on the therapeutic agent (inertial cavitation, acoustic streaming, and the formation of convective velocities) [16].

An innovative and effective platform for transdermal drug delivery may be achieved by combining ultrasound and microneedles. When combined with microneedles, sonophoresis has increased the efficiency with which several drugs are delivered. Microporation, when combined with an ultrasonic driving force, may increase the range, quantity, and rate of transdermal drug delivery. In recent experiments, microneedles and ultrasound have been utilized together to improve the skin permeation of various macromolecules [21, 22]. Sonophoresis has attracted much attention as a method to enhance the transdermal delivery of hydrophilic compounds such as proteins and peptides [23]. The combination of microneedles and sonophoresis has been reported to effectively improve transdermal delivery of calcein and BSA [24] and glycerol [25]. Nevertheless, this field of study is only being initiated, and there is now just a modest amount of information accessible [1].

To puncture the skin and deliver ultrasound simultaneously, researchers may utilize hollow microneedles, which should be positioned underneath the ultrasonic field. Some skin permeability increases may be provided by increasing the flow rate through convection. Ultrasound cavitation may be used in conjunction with solid microneedles as well. The increased permeability may be achieved by the use of solid microneedles to create microchannels in the skin. High-intensity ultrasound applied to the microneedles-treated site will cause ultrasonic cavitation to generate superior skin permeability. This is an excellent strategy for sustained transdermal drug delivery, and it works particularly well for the transport of macromolecules. In addition, low-intensity ultrasound may be used in tandem with dissolving microneedles to generate the optimum thermal impact. Dissolving microneedles can penetrate the skin and release the drug load at a steady rate dependent on the surrounding temperature. Ultrasound may be used for precise local heating. The drug release kinetics may be altered by adjusting the local temperature. If this strategy can be optimized, it will improve drug delivery rates and allow for more precise dosing [26].

11.2.3 Microneedles and Near-infrared Light

Microneedles made of a polymer–nanostructure combination that responds to near-infrared light are an intriguing and potentially beneficial method to enhance and control transdermal drug delivery [27]. Lanthanum hexaboride (LaB6@SiO$_2$) nanostructures were integrated into polycaprolactone microneedles to absorb near-infrared light effectively. Microneedles exposed to NIR light melted at 50°C due to light-to-heat transmission facilitated by LaB6@SiO$_2$ nanostructures. One benefit of this method is that it allows for the external triggering of the drug release via near-infrared light [28].

11.2.4 Microneedles and Electroporation

Electroporation (also known as electropermeabilization) entails applying high-intensity electric field pulses (≥50V) for a particularly short time (milliseconds) to induce a transitory, localized disturbance in the stratum corneum, thereby forming temporary aqueous pathways through lipid bilayer membranes and thereby permeabilizing skin for enhanced drug delivery [29]. The resulting aqueous channels facilitate drug permeation through the disrupted stratum corneum layer. *In vitro* electroporation of stratum corneum was carried out using a transmembrane potential of up to 1 kV for 10–500 ms [30]. The application of high-voltage electric pulses improves electrophoretic mobility and molecular diffusivity by temporarily altering the stratum corneum. Some factors that might impact drug delivery include the waveform, rate, and the number of pulses. There is evidence that this method increases the transdermal delivery of drugs of varying sizes and lipophilicity. In the last several decades, this method has become standard practice for transporting genes, DNA, macromolecules, and other hydrophilic substances [16]. Small molecules, macromolecules (i.e., proteins, peptides, and oligonucleotides), and biomolecules may all be successfully delivered into the skin using electroporation [31].

The removal of electrodes in electroporation could be achieved by pairing them with microneedles, which acted as microelectrodes. Combined, they reinforce each other, allowing more drugs to pass through the skin [32]. Nevertheless, the synergistic impact of combining microneedles with electroporation to increase transdermal drug delivery is still not well-understood and researched [2]. The combination of microneedles and electroporation has increased the transdermal delivery of various molecules such as dextran [31], DNA [33], fluorescein isothiocyanate dextran [31], and smallpox DNA vaccine [34].

11.2.5 Microneedles and Gene Guns

Gene guns, also known as "particle bombardment" or "biolistic delivery" devices, are particle accelerators capable of propelling DNA-loaded microparticles to high enough velocities to penetrate deep into the target tissue and induce gene transfection therein. The depths of skin penetration obtained could be adjusted by modifying the gas pressure, gene gun type, particle size, velocity, and density [35]. Gene guns have been used to transfect cells with genes by penetrating muscle tissue and releasing microparticles encapsulated with deoxyribonucleic acid (DNA). Microparticles may penetrate deep into the epidermis, and their maximal depth of penetration can pass through the stratum corneum [36–38]. The epidermis layer is often recognized as the target area for gene transfer owing to its accessibility [36, 37, 39]. But because most gene guns need a high level of pressure to function, the impaction of the pressured gas on the skin might be potentially harmful to the tissue [35].

Lately, Zhang et al. suggested a novel strategy of microneedle-mediated microparticle delivery, in which microneedles are combined with a particle delivery system. The use of microneedles in conjunction with gene guns shows promise since this approach can lower the pressures required to operate the gene guns and hence lessen the risk of tissue or cell disruption. The microchannels created by solid microneedles offer a favorable setting for the penetration of fast-moving microparticles into the skin tissue. Because the channels provide a low-resistance route for microparticle penetration, their penetration depths are superior to those achieved with a needle-free biolistic microparticle delivery system [35].

11.2.6 Microneedles and Vesicles

Over the last decade, researchers have investigated the potential of nanoparticles and microparticles as drug-delivery vehicles. The size, physical, and chemical characteristics of these systems differ from their materials, which may range from lipids and carbohydrates to polymers [40]. The advantages of particulate systems over traditional administration methods include sustained drug release, site-specific action via targeted delivery, and increased bioavailability [40–42]. Particulate systems for vaccination may be beneficial because of their intrinsic immunogenic qualities, as shown by various research works [43]. As an attractive feature, they prevent the antigen from degrading and may stabilize it [44–46]. They are also capable of delivering the encapsulated vaccine at a controlled release rate, should that be required. The efficacy might be affected by a number of variables, such as the physical and chemical characteristics of the antigen or particle structure and properties. There have been a number of published research on the topic of using lipid vesicles for transdermal drug delivery. Nevertheless, these systems are mired in controversy due to their mechanism, in which the accumulation of the drug-encapsulated particles in the stratum corneum hinders their penetration into deeper skin layers for effective transdermal delivery.

Increased transdermal drug delivery may be achievable when microneedles are used in combination with these vesicular systems. Liposomes may be deposited at various depths into the skin, dependent on the dimensions, geometries, and loading of the microneedles used. Vesicles may be delivered to the outermost layer of skin (the stratum corneum) using shorter microneedles, or they can be deposited deeply in underlying skin layers using longer microneedles [32]. Microchannels formed by the microneedles have been found to be significantly large to facilitate the unobstructed movement of drug-loaded vesicles into the skin, thus considerably improving transdermal drug delivery. Even large microparticles may be transported into the skin with the assistance of suitable microneedle design and insertion procedures. The integration of vesicles and microneedles into a single vaccine delivery system has enormous potential. This strategy shows a lot of promise due to the benefits of particle formulations, such as antigen stability, depot release, and the capacity to stimulate an immune response. More research into formulation development and microneedle production is required to make this a practical method for administering vaccines [1]. Transdermal delivery of numerous molecules has been enhanced using this combinatorial strategy, such as lipophilic fluorescent compound, docetaxel [47], mannitol [48], calcein, insulin, BSA [49], fluorescein isothiocyanate-tagged nanoparticles, coumarin 6 [50], and insulin [12, 51, 52].

11.2.7 Microneedles and Actuation

Inserting a microneedle array into the skin requires precise control of application force, which must be kept below the microneedle's fracturing force. For the microneedles to be effective, there must be a fair balance between their dimensions and structural integrity. The application force of microneedles may be decreased by using a vibration actuation in conjunction with microneedles. The influence of vibratory actuation on the insertion force of microneedles was investigated, and a 70% decrease in the insertion force was achieved [53]. This combinatorial approach was used in a study where the application of vibration actuation facilitated the insertion of microneedles made from metals and polymers with a low value of Young's modulus.

11.2.8 Microneedles and Micropumps

The combination of microneedles and micropumps provides accurate, controlled drug administration since the pumps govern the fluid flow rate and pressure necessary for administering the drug solution. To manage fluid extraction for diagnostic testing and administer the medication according to metabolite amounts, this combinatorial approach was used to build an integrated system containing microvalves and micropumps [54].

11.3 Conclusions

Microneedles have been the subject of several scientific investigations, and the results have demonstrated that they have great promise as transdermal delivery methods. Their primary advantages over traditional delivery methods are that they are safe, simple, convenient, and noninvasive; hence, they have garnered a lot of attention recently. Because of the success of microneedles in penetrating the stratum corneum, a wide variety of medications are now amenable to transdermal and intradermal delivery [32]. A lot of effort has been put into developing new techniques and investigating the potential uses of microneedles. Microneedles have various applications in phlebotomy, diagnostics, and cosmeceuticals, in addition to their central position in the delivery of several pharmaceutical molecules, particularly small molecules, macromolecules, and biopharmaceuticals.

Recent efforts have focused on integrating microneedles with other physical enhancement technologies, which may further expand the range of substances that can be administered transdermally, even though microneedles themselves have demonstrated to be successful in delivering molecules throughout a broad molecular weight range. In most situations, the findings indicate a synergistic impact, which is promising. Integrating microneedles with various physical techniques allows fine-grained control of the drug release kinetics. The use of hollow microneedle-based electrodes to facilitate drug delivery by electroporation has been the subject of only a small number of published studies. Protecting therapeutic agents by placing them in a particulate system might also lead to an extended and controlled drug release. Increased transdermal flux and significantly shorter lag time are achieved when vesicles and microneedles are used together. Interest in combinatorial strategies, which dramatically improve skin permeability, is considerable. With the greatest potential for scientific investigation, ultrasound paired with microneedles has been rapidly evolving over the last decade, and more studies are expected to be undertaken in the future if the present trend holds. The greatest contribution is currently shown by the conjunction of iontophoresis and electroporation with microneedles, indicating that this is the area where most combinational investigations are centered [26]. Controlled drug delivery may be achieved by combining microneedles with particulate systems such as nanoparticles, microparticles, etc. Combining microneedles with micropumps has allowed for precise drug administration. Conclusively, the synergistic impact of integrating microneedles with other physical enhancement techniques has been demonstrated to more effectively deliver drugs and other therapeutic agents into and across the skin.

References

[1] Stoeber B, Sivamani RK, Maibach HI. Microneedling in clinical practice. Boca Raton, Florida: CRC Press; 2020.

[2] G Nava-Arzaluz M, Calderon-Lojero I, Quintanar-Guerrero D, et al. Microneedles as transdermal delivery systems: combination with other enhancing strategies. Curr Drug Deliv. 2012;9:57–73.

[3] Kalia YN, Naik A, Garrison J, et al. Iontophoretic drug delivery. Adv Drug Deliv Rev. 2004;56:619–658.

[4] Bok M, Zhao Z-J, Jeon S, et al. Ultrasonically and iontophoretically enhanced drug-delivery system based on dissolving microneedle patches. Sci Rep. 2020;10:2027.

[5] Batheja P, Priya B, Thakur R, et al. Transdermal iontophoresis. Expert Opin Drug Deliv. 2006;3:127–138.

[6] Guy RH, Kalia YN, Delgado-Charro MB, et al. Iontophoresis: electrorepulsion and electroosmosis. J Control Release. 2000;64:129–132.

[7] Cázares-Delgadillo J, Naik A, Ganem-Rondero A, et al. Transdermal delivery of cytochrome C—A 12.4 kDa protein—across intact skin by constant–current iontophoresis. Pharm Res. 2007;24:1360–1368.

[8] Katikaneni S, Badkar A, Nema S, et al. Molecular charge mediated transport of a 13 kD protein across microporated skin. Int J Pharm. 2009;378:93–100.

[9] Vemulapalli V, Yang Y, Friden PM, et al. Synergistic effect of iontophoresis and soluble microneedles for transdermal delivery of methotrexate. J Pharm Pharmacol. 2008;60:27–33.

[10] Vemulapalli V, Bai Y, Kalluri H, et al. In vivo iontophoretic delivery of salmon calcitonin across microporated skin. J Pharm Sci. 2012;101:2861–2869.

[11] Wu X-M, Todo H, Sugibayashi K. Enhancement of skin permeation of high molecular compounds by a combination of microneedle pretreatment and iontophoresis. J Control Release. 2007;118:189–195.

[12] Chen H, Zhu H, Zheng J, et al. Iontophoresis-driven penetration of nanovesicles through microneedle-induced skin microchannels for enhancing transdermal delivery of insulin. J Control Release. 2009;139:63–72.

[13] Lanke SSS, Kolli CS, Strom JG, et al. Enhanced transdermal delivery of low molecular weight heparin by barrier perturbation. Int J Pharm. 2009;365:26–33.

[14] Badkar AV, Smith AM, Eppstein JA, et al. Transdermal delivery of interferon alpha-2B using microporation and iontophoresis in hairless rats. Pharm Res. 2007;24:1389–1395.

[15] Lin W, Cormier M, Samiee A, et al. Transdermal delivery of antisense oligonucleotides with microprojection patch (Macroflux®) technology. Pharm Res. 2001;18:1789–1793.

[16] Prausnitz MR, Langer R. Transdermal drug delivery. Nat Biotechnol. 2008;26:1261–1268.

[17] Garland MJ, Caffarel-Salvador E, Migalska K, et al. Dissolving polymeric microneedle arrays for electrically assisted transdermal drug delivery. J Control Release. 2012;159:52–59.

[18] Katikaneni S, Li G, Badkar A, et al. Transdermal delivery of a approximately 13 kDa protein-an in vivo comparison of physical enhancement methods. J Drug Target. 2010;18:141–147.

[19] Kumar V, Banga AK. Modulated iontophoretic delivery of small and large molecules through microchannels. Int J Pharm. 2012;434:106–114.

[20] Sachdeva VK, Banga A. Microneedles and their applications. Recent Pat Drug Deliv Formul. 2011;5:95–132.

[21] Han T, Das DB. Permeability enhancement for transdermal delivery of large molecule using low-frequency sonophoresis combined with microneedles. J Pharm Sci. 2013;102:3614–3622.

[22] Nayak A, Babla H, Han T, et al. Lidocaine carboxymethylcellulose with gelatine co-polymer hydrogel delivery by combined microneedle and ultrasound. Drug Deliv. 2016;23:658–669.

[23] Rao R, Nanda S. Sonophoresis: recent advancements and future trends. J Pharm Pharmacol. 2009;61:689–705.

[24] Chen B, Wei J, Iliescu C. Sonophoretic enhanced microneedles array (SEMA)—Improving the efficiency of transdermal drug delivery. Sens Actuators B Chem. 2010;145:54–60.

[25] Yoon J, Park D, Son T, et al. A physical method to enhance transdermal delivery of a tissue optical clearing agent: combination of microneedling and sonophoresis. Lasers Surg Med. 2010;42:412–417.

[26] Han T, Das DB. Potential of combined ultrasound and microneedles for enhanced transdermal drug permeation: a review. Eur J Pharm Biopharm. 2015;89:312–328.

[27] Chen M-C, Ling M-H, Wang K-W, et al. Near-infrared light-responsive composite microneedles for on-demand transdermal drug delivery. Biomacromolecules. 2015;16:1598–1607.

[28] Ita K. Transdermal delivery of drugs with microneedles-potential and challenges. Pharmaceutics. 2015;7:90–105.

[29] Singh TR, Garland MJ, Cassidy CM, et al. Microporation techniques for enhanced delivery of therapeutic agents. Recent Pat Drug Deliv Formul. 2010;4:1–17.

[30] Naik A, Kalia YN, Guy RH. Transdermal drug delivery: overcoming the skin's barrier function. Pharm Sci Technol Today. 2000;3:318–326.

[31] Yan K, Todo H, Sugibayashi K. Transdermal drug delivery by in-skin electroporation using a microneedle array. Int J Pharm. 2010;397:77–83.

[32] Nayak S, Suryawanshi S, Bhaskar V. Microneedle technology for transdermal drug delivery: applications and combination with other enhancing techniques. J Drug Deliv Ther. 2016;6:65–83.

[33] Daugimont L, Baron N, Vandermeulen G, et al. Hollow microneedle arrays for intradermal drug delivery and DNA electroporation. J Membr Biol. 2010;236:117–125.

[34] Hooper JW, Golden JW, Ferro AM, et al. Smallpox DNA vaccine delivered by novel skin electroporation device protects mice against intranasal poxvirus challenge. Vaccine. 2007;25:1814–1823.

[35] Zhang D, Das DB, Rielly CD. Potential of microneedle-assisted micro-particle delivery by gene guns: a review. Drug Deliv. 2014;21:571–587.

[36] Liu Y, Kendall MAF. Numerical simulation of heat transfer from a transonic jet impinging on skin for needle-free powdered drug and vaccine delivery. Proc Inst Mech Eng Part C J Mech Eng Sci. 2004;218:1373–1383.

[37] Quinlan NJ, Kendall MAF, Bellhouse BJ, et al. Investigations of gas and particle dynamics in first generation needle-free drug delivery devices. Shock Waves. 2001;10:395–404.

[38] Yager EJ, Stagnar C, Gopalakrishnan R, et al. Optimizing particle-mediated epidermal delivery of an influenza DNA vaccine in ferrets. In: Biolistic DNA delivery. New York, New York: Springer; 2013. p. 223–237.

[39] Soliman SM. Micro-particles and gas dynamics in an Axi-symmetric supersonic nozzle. Ohio: University of Cincinnati; 2011.

[40] Prow TW, Grice JE, Lin LL, et al. Nanoparticles and microparticles for skin drug delivery. Adv Drug Deliv Rev. 2011;63:470–491.

[41] Donnelly RF, Singh TRR, Morrow DI, et al. Microneedle-mediated transdermal and intradermal drug delivery. New Jersey: John Wiley & Sons; 2012.

[42] Patravale V, Dandekar P, Jain R. Nanoparticulate drug delivery: perspectives on the transition from laboratory to market. Amsterdam, NL: Elsevier; 2012.

[43] Storni T, Kündig TM, Senti G, et al. Immunity in response to particulate antigen-delivery systems. Adv Drug Deliv Rev. 2005;57:333–355.

[44] Gutierro I, Hernandez RM, Igartua M, et al. Size dependent immune response after subcutaneous, oral and intranasal administration of BSA loaded nanospheres. Vaccine. 2002;21:67–77.

[45] Jaganathan KS, Vyas SP. Strong systemic and mucosal immune responses to surface-modified PLGA microspheres containing recombinant hepatitis B antigen administered intranasally. Vaccine. 2006;24:4201–4211.

[46] Mahapatro A, Singh DK. Biodegradable nanoparticles are excellent vehicle for site directed in-vivo delivery of drugs and vaccines. J Nanobiotechnology. 2011;9:1–11.

[47] Qiu Y, Gao Y, Hu K, et al. Enhancement of skin permeation of docetaxel: a novel approach combining microneedle and elastic liposomes. J Control Release. 2008;129:144–150.

[48] Badran MM, Kuntsche J, Fahr A. Skin penetration enhancement by a microneedle device (Dermaroller®) in vitro: dependency on needle size and applied formulation. Eur J Pharm Sci. 2009;36:511–523.

[49] McAllister DV, Wang PM, Davis SP, et al. Microfabricated needles for transdermal delivery of macromolecules and nanoparticles: fabrication methods and transport studies. Proc Natl Acad Sci. 2003;100:13755–13760.

[50] Zhang W, Gao J, Zhu Q, et al. Penetration and distribution of PLGA nanoparticles in the human skin treated with microneedles. Int J Pharm. 2010;402:205–212.

[51] Ito Y, Hagiwara E, Saeki A, et al. Sustained-release self-dissolving micropiles for percutaneous absorption of insulin in mice. J Drug Target. 2007;15:323–326.

[52] Yu J, Zhang Y, Ye Y, et al. Microneedle-array patches loaded with hypoxia-sensitive vesicles provide fast glucose-responsive insulin delivery. Proc Natl Acad Sci. 2015;112:8260–8265.

[53] Yang M, Zahn JD. Microneedle insertion force reduction using vibratory actuation. Biomed Microdevices. 2004;6:177–182.

[54] Zahn JD, Pisano AP, Liepmann D. Continuous on-chip micropumping for microneedle enhanced drug delivery. Biomed Microdevices. 2004;6:183–190.

12

Microneedles in Diagnostic

12.1 Microneedles for Interstitial Skin Fluid Sampling

Novel diagnostic technologies that can promptly, sensitively, and correctly identify and monitor significant conditions of societal concern are essential for efficient healthcare administration. While there is a lot of research demonstrating microneedles technology's capacity to improve transdermal drug delivery, in the last five years, this technology has also been utilized to collect and process information from interstitial skin fluid (ISF) and serve as a noninvasive technique of health monitoring. Individualized diagnostics and point-of-care (POC) testing would benefit significantly from skin monitoring of targeted substances utilizing the microneedles technology [1]. Individualized diagnostics and point-of-care testing would benefit greatly from skin monitoring of targeted substances using the microneedles technology. There has been a significant increase in research on the viability of employing microneedles as sampling devices. The sampling of ISF and blood has been explored with the use of microneedles [2]. Although a few investigations have established proof of concept for employing microneedles to collect interstitial fluid or blood from human subjects without substantial discomfort, a completely integrated system has not yet been shown *in vitro* or *in vivo*, much alone brought to market [3, 4]. Measurements and monitoring of the levels of glucose, hemoglobin, critical ions, cholesterol, bilirubin, metabolic enzymes, heparin, hormones, gases, pH, alcohol, narcotics, nicotine metabolites, proteins, toxins, and other analyzable substances in the blood and ISF could be markedly helpful. Diseases are correctly diagnosed based on these clinically relevant analytes. As ISF is rich in relevant biomarkers, including K^+ and Na^+ ions, nitrogen oxides, and glucose, the assessment may be as accurate as that of blood [5].

The composition of ISF and blood vary in response to different disorders. Analyte levels in ISF may serve as a measure of health condition [6]. Owing to several noted risks associated with blood testing, it may be preferable to monitor patients using biomarkers contained within ISF rather than whole blood. But whole blood may frequently provide more information about the situation when utilized for quantitative examination of analyte levels. Since hydrostatic and osmotic forces govern the flow of solutes from blood to the ISF, it has been revealed that the levels of small molecules, electrolytes, and proteins in the ISF strongly correlate with those of plasma [7–9]. Furthermore, the benefit of ISF over blood sampling is a significant decrease in the desired penetration depth, from 400–900 to 50–150 μm, which may lead to reduced pain or skin reactions [10]. Although several biomarkers could be collected from the epidermis, their quantities are believed to be significantly greater in the dermis layer, where blood capillaries are located. Therefore, microneedles penetrating deeper skin layers should be in contact with a higher level of biomarkers, possibly allowing for the identification of biomarkers at low concentrations [11]. It

DOI: 10.1201/9780429294433-12

was shown that the diagnostic capacity of microneedles is strongly correlated to the penetration depth of microneedles into the skin and the application duration. Notably, several drugs have been shown to have a delayed effect on ISF levels as they first migrate to and establish equilibrium in different body parts [12].

The use of microneedles has not only demonstrated the potential for a painless sampling of ISF but also manipulation of the technique for full blood sampling. Alterations in microneedles geometry, dimensions, and construction material have been proposed to adapt the system for use with either ISF or blood [2]. Take the impact of the depth at which microneedles are inserted into the skin as an instance: studies have revealed that ISF may be sampled at penetration depths as shallow as 50–150 μm, while blood can be sampled at microneedle penetration depths of up to 1,000–2,000 μm [13–15]. Since microneedles cause less pain and skin irritation than conventional needles, they are well-accepted by patients, allowing for convenient and continuous health monitoring [16]. Combining microneedles with specific analytical methods allows for the quantitative measurement of parameters of clinical significance [17]. Therefore, the application of microneedles for ISF sampling is an advanced method for noninvasively analyzing a wide range of health-associated factors by penetrating the stratum corneum layer without triggering the stimulation of nerve fibers for pain sensation. Effective detection of a shift in glycemic levels, accompanied by insulin administration within 20 min, was possible with a microneedles-based vacuum pump-assisted ISF device. As a promising alternative to more intrusive methods like the suction-blister technique and micropipette insert, microneedles have been used for disease detection and metabolic analysis due to their capacity to collect ISF [18, 19]. Since the ISF's composition is comparable to the plasma, it is conceivable that component alterations in the ISF may serve as proxies for any corresponding changes in the body [20, 21]. Without causing discomfort, targeted molecules in the epidermis and dermis may be detected and monitored using microneedle systems. Microneedles can, crucially, be applied by users or patients without the requirement of trained healthcare professionals [22]. Although microneedle application for diagnostic purposes has been around for quite some time now for their usage in fields like glucose level assessment and monitoring, their utilization in the evolving field of infectious disease diagnosis appears promising. Recent years have noticed incredible advancements in microneedle diagnostic technologies, which have been driven by developments in associated technology.

However, some concerns about microneedles-based ISF sampling have been noted. Long-term or recurring ISF or blood sampling is necessary for effective health monitoring. What long-term use of microneedles devices will impact the skin physiologically is a major question mark. Once microneedles puncture the stratum corneum, the body's natural wound-healing mechanism is stimulated. Surprisingly, they are correlated with improved local blood flow and cytokine recruitment, which in turn alters the level of biomarkers in the skin [23]. Microneedles should indeed be left in place for a sufficient duration to allow for appropriate binding with targeted biomarkers, but the sampling period should be kept to a minimum to prevent changes to the ISF composition brought on by wound healing [24].

In general, the collected ISF samples still need purification to identify the analyte of interest before the analysis. One potential benefit is that the analysis might be conducted using the already-existing analytical instrument, making its widespread implementation less of a challenge. However, it will need experienced employees and centralized analysis resources, which might slow down the diagnostic process. A lab-on-a-chip microneedle diagnostic system with built-in analytics is preferred to facilitate the decentralization of the analytical process. Microneedle systems with inbuilt colorimetric analytical tools hold great promise as a rapid, cheap, and convenient method for detecting a wide variety of metabolites. This has already been verified for a few common molecules like glucose and cholesterol.

Several researchers have called for more control over the volume of extracted fluid, arguing that passive diffusion was unable to extract enough fluid at a user-acceptable rate or in significant quantities to provide reliable measurement of the targeted analytes. This obstacle has been addressed by the use of a vacuum to facilitate the removal of ISF and whole blood [25]. Many other techniques for fluid sampling have been developed.

The quantity obtained for analysis is crucial when sampling ISF using microneedles due to their miniature size and the properties of ISF, which preclude the collection of significant quantities [26]. The manual removal of ISF with solid microneedles provides an increased sample volume (up to 10 μL) that may be sent out for further testing. Low-volume studies benefit from the more complicated detecting systems found in hollow microneedles, which are typically used to sample quantities of less than 1 μL. Microneedles made from swelling hydrogel-forming materials are often only capable of sampling ISF volumes of 1–2 μL, which must be removed and evaluated externally. Unless integrated sensing systems are included in microneedles structure or materials with increased fluid-absorbing capabilities are employed, these microneedles may be limited in scenarios where low abundant analytes are evaluated, such as in therapeutic drug monitoring [24]. Large sample quantities are necessary for most modern lab-based analytical methods or commercially accessible testing kits [27]. Extending the microneedle length and penetration to collect greater volumes directly from deeper tissues is technically achievable but does so at the expense of the technique's minimal invasiveness and self-administration.

12.2 Conventional Therapeutic Monitoring

The assessment of drug or endogenous substance levels in a patient's ISF or blood is beneficial for doctors in making diagnoses and fine-tuning treatments [2]. The following are some medical situations in which therapeutic monitoring is frequently employed:

- Acute and chronic diseases require urgent medical attention.
- Identify infectious diseases and cancers.
- For therapeutic agents with a narrow therapeutic window to avoid suboptimal dosing or possible toxicity.
- When clinical response may be lacking due to pharmacodynamic variability.
- As there are significant individual differences in pharmacokinetic profile, it is necessary to tailor therapy to each patient.
- More stringent drug-level monitoring is required for particularly susceptible patient groups.
- Track the compliance of patients with long-term treatments

Needle-based blood sampling is commonly used for laboratory tests due to its high efficiency and cheap cost. This invasive method generally uses hypodermic needles or lancets. Nevertheless, these invasive and laborious techniques have several significant drawbacks, including the pain and bleeding they cause to the patients, the necessity for a relatively large quantity of samples, the requirement for trained medical personnel, and the creation of sharp waste [3, 28]. Underneath the glitz and glamour, however, lie persistent issues, such as the widespread practice of reusing needles that have not been properly disinfected, which poses a significant hazard to the spread of blood-borne diseases. Hypodermic needles and syringes provide unique challenges for self-administration at home by inexperienced patients due to concerns about patient safety and the disposal of potentially hazardous medical waste. Pain and discomfort from puncture wounds may occur with regular use of even the most user-friendly blood glucose monitor [29].

The disadvantages of conventional therapeutic monitoring are noted as follows:

- Expensive cost of required instrument for analysis and trained medical personnel
- Laborious procedure
- Use of invasive hypodermic needles
- Risk of infection

There is a compelling demand for the creation of noninvasive or minimally invasive procedures that would be more well-tolerated and accepted by patients and enable speedy testing without the need to collect blood. The identification of illegal drugs in addicts or drivers, as well as the improvement of disease management, prompt identification of alarmingly high or low drug concentrations, and monitoring of compliance with prescribed treatment schedules, all would result from this [2].

12.3 Microneedle Sensors

Microneedles have been employed as a sensor for critical therapeutic signals. Electrolytes account for an electric potential in the ISF of the epidermis, which is related to the functioning of electronically controlled tissues like the heart and muscle tissues. Biosignals may be monitored by the assessment of this electric potential. A combination of microneedles with wearable point-of-care testing has great potential for facilitating the monitoring and sampling process on patients and delivering precise information on biomarker, drug, or analyte levels in a short period. Treatment results for patients will undoubtedly benefit from this. With the substantial financial motive and the potential to improve patient care, industry partners in the medical devices and sensor fields are expected to go forward with research and development [12].

Though most studies so far have focused on collecting ISF or blood for analyte identification and measurement, a few studies have described microneedles as electrodes or sensors for measuring biological electrical signals. Since microneedles can be inserted effortlessly into the skin, they might be used as *in situ* sensing devices to provide the point-of-care assessment. Applying an electrochemical coating on the microneedles is one way to equip them with an electric function. Several designs have been developed and patented to analyze the obtained sample concurrently utilizing sensor systems, including hollow or other types of microneedles for collecting blood, lymph, or ISF samples. A novel technique has evolved for measuring analyte levels inside the skin (*in situ*) utilizing microneedles. This method involves functionalizing the needles' surfaces, typically by attaching an immobilized enzyme. A redox reaction may occur at the needle's surface following interaction with the targeted analytes. This way, the microneedles' surfaces could serve as electrodes, producing an electrical signal whose strength is directly proportional to the analyte quantity [24]. Microneedle-based electrochemical sensors can assess and monitor biomarkers, metabolites, drug release, and other properties of the ISF [30]. Notable, efficient recovery is often required if the microneedles system is used to collect bodily fluids, necessitating subsequent off-line examination in a laboratory setting. Microneedles may have electrodes integrated into their structure, or they can be designed to function as electrodes directly by the use of electrically conductive materials in their construction. Coating, mixing, or covalent bonding may be used to fix the sensing agents on microneedles. As the chemical reaction occurs, it may be exploited to generate an electrical signal that can be read by a detector [30–32]. Microsensors, microheaters, and other related sensing devices may be incorporated directly into the microneedle system, opening up new possibilities for its usage as a diagnostic tool. Consequently, physiological monitoring systems, biological detection, electroencephalographs, and brain wave monitoring devices can benefit from the application of microneedle arrays with appropriately integrated microelectronics components [33]. Since microneedles may penetrate to a depth of about 1 mm into skin tissue, they can access the blood and ISF, which are typically the desired target of the biosensing system. Except in cases when a disposable sensor is required, having a sensor that could be used more than once and provides precise readings for the analytes of relevance would be ideal in a sensing device. An array of miniaturizable analytical techniques might serve as the basis of a sensor [34]. Integration of data collecting, processing, and readout components into the structure of microneedle sensing systems might have significant long-term and societal benefits for patients. To be fully functional, microneedle biosensors need to be designed with certain factors in mind. These factors include ease of production, compactness, low cost, and sufficient reliability [29]. Microneedles, which are frequently employed to administer therapeutic agents, may also be used to administer diagnostic chemicals in a targeted and painless way. Various microneedle types (i.e., hollow, coated, and dissolving microneedles) have been studied for use in this context as potential vehicles for administering various diagnostic agents. Electrodes in an electrochemical cell can be built as solid microneedles, whereas hollow microneedles are utilized to collect and route bodily fluids to the electrodes [22]. These methods have primarily been investigated to monitor small molecules such as glucose, lactate, uric acid, nitric oxide, ascorbic acid, cholesterol, and levodopa [3, 16].

The level of sensitivity offered by microneedle sensors is crucial. Increasing the electroactive surface area and the electron transfer rate is a common strategy for enhancing sensitivity. The materials used in the microneedles should be able to either conduct electricity or react electrochemically. Solid microneedles made of silicon or glass with a metal coating have been used to construct electrodes for biopotential sensing. Numerous factors, including the design, dimensions, and geometry of microneedles, the functionality of the sensor, the effective incorporation of the two components into the same system, adequate contact between the sensor and the skin, and patient compliance, are crucial to the success of such microneedles-based sensing systems [33]. Remarkably, self-disabling microneedles that become soft upon absorption of skin ISF would be ideal for monitoring and diagnostic applications since they would prevent the spread of infection and needlestick injuries and complicate sharp waste disposal [2].

12.3.1 Advantages of Microneedles-based Sensors

Significant interest has lately been shown in microneedle systems for bodily fluid sampling and biomarker monitoring using colorimetric reactions. This is because these systems eliminate the requirement for sophisticated laboratory instruments and can eventually be used for self-diagnosis in the comfort of one's home setting [35–37]. For a successful detection of analytes in ISF, the microneedles-based ISF sampling must collect a minimum of a few picoliters of skin fluid [38, 39], while a microneedles-based sensor system advantageously can access plenty of biofluids beneath the skin's surface. Microneedles are considered suitable biosensing devices for monitoring diverse analytes such as macromolecules, metabolites, and pharmaceuticals. In addition, this innovative tool is bringing to light ISF as a repository of biomarkers for POC testing, a source that has been largely disregarded in the past. Particularly in dermatological diseases, ISF includes several biomarkers not present in blood [40, 41] or that are more abundant in ISF than in blood [29]. Microneedle devices may be used to collect just the analytes of interest from the skin, with no noticeable loss of biofluid. When compared to biofluid extraction, the necessity for sample purification is avoided using this microneedles technology. Microneedles provide several benefits over traditional wet and dry electrodes for measuring biopotentials. The primary benefit is not having to use conductive gels or abrade the skin to make contact with the skin. It is evident that the gel application may induce edema, skin reactions, and evaporation with time, restricting its application for continuous monitoring; nevertheless, the skin abrasion is laborious and unpleasant for the patients [42]. Furthermore, microneedles-based sensors do not require as much skin area for application because of their diminutive size. Microneedles show promise as a point-of-care technology for continuous biosignal assessment due to their quick implementation, user-friendliness, and lack of need for trained professionals. To be extensively incorporated into clinical settings, microneedle sensors must be capable of functioning reliably over long periods, and their manufacture has to be inexpensive. Due to the unique structures that can be readily generated by adjusting the manufacturing settings, this cutting-edge microneedles technology is highly desirable for diagnostic applications. Recent advances in microneedles-based electrochemical biosensors indicate that this flexible and inexpensive technology will form the backbone of the forthcoming generation of products that will capture sizable chunks of the market in the fields of clinical diagnostics [30]. Potentially, microneedles-based sensing function might lessen demands on healthcare providers and facilities, enhance the effectiveness of treatment, and encourage patients to adhere to their doctors' orders. Researchers are increasingly interested in microneedles-based POC testings because of its incredible potential for noninvasive detection of a wide range of analytes. The detecting capabilities of microneedles have recently been enhanced by an innovative synergy between microneedles and wearable technology [29].

12.3.2 Concerns of Microneedles-based Sensors

There are still barriers to be overcome when conducting biosensing with microneedles; hence new approaches to their design are required. The use of microneedles in monitoring and diagnosis will likely result in their classification as medical devices [2]. Sterilization is a heavily debated topic in the field of drug delivery using microneedles. Still, authorities have not confirmed whether or not sterility is required for these microneedles systems [43]. Microneedles products are getting closer to approval; thus, regulatory obstacles like sterility or low bioburden manufacturing has to be addressed [44].

It has been proposed that microneedles will not significantly contaminate the skin due to negligible microbial penetration via microneedles-created microchannels. Since the interstitial skin fluid fills the microchannels, the skin-colonizing bacteria may be more likely to persist on the skin's outermost stratum corneum layer. Furthermore, the skin is a strongly immunocompetent tissue, with a plethora of immune cells capable of engulfing and detecting invading microorganisms before they can cause an infection [45]. The skin's nonimmune enzymes may also aid in the defense against pathogenic microorganisms. Besides, transferring from the laboratory to the users involves understanding sterilization and waste disposal. Misuse and improper disposal nevertheless carry the risk of infection, even with minimally invasive skin disruption [46, 47]. Manufacturers must either (i) include a disinfectant in the microneedle package, (ii) apply a self-sterilizing coating onto the microneedles, or (iii) investigate a secondary housing for removing or impairing microneedles after usage to reduce the risk of infection [48, 49].

Furthermore, it is recommended that inert or biocompatible materials be favored for microneedle device manufacturing despite a minor compromise in analytical performance [30]. Microneedles' ability to absorb bodily fluids is also being actively researched by developing novel and appropriate materials. Critical progress will be made with the fabrication of microneedles that can capture and monitor molecules from bodily fluids. The electrical conductivity to amplify the signal, and the protective measures of the bioprobe, both of which are essential in biomarker detection, are two more major challenges to resolve [50]. Furthermore, biofouling at the tissue–device contact must be resolved before a microneedles-based *in situ* sensing device can be constructed [51].

To enhance the efficacy of transdermal sensing devices, the device must have sufficient stretchability and flexibility to ensure a conformal interface between the device and the skin. The device's flexibility and deformability allow for the elimination of local detachment and gaps between the device and the skin caused by the curvilinear structure of the skin and the body's motions [52]. Sensing devices monitor physiological, electrophysiological, and biochemical signals from the skin and benefit significantly from the precision afforded by conformal contact because of the reduced motion-related interference. Hence, conformally affixed biosensors allow for accurate real-time detection of a physiological indicator without impeding the user's freedom of movement. Moreover, as adequate extraction of bodily fluids needs a prolonged period, sufficient device-skin adhesion might be required in the present designs. The efficiency of skin extraction may be diminished if the microneedles on a patch loosen from their physical adhesion and fall off.

Moreover, the majority of studies using microneedle biosensors were performed on animals (i.e., mice, rats, and rabbits). Microneedles may need modifications to their dimensions and geometries to accommodate the unique anatomical and physiological properties of human skin before they can be successfully applied to humans. Besides, short-term and long-term patient safety concerns may be distinguished among the complications. It is widely accepted that using microneedles for a limited time will not pose any significant issues, although there are some reservations about using them repeatedly or for extended periods. Patients should be taught manual self-administration skills if microneedles are to be used in a long-term schedule.

Regulatory agencies have raised biosafety concerns about the potential for microneedles to leave broken pieces of silicon or metal in the skin after they are removed [44]. The FDA has only provided a draft guidance outlining whether a microneedles product is a device and hence subject to regulation. Furthermore, the FDA has not yet decided how to classify microneedles devices. Due to the requirement to address challenges such as dependability, biosafety, and complicated designs of microneedle sensing devices before clinical trials can be conducted, commercialization of these devices may take several years, if not a decade. Penetration depth, uniformity, testing period, and even mechanical properties are all relevant in microneedles testing [53, 54]. These variables differ from patient to patient due to their age, weight, body region, handling techniques, and microneedle structure.

12.4 Microneedle Designs

Numerous microneedle designs have been developed, each featuring a suited microneedle for collecting blood, lymph, or interstitial fluid from a patient into a sampling chamber and a built-in sensor for analyzing the analyte level in the sample. Several microneedles-based monitoring strategies have been reported, such as employing solid microneedles for skin pretreatment prior to ISF sampling or integrated sensing systems that eliminate the necessity for fluid removal. Efficient and reliable skin penetration without breakage and the ability to accurately detect the analytes of interest are prerequisites for every microneedles-based diagnostic system [2].

Microneedles of different configurations have been documented for use in ISF sampling. These include hollow microneedles, solid microneedles, and swelling microneedles (Fig. 12.1). While hollow microneedles use the capillary mechanism to capture ISF, swelling microneedles rely on fluid absorption into the microneedle structure [29]. Hydrophilic groups and crosslinking network structure allow it to swell and absorb ISF. The ISF absorbed by the swelling microneedles was collected by centrifugation and then measured by off-site analytes. Both glucose and cholesterol results were consistent with the gold standard. *In situ* analysis of ISF is also possible with the integration of a collector and a sensing component into a single device. These microneedles have been made utilizing a wide variety of microfabrication processes, and their materials of construction have ranged from metals and ceramics to polymers of varying compositions.

Microneedles have been designed in several different forms for use in diagnostic and monitoring purposes; broadly speaking, they fall into one of five groups: (i) microneedles for minimally invasive ISF extraction; (ii) microneedles for specific detection of biomarkers of interest; (iii) microneedles for real-time *in situ* analyte monitoring; (iv) microneedles for dermal biopotential assessments; and (v) microneedles for delivering diagnostic agents [24]. Methods of using microneedles for diagnostic applications include (i) collecting analytes from ISF or blood for subsequent testing and (ii) modifying microneedles into sensors for analysis close to or right at the point of care. The second approach is currently preferred in light of its ease of use, speed, and effectiveness. Both strategies are reshaping our visions for the future of clinical diagnosis [29]. The mechanism of action of microneedles-based diagnostic systems heavily depends on the analytes of interest, affecting the analytical method used for the analysis. Electrochemical sensors, which primarily comprise sensing components and conductive electrodes, must be integrated with or changed into microneedles for continuous monitoring. The majority of electrochemical microneedle sensors rely on enzymes.

The discomfort associated with ISF extraction is substantially reduced when the length of the microneedles is shortened from 1,000–2,000 µm to 100–800 µm. Compared to longer needles, shorter microneedles for ISF sampling provide more design and material options due to their increased mechanical strength and shear capacity [55, 56]. According to the literature, microneedle arrays intended for blood collection should penetrate skin significantly deeper, with penetration depths of 1,000–1,500 µm recommended as required for efficient blood removal [13–15].

Several factors have been reported to determine the success of the microneedles-based diagnostic system, such as the microneedles' size and shape, sensor configuration, efficient integration with the microneedle, the ability to make an effective interface with the skin, and the patient's acceptability. It is obvious that sensors are essential for devices meant to detect analytes in bodily fluids. Except if the sensor is intended for one-time use

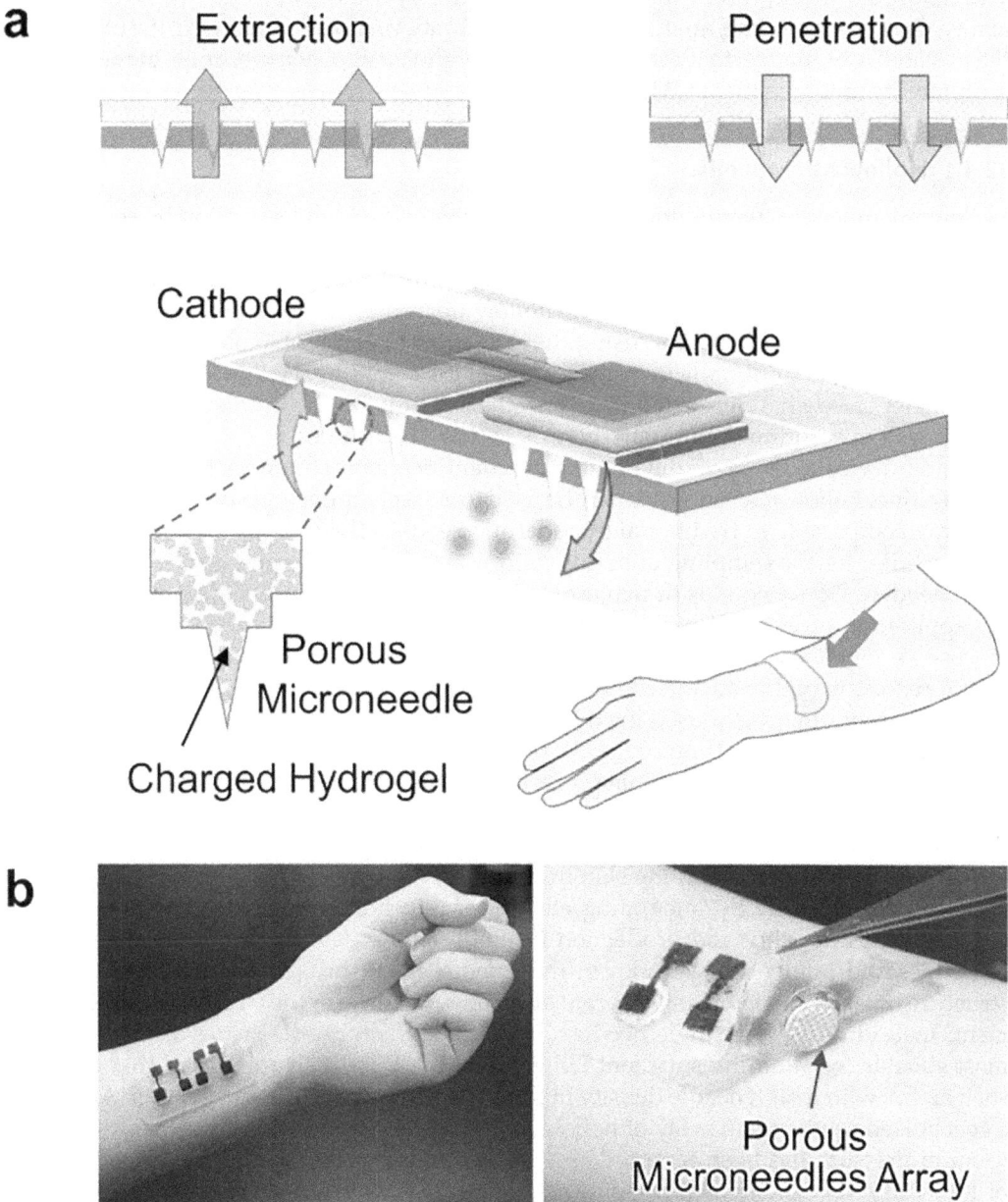

FIGURE 12.1
Schematic representation of (a) electroosmotic penetration/extraction for efficient drug delivery and analysis of ISF with porous microneedles, and (b) combination of the biobattery and porous microneedles. Images reprinted with permission from [83].

only, the sensor should be reusable and capable of providing accurate and reliable results when analyzing a given analyte. These sensing devices may use various analytical methods, such as potentiometric, physiochemical, thermal, spectroscopic, calorimetric, optical, light scattering, gravimetric, amperometric, electronic, or electrochemical systems. The calibration, sensitivity, and consistency of the sensor would contribute to the data's reliability. Cost, starting time, analysis duration, calibration, insertion location, tissue healing, the possibility of inadvertent errors, and disposability will play major roles in the device's acceptability among patients [33].

12.4.1 Hollow Microneedles

Hollow microneedles were initially designed for painless blood sampling by several processes, such as passive diffusion, capillary force, and vacuum suction, with the concept originating from the mosquito's process of drawing blood from human skin [15, 57, 58]. Even though there are already cases of using hollow microneedles for blood draws [59], more research has been conducted on using these needles to extract ISF due to the lower penetration depth and minimally invasive feature of ISF sampling. Hollow microneedles with micrometer-sized channels extending from the substrate to the needle tip enable fluid to be removed in a minimally invasive way [3, 15, 60]. The needles' tips are often attached to a sensing device to facilitate the immediate quantification of analytes from the extracted ISF [24]. Since hollow microneedles may be used to extract the desired volume of bodily fluid in a way comparable to traditional hypodermic needles, the investigation into the use of these needles for the sampling of bodily fluid was undertaken earlier than other kinds of microneedles. ISF or blood is drawn into hollow microneedles by capillary mechanism or the application of external negative pressure. With this method, proteins [61], ions [62], glucose [4, 15, 63–66], and other analytes [67, 68] in blood or ISF may be measured and monitored using highly advanced hollow microneedles-based sensing devices.

The electrodes may be housed inside hollow microneedles, allowing for convenient and effective integration [69–71]. Since the electrode materials are not appropriate for microneedles manufacturing by conventional processes, the hollow microneedles are used as physical supports for the contained sensor to penetrate the skin and retain the electrodes within the microneedles structure. This method offers the benefit that the attached enzymes and the sensors are shielded from the skin insertion and the measuring processes [72]. While sensing systems made by integrating electrodes into hollow microneedles demonstrate electrodes functionality and production flexibility, these devices do not include counter electrodes and reference electrodes in the same system; thus, a two- or three-electrode structure must be created using external electrodes to perform the electrochemical assessment. Instead of using a single needle, out-of-plane microneedle arrays are regarded as most suitable for attaining sufficient ISF volume [14]. It has been proposed that utilizing such arrays with a high needle density might provide acceptable flow rates [73]. Attaching a specialized sensor to an array of hollow microneedles enables on-device analysis. Also, vacuum pressure has been reported as a tool to facilitate fluid sampling [25]. Flow rates of 1–100 mL/h are mentioned by some as required for hollow microneedles regardless of the fluid being collected; hence the pressure that drives fluid flow into and across hollow microneedles must be taken into account to ensure appropriate fluid extraction [14]. Some concerns about hollow microneedles for fluid sampling have been reported. The risk of clogging is a typical challenge with hollow microneedle designs. To solve the issue of skin pieces clogging the channels of hollow microneedles during fluid collection, researchers have looked at modifying the configuration of the needle. This has been accomplished by constructing microneedles capable of successfully penetrating the skin by slightly shifting the channel off from the needle tip [14]. Another potential downside with nonbiodegradable and incompatible hollow microneedles is that they might fracture and remain in the skin tissue [2].

12.4.2 Solid Microneedles

Since its introduction over 15 years ago, investigators have relied heavily on solid microneedles for biopotential assessments. Piercing the stratum corneum layer with solid microneedles and then extracting the ISF (with a cloth, a sheet of paper, or a vacuum container) is one of the easiest ways to obtain ISF. Skin sweat was observed to interfere with the analysis, and sample intervals of up to 20 min were necessary to collect sufficient ISF; therefore, this approach has significant drawbacks [4]. Also, the analyte concentration is usually diluted in solid microneedle devices because of the downstream procedures required to release the target analyte. For low-abundance analytes, it may be difficult to couple these microneedles-based sampling devices with existing analytical apparatus [22]. Despite the limitations inherent to the application of solid microneedles, this technique has the potential to assess a broader range of analytes in the skin. Suppose it can be verified that the level of a drug in ISF is comparable to its concentration in blood. This noninvasive technique might be used to study the drug's pharmacokinetic profile [24]. As a result of their less complicated structure, solid microneedles are more likely to be inexpensive and simple to collect large fluid quantities.

12.4.3 Swelling Microneedles

Swelling microneedle arrays have recently been presented as another kind of microneedles for ISF sampling. These microneedles made from crosslinked hydrophilic polymers enable them to absorb bodily fluid without dissolving. Due to their biocompatibility and flexibility, swelling hydrogels have attracted much interest in microneedles [74, 75]. Once inserted into the skin, swelling hydrogel-forming microneedles expand naturally, which is beneficial for absorbing bodily fluids. The hydrogel matrix may be able to capture and conceal retrieved fluid for use in following analytical tests [76]. After being inserted into the skin, ISF diffuses into the dry solid microneedles, creating a soft hydrogel porous structure, after which it must be removed and extracted during downstream processing by centrifugation or solvent immersion to be used for analysis. Microneedles may be equipped with inbuilt sensors that monitor the target analyte. They can be withdrawn from the skin after a few minutes of insertion to allow the analyte to "wash out" in a particular medium before the offsite analysis [2]. While the analytes in swelling microneedles necessitate an extra step during the analysis, the primary fabrication process of micromolding is simple and inexpensive. The microneedles' large sample volume makes them particularly suitable for collecting ISF [77, 78]. In contrast to solid and hollow microneedles, these swelling microneedles immediately disable themselves after usage, leaving behind no hazardous waste [24]. For the swelling microneedle array to be appropriately removed from the skin, the material must have sufficient mechanical robustness to keep the needle tips affixed to the array structure [79].

12.4.4 Porous Microneedles

Based on the shape and dimensions of the pores in the microneedle structure and their hydrophilic properties, porous microneedles may capture ISF through a capillary mechanism. Similar to swelling microneedles, porous microneedles require centrifugation or dipping in a release medium to isolate the absorbed analytes, which adds an extra step to the analytical process [72]. The ISF is transported from the microneedles–skin contact to the array substrate through a dense network of continual capillaries and interconnected pores.

Porous microneedles with a pore diameter in the nanometer or micrometer range were generally fabricated using ceramics and metals [80–82]. Interestingly, Kusama et al. combined the application of porous microneedles with iontophoresis for effective ISF extraction (Fig. 12.1) [83].

12.5 Combination of Sensors and Drug Delivery in Microneedles

Microneedles system can deliver and remove molecules of interest across the skin in a noninvasive way, which creates the potential to develop a closed-loop responsive device in which a drug delivery component releases a therapeutic agent in accordance with the biosignals captured by a microneedles-based monitoring component [2]. If the elements used for treatment and diagnosis can be combined into a single bio-feedback system, it would be incredibly valuable (Fig. 12.2). The pharmacokinetic and pharmacodynamic profile of the medicine may be correlated and controlled with the use of such a system, allowing for more effective patient monitoring and treatment [33]. As a smart microneedle array integrates the sensors, actuators, and optimized drug formulation into a comprehensive feedback loop of individualized therapy, this system represents the pinnacle of sophisticated transdermal drug delivery. Actuators regulate the drug's release rate and dosage in response to input from sensors, which monitor the patient's vital signs and activate the drug administration at the appropriate time. An automated microneedle system could react according to the development of a disease without any further medical intervention, relieving symptoms as they develop. The on/off trigger for medication delivery is made simple for patients using microneedles that respond to external inputs (such as heat, laser, and mechanical stress) [85, 86]. To provide a closed-loop insulin delivery system, insulin-loaded microneedles with glucose-monitoring components are beneficial for individuals with diabetes who are burdened with regular checking of blood glucose levels and prompt insulin administration in the diabetes self-management plan [87, 88].

The concept behind this may seem simple, but putting it into practice will need some forethought. Patient safety must be considered, requiring serious scrutiny of a wide range of issues, including electronic defects, programming errors, physical and electronic damage, and patient data security [2]. As a result of its variability and complexity, the human body defies typical generalizations. Poor spatiotemporal controllability and difficulty in precisely controlling the quantity of drugs delivered are challenges of drug release in response to the magnitude of physiological stimulus biosignals [86].

12.6 Conclusions

Microneedles undoubtedly represent the optimum technique when it comes to noninvasive novel technologies that allow for accurate, real-time health monitoring. This can promote disease prevention by facilitating the early diagnosis and identification of health-related concerns [24]. Increased use of microneedles-based biosensors has resulted from the development of material, system design, and detection mechanisms during the last several decades. Depending on the intended diagnostic use, microneedles may take on

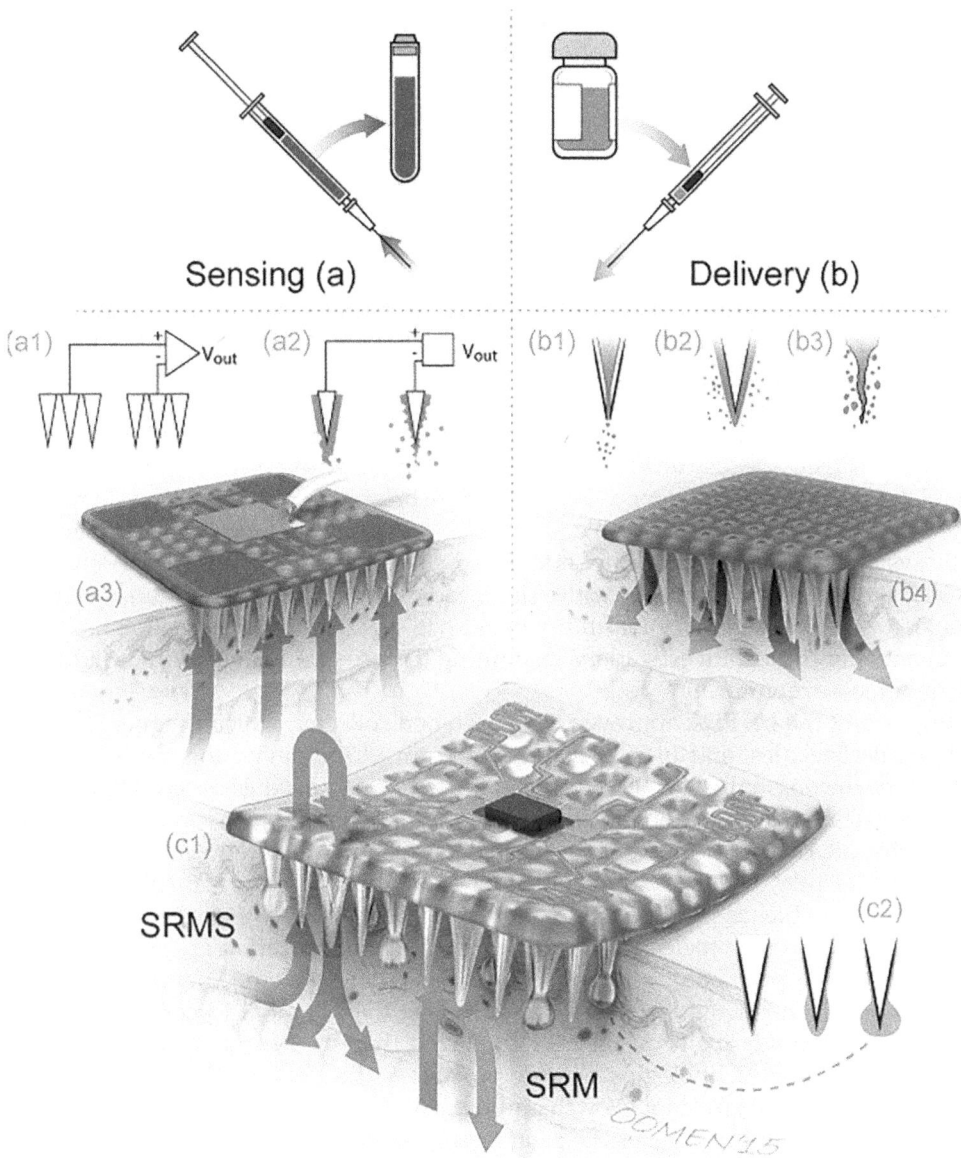

FIGURE 12.2

Development of microneedles-based devices for biosensing and transdermal drug delivery. From (a) the use of conventional hypodermic needles and syringes to draw blood for laboratory assessment and (b) administer therapeutic agents. As of now, (a1) biopotential, (a2) electrochemical signals, and (a3) microneedles-based biosensors are utilized for biosensing, and (b1) hollow, (b2) coated, and (b3) dissolving (b4) microneedle patches are employed for transdermal and intradermal drug delivery. These combined methods create (c1) a biofunctional microneedle patch for stimulus-sensitive drug delivery, complete with (c2) swelling microneedles to facilitate patch–skin attachment. To provide controlled drug release from a second patch, stimulus-responsive microneedle systems may monitor a biosignal via a microneedles-based sensor. Alternatively, microneedles that degrade in response to a stimulus might be developed to deliver encapsulated medications [84].

various forms, including hollow, solid, or swelling microneedles. Twenty-five analytes may be monitored using microneedle sensors utilizing multiple detection methods. Glucose, proteins, ions, drugs, metabolites, biopotentials, and plant DNA are only some of the target analytes that might be measured and monitored [89]. The microneedles-based system has led to the development of point-of-care/lab-on-chip diagnostic procedures. Microneedles diagnostic devices can replace laborious and invasive monitoring techniques, thus improving the quality of life for patients with a wide range of health conditions.

12.7 Future of Microneedle for Diagnosis

The use of microneedles-based sensors as point-of-care testing (POCT) is in its early stages. For measuring glucose levels in the ISF, only long needle-based sensors have been commercially available (Medtronic Guardian™ Sensor and Abbott's Libre system [90]). Marketed microneedles devices for blood and ISF sampling include the TAP (Seventh Sense Biosystems, Inc.) [91], the HemoLink (Tasso, Inc.), and the ISF absorber (Renephra Ltd.). These tools penetrate the skin with microneedles and employ a vacuum suction to extract blood and ISF gently. The feasibility of analyte sensing by ISF extraction has been shown in ongoing clinical investigations examining the use of microneedles for fluid collection and glucose monitoring.

Notably, in 2017, the US FDA approved the TAP blood collector, which is equipped with a set of 30 microneedles, and in 2018 the EMA approved the device for use in Europe. This opens up the possibility for the widespread use of microneedles-based bioassay. As microneedle technologies continue to evolve, microneedles-based bioassays will provide a less invasive alternative to conventional detection techniques in clinical settings and play an essential role in the evolution of individualized healthcare [76]. The study of microneedles-based biosensors is expected to increase significantly over the next decade. Microneedle biosensors, optoelectronics, and wireless communication are converging to provide a novel and promising platform for the healthcare system. Microneedle-based next-generation diagnostic and delivery systems have the potential to combine several components into a single platform for individualized therapy. Microneedle-based diagnostic and therapeutic technologies provide advantages to patients. Microneedles are expected to experience significant growth and increased prospects in the future because of their low cost and noninvasiveness [92]. One might foresee microneedles-based biosensors playing a crucial role in a future healthcare system. The following capabilities become available when the wearable devices are equipped with smart sensors, therapeutic modules, and wireless systems: (i) the sensors can monitor disease-associated biomarkers and publish patient information on the shared server; (ii) remote physicians or artificial intelligence can make a timely and accurate diagnosis from the collected information on the server; (iii) the diagnosis can result in medical treatments like the drug delivery directly to the patients. Decentralizing healthcare would benefit patients by making it simpler for them to control their personal health, which may also assist in alleviating the shortage of healthcare professionals. Collaboration between academic institutions, businesses, and governments is necessary to develop these breakthroughs into marketable healthcare products [29].

References

[1] Hosu O, Mirel S, Săndulescu R, et al. Minireview: smart tattoo, microneedle, point-of-care, and phone-based biosensors for medical screening, diagnosis, and monitoring. Anal Lett. 2019;52:78–92.

[2] Donnelly RF, Mooney K, Caffarel-Salvador E, et al. Microneedle-mediated minimally invasive patient monitoring. Ther Drug Monit. 2014;36:10–17.

[3] Smart WH, Subramanian K. The use of silicon microfabrication technology in painless blood glucose monitoring. Diabetes Technol Ther. 2000;2:549–559.

[4] Wang PM, Cornwell M, Prausnitz MR. Minimally invasive extraction of dermal interstitial fluid for glucose monitoring using microneedles. Diabetes Technol Ther. 2005;7:131–141.

[5] Fogh-Andersen N, Altura BM, Altura BT, et al. Composition of interstitial fluid. Clin Chem. 1995;41:1522–1525.

[6] Cobelli C, Schiavon M, Dalla Man C, et al. Interstitial fluid glucose is not just a shifted-in-time but a distorted mirror of blood glucose: insight from an in silico study. Diabetes Technol Ther. 2016;18:505–511.

[7] Rebrin K, Steil GM. Can interstitial glucose assessment replace blood glucose measurements? Diabetes Technol Ther. 2000;2:461–472.

[8] Stout PJ, Peled N, Erickson BJ, et al. Comparison of glucose levels in dermal interstitial fluid and finger capillary blood. Diabetes Technol Ther. 2001;3:81–90.

[9] Tran BQ, Miller PR, Taylor RM, et al. Proteomic characterization of dermal interstitial fluid extracted using a novel microneedle-assisted technique. J Proteome Res. 2018;17:479–485.

[10] Khanna P, Strom JA, Malone JI, et al. Microneedle-based automated therapy for diabetes mellitus. J Diabetes Sci Technol. 2008;2:1122–1129.

[11] Coffey JW, Corrie SR, Kendall MAF. Early circulating biomarker detection using a wearable microprojection array skin patch. Biomaterials. 2013;34:9572–9583.

[12] Courtenay AJ, Abbate MT, McCrudden MT, et al. Minimally-invasive patient monitoring and diagnosis using microneedles. Microneedles Drug Vaccine Deliv Patient Monit. 2018;207–234.

[13] Chaudhri BP, Ceyssens F, De Moor P, et al. A high aspect ratio SU-8 fabrication technique for hollow microneedles for transdermal drug delivery and blood extraction. J Micromechanics Microengineering. 2010;20:064006.

[14] Gardeniers HJ, Luttge R, Berenschot EJ, et al. Silicon micromachined hollow microneedles for transdermal liquid transport. J Microelectromechanical Syst. 2003;12:855–862.

[15] Mukerjee EV, Collins SD, Isseroff RR, et al. Microneedle array for transdermal biological fluid extraction and in situ analysis. Sens Actuators Phys. 2004;114:267–275.

[16] Bollella P, Sharma S, Cass AEG, et al. Minimally-invasive microneedle-based biosensor array for simultaneous lactate and glucose monitoring in artificial interstitial fluid. Electroanalysis. 2019;31:374–382.

[17] Xie L, Zeng H, Sun J, et al. Engineering microneedles for therapy and diagnosis: a survey. Micromachines. 2020;11:271.

[18] McAllister DV, Wang PM, Davis SP, et al. Microfabricated needles for transdermal delivery of macromolecules and nanoparticles: fabrication methods and transport studies. Proc Natl Acad Sci. 2003;100:13755–13760.

[19] Zheng G, Patolsky F, Cui Y, et al. Multiplexed electrical detection of cancer markers with nanowire sensor arrays. Nat Biotechnol. 2005;23:1294–1301.

[20] El-Laboudi A, Oliver NS, Cass A, et al. Use of microneedle array devices for continuous glucose monitoring: a review. Diabetes Technol Ther. 2013;15:101–115.

[21] Ventrelli L, Marsilio Strambini L, Barillaro G. Microneedles for transdermal biosensing: current picture and future direction. Adv Healthc Mater. 2015;4:2606–2640.

[22] Dixon RV, Lau WM, Moghimi SM, et al. The diagnostic potential of microneedles in infectious diseases. Precis Nanomedicine. 2020;3:629–640.

[23] Gupta J, Gill HS, Andrews SN, et al. Kinetics of skin resealing after insertion of microneedles in human subjects. J Control Release. 2011;154:148–155.

[24] Babity S, Roohnikan M, Brambilla D. Advances in the design of transdermal microneedles for diagnostic and monitoring applications. Small. 2018;14:1803186.

[25] Tsuchiya K, Jinnin S, Yamamoto H, et al. Design and development of a biocompatible painless microneedle by the ion sputtering deposition method. Precis Eng. 2010;34:461–466.

[26] Samant PP, Prausnitz MR. Mechanisms of sampling interstitial fluid from skin using a microneedle patch. Proc Natl Acad Sci. 2018;115:4583–4588.

[27] Dale JC, Ruby SG. Specimen collection volumes for laboratory tests: a College of American Pathologists study of 140 laboratories. Arch Pathol Lab Med. 2003;127:162–168.

[28] Yao W, Tao C, Zou J, et al. Flexible two-layer dissolving and safing microneedle transdermal of neurotoxin: a biocomfortable attempt to treat Rheumatoid Arthritis. Int J Pharm. 2019;563:91–100.

[29] Liu G-S, Kong Y, Wang Y, et al. Microneedles for transdermal diagnostics: recent advances and new horizons. Biomaterials. 2020;232:119740.

[30] Dardano P, Rea I, De Stefano L. Microneedles-based electrochemical sensors: new tools for advanced biosensing. Curr Opin Electrochem. 2019;17:121–127.

[31] Liu F, Lin Z, Jin Q, et al. Protection of nanostructures-integrated microneedle biosensor using dissolvable polymer coating. ACS Appl Mater Interfaces. 2019;11:4809–4819.

[32] Skaria E, Patel BA, Flint MS, et al. Poly (lactic acid)/carbon nanotube composite microneedle arrays for dermal biosensing. Anal Chem. 2019;91:4436–4443.

[33] Sachdeva VK, Banga A. Microneedles and their applications. Recent Pat Drug Deliv Formul. 2011;5:95–132.

[34] Yuzhakov VV, Gartstein V, Owens GD. Microneedle apparatus used for marking skin and for dispensing semi-permanent subcutaneous makeup. Google Patents; 2003. [Internet] [cited 2016 Aug 23]. Available from: www.google.com/patents/US6565532.

[35] Bandodkar AJ, Gutruf P, Choi J, et al. Battery-free, skin-interfaced microfluidic/electronic systems for simultaneous electrochemical, colorimetric, and volumetric analysis of sweat. Sci Adv. 2019;5:eaav3294.

[36] Chen L, Zhang C, Xiao J, et al. Local extraction and detection of early stage breast cancers through a microneedle and nano-Ag/MBL film based painless and blood-free strategy. Mater Sci Eng C. 2020;109:110402.

[37] Tejavibulya N, Colburn DA, Marcogliese FA, et al. Hydrogel microfilaments toward intradermal health monitoring. Iscience. 2019;21:328–340.

[38] Loewenstein D, Stake C, Cichon M. Assessment of using fingerstick blood sample with i-STAT point-of-care device for cardiac troponin I assay. Am J Emerg Med. 2013;31:1236–1239.

[39] Parikh P, Mochari H, Mosca L. Clinical utility of a fingerstick technology to identify individuals with abnormal blood lipids and high-sensitivity c-reactive protein levels. Am J Health Promot. 2009;23:279–282.

[40] Miller PR, Taylor RM, Tran BQ, et al. Extraction and biomolecular analysis of dermal interstitial fluid collected with hollow microneedles. Commun Biol. 2018;1:1–11.

[41] Watanabe R, Gehad A, Yang C, et al. Human skin is protected by four functionally and phenotypically discrete populations of resident and recirculating memory T cells. Sci Transl Med. 2015;7:279ra39–279ra39.

[42] Forvi E, Bedoni M, Carabalona R, et al. Preliminary technological assessment of microneedles-based dry electrodes for biopotential monitoring in clinical examinations. Sens Actuators Phys. 2012;180:177–186.

[43] McCrudden MTC, Alkilani AZ, Courtenay AJ, et al. Considerations in the sterile manufacture of polymeric microneedle arrays. Drug Deliv Transl Res. 2015;5:3–14.

[44] Donnelly RF, Woolfson AD. Patient safety and beyond: what should we expect from microneedle arrays in the transdermal delivery arena? Ther Deliv. 2014;5:653–662.

[45] Zaric M, Lyubomska O, Touzelet O, et al. Skin dendritic cell targeting via microneedle arrays laden with antigen-encapsulated poly-D,L-lactide-co-glycolide nanoparticles induces efficient antitumor and antiviral immune responses. ACS Nano. 2013;7:2042–2055.

[46] Donnelly RF, Singh TRR, Tunney MM, et al. Microneedle arrays allow lower microbial penetration than hypodermic needles in vitro. Pharm Res. 2009;26:2513–2522.

[47] McConville A, Hegarty C, Davis J. Mini-review: assessing the potential impact of microneedle technologies on home healthcare applications. Med. 2018;5:50.

[48] Donnelly RF, Singh TRR, Alkilani AZ, et al. Hydrogel-forming microneedle arrays exhibit antimicrobial properties: potential for enhanced patient safety. Int J Pharm. 2013;451:76–91.

[49] García LEG, MacGregor MN, Visalakshan RM, et al. Self-sterilizing antibacterial silver-loaded microneedles. Chem Commun. 2019;55:171–174.

[50] Sharma S, El-Laboudi A, Reddy M, et al. A pilot study in humans of microneedle sensor arrays for continuous glucose monitoring. Anal Methods. 2018;10:2088–2095.

[51] Cass AE, Sharma S. Microneedle enzyme sensor arrays for continuous in vivo monitoring. In: Richard B. Thompson, Carol A. Fierke, editors. Methods in enzymology. Amsterdam, NL: Elsevier; 2017. p. 413–427.

[52] Kim D-H, Lu N, Ma R, et al. Epidermal electronics. Sci. 2011;333:838–843.

[53] Coffey JW, Meliga SC, Corrie SR, et al. Dynamic application of microprojection arrays to skin induces circulating protein extravasation for enhanced biomarker capture and detection. Biomaterials. 2016;84:130–143.

[54] Coffey JW, Corrie SR, Kendall MA. Rapid and selective sampling of IgG from skin in less than 1 min using a high surface area wearable immunoassay patch. Biomaterials. 2018;170:49–57.

[55] Kim K, Park DS, Lu HM, et al. A tapered hollow metallic microneedle array using backside exposure of SU-8. J Micromechanics Microengineering. 2004;14:597.

[56] Park J-H, Allen MG, Prausnitz MR. Biodegradable polymer microneedles: fabrication, mechanics and transdermal drug delivery. J Control Release. 2005;104:51–66.

[57] Paik S-J, Byun S, Lim J-M, et al. In-plane single-crystal-silicon microneedles for minimally invasive microfluid systems. Sens Actuators Phys. 2004;114:276–284.

[58] Strambini LM, Longo A, Diligenti A, et al. A minimally invasive microchip for transdermal injection/sampling applications. Lab Chip. 2012;12:3370–3379.

[59] Liu R, Wang XH, Tang F, et al. An in-plane microneedles used for sampling and glucose analysis. 13th Int Conf Solid-State Sens Actuators Microsyst. 2005. p. 1517–1520.

[60] Kobayashi K, Suzuki H. A sampling mechanism employing the phase transition of a gel and its application to a micro analysis system imitating a mosquito. Sens Actuators B Chem. 2001;80:1–8.

[61] Miller P, Moorman M, Manginell R, et al. Towards an integrated microneedle total analysis chip for protein detection. Electroanalysis. 2016;28:1305–1310.

[62] Miller PR, Xiao X, Brener I, et al. Microneedle-based transdermal sensor for on-chip potentiometric determination of K(+). Adv Healthc Mater. 2014;3:876–881.

[63] Chua B, Desai SP, Tierney MJ, et al. Effect of microneedles shape on skin penetration and minimally invasive continuous glucose monitoring in vivo. Sens Actuators Phys. 2013;203:373–381.

[64] Li CG, Joung H-A, Noh H, et al. One-touch-activated blood multidiagnostic system using a minimally invasive hollow microneedle integrated with a paper-based sensor. Lab Chip. 2015;15:3286–3292.

[65] Nicholas D, Logan KA, Sheng Y, et al. Rapid paper based colorimetric detection of glucose using a hollow microneedle device. Int J Pharm. 2018;547:244–249.

[66] Strambini LM, Longo A, Scarano S, et al. Self-powered microneedle-based biosensors for pain-free high-accuracy measurement of glycaemia in interstitial fluid. Biosens Bioelectron. 2015;66:162–168.

[67] Ranamukhaarachchi SA, Padeste C, Dübner M, et al. Integrated hollow microneedle-optofluidic biosensor for therapeutic drug monitoring in sub-nanoliter volumes. Sci Rep. 2016;6:29075.

[68] Yu LM, Tay FEH, Guo DG, et al. A microfabricated electrode with hollow microneedles for ECG measurement. Sens Actuators Phys. 2009;151:17–22.

[69] Ciui B, Martin A, Mishra RK, et al. Wearable wireless tyrosinase bandage and microneedle sensors: toward melanoma screening. Adv Healthc Mater. 2018;7:1701264.

[70] Mishra RK, Mohan AMV, Soto F, et al. A microneedle biosensor for minimally-invasive transdermal detection of nerve agents. Analyst. 2017;142:918–924.

[71] Mohan AMV, Windmiller JR, Mishra RK, et al. Continuous minimally-invasive alcohol monitoring using microneedle sensor arrays. Biosens Bioelectron. 2017;91:574–579.

[72] Takeuchi K, Kim B. Functionalized microneedles for continuous glucose monitoring. Nano Converg. 2018;5:28.

[73] Groenendaal W, Von Basum G, Schmidt KA, et al. Quantifying the composition of human skin for glucose sensor development. Los Angeles, CA: Sage Publications; 2010.

[74] Chang H, Zheng M, Chew SWT, et al. Advances in the formulations of microneedles for manifold biomedical applications. Adv Mater Technol. 2020;5:1900552.

[75] Ito Y, Inagaki Y, Kobuchi S, et al. Therapeutic drug monitoring of vancomycin in dermal interstitial fluid using dissolving microneedles. Int J Med Sci. 2016;13:271.

[76] Zhu J, Zhou X, Libanori A, et al. Microneedle-based bioassays. Nanoscale Adv. 2020;2:4295–4304.

[77] Caffarel-Salvador E, Brady AJ, Eltayib E, et al. Hydrogel-forming microneedle arrays allow detection of drugs and glucose in vivo: potential for use in diagnosis and therapeutic drug monitoring. PloS One. 2015;10:e0145644.

[78] Chang H, Zheng M, Yu X, et al. A swellable microneedle patch to rapidly extract skin interstitial fluid for timely metabolic analysis. Adv Mater. 2017;29:1702243.

[79] Lutton REM, Larrañeta E, Kearney M-C, et al. A novel scalable manufacturing process for the production of hydrogel-forming microneedle arrays. Int J Pharm. 2015;494:417–429.

[80] Cahill EM, Keaveney S, Stuettgen V, et al. Metallic microneedles with interconnected porosity: a scalable platform for biosensing and drug delivery. Acta Biomater. 2018;80:401–411.

[81] Gholami S, Mohebi M-M, Hajizadeh-Saffar E, et al. Fabrication of microporous inorganic microneedles by centrifugal casting method for transdermal extraction and delivery. Int J Pharm. 2019;558:299–310.

[82] Verhoeven M, Bystrova S, Winnubst L, et al. Applying ceramic nanoporous microneedle arrays as a transport interface in egg plants and an ex-vivo human skin model. Microelectron Eng. 2012;98:659–662.

[83] Kusama S, Sato K, Matsui Y, et al. Transdermal electroosmotic flow generated by a porous microneedle array patch. Nat Commun. 2021;12:658.

[84] Cahill EM, O'Cearbhaill ED. Toward biofunctional microneedles for stimulus responsive drug delivery. Bioconjug Chem. 2015;26:1289–1296.

[85] Chen M-C, Lin Z-W, Ling M-H. Near-infrared light-activatable microneedle system for treating superficial tumors by combination of chemotherapy and photothermal therapy. ACS Nano. 2016;10:93–101.

[86] Di J, Yao S, Ye Y, et al. Stretch-triggered drug delivery from wearable elastomer films containing therapeutic depots. ACS Nano. 2015;9:9407–9415.

[87] Mo R, Jiang T, Di J, et al. Emerging micro-and nanotechnology based synthetic approaches for insulin delivery. Chem Soc Rev. 2014;43:3595–3629.

[88] Veiseh O, Tang BC, Whitehead KA, et al. Managing diabetes with nanomedicine: challenges and opportunities. Nat Rev Drug Discov. 2015;14:45–57.

[89] Paul R, Saville AC, Hansel JC, et al. Extraction of plant DNA by microneedle patch for rapid detection of plant diseases. ACS Nano. 2019;13:6540–6549.

[90] Girardin CM, Huot C, Gonthier M, et al. Continuous glucose monitoring: a review of biochemical perspectives and clinical use in type 1 diabetes. Clin Biochem. 2009;42:136–142.

[91] Blicharz TM, Gong P, Bunner BM, et al. Microneedle-based device for the one-step painless collection of capillary blood samples. Nat Biomed Eng. 2018;2:151–157.

[92] Alimardani V, Abolmaali SS, Tamaddon AM, et al. Recent advances on microneedle arrays-mediated technology in cancer diagnosis and therapy. Drug Deliv Transl Res. 2021;11:788–816.

13

Other Applications of Microneedles

13.1 Introduction

Microneedles have been extensively researched for their applications in transdermal and intradermal drugs and vaccine delivery. Numerous uses of the microneedles-based system in the cosmetic field have also been recognized. Besides, disrupting the barrier function of various epithelial tissues using microneedles (such as the gastrointestinal tract [1], sclera [2, 3], and endothelium [4], buccal, nasal, and vaginal mucosa) is also being studied to enhance drug delivery to targeted sites (Table 13.1). Microneedles are versatile enough to be employed in inkjet printing, cell surgery, microdialysis, gene therapy, and cancer treatment. The suprachoroidal space is a potential drug delivery site being investigated in conjunction with microneedles [5].

13.2 Oral Route of Administration

13.2.1 Introduction of Microneedles for Oral Drug Delivery

The applications of microneedles for oral drug administration are driven by (1) the possibility for the technology capable of delivering a wide variety of medications with minimum effort for formulation development orally; (2) the properties of the gastrointestinal (GI) tract allowing for minimally invasive microinjection; (3) the capability of the GI tract to endure the transportation of sharp objects and mucosal disturbance as demonstrated by the minimal rate or absence of issues related to microscopic sharp object ingestion [15]. There has reportedly been a surge in this area due to this trigger. Several researchers have proposed that microneedles might be used to administer pharmaceuticals and biologics orally. This has led to an increase in both granted and ongoing patent applications, demonstrating this sector's growing importance. Nevertheless, at the current time, this endeavor is more commercial than academic, as indicated by a large number of patent applications in this field and the scant number of published research that comprehensively evaluate the safety and efficiency of this technology [16] Oral mucosal vaccination, oral cancer therapy, and drug delivery to the gastrointestinal tract using a microneedle pill are a few of the areas where microneedles have recently been studied [17]. Vaccines delivered through microneedle patches have been researched for use in the gastrointestinal system and the mouth cavity. Vaccine delivery to a region rich in mucosal antigen-presenting cells frequently elicits mucosal immune responses at remote locations, leading to more

DOI: 10.1201/9780429294433-13

TABLE 13.1

Microneedle-mediated Drug Delivery into Various Tissues

Internal Tissues	External Tissues
Mouth [6]	Skin [7–9]
Vagina [10]	Eye [2]
Gastrointestinal tract [1]	Fingernail [11]
Vascular wall [12]	Anus [13]
	Scalp [14]

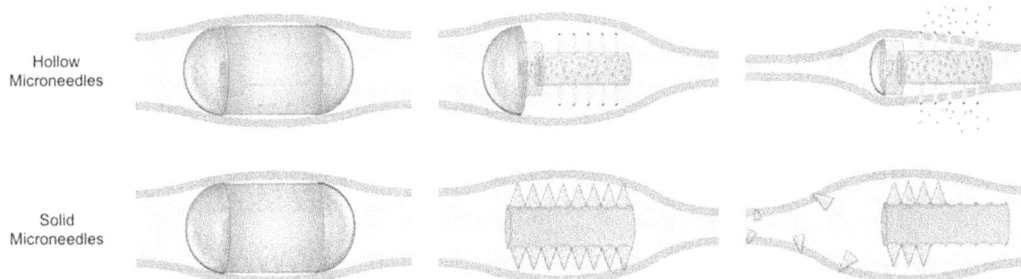

FIGURE 13.1

Schematic representation of a therapeutic microneedle pill. Microneedles, either hollow or solid types, could be employed. Both types of pills use a pH-responsive coating to make them more ingestible (left). The pill's covering disintegrates once it reaches the target area of the gastrointestinal system, exposing the microneedles inside (middle). The loaded drug is then released via the hollow microneedles (top right) when the drug reservoir is squeezed via peristalsis. Solid microneedles (bottom right) have the drug already incorporated into their structure. Depending on the needle's composition, they can pierce the tissue, separate from the pill, and gradually release the drug payload. Images reprinted with permission from [1].

robust immunity. One proposed method for enhancing oral mucosal vaccination is the reversible rupture of this mucosal barrier using microneedles, allowing for more efficient delivery of the vaccine to the antigen-presenting cells of the tissue [17]. Recent studies have reported that liposomes loaded with model antigens (i.e., hepatitis B antigen and bovine serum albumin) may be delivered into the oral mucosa using hollow microneedles to elicit a strong immune response [18, 19]. Microneedle pill technology, which is used for the oral administration of biologics, is predicated on the rationale that hollow or solid microneedles may penetrate and bypass the intestinal mucosa [17]. The loaded drug is then discharged from the reservoir or the microneedles when the mucosal barrier has been disrupted. Remarkably, needle geometry and dimensions may have a significant impact on the pill's resident duration within the GI tract and may facilitate sustained drug release, hence lowering the necessary dose frequency of several medications [20] (Fig. 13.1). The safety and viability of these methods may be improved with more preclinical studies in pigs and other large animals. Safety and effectiveness must be prioritized; thus, research into new formulations, such as polymer-based systems, to enhance the stability of the therapeutic agents and preserve sufficient mechanical strength is crucial [15].

Rani Therapeutics LLC is working on a microneedle pill that could be swallowed. Their technique, known as the "Rani Pill" or "robotic pill," maintains in capsule form in the stomach until dissolving in the small intestine due to a shift in pH [16]. Actuators in this system are responsible for dislodging drug-loaded needles from the pill and inserting them into the tissue. According to recently published research, insulin and adalimumab have been found to be effectively delivered orally. The early findings show the tolerance of passage of such a device, and the safety of such a technology is crucial for its widespread application; as per Rani's documented preclinical research, insulin and adalimumab exhibit more than 50% bioavailability in swine. Several major pharmaceutical companies, such as Novartis and AstraZeneca, have invested $142 million in Rani in preparation for human clinical trials of the company's microneedle pill.

Different types of microneedles have been employed to deliver therapeutic agents into oral mucosa. Delivering antigen-loaded liposomes into the oral mucosa by hollow microneedles has been shown to elicit a strong immune response [18, 19]. There has been some success in using coated microneedles for oral immunization. Strong IgA responses in saliva were triggered when these microneedles patches coated with ovalbumin were orally administered. Furthermore, similar responses were obtained after microneedle insertion into the oral cavity after intramuscular delivery of HIV model antigens [6]. For dissolving polymeric microneedles, even a low moisture level in the mouth's wet environment might drastically diminish the sharpness and mechanical strength of the microneedle tip. While it has been shown that dissolving microneedles may penetrate wet tissues like the cornea and sclera, the microneedle material must be properly engineered to ensure successful needle penetration before needle dissolution [21].

The pain might be a concern, considering the mucosa's susceptibility to injury. Given saliva may trigger drug release in advance of when it is expected and may impede polymeric microneedles' capacity to penetrate the mucosal barrier, it will be vital that microneedles not be subjected to large volumes of saliva before their application. If long-term drug delivery is desired, the microneedle array substrate should have mucoadhesive features to hold the needles in place. The device's opposite side should be covered with a moisture-impermeable backing layer to prevent the needles from dissolving too rapidly. The mucosal cavity is a source of microorganisms; therefore, it is also critical to consider the safety aspect. Because of the potential for either local or systemic infection, such microorganisms should not pass through a disrupted mucosal barrier. The industry may become interested when more research is presented and technology advances. This is crucial for the development of the technology toward commercialization and, most significantly, patient benefit [17]. There is a propensity to jump to the conclusion that this technology will instantly revolutionize the administration of biological treatments by eliminating the need for needles. Whether the technology behind microneedle pills can make the leap from the laboratories to the clinical settings and win over a large patient population is still up in the air. There is a wide range in intraluminal intestinal pressure [17] from patient to patient, and diet may affect the drug absorption rate and the device's efficiency (especially viscous and particulate food items). A poorly designed delivery system may do more harm than good when applied to a compound like insulin, which needs precise dosage. Drug absorption and therapeutic response will vary from patient to patient if they have to take these pills regularly. Especially for biologics necessitating frequently repeated administration and chronic usage, safety, efficacy, reliability, and cost pose a significant obstacle to the approval and acceptance of technology [16].

The importance of the dosing site is not sufficiently understood, which is a significant limitation of oral mucosal microneedles-assisted vaccine administration. Microneedles have the potential to deliver vaccines through the oral mucosa, although this feature has not yet been thoroughly explored in previous investigations. Another major knowledge gap is the impact of microneedles-assisted vaccine delivery on innate and cellular immunity in the oral mucosa. Improvements and developments are also necessary for the use of adjuvants in oral microneedle systems. The delivery capabilities of microneedles may also aid in understanding adjuvant function in the oral mucosa. Although immunological responses have been elicited without adjuvants that are equivalent to intramuscular injection [6, 22], it is possible that the inclusion of adjuvants in the oral microneedle systems would significantly enhance the quality and quantity of mucosal and systemic immune responses.

Researchers must investigate various parameters associated with oral mucosal vaccination and use relevant animal models. Mice and rabbits have only been used so far in research involving microneedles-based vaccination to the oral mucosa. Because of the limitations of the small animal models, the types and numbers of mucosal locations that could be studied were restricted. If vaccines could be administered to several locations in the oral mucosa, it would be feasible to conduct more sophisticated investigations of the impact of delivery locations on immune responses. To more accurately evaluate the possibility of this vaccine delivery strategy for inducing immunogenicity in human subjects, it should be applied to nonhuman primate species [22].

13.2.2 Case Studies of Microneedles for Oral Drug Delivery

Ma and colleagues initially investigated the microneedle-mediated delivery of vaccines to the oral mucosa in a 2014 publication [6]. One row of coated solid microneedles was inserted into the rabbits' inner lip or dorsal tongue. Researchers showed that they could successfully deliver sulforhodamine into the lip (63.9% efficiency) and the tongue (91.2% efficiency). Tissue histology studies confirmed that coated microneedles entered the oral cavity via the lips and tongue. Approximately 400 μm, or 57% of the needle length, was inserted into the tissue [23, 24]. Researchers found both lip and tongue tissues were efficient sites for delivering vaccines in an experiment using ovalbumin as a prototype antigen. Notably, both locations generated a substantial increase in secretory IgA in saliva compared to pre-immunization saliva. Microneedles-assisted delivery of a virus-like particle and a DNA vaccine into the oral cavity was compared with intramuscular injection. Both intramuscular and oral microneedle delivery resulted in a substantial elevation of antigen-specific IgG in serum. Furthermore, there was a significant increment of antigen-specific IgA response in saliva only in the group that received vaccines via the oral cavity using microneedles treatment [17].

In a different experiment, 25 μg of ovalbumin (OVA) was coated on five microneedle arrays. The researchers assessed the adaptive immune responses triggered by the delivery of 125 μg OVA into the lip against that into the dorsal tongue. Drugs administered into the tongue or the lip demonstrated equivalent efficacy. A virus-like particle and HIV antigens encoded in plasmid DNA induced immune responses that were comparable to those induced by OVA [22]. This team has also studied microneedle-mediated drug delivery to the oral cavity to investigate the effects of salivary washout on drug delivery [25]. Microneedles could transport biologics directly into oral tissues, but they still leave openings through which saliva can wash away or dilute the delivered drug. The concept of microneedles for buccal delivery has been described by Caffarel-Salvador et al. (Fig. 13.2) [26]. In an investigation, microneedle arrays have been studied by McNeilly and coworkers for their application in delivering vaccines to the buccal mucosa of mice. Commercial Fluvax influenza vaccine (37 ng) was used to coat the needles. As a result, the device delivered the Fluvax vaccine into the buccal tissue to a mean depth of 47.8 μm. Microneedle arrays only had a 30% success rate in terms of vaccine administration, with 10% reaching the tissue surface and 60% remaining on the needles [22, 27].

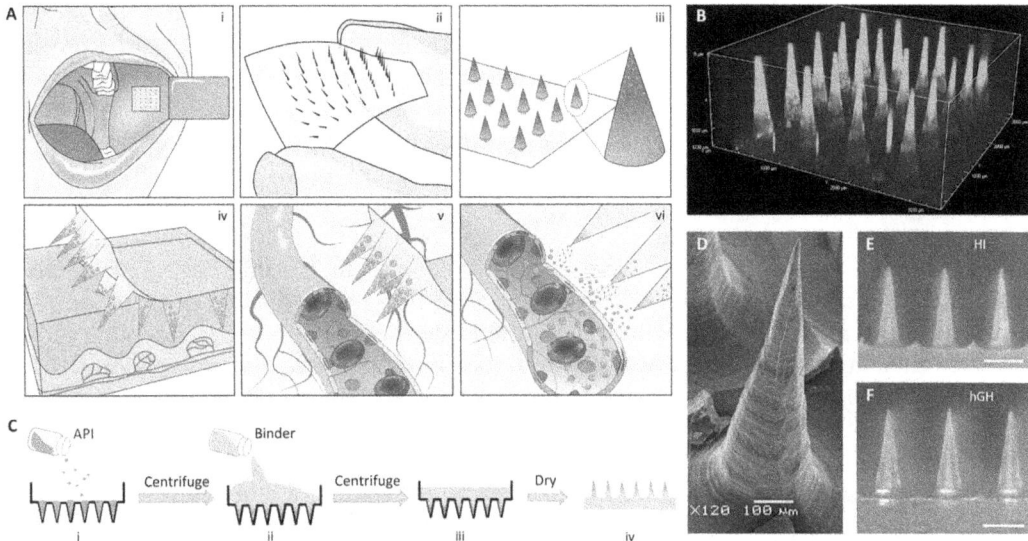

FIGURE 13.2
Microneedle-mediated buccal delivery: concept and fabrication. (A) Application of microneedle patch into buccal tissue: (i) application process, (ii) microneedle patch, (iii) API loaded in microneedle tips, (iv) microneedles penetration into buccal tissue, (v) in the vicinity of blood capillaries, and (vi) API release from microneedles patch. (B) Confocal image of FITC-dextran-loaded microneedles. (C) Fabrication of microneedle array. (D) SEM image of a single microneedle. (E and F) Optical image of drug-loaded microneedles. Images reprinted with permission from [26].

Oral mucosal drug delivery using dissolving microneedles has also been documented. Liposomes containing hepatitis B surface antigens (HBs) or bovine serum albumin (BSA) antigens were encapsulated in poly(vinylpyrrolidone) polymeric microneedles [18]. The oral mucosa of mice was given either 4 μg of bovine serum albumin (BSA) or 0.5 μg of HBs using the drug-coated microneedles [22]. Microneedle-mediated delivery of liposomes to the oral mucosa yielded greater levels of serum IgG antibodies than topical oral mucosa delivery for any given antigen, although lower levels of serum IgG antibodies in comparison with subcutaneous and dermal delivery methods.

Wang and collaborators endeavored to develop a mucosal vaccine delivery system for hepatitis B virus (HBV) treatment that is efficient, user-friendly, and long-lasting [18]. The researchers fabricated HBsAg-encapsulated mannose-PEG-cholesterol/lipid A-liposomes (HBsAg-MLLs) by emulsification–lyophilization and then poured them into microneedle molds and let them dry to construct microneedle structure. These drug-loaded microneedles could be stored for up to three days at 40°C without noticeable degradation and had strong mechanical properties to penetrate pig skin. Rapid dissolution of microneedles upon exposure to water allowed for the recovery of HBsAg-MLLs with no discernible modification in particle size or antigen association efficiency. Inducing a multimodal immunological response against HBV infection could be feasible with the assistance of this innovative microneedle design [17]. It is credible to wonder whether the saliva in the microneedle application area in the oral cavity might cause a significant loss of the delivered drugs or vaccines and if saliva can impact microneedles penetration into the tissue. Solid microneedles coated with sulforhodamine (SRD) were inserted into pig buccal tissue in an *in vitro* study performed by Serpe and coworkers [25]. The microscopy results confirmed that SRD was effectively deposited into the tissue. Albeit with PBS on the microneedle-treated site, some drugs were retained in the tissue after 24 h. Therefore, coated microneedles may be used to deliver drugs and vaccines into the mucosal tissues, although they can be washed away by saliva to a certain extent.

Lately, proof-of-concept tests using pH-responsive microneedles-based capsules in the pig gastrointestinal tract have been conducted *in vivo*. In this study, the delivery profile of insulin was investigated after it was injected through microneedles into different regions of the gastrointestinal system and compared to delivery via the more conventional subcutaneous route. When triggered in the gastrointestinal system, the microneedles puncture the epithelium and then discharge the loaded drug through peristaltic pressure applied to the drug reservoir. When insulin was injected into the stomach and duodenum, rather than subcutaneously, the onset duration to notice a hypoglycemic effect was drastically shortened. To be more precise, the onset time was shortened by nearly 20 min as compared to subcutaneous delivery [1].

Drugs may be delivered through the intestinal epithelium and into the systemic circulation without the requirement for hypodermic injection due to a microneedle pill design presented by Abramson and associates [28]. To create a luminal unfolding microneedle injector (LUMI), the scientists attached a patch of microneedles of 0.5 cm² to the tip of each of three movable arms that extended from a central base. Each patch contains 32 microneedles produced from a biodegradable polymer with a drug payload. The LUMI's arms are packed together, and the whole assembly is put bottom-down within a capsule with a depressed spring attached to the base. The LUMI system is released from the capsule once it has been ingested and has reached the gut, when the polymeric structure containing the spring dissolves, triggering the release. As the LUMI arms extend outward, microneedle patches are forced on the intestinal lining to penetrate the epithelial tissue, where they disintegrate and discharge the drug payload. Microneedle insertion into the intestinal epithelium without significant tissue puncture was achieved in *ex vivo* trials by adjusting the force or pressure of microneedles application. Continued research will need to evaluate whether the injury caused by LUMI microneedle release and insertion is unpleasant.

A model device's efficacy and transit rate through a pig's digestive system has also been investigated. Endoscopic insertion of a model device measuring 2 cm in length and 1 cm in diameter with radially projecting 25G stainless steel needles was performed in the stomachs of Yorkshire pigs, and their radiographic development was recorded. The results indicated that the transit time varied in the range of 7–56 days. More significantly, the capsule was successfully administered, and there were no reported adverse effects from the animal's physiology. There was no sign of injury on gross or histological evaluation after the device's passage [15].

13.2.3 Conclusion of Microneedles in Oral Delivery

There is a lack of effective oral mucosa vaccination technologies, making it challenging to investigate the impact of formulation composition, dose, release profile, and immunological responses. Although the many benefits of microneedles for transdermal and intradermal drug delivery have been well-documented, there is a critical lack of evidence for their use in oral mucosa. The use of adjuvants, evaluation of immune responses, and comparison between different oral mucosal sites are promising avenues for future research. Extensive evaluation of long-term safety, as well as the development of mass production feasibility, is crucial for determining the complete capacity of these technologies for regular usage in the clinic. Dosage considerations, physiological and therapeutic benefits (or drawbacks) of oral administration versus conventional injections, and the product cost should be considered when matching the biologics with the appropriate delivery method. Oral delivery systems for biologics in clinical settings have a bright future owing to the accelerated development of related technologies [16].

13.3 Ocular Route of Administration

13.3.1 Introduction of Ocular Drug Delivery

Several methods for administering drugs to the eye include intravitreal injections, surgical implantation of drug carriers, systemic administration, and topical application [29]. Each method has its benefits but inevitably has its limits and drawbacks. For instance, the blood-ocular barrier significantly reduces the penetration of systemically delivered drugs, requiring a very high dose that may be detrimental or result in severe adverse effects [30]. Among the barriers to drug absorption in the eye is the corneal epithelium, which makes ocular drug bioavailability relatively low with topical delivery of pharmaceuticals (i.e., eye drops). As with any other kind of surgery, sustained-release drug vehicles implanted surgically are very intrusive and are only conducted when there are no other viable options [17].

Traditional past strategies for treating eye issues included eye drops, laser therapy, injections, and even surgery. These have shown some efficacy but come with complications, including adverse effects, bleeding, and visual loss, and ultimately fall short of providing lasting treatment [31]. Traditionally, topical drug formulations (such as ointments, gels, and solutions) have been commonly used to treat eye diseases as they are effective in penetrating the anterior portion of the eye, may be self-administered, and have excellent patient compliance. The barrier function of the cornea and the lacrimal fluid that washes away topically applied drugs from the eye surface makes it difficult for eye drops and ointments to have any significant therapeutic impact. In addition, part of the administered drug in the standard topical formulations may be absorbed into the blood capillaries of a highly vascularized conjunctiva, thus reducing the drug's bioavailability and increasing the risk of adverse systemic effects [17].

Direct injections of drug formulation into the eyeball or the surrounding tissues using conventional hypodermic needles is standard practice for achieving targeted ocular drug delivery. Injections are employed to address various ocular conditions, including those affecting the anterior and posterior regions of the eye. They are preferred over systemic drug delivery since they allow more precise drug delivery to the affected areas [17]. When practical, it is advisable to refrain from injecting pharmaceutical products directly into the eye using hypodermic needles since doing so may cause considerable pain and injury to the fragile ocular and periocular tissues. The use of hypodermic needles-based injections poses additional risks, including elevation of intraocular pressure, bacterial infection, mechanical tissue disruption, inflammation, retinal detachment, and local bleeding. Moreover, intraocular injections are technically challenging and need the expertise of medical professionals. The risk of serious ocular issues and low patient acceptability seems to rise with the frequency and duration of conventional ocular needle injections. As a result, there is a pressing necessity for less intrusive methods that improve patient compliance and facilitate localized and targeted drug administration to the eye [32].

13.3.2 Microneedles Applications in Ocular Drug Delivery

Recently, microneedles have been advocated as a viable, less invasive alternative to the previously mentioned drug delivery methods utilized in ocular therapy [2]. Instead of using large, long, and invasive hypodermic needles for intraocular injections, microneedles may provide several benefits. The use of invasive hypodermic needles to provide ocular injections may be eliminated with microneedles in the length range of 25–2,000 μm.

Compared to traditional hypodermic injections, this microneedle method causes less discomfort and minimal tissue damage and eliminates the risk of bacterial infection. Self-administration is also a feasible option, which improves patient compliance, and the procedure reduces administration pain. In addition, since microneedles are applied precisely where they ought to be, ocular therapy is both dose-sparing and highly bioavailable, even though it must pass through the physiological barriers of the eye. To insert microneedles into the cornea requires just a miniature disruption and, as a result, causes little microinjury to the eye. Several studies' findings imply that the ocular application of microneedles may be well-tolerated. Numerous evaluations have also shown that microneedles are safe and effective for ocular treatment, with no significant side effects recorded, including discomfort, inflammation, redness, or vision loss [2, 33–35]. However, further research is required to determine the procedure's safety [32].

There has been relatively little study into the use of microneedles for ocular drug delivery; therefore, the approach is still somewhat novel. The use of microneedles as a therapeutic strategy for anterior and posterior eye sections is now under investigation [36]. Microneedles may provide localized drug delivery inside ocular tissues, including the sclera, stroma, and suprachoroidal region, because their sizes are sufficiently long to bypass ocular barriers of the anterior and posterior parts of the eye [37]. Several experiments have shown that coated, dissolving, and hollow microneedles are promising for ocular drug delivery. Microneedles might penetrate ocular tissues, including conjunctiva, sclera, and cornea, to deliver drugs to the rear or front regions of the eye. It has been suggested that microneedles be used to remove fluid from the eye cavity in order to alleviate glaucoma [38]. Typically, the cornea, sclera, or suprachoroidal space (SCS) is frequently where microneedles are inserted during eye therapy. Drugs administered in this way have a greater chance of penetrating the cornea and sclera and being deposited or released in the anterior or posterior region of the eye [39].

It is envisaged that microneedles would provide a safer and more convenient alternative to traditional hypodermic needles for accessing the SCS. Patient compliance issues generated by intravitreal injections and bioavailability shortfalls induced by periocular drug delivery may be prevented if drug solutions are injected into this SCS space, where they can flow circularly around the eye and potentially reach the macula if the injection location is adjacent to the limbus [40, 41]. If the drug formulation is precisely delivered to the SCS, it should cause less damage to the retina's supporting layers. Drug delivery via the SCS is a promising field of ophthalmic research that might benefit from the use of microneedles. SCS drug delivery calls for the drug product to be positioned in the space just below the sclera and over the choroid. Needles utilized for this function should preferably be of a length equivalent to scleral thickness (<1 mm) so as not to penetrate the choroidal vasculature or underlying tissue. Due to this requirement, needle lengths must be reduced to the micrometer range or much less than 1 mm [42].

Research about microneedle-mediated ocular drug delivery performed by the Prausnitz Group suggests that the following four criteria should be included in any viable method for administering drugs to the retina [3]:

- Noninvasive or minimally invasive and safe.
- Enable targeted delivery with high bioavailability and minimal side effects and toxicity risk.
- Facilitate sustained drug delivery to reduce dosing frequency and improve therapeutic control.
- Simple, convenient, requiring only a routine practice or, ideally, allowing for self-administration.

Although all four types of microneedles (solid, coated, hollow, and dissolving microneedles) are applicable to ocular drug delivery, the focus has been on hollow, dissolving, and coated microneedles. When using solid microneedles, two separate steps must be taken. Ocular drug permeation may be improved by inserting an array of solid microneedles into the eye and then removing them to create numerous micrometer-sized channels in the tissue. Subsequently, the second step involves the application of a topical preparation to the location where microneedles were used. The active ingredients in this formulation are delivered into and across the tissue by passive diffusion via the microneedles-created microchannels. Coating the microneedles with a suitable drug formulation (coated microneedles) makes it possible to localize the drug inside the ocular tissue after they have been inserted into the eye. Intriguingly, in an *in vitro* experiment designed to test posterior segment delivery, these coated microneedles successfully delivered various compounds such as sulforhodamine, protein, and DNA [32]. As the name implies, hollow microneedles are hollow micrometer-sized needles that, once inserted, provide the injection of a drug formulation (i.e., a drug solution or nano/microparticle drug fluid) into the ocular tissue for localized or prolonged drug delivery. Various drugs were also injected into the suprachoroidal area using hollow microneedles [32]. Another interesting strategy for ocular drug delivery is the use of polymeric dissolving microneedles. These microneedles are composed of a biodegradable and biocompatible matrix that contains the active ingredient. This sort of microneedle is often fabricated using micromolding methods [37, 43]. Once the needles have been inserted, the matrix material dissolves or degrades in the tissue, releasing the drug payload [32]. Dissolving microneedles can reduce the use of solid materials and prevent unintentional retinal injury compared to solid or hollow microneedles. In addition, dissolving microneedles could either dissolve quickly inside the treated tissue or remain as a drug reservoir for sustained drug delivery [37]. Dissolving microneedles, in contrast to hypodermic needles used for intravitreal injections, produce no sharps waste after usage since they dissolve completely in the fluid of the ocular tissue.

The utilization of microneedles in drug delivery to the eye is becoming more prevalent. Nevertheless, there are few studies in the research literature on the biosafety of microneedles for such purposes. The microneedle approach is generally safe but does not yet meet all of the standards for typically safe ocular treatment. This makes the potential for the nondissolving microneedle to break within the eye a serious cause for concern. A few challenges must be resolved before microneedles ocular delivery may be used, including sterility, needle fracture, accidental injury, the administration technique, and others. It is agreeable that transferring the highly sophisticated procedure of microneedles-based drug administration from the clinic to the home setting is a significant difficulty and that much more work is necessary for this area.

Microneedle insertion's influence on intraocular pressure is another critical aspect that has to be thoroughly studied. Few studies have investigated whether microneedle insertion forces contribute to an increase in intraocular pressure (IOP). Microneedle injection has been shown to generate a temporary rise in IOP, peaking at 35 ± 3 mmHg and decaying in less than 1 h, which is comparable to the IOP rise created by intravitreal injection (30 mmHg) [44]. The transient increment in IOP generated by microneedle insertion is considered safe since the conventional injection is well-tolerated in patients when just a topical anesthetic is used [33]. However, further research is required to verify the microneedles' long-term safety and to quantify the ocular tissues' recovery rate from the stress brought on by the microneedles application [45].

Due to tissue resistance and needle dimensions, the magnitude of the force necessary for microneedles to administer the drug is also crucial [3, 46, 47]. Microneedles have the potential to be a game-changing platform for ocular drug delivery; however, they may be hampered by challenges related to the reliability and repeatability of microneedle insertion into ocular tissues. Very few research efforts have focused on this challenge and developed novel techniques for microneedles application [32]. Most healthcare professionals would rather have some assistance when carrying out an intraocular injection. To facilitate accurate positioning and injection, some experts have gone so far as to create syringe/needle supports. InVitria (FCI), SCS microinjector (Clearside Biomedical), and SpEye (Alyko Medicals) are just a few examples of guarded injectable devices [42]. The microneedles pen, a spring-loaded microneedles application device, was specially constructed to increase the accuracy and reliability of microneedle insertion by making the needles simpler to handle and allowing for their effective penetration into the targeted ocular tissue with little tip fracture.

13.3.3 Case Studies of Microneedles for Ocular Drug Delivery

Investigators have been inserting hollow microneedles into the human sclera (intrascleral) for the last decade, with preliminary *in vitro* and *in vivo* research conducted on rabbit and pig eyes. Even though this research has focused on using microneedles to administer drugs into SCS, it would be possible to adapt their technique for use in other eye regions. Microparticle and nanoparticle suspensions with varying particle sizes were injected into the eye [3]. Based on the findings of this study, microneedles may provide a noninvasive way to bypass the eye's physical barriers, thus delivering therapeutic molecules and particulate systems to specific targeted sites in the eye. In another study, nanoparticle and microparticle suspensions were successfully delivered to the back of the eye through a minimally invasive injection using a single hollow borosilicate microneedle, as described by Patel et al. [3]. This experiment used entire eyeballs from rabbits, pigs, and humans as an *ex vivo* model. The researchers discovered that hollow microneedles might be inserted into the sclera. However, injection of drug solution into the tissue was exceedingly sluggish without retraction, while injection of 10–35 μL was possible after partial retraction of the microneedle across a distance of 200–300 μm. The impacts of scleral thickness and injection pressure on drug delivery were negligible. Neither the sulforhodamine B solution nor the FlouoSpheres suspensions failed to reach their targets, as revealed by the authors. Effective drug administration into the suprachoroidal space was observed at microneedle lengths of 800–1,000 μm and pressures of 250–300 kPa.

Researchers also visualized the insertion of solid metal microneedles coated with model drugs, protein, and DNA into human cadaver sclera [2]. The sodium fluorescein-coated microneedles were applied to the rabbit cornea *in vivo*. The fluorescein level in the front of the rabbit's eye was monitored for a day after the needle's insertion and removal. Solid microneedles coated with pilocarpine were used in a similar way to observe the pupils of rabbits. The coating layer quickly dissolved inside the scleral tissue, and *in vitro* insertion experiments indicated that microneedles were mechanically robust enough to puncture human cadaver sclera. The quantity of fluorescein in the anterior chamber was 60-fold higher after *in vivo* administration using fluorescein-coated microneedles than after topical treatment. A 45-fold increase in bioavailability was observed when pilocarpine was coated on microneedles as compared to topical administration [2]. Utilizing 33-G hollow microneedles of 850 µm length, Gilger and colleagues reported effective triamcinolone acetonide (TA) delivery in the SCS *in vivo*. The investigators showed that 0.2 mg of TA administered by microneedles into the SCS was equally as effective in reducing inflammation as 2.0 mg of TA provided via intravitreal injection in animals with acute posterior uveitis inflammation. In this *in vivo* experiment, no adverse side effects were reported, including increased intraocular pressure (IOP), toxicity, or bleeding [48].

For drug delivery into the SCS, effectiveness and safety have recently been evaluated in humans using microneedles shorter than a millimeter and diameters comparable to those of presently employed intravitreal needles. In these research studies, a microinjector device manufactured by Clearside Biomedical, Inc., has been utilized to administer a 100 mL volume of TA drug solution. If sufficiently robust nanoscale needles capable of penetrating eye tissues can be produced, intraocular injections with nanoneedles may one day be possible [40]. Injecting triamcinolone acetonide solution (TA) into the SCS of pigs, Clearside Biomedical, Inc., tested the effectiveness of suprachoroidal delivery utilizing hollow microneedles for the treatment of acute posterior segment uveitis. Low (0.2 mg) and high (2.0 mg) doses of TA injected through microneedles were shown to be equally efficacious as intravitreal injection of the greater TA dose, with the distribution across the eyeball mainly depending on the injected volume [48]. Following this, the company conducted a phase II clinical study to assess the safety and effectiveness of its patented product (Zuprata™), delivered TA suprachoroidal through 1,000 µm microneedles in patients with macular edema [49]. Clearside Biomedical, Inc., has also concluded a phase II clinical trial (TANZANITE) demonstrating that concurrent delivery of suprachoroidal CLS-TA with intravitreal aflibercept resulted in superior visual gain than intravitreal aflibercept alone. Lastly, the business is looking at using a tyrosine kinase inhibitor (Axitinib™) delivered suprachoroidally to treat wet age-related macular degeneration.

Kim and associates studied intrastromal delivery of bevacizumab to treat central nervous system tumors using a single coated stainless steel microneedle of 400 µm in length [50]. Compared to 2,500 µg given through subconjunctival injection and 52,500 µg provided topically by eye drops, only 4.4 µg of bevacizumab was sufficient to induce the equivalent therapeutic efficacy, demonstrating a considerable benefit of localized drug administration utilizing microneedles.

To fabricate polyvinylpyrrolidone (PVP)-based dissolving microneedles, Thakur and colleagues used a simple and inexpensive micromolding technique [21]. They tested the material's biocompatibility by exposing it to retinal cells to determine whether the use of PVP-based dissolving microneedles was safe [34]. In the *in vitro* tests, PVP microneedles were biocompatible with retinal cells, with more than 83% viability at PVP levels below 2 mg/mL [32]. According to the research findings, it can be concluded that PVP microneedles have sufficient strength to penetrate scleral and corneal tissues and that they quickly dissolve in less than 3 min after the insertion. The dissolving microneedles significantly improved the penetration of the model drugs through the cornea and sclera compared to topically administered aqueous solutions. According to the observations, these microneedles could swiftly dissolve inside the sclera to create a drug depot and easily enter the outer scleral layers, facilitating the intrascleral penetration of large molecules (dextrans with a molecular weight of 70 and 150 kDa). Dissolving microneedles were produced out of biodegradable polylactic acid (PLA) and filled with 10% methotrexate to treat primary vitreoretinal lymphoma. These microneedles were then administered intrasclerally. Preliminary toxicity tests found that the dissolving microneedles were safe to use (with no toxicity and inflammation events), allowing for extended drug release from deep lamellar scleral pockets in rabbit eyes [34]. Researchers have shown that hollow microneedles can be used to administer drugs continuously into the sclera through *in situ* poloxamer-based gels. The duration that fluorescein sodium was released from the gel after being applied to the scleral tissue ranged from 24 h to several days [51].

13.3.4 Conclusion of Microneedles for Ocular Drug Delivery

Recent years have seen phenomenal growth in both interest and engagement in the microneedles sector, leading to accelerated advances in understanding the technology that is driving more industry involvement. Microneedle-mediated ocular drug delivery is a potential study area despite the lack of information so far. Minimally invasive microneedles ocular drug delivery might provide various benefits to solve the present challenges around hypodermic needle injections. When compared to hypodermic needles, microneedles provide a less invasive option that results in fewer adverse effects and the use of lower doses of the drug. Advantages of microneedles over conventional hypodermic needles include reduced pain sensation, reduced risk of infection, and more precise control over the delivered dose. Furthermore, the barrier function of ocular tissues is not severely compromised, and any damage is rapidly healed.

Microneedles may help localize drug delivery in the targeted ocular tissue, which will circumvent the barrier and enable therapeutic drug concentrations to be sustained in the eye for extended periods. Microneedles may offer effective therapy for both anterior and posterior diseases. Nevertheless, the needles' dimensions should be controlled to minimize accidental injury to surrounding tissues while effectively bypassing the ocular barrier. Extensive studies are required to develop an acceptable applicator for microneedle ocular delivery. Safety of microneedles ocular drug delivery also needs more investigation since, so far, insufficient research has been conducted in this area. Specifically, safety associated with microneedles insertion force, tissue type, penetration depth, application duration, drug formulation, and acceptable animal model requires additional research. Ultimately, microneedles can transform the way drugs are delivered into the eye. However, the limits and problems of microneedle applications require more study to facilitate their extensive clinical applications [32]. When manufacturing techniques are completely developed, optimized, and validated, and regulatory hurdles are addressed, the maximum potential of microneedles can be realized. Regulatory agencies, industries, and universities should collaborate to achieve this goal which would have profound consequences for the healthcare system and the patients.

13.4 Other Applications of Microneedles

13.4.1 Vaginal Drug Delivery

Vaginal vaccination may be effective as it could be delivered to antigen-presenting cells in the vaginal mucosa. By delivering antigens through microneedles into the vaginal tissue, Wang and coworkers [10] obtained strong antigen-specific immune responses at systemic and mucosal levels.

13.4.2 Transungual Drug Delivery

As reported by Chiu and colleagues, solid microneedles treatment could provide extended topical drug delivery into the nail. Unlike topical drug delivery without microneedles, where the highly keratinized nail barrier impedes drug permeation, microneedle-treated nails allow for efficient drug diffusion deep into the nail [11]. Evidence suggests that the reported method of microneedles-based nail poration, followed by the application of a topical drug formulation, is a potential avenue for further research.

13.4.3 Drug Delivery to the Anal Sphincter Muscles

The administration of phenylephrine (PE) into the anal sphincter muscle has been shown to be effective in treating fecal incontinence. As PE delivery to the anal sphincter muscle is usually insufficient after topical gel administration, Baek and coworkers fabricated a microneedle patch to improve the drug bioavailability [13]. This method of drug delivery resulted in a tenfold enhancement in PE delivery, leading to markedly higher resting anal sphincter pressure than following treatment with topical gel alone.

13.4.4 Drug Delivery to Blood Vessels

Insufficient drug delivery into blood vessel walls may restrict therapeutic efficacy for cardiovascular diseases. Choi and colleagues developed microneedle patches with a curved substrate to treat atherosclerotic blood vessels [12]. The technique was designed to overcome the drawbacks of drug-eluting stents (which damage the endothelium lining the blood vessels) and cuff-style external devices (which only provide slow drug penetration and complicated drug distribution in the targeted tissue). The curved substrate of the patch was folded around the affected blood vessel, penetrating the barrier tunica adventitia and releasing the medication swiftly into the target vascular tissue.

13.4.5 Injection in Living Cells

Biomaterials (i.e., DNA, RNA, protein, virus particles, etc.) may be introduced into a plant or animal cell *in vivo* using an array of silicon microneedles, as described by Ginaven et al. This has the potential to improve human gene therapy in the areas of gene delivery, gene expression, transgenic organism generation, and somatic cell transformation. The researchers employed solid microneedles coated with the delivered material to transport the biological material of interest into the target cell. The patent also describes a basic device design that demonstrates the effectiveness of the microneedles for this application [31].

13.4.6 Microneedles in Animal Identification

The microneedles-based technology allows for noninvasive epidermal permanent marking (colored mark, pattern, or number), which might be particularly useful for rapid identification and keeping a record of animals during studies. In addition, the recognition and monitoring could be performed within the facilities and in the open areas if a microneedle device could be utilized to implant a microelectronic device into the animals [31].

13.5 Conclusions

Drug delivery directly to diseased tissues has attracted a lot of attention because it has the potential to increase therapeutic efficacy, decrease adverse effects, and circumvent obstacles that systemic drug delivery must overcome on the way to the targeted site. Microneedles patches provide a simple yet effective alternative for making biological barriers transiently susceptible to drugs after the physical treatment. They can be used on tissues accessible by an external device and contain a thin protective layer on the tissue surface. The application of microneedles onto certain types of tissues presents new challenges because these tissues are usually moist (microneedles must not disintegrate or lose their mechanical strength due to moisture absorption before the insertion), soft (microneedles must have a suitable design and insertion method), and vulnerable to discomfort and injury (microneedle application by competent healthcare providers). Novel microneedle designs taking into consideration the structure, biology, and mechanical properties of the targeted tissues, as well as the physicochemical properties and quantities of drugs to be given and the specific disease to be treated, will be necessary for developing microneedles for safe and efficient application in the tissues.

References

[1] Traverso G, Schoellhammer CM, Schroeder A, et al. Microneedles for drug delivery via the gastrointestinal tract. J Pharm Sci. 2015;104:362–367.
[2] Jiang J, Gill HS, Ghate D, et al. Coated microneedles for drug delivery to the eye. Invest Ophthalmol Vis Sci. 2007;48:4038–4043.
[3] Patel SR, Lin AS, Edelhauser HF, et al. Suprachoroidal drug delivery to the back of the eye using hollow microneedles. Pharm Res. 2011;28:166–176.
[4] Ikeno F, Lyons J, Kaneda H, et al. Novel percutaneous adventitial drug delivery system for regional vascular treatment. Catheter Cardiovasc Interv. 2004;63:222–230.
[5] Lee CY, You YS, Lee SH, et al. Tower microneedle minimizes vitreal reflux in intravitreal injection. Biomed Microdevices. 2013;15:841–848.
[6] Ma Y, Tao W, Krebs SJ, et al. Vaccine delivery to the oral cavity using coated microneedles induces systemic and mucosal immunity. Pharm Res. 2014;31:2393–2403.
[7] Hong JY, Ko EJ, Choi SY, et al. Efficacy and safety of a novel, soluble microneedle patch for the improvement of facial wrinkle. J Cosmet Dermatol. 2018;17:235–241.
[8] Kellerman DJ, Ameri M, Tepper SJ. Rapid systemic delivery of zolmitriptan using an adhesive dermally applied microarray. Pain Manag. 2017;7:559–567.

[9] Rouphael NG, Paine M, Mosley R, et al. The safety, immunogenicity, and acceptability of inactivated influenza vaccine delivered by microneedle patch (TIV-MNP 2015): a randomised, partly blinded, placebo-controlled, phase 1 trial. The Lancet. 2017;390:649–658.

[10] Wang N, Zhen Y, Jin Y, et al. Combining different types of multifunctional liposomes loaded with ammonium bicarbonate to fabricate microneedle arrays as a vaginal mucosal vaccine adjuvant-dual delivery system (VADDS). J Control Release. 2017;246:12–29.

[11] Chiu WS, Belsey NA, Garrett NL, et al. Drug delivery into microneedle-porated nails from nanoparticle reservoirs. J Control Release. 2015;220, Part A:98–106.

[12] Choi CK, Kim JB, Jang EH, et al. Curved biodegradable microneedles for vascular drug delivery. Small. 2012;8:2483–2488.

[13] Baek C, Han M, Min J, et al. Local transdermal delivery of phenylephrine to the anal sphincter muscle using microneedles. J Control Release. 2011;154:138–147.

[14] Dhurat R, Sukesh M, Avhad G, et al. A randomized evaluator blinded study of effect of microneedling in androgenetic alopecia: a pilot study. Int J Trichology. 2013;5:6–11.

[15] Schoellhammer CM, Langer R, Traverso G. Of microneedles and ultrasound: physical modes of gastrointestinal macromolecule delivery. Tissue Barriers. 2016;e1150235.

[16] Vllasaliu D, Thanou M, Stolnik S, et al. Recent advances in oral delivery of biologics: nanomedicine and physical modes of delivery. Expert Opin Drug Deliv. 2018;15:759–770.

[17] Rzhevskiy AS, Singh TRR, Donnelly RF, et al. Microneedles as the technique of drug delivery enhancement in diverse organs and tissues. J Control Release. 2018;270:184–202.

[18] Wang T, Zhen Y, Ma X, et al. Mannosylated and lipid A-incorporating cationic liposomes constituting microneedle arrays as an effective oral mucosal HBV vaccine applicable in the controlled temperature chain. Colloids Surf B Biointerfaces. 2015;126:520–530.

[19] Zhen Y, Wang N, Gao Z, et al. Multifunctional liposomes constituting microneedles induced robust systemic and mucosal immunoresponses against the loaded antigens via oral mucosal vaccination. Vaccine. 2015;33:4330–4340.

[20] Traverso G, Langer R. Perspective: special delivery for the gut. Nature. 2015;519:S19–S19.

[21] Thakur RRS, Tekko IA, Al-Shammari F, et al. Rapidly dissolving polymeric microneedles for minimally invasive intraocular drug delivery. Drug Deliv Transl Res. 2016;6:800–815.

[22] Creighton RL, Woodrow KA. Microneedle-mediated vaccine delivery to the oral mucosa. Adv Healthc Mater. 2019;8:1801180.

[23] Lee JW, Park J-H, Prausnitz MR. Dissolving microneedles for transdermal drug delivery. Biomaterials. 2008;29:2113–2124.

[24] Sullivan SP, Koutsonanos DG, Del Pilar Martin M, et al. Dissolving polymer microneedle patches for influenza vaccination. Nat Med. 2010;16:915–920.

[25] Serpe L, Jain A, Macedo CG de, et al. Influence of salivary washout on drug delivery to the oral cavity using coated microneedles: an in vitro evaluation. Eur J Pharm Sci. 2016;93:215–223.

[26] Caffarel-Salvador E, Kim S, Soares V, et al. A microneedle platform for buccal macromolecule delivery. Sci Adv. 2021;7:eabe2620.

[27] Nolan T, Richmond PC, McVernon J, et al. Safety and immunogenicity of an inactivated thimerosal-free influenza vaccine in infants and children. Influenza Other Respir Viruses. 2009;3:315–325.

[28] Abramson A, Caffarel-Salvador E, Soares V, et al. A luminal unfolding microneedle injector for oral delivery of macromolecules. Nat Med. 2019;25:1512–1518.

[29] Gaudana R, Ananthula HK, Parenky A, et al. Ocular drug delivery. AAPS J. 2010;12:348–360.

[30] Cunha-Vaz J, Marques FB, Fernandes R, et al. Drug transport across blood-ocular barriers and pharmacokinetics. In: Thirumurthy Velpadian, editors. Pharmalology ocular therapeutics. New York: Springer; 2016. p. 37–63.

[31] Sachdeva VK, Banga A. Microneedles and their applications. Recent Pat Drug Deliv Formul. 2011;5:95–132.

[32] Donnelly RF, Singh TRR, Larrañeta E, et al. Microneedles for drug and vaccine delivery and patient monitoring. Hoboken, New Jersey: John Wiley & Sons; 2018.

[33] Kim YC, Edelhauser HF, Prausnitz MR. Targeted delivery of antiglaucoma drugs to the supraciliary space using microneedles. Invest Ophthalmol Vis Sci. 2014;55:7387–7397.

[34] Palakurthi NK, Correa ZM, Augsburger JJ, et al. Toxicity of a biodegradable microneedle implant loaded with methotrexate as a sustained release device in normal rabbit eye: a pilot study. J Ocul Pharmacol Ther. 2011;27:151–156.

[35] Patel SR, Berezovsky DE, McCarey BE, et al. Targeted administration into the suprachoroidal space using a microneedle for drug delivery to the posterior segment of the eye. Invest Ophthalmol Vis Sci. 2012;53:4433–4441.

[36] Davis B. Recent advances in drug delivery to the retina. Acta Ophthalmol (Copenh). 2015;93.

[37] Thakur Singh RR, Tekko I, McAvoy K, et al. Minimally invasive microneedles for ocular drug delivery. Expert Opin Drug Deliv. 2017;14:525–537.

[38] Prausnitz MR, Allen MG, McAllister DV, et al. Microneedle device for transport of molecules across tissue. Google Patents; 2003. [Internet] [cited 2016 Aug 23]. Available from: www.google.com/patents/US6503231.

[39] Fischbarg J. The biology of the eye. Amsterdam, NL: Elsevier; 2005.

[40] Kim Y-C, Park J-H, Prausnitz MR. Microneedles for drug and vaccine delivery. Adv Drug Deliv Rev. 2012;64:1547–1568.

[41] Rai UDJP, Young SA, Thrimawithana TR, et al. The suprachoroidal pathway: a new drug delivery route to the back of the eye. Drug Discov Today. 2015;20:491–495.

[42] Hartman RR, Kompella UB. Intravitreal, subretinal, and suprachoroidal injections: evolution of microneedles for drug delivery. J Ocul Pharmacol Ther. 2018;34:141–153.

[43] Quinn HL, Bonham L, Hughes CM, et al. Design of a dissolving microneedle platform for transdermal delivery of a fixed-dose combination of cardiovascular drugs. J Pharm Sci. 2015;104:3490–3500.

[44] Chehab HE, Le Corre A, Agard E, et al. Effect of topical pressure-lowering medication on prevention of intraocular pressure spikes after intravitreal injection. Eur J Ophthalmol. 2013;23:277–283.

[45] Huang D, Chen Y-S, Rupenthal ID. Overcoming ocular drug delivery barriers through the use of physical forces. Adv Drug Deliv Rev. 2018;126:96–112.

[46] Jiang J, Moore JS, Edelhauser HF, et al. Intrascleral drug delivery to the eye using hollow microneedles. Pharm Res. 2009;26:395–403.

[47] Patel SR, Edelhauser HF, Prausnitz MR. Targeted drug delivery to the eye enabled by microneedles. In: Uday B. Kompella, Henry F. Edelhauser, editors. Drug product development for the back of the eye. New York: Springer; 2011. p. 331–360.

[48] Gilger BC, Abarca EM, Salmon JH, et al. Treatment of acute posterior uveitis in a porcine model by injection of triamcinolone acetonide into the suprachoroidal space using microneedles. Invest Ophthalmol Vis Sci. 2013;54:2483–2492.

[49] Yeh S, Kurup SK, Wang RC, et al. Suprachoroidal injection of triamcinolone acetonide, CLS-TA, for macular edema due to noninfectious uveitis: a randomized, phase 2 study (DOGWOOD). Retina. 2019;39:1880–1888.

[50] Kim Y-M, Lim J-O, Kim H-K, et al. A novel design of one-side coated biodegradable intrascleral implant for the sustained release of triamcinolone acetonide. Eur J Pharm Biopharm. 2008;70:179–186.

[51] Thakur RRS, Fallows SJ, McMillan HL, et al. Microneedle-mediated intrascleral delivery of in situ forming thermoresponsive implants for sustained ocular drug delivery. J Pharm Pharmacol. 2014;66:584–595.

14

Development Issues and Commercialization of Microneedles

14.1 Introduction of Microneedle Commercialization

Microneedle delivery systems have been developed more recently than transdermal systems, which have been around for over 30 years, or deeper tissue injection systems, which have been in use for over a century. The global transdermal drug delivery industry is expected to reach $95.57 billion by 2025, while the biopharmaceuticals market will reach $388 billion by 2024. Current medical needs have increased demand for protein and peptide-based drugs with high molecular weight, high dosage, and low potency. Microneedles have been identified as a promising technology platform for the transdermal delivery of various compounds (Fig. 14.1). Currently, only microneedle-based devices are available, not microneedle array-based drug delivery products. The market is expected to see around 13 microneedles goods launched in the next few years, with 485 million units of sales forecasted by 2030. Microneedle patches are estimated to cost between $0.50 and $1.00 per unit, and the market value will reach $266 million by 2030. Lohmann Therapy Systems AG (LTS), the world's largest transdermal patch manufacturer, has entered the microneedle field. They may have a tremendous influence if they could produce microneedle products at the same volume as transdermal patches.

Ideal microneedles should have a length of 50–900 μm and a tip diameter of 1 μm [2, 3]. Microneedles must be able to penetrate deeply into the skin without breaking. Microneedles should have optimal dimensions and geometries to sustain insertion forces of around 10 N, being strong and mechanically stable [4]. These are also designed for controlled drug delivery at a set rate. Hollow microneedles should be durable and leak-proof while delivering liquid drug formulations. Microneedle patches must adhere to the skin as firmly as regular transdermal patches. Comparable to a hypodermic needle, microneedles should provide rapid action and efficient medication administration. Microneedles should facilitate self-medication and tailored medicines.

Microneedles enable transdermal delivery of agents which are unable to passively permeate the stratum corneum, such as proteins, peptides, and biological molecules. Microneedles are a cost-effective transdermal drug delivery technology that is as effective as an intramuscular injection while being more convenient. Safety, ease of use, manufacturing, storage, administration, and effectiveness are critical pharmacoeconomic factors of microneedles. Currently, most clinical trials have used microneedles for vaccination and insulin administration. Other treatments require further research. Microneedles have a comparable success rate to traditional treatments; however, it varies depending on the drugs. Unlike syringe needles, microneedles lessen patient pain and anxiety, thus being ideal for children.

DOI: 10.1201/9780429294433-14

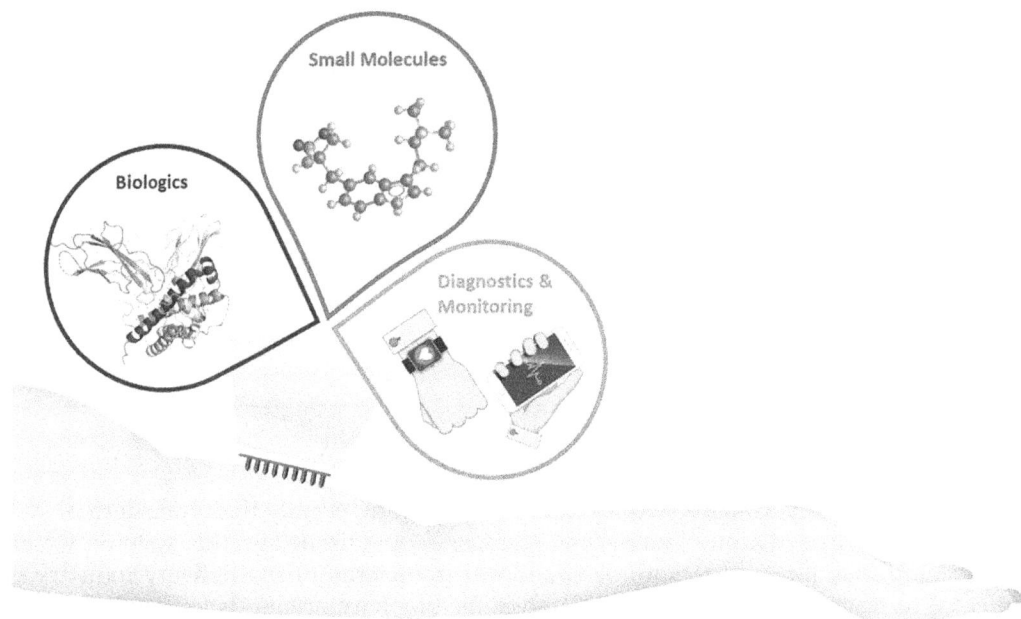

FIGURE 14.1
Microneedle applications in diagnosis delivery of various therapeutic agents (i.e., small molecules and macro-molecules). Image reprinted with permission from [1].

Microneedle system has certain safety concerns: mechanical strength, drug release, bioavailability, painlessness, and manufacturability have impacts on microneedle performance. Also, microneedle designs should have sufficient skin insertion, complete dissolution, and drug-loading capacity. As microneedles are miniature, mechanical strength is required for successful skin insertion without fracturing. There is no way to remove materials delivered with the drug after microneedles are inserted into the skin. Thus, the design of microneedle systems must consider the materials' biocompatibility and safety, which must be similar to the intramuscular delivery systems. To successfully administer therapeutic agents using microneedles, mechanical, chemical, and biological safety must be considered.

Cost comparisons vary depending on microneedle types. Metal microneedles require different manufacturing procedures than polymer microneedles; hence their costs will vary significantly. Microneedles could compete on price with typically expensive biologicals. Vaccination prices are heavily impacted by administration expenses rather than vaccine costs. Since microneedles are self-administered, they are cheaper than injectables. The cost saving by increasing patient adherence and vaccination willingness must be considered. In general, novel technology is more expensive until it becomes more popular.

Preclinical evidence on microneedle delivery devices is substantial, and some clinical trials have displayed equivalent pharmacokinetics profiles to existing injection systems. The systems are designed to focus on patients' needs, human factors, and usability. Technical development makes use of current understandings of transdermal and injectable systems. Most clinical trials employed microneedle injectable systems and microneedle array-based patches to compare microneedle delivery systems to traditional drug delivery systems. Many clinical investigations have indicated rapid onset pharmacokinetic effects and improved pain-scores of microneedles than standard subcutaneous administration.

14.2 Economic Evaluation of Microneedles

14.2.1 Introduction of Economic Aspects of Microneedles

By 2013, the microneedle market had grown to $24 billion [5]. By 2025, the estimated value of the worldwide transdermal drug delivery market is $95 billion. According to a recent Future Market Insight analysis, the microneedle drug delivery system market will reach $1.2 billion by 2030, growing at a 6.6% compound annual growth rate. For microneedles to be cost-effective, they must be inserted reliably on the first try and offer equivalent efficacy to conventional treatments. The effectiveness, compliance, and uptake of microneedles must be improved to make them more cost-effective than existing medicines. DebioJect and VaxMAT are examples of microneedle drug delivery systems that provide a glimpse into the future. Several companies have demonstrated that microneedle technology can be scaled up from the lab to large-scale manufacturing.

In the cosmetic industry, microneedles have long been recognized as a treatment option, with many devices available for home usage. Regulatory procedures and standards are required, which consume time and cost for the finished product. Evaluating innovative technologies from an economic standpoint while still developing will promote market adoption. The cosmetic sector is boosting microneedle acceptability and mass production. Besides, the self-administration of microneedles can also reduce vaccination costs. Further research is required to provide an economic analysis of self-vaccination and investigate how this strategy could be used globally in various healthcare payer systems. Minimally invasive influenza vaccine technology—microneedles—has numerous potential benefits; the economic value will be determined by the pricing, self-administration, and vaccination success rates. Microneedle patch technology may lower healthcare expenses and increase vaccination coverage in hard-to-reach communities. However, any microneedle manufacturer must invest substantially to develop this novel technology.

14.2.2 Factors Affecting the Cost of Microneedles

Depending on microneedle types, patients or others may be able to reuse the needles. Silicon, metal, and ceramic microneedles are removed intact from the skin after usage and might be reinserted if not properly discarded. Thus, a fail-safe or self-destructing disposal system may be necessary; however, it will add to the cost of microneedles.

For the microneedle patch to be cost-effective, it must be accepted as a novel technology compared to conventional vaccine delivery techniques. Medicine adherence and vaccine coverage enhance microneedle cost-effectiveness. The application of microneedles must be simple and straightforward, with or without an applicator. Hand application avoids the cost, size, and complexity of applicators; however, it reduces patients' confidence in an accurate way to apply microneedles [6]. Painless microneedles increase patient adherence and treatment willingness. Patient compliance markedly improves cost savings, as shown in numerous vaccine trials, but no study has been performed on how diagnostic microneedles affect patient compliance. Adhikari et al. reported that measles prevalence affects the cost-effectiveness of vaccination [7]. A significant cost would be saved in a population with a high incidence of measles. Also, the cost-reducing effect will be maximized if this microneedle system is used on a large scale. Furthermore, advertising and promotional campaigns will also impact the uptake and rate of vaccination.

Administration expenses rather than vaccine costs heavily influence vaccination prices. Medicare and Medicaid reimburse twice as much for administration as for vaccines ($26.20 versus $12.40). Microneedles are designed to be self-administered, resulting in significant cost savings. Moreover, biologicals are generally administered by a doctor or nurse, whereas patients can self-administer microneedles at home, thus saving a lot of money [8, 9]. Improved vaccine coverage will decrease influenza-associated hospitalizations, fatalities, and lost productivity.

An investigation revealed that microneedles could persuade 30% of typically unvaccinated volunteers to vaccinate. The advantage of microneedle self-administration increased the intent to vaccinate to 38% [10]. Adhikari et al. investigated the cost-effectiveness of microneedle patches for measles vaccination campaigns. Generally, microneedles were expected to withstand high temperatures and not need a cold-chain supply. Subcutaneous vaccination costs $1.65 against $0.95 for the microneedle vaccine. Adhikari and coworkers estimated the average cost of preventing one measles case with a microneedle patch at $1.66 compared to $2.64 using standard subcutaneous vaccination. The authors found that microneedles can lower costs based on user acceptance and vaccination efficacy [7].

Biologicals are generally expensive products, and microneedles could likely compete on price, whereas competing against creams and tablets would be difficult. Studies have revealed that microneedle systems can administer a combination of therapeutic agents to save the cost of drugs and administration. Quinn and coworkers (2015) have developed a dissolving polymeric microneedle system that could deliver a combination of three cardiovascular drugs (aspirin, lisinopril dihydrate, and atorvastatin calcium trihydrate) across porcine skin *in vitro* [11]. To evaluate cost-effectiveness, the treatment efficacy must be compared: (i) Do microneedles treat the condition more effectively? (ii) Do they provide greater vaccination coverage?

The cost of microneedles could be saved by improving commercial scalability and robustness. Microneedles cost is predicted to be comparable to injectable medicines [12]. The vaccine contributes to parts of the product cost. The cost of vaccine products using microneedle technology could be lower than the conventional vaccine vials or prefilled syringes. Microneedles are made from common low-cost biomedical-grade materials of minute quantities (less than 1 g), while the backing, adhesive, and packaging are made of conventional materials commonly used in transdermal patches or the like [13]. Furthermore, polymeric needles could be produced using the low-cost casting method. However, biologics or macromolecules may be a significant component of microneedle cost. For example, the mean annual cost per patient for maintenance dosing in rheumatoid arthritis treatment is $46,532 for Abatacept, $44,973 for Infliximab, $36,663 for Rituximab, and $36,821 for Tocilizumab [14]. Since microneedles puncture the skin, they must be sterile. Aseptic compounding might increase the product cost, while terminal sterilization can degrade the active ingredients. Coated microneedles generally consist of low-cost metal, polymer, or silicon microneedle structures onto which a vaccine formulation is coated by dipping or spraying. The polymeric formulation is cast onto a low-cost mold, dried, and packed to manufacture dissolving microneedles. The process of casting, dipping, spraying, coating, drying, and packing are commonly compatible with standard pharmaceutical manufacturing facilities and equipment. A primary portion of microneedle cost belongs to the requirement of aseptic conditions, which is comparable to the cost of producing vaccines in vials and syringes [13]. 3M provides an FDA-to-be-approved solid microneedle device (sMTS) for sale as a stand-alone device without any active ingredients. They are capable of manufacturing 10,000 patches per day with GMP aseptic coating conditions [15]. The necessity for sterile or low-bioburden manufacturing and the regulatory-acceptable processes remains unclear. As vaccination patches are applied to non-sterile skin, low bioburden manufacturing eliminates the costly requirement for sterility yet keeps organisms in the finished product to a minimum level. Low-bioburden production would allow substantial cost-saving since sterile production requires expensive machines and equipment. The cost of vaccination patches will be determined by the production and design of microneedles. Microneedles have been produced with various materials, processes, designs, and configurations; solid and hollow microneedles (silicone or metals) require different production techniques than polymeric microneedles; hence the cost will vary significantly. For instance, mechanically strong and biocompatible microneedles could be produced with excellent accuracy and minimum cost using the microelectromechanical systems process.

14.2.3 Reduced Cost of Vaccination

Microneedles have been the focus of numerous studies, which have shown that they might reduce vaccination costs. Using a susceptible-exposed-infectious-recovered transmission model [8], researchers estimated the financial value of introducing microneedle patches into the present influenza vaccination market in the United States. With healthcare professional administration, the incremental cost-effectiveness ratios (ICERs) are below or equivalent to $23k per quality-adjusted life years, and the market share is between 10% and 60%. Contrarily, self-administration ICERs are lower than $1,400. The administration of flu vaccines is more expensive than the vaccine itself in the United States, with the Centers for Medicare and Medicaid Services (CMS) reimbursing $12.40 for the vaccine compared to $26.20 for the vaccine administration. There will undoubtedly be substantial upfront expenses involved with developing and executing the new manufacturing process, but in the long run, the price of a microneedle patch for influenza vaccination is predicted to be comparable to the dosage cost for intramuscular vaccination. Self-vaccination is projected to cost about $5.50 in 2012 [16], which is comparable to the cost of storing, selling, and recording one influenza vaccine at a drugstore. Therefore, self-vaccination has the potential to save healthcare payers a lot of money, provided that adjustments to dose cost, reimbursement, and distribution can be made without too much complexity. The total cost of vaccination must include not only the price of the vaccine but also the expenses incurred in delivering the vaccine to the patient. Microneedle-based vaccines could be more expensive than traditional vaccines, but the savings in logistics, such as the direct costs of vaccine delivery and the indirect costs of poor vaccination safety, effectiveness, and coverage, could more than make up for the difference. Microneedle patches have the potential to lower vaccination costs by improving vaccine efficacy, decreasing the necessity for medically trained personnel, streamlining the vaccine supply chain, decreasing the risk of sharps injury, reducing vaccine waste, and doing away with the requirement for vaccine reconstitution [13]. By employing a compartment model coupled with a Monte Carlo simulation, Lee and colleagues assessed the potential economic and epidemiologic benefit of introducing microneedles to the US influenza vaccination market. The research analyzed the market share of microneedles and their pricing, effectiveness, and usage across various vaccination scenarios, including self-administration, vaccine efficacy, and compliance. Throughout all evaluated situations where healthcare practitioners administered the microneedles, the findings indicated that the microneedles would be cost-effective, with the exception of the low market share (10%) case. Market shares for microneedles ranged from 10% to 60%, while prices ranged from $9.50 to $30. If the reduction in self-administration success is minimal or if the improvement in compliance is sufficient to offset it, then microneedles could be cost-effective in all self-administration situations [8]. Research supported by the Centers for Disease Control and Prevention in the United States found that the cost of administering a measles vaccination using a microneedle patch was significantly lower than that of administering a conventional subcutaneous vaccine. Spreadsheet-based incidence-of-measles vaccination model was employed to assess expenditures of a two-dose measles vaccination campaign among a hypothetical population of 1 million children utilizing the microneedles patch compared with conventional syringe-and-needle delivery. Measles vaccination was priced at $0.95 for the first dose provided through the use of a microneedle patch, especially in contrast to $1.65 for the first dose received via the subcutaneous route, with the cost-effectiveness being based on the assumption that microneedles-based vaccines would be more thermostable and require no expensive cold-chain storage and transportation. The cost of vaccinating using a microneedle patch was projected to be $1.66 per measles case, a substantial saving over the cost of vaccinating subcutaneously, which was calculated at $2.64 per each case. Ultimately, overall vaccination program expenses were estimated at $1.5 million, or 50% less than the previous estimate of $2.5 million [17].

14.3 Safety and Acceptability of Microneedles

14.3.1 Safety of Microneedles

Little is known now concerning the regulatory perspectives on the safety of microneedle devices' long-term use. Specifically, research is required to determine how often microporation may be performed to assist skin barrier restoration. Nevertheless, it is expected that microneedle technology would be demonstrated to have a favorable safety profile due to the minimally invasive feature of the microchannels generated inside the skin post microneedles insertion, especially in contrast to the injection with hypodermic needles, and very seldom have microneedles been used in the exact locations on the same patient more than once over their lifetime. While it is evident that microneedles are minimally invasive in disrupting skin structure, the minuscule size of microchannels is generally believed to be innocuous. The possibility of painful sensation and bleeding is very low because microneedles treatment does not significantly disrupt the sensory nerves and blood capillaries in the skin dermis. Microneedles have been shown to be safe and effective in a number of different research studies [18]. Inactivated influenza vaccination was evaluated for its safety, immunogenicity, and acceptability in phase I placebo-controlled investigation that used a microneedle patch to administer the vaccine. In addition to producing strong antibody responses on par with the intramuscular method, the vaccination patch was found to be well-tolerated, with no significant side effects recorded [19]. No infections have been documented in the short-term safety investigations that have been performed thus far. In addition, individuals have been using cosmetic microneedles devices frequently without sterilizing them between usage and without experiencing any negative side effects. However, further research is necessary on the immunological effects of prolonged microneedles usage [20]. Most people feel that microneedles are safe for short-term use, but repeated applications, depending on their size and number of needles, might result in erythema and irritation.

14.3.1.1 Mechanical Safety

When microneedles are mechanically safe, they can be inserted into the skin without fracturing. Skin injury and inadequate drug dosing are also potential consequences of the mechanical failure of microneedles. Needle sharpness, aspect ratio, and material strength all play a role in ensuring mechanical safety [21, 22]. Utilizing the microfabrication technique, numerous microneedle geometries may be designed and manufactured from a variety of materials. The possibility of compression failure increases when microneedles are short, and the aspect ratio is less than 3 [22, 23]. Furthermore, the brittleness of silicon has prompted safety concerns owing to the risk of needles fracturing under the skin [24, 25]. Because of their shell form, hollow microneedles are mechanically susceptible to buckling. An increment in the wall thickness improves the amount of force that hollow microneedles can withstand [26]. Flow in microfluidic devices is another potential issue. The limited flow generated by condensed tissue may lead to undesirable flow parameters of hollow microneedles, which have a diameter and length of a few hundred micrometers. There is also the issue of drug leakage onto the skin's surface when using hollow microneedles. Drug solutions have been infused through the skin using a single hollow microneedle at flow rates of 15–96 mL/h. The flow rate might be enhanced by as much as 11.6 times by partially retracting the microneedles. In addition, increasing the insertion depth, raising the infusion force, and using a beveled microneedle tip all contributed to a higher infusion flow rate [27, 28]. The flow rate also depends on the axial pressure, fluid viscosity, needle length, diameter, and angle of the needles' tips [29]. It is crucial to understand the microfluidic characteristics of hollow microneedles in conjunction with their material and mechanical safety profiles.

14.3.1.2 Toxicity

The potential for toxicity posed by various microneedle designs varies. The material of the construction of dissolving microneedles is another factor to consider for possible toxicity. Microneedles made from a variety of water-soluble polymers have been employed in clinical applications. Dissolving microneedles are constructed from biocompatible, biodegradable, water-soluble polymers that break down gradually after being inserted under the skin. As a result, microneedles do not produce any potential biohazardous sharps waste, only an adhesive backing that could be disposed of with regular trash. Using dissolving microneedles reduces the risk of injury, debris pollution, and disease transmission from discarded needles. Microneedle materials left in the skin for a prolonged period generate some safety issues. However, repeated application of dissolving microneedles does not pose any safety concerns due to the safe materials employed [30]. The polymer's molecular weight should be considered when using a dissolving and nonbiodegradable polymer as microneedle material [31]. Microneedles made of polylactic acid and preloaded with methotrexate were inserted in rabbit eyes, and their toxicity was studied [32]. There was no evidence of either acute inflammation or infection at the application location. Thus, microneedles made of biodegradable materials allowed for nontoxic and extended drug delivery. Swelling microneedles are constructed from hydrolyzed poly(methyl vinyl ether-*co*-maleic anhydride) and poly(ethylene glycol) [33, 34] and crosslinked hyaluronic acid [35–37]. The matrix material is biocompatible, and enzymes may break down hyaluronic acid. However, the safety profile of crosslinking additives has to be considered. Although the polymers used to make microneedles are generally regarded as biocompatible and safe, further research on their skin application and the effect of repetitive use is necessary. Repeated usage of microneedles, especially dissolving microneedles, might have unintended consequences, such as the accumulation of polymer in the skin. For instance, the dissolving microneedles studied by McCrudden and colleagues would leave behind 5–10 mg of polymer/cm² in the skin tissue [38]. If the average patch were 10 cm² in size, then 50–100 mg of polymer would be placed into the skin on each application. Vaccines are an exception to the concern since they only need to be administered once, but the majority of therapeutic agents, especially biologics, need to be delivered several times. Having a microneedle device that can be withdrawn from the skin without causing any polymer deposition makes hydrogel-forming microneedles a viable option. As their usage is less frequent, dissolving microneedles may be preferable for vaccination because they mitigate the problem of repetitive polymer accumulation inside the skin [39].

Coated microneedles can be safely discarded after drug administration; they pose less of a hazard to patients than other microneedle types. Nevertheless, coated microneedles may cause cross-contamination [31]. Unfortunately, even when using a coated microneedle, sharps waste still remains. Yet, reusing microneedles is improbable because of the need for specialized coating equipment to reload the drug on the needles. Since it takes a lot of effort to get a microneedle to puncture the skin with a controlled-force application, unintentional exposure to used microneedles is also believed to be lesser than conventional hypodermic needles [13].

Repeated microneedles-assisted drug administration may provoke an immunological response if the body somehow recognizes the therapeutic protein, peptide, or antibody as an antigen [40, 41]. Drug delivery through the dermal path exposes the therapeutic agents to many immune cells in the skin tissue associated with the innate immune system, including Langerhans cells in the epidermis and dendritic cells in the dermis layers [42, 43]. This is in contrast to the goal of "humanization," which is to make biological therapies nonimmunogenic. These immune cells may be found in lesser numbers in subcutaneous tissue or muscle, which are the typical target of protein-based medicines. Although it appears that protein and peptide drugs administered via microneedles are least likely to cause undesirable immunogenic impacts, long-term studies investigating the immune response following repeated insertion of biological drugs-loaded microneedles are necessary before clinical acceptance can be confirmed, and will undoubtedly have to be verified on individual drug [39].

14.3.1.3 Anxiety

Conventional hypodermic needles instilled so much anxiety in several patients that they passed out. Sixty percent of pediatric and 50% of adult patients were needle phobic, with children exhibiting higher aversion and stress [44]. Most pediatricians (83.7%) believed that needle phobia is a significant clinical concern and that needle use in children can negatively impact future interactions with healthcare professionals [45]. When a medication is administered frequently, mild to moderate anxiety is desirable. The difficulty and appearance of blood collection inspire fear and disapproval. Due to its miniature size, microneedle monitoring, on the other hand, was appealing to all volunteers independent of age, gender, medical history, or school [46]. Microneedle anxiety has been mitigated by a variety of methods [44]. Numerous companies produced extremely fine needles (less than 31 gauge), such as the Fine Plus and the 33-gauge NanoPass, for reducing anxiety [47]. In one trial, 86 children reported microneedles which were visually acceptable and less frightening [46]. Notably, the microneedle approach avoids a slew of safety concerns and patient phobia issues, especially for children [48]. Microneedles' potential to alleviate injection anxiety is a highly desirable feature [49].

14.3.1.4 Infection

By nature, devices based on microneedles are designed to disrupt the stratum corneum and could allow bacteria and other pathogens to potentially enter the skin. They pose a risk of infecting the skin's healthy dermis and epidermis, which are generally sterile and free of pathogenic microorganisms. Nevertheless, microneedle-created channels are not conducive to microbial entry [50, 51]. Microneedles have been demonstrated to cause only minimal, superficial microinjuries; therefore, the potential for infection is minimal [50]. Microneedles are devoid of any microorganisms that might cause local or systemic infection. Minimizing bioburden is crucial for avoiding immune reaction upon micronee-dles treatment because of the abundance of immune cells in the viable epidermis and dermis, as well as the skin's nonimmune, enzyme-based defenses [52, 53]. Microorganisms may be less likely to leave the hydrophobic stratum corneum layer due to the hydrophilic properties of the microchannels. No incidences of microneedles-producing epidermal or systemic infections have ever been reported. To what extent skin cleansing prior to microneedle insertion is essential is an important open question. It would be preferable if this cleansing step weren't required since it would cause inconvenience for patients and make it seem like they are self-administering an injection rather than applying a stan-dard transdermal patch at home. Hydrogel-forming swelling microneedles have even exhibited antibacterial characteristics. The use of microneedles to pierce the skin results in substantially less microbial entry than that caused by a standard hypodermic needle [52]. Therefore, microneedles insertion seldom results in the skin or soft tissue infections. Furthermore, owing to the minute size of the device, it is highly improbable that micronee-dles would ever puncture the same spots on the skin, which further improves the possibil-ity that microneedles have a favorable safety profile [54].

According to research conducted by Donnelly et al., microneedle insertion led to substantially less microbial penetration than a hypodermic needle, and no pathogenic microorganisms entered the viable epidermis in microneedle-treated skin. Hence, in immune-competent individuals, it is safe to say that the proper insertion of a microneedle array to the skin will not result in either localized or systemic infection [50]. Some research-ers have investigated the microbial content within hydrogel-forming swelling micronee-dles and the possibility of microbe entry into the skin after microneedle treatment [52]. Following microneedles application, no microbes were able to penetrate the epidermis in this study. There were no detectable viable microorganisms in the microneedles' poly-meric matrix, which resulted in the conclusion that the drying method used to produce the microneedles and the following heating (80°C, 24 h) to stimulate chemical crosslinking were most likely the primary reasons for the absence of the microorganisms [55]. When appropriately used, microneedles have never been reported to cause skin or systemic infec-tions [50]. This might be because of the skin's powerful ability to stimulate the immune system [56] or because of the skin-derived proteases, including skin esterase and serine proteases, which break down invading microbes enzymatically [57]. Microneedle-created microinjuries in the skin rapidly heal, according to research [58], making it impossible for bacteria like *E. coli* to enter the body. One research found that wounds from microneedles treatment healed within 15 min when the skin was dry but stayed open for more than 48 h when the skin was moist. In contrast to skin regions treated with dissolving microneedles, skin perforated with solid microneedles regained its barrier function within 2 h. Between 3 h and 40 h, depending on microneedle geometry and dimensions, was the skin resealing period [59]. The risk of contamination from microneedles has to be taken into consideration. One research managed to mitigate this concern by utilizing microneedles that dissolve quickly [49].

Regulatory agencies will arrive at major judgments based on the information they collect. Devices built on microneedles may be classified as drug delivery systems, consumer products, or medical equipment, depending on their intended use. If microneedles are seen as injections rather than topical, transdermal, and intradermal delivery, then the requirement for sterilization, aseptic manufacturing, or just a minimal bioburden in the finished product will be obvious. Product pyrogen content and microbial count may have to be determined.

14.3.1.5 Skin Irritation

A skin reaction such as inflammation, irritation, or erythema may occur during or after microneedle therapy if foreign objects or biological incompatibilities are present. When using microneedle-assisted drug delivery, skin irritation or reaction is a possible risk since the stratum corneum is disrupted. Many human studies have evaluated the biosafety of microneedle applications. Generally, microneedles have been proven to be safe and have very minimal side effects. When utilizing microneedles, dermal tolerance was observed, with moderate erythema being the major notice [60]. Clinical studies on a small scale have shown that employing a microneedle-based system is a minimally invasive option, with patients reporting no pain, mild irritation, and total skin healing within just a few hours. Erythema, seemingly caused by skin irritation from the microneedles, was the most prevalent negative effect among those who were given the treatment. These findings show that while microneedles were a safe and well-tolerated therapy, they may often trigger minimal local adverse effects due to skin irritation [61]. Short-term usage of microneedles is considered safe; however, depending on their dimensions and the number of needles, long-term use might generate erythema and pain. As the materials of polymeric microneedles are often taken from other sectors of the pharmaceutical industry, where ingredient compatibility has been ensured, microneedle-based techniques seldom exhibit low biocompatibility or allergic reactions. On the other hand, hollow and solid microneedles may have their own variety of complications. Microneedle treatment for skin rejuvenation has been linked to reports of allergic granulomatous reactions and systemic hypersensitivity in the cosmetics industry [62]. Whatever the length of time the microneedles were kept in skin tissue, it is well-documented that the skin's barrier function recovers fully within a few hours after microneedles removal. Skin redness and the skin's barrier function impairment are temporary and transient [63]. Some individuals may face issues of post-microneedle-removal skin irritation or erythema. It will be important in the future to design microneedles products with mild side effects and to adequately prepare patients for such events [61]. As a result of microneedle fragments still being lodged under the skin, the biological safety of microneedles may be compromised. The Food and Drug Administration (FDA) has acknowledged microneedles as medical devices, although it is concerned about microneedles-created microinjuries in skin tissue. Therefore, the Food and Drug Administration has drafted a guideline where the length of microneedles is utilized to determine their suitability for medical applications. Typically, only microneedles shorter than 300 μm are safe for cosmetic usage [31]. In general, only when microneedles are applied incorrectly, i.e., in conjunction with cosmetic preparations that were not designed for application to microneedles-disrupted skin, side effects such as skin irritation and intradermal granulomas may occur [62].

Microneedle length, material, and drug load all had substantial effects on the possibilities of skin irritation. The needle length is of primary interest. The degree of induced redness varies with the length of the microneedles. The redness values were markedly higher after treatment with 400-μm solid microneedles than after treatment with 200-μm microneedles. Yet, even with 400-μm microneedles, irritation was still very short-lived, lingering for less than 2 h [64]. When using microneedles as long as 400 μm, the skin redness faded within 90 min. Blood spots appeared on the skin after using microneedles longer than 550 μm [64], and it took the skin around 60 min to stop bleeding after the needles were removed. No erythema was observed when using microneedles shorter than 100 μm [65]. These findings lead to the conclusion that the time required to get rid of the redness increased proportionally with the duration of microneedles insertion [66]. When 700-μm microneedles were used on human face skin, no matter the patient's age or skin type, the skin reaction score was recorded as 1. Microneedling devices seem to be risk-free for people of both sexes, ages, and skin tones. When the microneedles are applied to the face, a minor erythema develops that fades away quickly [67]. Hyaluronic acid microneedles of varying lengths were the focus of another investigation. Mild to moderate erythema was caused by the 800-μm hyaluronic acid microneedles, although this side effect dissipated over the course of a few days. Minor erythema was produced by the 200- and 300-μm hyaluronic acid microneedles, but it went away within a few hours [68]. Slight erythema was also observed on microneedle patches containing carboxymethyl cellulose (CMC) and CMC/trehalose. It took 48 h for the erythema caused by CMC microneedles to recover to pre-microneedles treatment levels. Initial erythema was more severe with CMC microneedle patches as compared with CMC/trehalose patches [69].

Several studies have used skin redness after microneedles treatment as a quantitative measure of skin irritation [64, 66]. Microneedles containing hyaluronic acid (as the polymeric matrix) and alendronate (as the active ingredient) were applied to the skin and examined for irritation reaction using the Draize technique [70]. At 24 h, neither erythema nor edema was present following the application of a dissolving microneedle array devoid of alendronate, but mild erythema was reported after the administration of alendronate-encapsulated microneedles. The irritation associated with drug-loaded microneedles disappeared on the 15th day. Bal et al. used a chromameter to assess the skin irritation caused by the insertion of uncoated stainless steel microneedles of varying lengths into the skin of healthy subjects [64]. Researchers evaluated microneedles of different lengths, diameters, and geometries and found that, even though the length and shape did affect the level of irritation, it is minor and short-lived [64]. Researchers found that microneedle application caused minimal irritation compared to tape stripping (a common noninvasive method of disturbing the stratum corneum) and that the irritation was transient. Investigators Bal and colleagues studied how the length of microneedles affected skin irritation by monitoring blood flow and skin redness. Redness (erythema) is one of the most basic indications of inflammation. After the insertion of solid metal microneedles, researchers observed a time course of redness that peaked at 15 min and decreased to baseline levels after 90 min. The length of those microneedles (200, 300, and 400 μm) was directly correlated to the degree of redness they caused. Furthermore, there were no discernible blood flow variations after treatment with varying lengths of microneedles [64]. It was found that microneedle-mediated delivery of teriparatide was well-tolerated in a randomized, double-blind, placebo-controlled trial spanning six months. There were no reports of delayed hypersensitivity or skin infection, and the only adverse event was mild to moderate erythema at the insertion point. There have been occasional cases of localized skin reactions such as redness, swelling, and pinpoint bleeding in the treated area [71]. Abaloparatide is a peptide molecule currently being studied for the treatment of osteoporosis. In the phase II clinical trial, participants applied the drug-loaded coated microneedles every day for 24 weeks, offering an opportunity to evaluate the patient tolerance to repeated applications of coated microneedles. The study found that neither the medication nor the microneedles were responsible for the small percentage (3.6% of patients) who experienced adverse effects [60]. The microneedle group also showed a significantly higher rate of adherence to therapy than the control group over the 24-week trial, which is in line with the research's observations of a generally positive skin tolerance profile. An *in vivo* investigation evaluated the repeated insertion of polymeric microneedles to hairless mice and was conducted by Vicente-Perez and colleagues in 2017. The findings reveal that patients may safely utilize microneedles repeatedly without experiencing any negative effects. Using dissolving microneedles once a day for five weeks and hydrogel-forming microneedles twice a week for three weeks showed no significant change in skin appearance or barrier integrity and no noticeable disruption in serum biomarkers of infection, inflammation, or immunity, independent of microneedle composition, needle density, or treatment frequency [72]. Al-Kasasbeh and associates evaluated the clinical effect of repeated insertion of hydrogel-forming microneedles. In this work, the researchers inserted a microneedle array on the upper arm of human participants multiple times over the course of five days. The barrier function of the skin and the presence of systemic inflammatory biomarkers in the blood were used to evaluate the safety of repetitive application of microneedles. Results showed that repeated application of microneedles did not result in persistent skin irritation or sustained impairment of the skin's barrier integrity [39]. A group of investigators studied the efficacy of intradermal delivery for 2 mL of 5% dextrose solution in a 2015 clinical trial. Observations from 30 healthy participants indicated that the whole 2 mL volume could be administered intradermally through the hollow microneedle system. By the completion of the fluid injection, the patient's pain, erythema, and edema scores had all decreased to the mild-to-moderate level, almost returned to the baseline. Considering microneedles for vaccination would only be used once, this skin irritation would not be as pressing a concern as it would be for microneedles intended for repeated usage [56]. Similar to rotating insulin injection locations, alternating microneedles insertion spots may help reduce the severity of this issue.

14.3.1.6 Pain

The inability of microneedles to cause discomfort during injection is the desired quality. Using a visual analogue scale, investigators could statistically assess the degree of pain (VAS). Pain from microneedle applications is a major factor in whether or not users would comply with and embrace the technology. As the needle tips do not penetrate the dermis layers, which house the nerve fibers, microneedles considerably reduce the pain associated with injections. Therefore, microneedles effectively assist people with needle phobia. Iatrogenic pain in children has long been associated with vaccination injections [73]. Child and parent anguish, needle fear, lack of trust in medical professionals, refusal to take medicine as prescribed, and poor adherence to medical treatment all were consequences of this pain [74]. Topical anesthetic, music distraction, oral distraction in babies, posture tactics, pH adjustment, and other methods have been used to alleviate injection-related discomfort.

Microneedle-associated pain is affected by a variety of factors, including but not limited to microneedles length and the number of needles [59], needle tip angle [75], microneedle thickness [76] and width, needle fracture during the application, insertion site, microneedle type, and applicator. For solid, dissolving, coated, and hollow microneedles, microneedle length presents the most substantial influence on pain. A strong relationship between visual analogue scale (VAS) score and microneedle length has been reported. Research has shown that microneedles length has a substantially more significant impact on pain than the number of microneedles or needle density. While the number of microneedles was increased from 5 to 50, just a twofold increase in pain was experienced. Furthermore, microneedles with tip angles ranging from 20° to 90° were evaluated, and no correlation was found between tip angle and perceived discomfort. Analyses of pain's association with microneedle thickness and width yielded similar findings [75]. The infusion or injection of drug solution, i.e., the injection volume and flow rate, through hollow microneedles is a major contributor to the patient's pain level throughout the procedure. The dermis' tight structure makes it difficult for fluids to get into the skin. The skin expands to make space for a fluid volume of a few hundred microliters. Because of the skin's remarkable stretching and the fluid pressure exerted, the injection of significant amounts of fluid into the skin is painful. Tissue deformation and injury may occur at injection volumes of as little as 1 mL due to the significantly increased pressure built [77]. In one investigation, the effects of skin stretching of less than 1 mm, there was no marked impact of a 0.80 mL injection volume on pain. Reduced infusion pressure brought about by the decreased flow rate was responsible for alleviating pain. Pain is worsened by a higher flow rate of 1 mL/min [77]. It is believed that people who demonstrate intolerance to pain may be negatively affected by the application of the needle, making it essential to create technologies to alleviate the discomfort produced by microneedles [61]. The pain threshold may be modified not just by the microneedles but also by the applicator. An applicator has been designed and employed to facilitate the application of microneedles into the skin [78]. The insertion pressure of the microneedles was minimized by using a vibration mechanism. There was no difference in VAS scores for 280-μm microneedles applied using the applicator and 500-μm microneedles administered without the applicator. Conclusively, the usage of the applicator did not significantly elevate the level of discomfort. While the rubber and foam mounting of the applicator helped lessen the pain, it also impeded the microneedles' ability to effectively penetrate the skin [31].

Multiple studies have shown that the insertion of microneedles is a minimally invasive treatment. When compared to a 26-gauge hypodermic needle, Gill and colleagues found that microneedles cause considerably less pain. They found that this reduction in pain decreased with the number and length of microneedles [47, 75]. Specifically, the authors evaluated needles ranging in length from 480 μm to 1,450 μm and found that the pain levels caused by these needles ranged from 5% to 37% of those achieved with the hypodermic needle. Moreover, the pain level increased slightly, going from 5% to 25% (compared to a hypodermic needle) when the number of needles increased ten times. Bal and associates examined microneedles less than 550 μm in length for their ability to induce pain. They found incredibly low pain ratings across the board with no considerable differences [64]. One research compared the effectiveness of clinical administration with microneedles of 180 μm, 280 μm length, and standard 25-gauge hypodermic needles. Subjects who received 180-μm microneedles insertion described the sensation as similar to having someone push down firmly on their skin. According to the participants, the insertion of 280-μm microneedles was likened to the sensation of having someone grasp their arm. In contrast, practically all participants reported instant pain and discomfort while using the 25-gauge hypodermic needle [79]. Furthermore, 500–750-µm-long microneedles were 10–20 times less uncomfortable than traditional hypodermic needles [47]. From a few hundred micrometers to 1.5 mm in length, all microneedles were found to be less painful than the hypodermic needle, with pain ratings ranging from 5% to 40% lower than those recorded with the hypodermic needle [75]. In another investigation, when the length of the microneedles was varied from 180 µm to 1,000 µm, there was no noticeable alteration in the VAS score. The VAS value did rise when the microneedles' length increased to more than 1,000 µm. To lessen microneedle-related pain, shorter needles (less than 1,000 µm in length) may be proposed [31]. Similarly, in children with type 1 diabetes, Gupta and colleagues found that the use of hollow microneedles for insulin administration resulted in a faster onset of action and substantially less pain than traditional injection using hypodermic needles [80, 81]. Norman and associates reported that intradermal insulin administration utilizing a hollow microneedle device for children and adolescents led to reduced insertion discomfort and speedier onset and offset of effect [82].

14.3.2 Acceptability

14.3.2.1 Introduction of Microneedles Acceptability

The concept of "acceptability" is frequently used to describe the process of gauging whether an intervention will be accepted by its intended users and how effectively a novel intervention or its components may fulfill the demands of those users in their particular organizational context [83]. There may be financial repercussions for failing to include patients' viewpoints on the usage of the technologies. Further in-depth research is required to reassure patients of the safety and efficacy of this novel drug delivery technique; if that happens, this technology will gain widespread popularity [84]. Acceptance by healthcare providers (such as physicians, nurses, and pharmacists) and patients is crucial to the long-term commercial viability of microneedle-based products [85]. The potential for large-scale usage of microneedles is contingent on the level of public interest and confidence in this technology [49]. It is crucial that both doctors and patients be comfortable with the product and confident in their ability to use the microneedles array properly for successful treatment. Consequently, pain- and anxiety-reducing properties and user-friendliness are major benefits of microneedles. Since microneedles do not penetrate deeply enough to stimulate the nerve endings located in the skin, microneedles are generally well-accepted by patients [86]. Due to this, it is feasible to develop microneedles products that require a minimum, if any, training to use correctly for self-administration or use in areas with no or little access to skilled healthcare providers. Several studies indicate that typical patients will be able to use a microneedle device by themselves, either manually or with the assistance of an applicator, after receiving guidance from a healthcare practitioner [10, 87]. Interestingly, short microneedles could be applied without the supervision of a medical expert. Nevertheless, a qualified medical expert is required to apply long microneedles. Therefore, it would be crucial to forging ahead to attempt to understand the end users' perspectives. To guarantee the safe and effective usage of microneedles products, especially by patients in their homes, such investigations, when properly customized to collect the relevant demographics, will undoubtedly support the industry to take proper actions to deal with any concerns and create practical instructive labels and patient consultation [85]. Both general people and medical experts favored microneedles over hypodermic needle injections, indicating that the technology is well-received in the community [8, 88]. With the use of microneedle patches, immunization might be administered by personnel with limited medical training or even by patients themselves. Microneedles attracted the attention of children, who said they would be interested in using microneedles in the future if they were confident of the proper application, effectiveness, safety, and minimized pain. It has been proposed that using a microneedle patch instead of a standard hypodermic needle will make things more convenient for patients. It has been noted that microneedle technology is highly acceptable and suitable for use with children immunizations [49]. Because of their diminutive size, microneedles need little training to use. In the event of a worldwide pandemic or bioterrorism attack, when immediate treatment may rely on the victim's capacity to self-administer the device, the use of microneedles takes on added significance. Human trials using placebo microneedles have shown that naive persons with no previous experience with microneedles may effectively apply microneedles after being given just basic instructions [10, 87]. Patients have successfully utilized microneedles for drug administration at home with no adverse effects [71]. Assessment of influenza vaccination in the United States indicated that self-applied microneedles might increase immunization coverage and that the usage of microneedles was cost-effective in most situations evaluated [10]. Despite the lack of related guidelines, investigators working on microneedles patches for vaccination have shown that their prototypes are safe and well-received by patients [10, 89, 90], and there is now published literature to reveal the evaluations of microneedles acceptance [49]. Guidelines for vaccine-loaded microneedles patches that would be useful across the board go beyond just where to apply the patches; they also address issues such as how long the patch should be worn, how to best prepare the skin for the application, how to best care for the patch after being applied, and what kind of verification of delivery is required [91].

The foundation and standards generated by the licensing and successful commercialization of the first vaccine-loaded microneedles patch will present possibilities and problems for subsequent microneedles products. After an approved microneedles product gains widespread public acceptability and builds the ecosystem, there may be a surge in consumer demand for more microneedles-based patches. This means that the success or failure of the initial vaccination patch product, as well as any earlier success or failure with other (i.e., non-vaccine) microneedles patch–based therapies, will undoubtedly have an impact on the acceptability and market for succeeding vaccine patch products. The first vaccine patch product has the potential to boost population immunity and show considerable advantages if it increases the desire for vaccination and encourages more people to be vaccinated. Moreover, the first product to launch will set the initial regulatory path for this technology, packaging considerations (i.e., product protection, desiccants, waste disposal), and product acceptance within the healthcare system (e.g., prices, the convenience of use, administration time frames and skills required, storage, possible sharps, residual drug after administration, verification of drug delivery). Potentially new side effects (i.e., skin reactions, unintentional use or ingestion of a patch, packing, etc.) and any possible injuries related to application or misuse might be observed for the first time when the first vaccine patch is used widely. Since seasonal influenza is likely the first vaccine patch to be developed, it is crucial to be aware that factors irrelevant to the vaccine patch may affect the product. For instance, when the United States approved and adopted FluMist™, the FDA temporarily halted its authorized use in the US market [92] for reasons unrelated to the delivery method [91].

Multiple factors could affect microneedles' acceptability. The acceptability depends on the users' ability to follow the instructions, maintain the microneedle delivery system in place sufficiently long for the active ingredient to be delivered, and then properly discard the needles after use. High-dose delivery of low-potency medicines using larger microneedles patches (1–30 cm^2) might benefit from a feedback system since not only one thumb but several fingers are needed to apply the patch. One feature that might be crucial to the microneedles patch's success and widespread adoption is a shift in color that indicates when sufficient pressure has been applied evenly across the entire patch [93].

14.3.2.2 Driver of Microneedles Acceptability

The expected benefits of microneedles noted by healthcare practitioners and the public at large are the primary factor in increasing acceptance of microneedles products [94] minimal pain on the application; possibility for controlled delivery, possibility for self-administration; benefit for those with needle phobia; benefit for children; substitute to oral administration; lesser anxiety and distress; minimal chance of needlestick injuries; benefit for those with diabetes and chronic disease; a substantial increase in vaccination rates; lowered chance of bleeding; simplicity of disposal; the convenience of use, and attractive product design. The aforementioned advantages were the most significant elements impacting the perception of microneedles across demographics, including young children and the elderly [46, 88, 95]. Prescribing doctors must take every precaution to ensure their patients understand how to use microneedle products safely, lest side effects like minor erythema diminish their commitment to treatment [39]. The level of microneedle acceptance among medical experts should also be considered. It has been shown that the vast majority of people will defer to their healthcare providers for making the final healthcare choice. Increased immunogenicity and seroprotection [96, 97] and decreased risk of needlestick injuries [88] are two significant advantages recognized by healthcare practitioners. Acceptance by the end user is shown to be nuanced and multidimensional via qualitative research. Consequently, such research will surely help the industry take the required steps to address issues and create informative labeling and patient counseling measures to guarantee the safe and successful use of microneedles devices. Effective marketing is essential if the desired market share is maximized compared to more recognized and popular traditional delivery methods [39]. Studies by Caffarel-Salvador and coworkers (2015) and Mooney et al. (2015) revealed that almost all participants (93%) were unaware of microneedles, including 90% of pediatricians and 85.2% of the general public interviewees [45, 98]. For this reason, how microneedles are first presented to the public will significantly impact how well they are perceived.

14.3.2.3 Barriers to Microneedles Acceptability

Various barriers to microneedles acceptability have been reported. The lack of familiarity with microneedles technology [46, 88], the possibility of allergic reactions [46], and the use of the word "needle" in the product label [46] all were recognized as hurdles to the acceptance of microneedles. Efforts at research and development should center on these obstacles and seek to eliminate them via patient education, the production of hypoallergenic products, and the introduction of novel terminologies, such as "ImmuPatch," to replace the negative connotations coupled with the word "needle." The use of the term "needles" to depict the microneedles technology was not well-received by children since it evokes thoughts of painful hypodermic injections. They speculated that giving it a different name may enhance its popularity. It was also theorized that adding attractive, kid-friendly graphics on the microneedles patch package, such as cartoon characters, would help make the system more acceptable to children [46]. Healthcare professionals highlighted the threat of cross-contamination and the difficulty in ensuring proper drug delivery on microneedle insertion as two main obstacles to product acceptance [88]. To tackle these issues, researchers have focused on developing biodegradable formulations for use in medical devices. Once deposited into the skin, these polymers either swiftly disintegrate or exhibit morphological alterations that impede effective skin penetration if given to another person [99, 100], hence avoiding purposeful or unintentional cross-contamination. Incorporating a delivery indication or verification would likely increase manufacturing costs, thus attention must be given to minimize such increases. The following are some of the noticeable issues with microneedles that have been observed by healthcare providers and the general public [94]: slow delivery onset, inefficacy, difficulty to verify dose delivery, relatively high cost, misapplication, cross-contamination, inter-user variation in skin's physical properties, potential allergic reaction, or irritation. To ensure safe and effective use of microneedles, instruction and training will be required not just for medical professionals but also for patients [45]. Microneedle products provide the possibility of self-administration, but their correct usage is crucial to achieving the intended drug delivery; hence, microneedles must be designed to allow easy, convenient, and reliable patient self-administration. Bhatchelbert et al. (2012) found that patients' perceptions of the usefulness of various medical procedures and tools were significantly influenced by their interactions with healthcare providers and prior experiences with such procedures and equipment. Adolescents' viewpoints on vaccination were revealed to be related to previous experiences and the ideas of either parents or, more often, the information accessible via social networking and the internet [101]. The acceptance of microneedles may be heavily influenced by healthcare providers' perspectives and public perceptions of the devices as presented in the online and print media [94]. However, microneedles self-administration was viewed with skepticism, and the questioned parents reported a necessity to have a medical expert verify that they were applying the needles correctly [98]. A further criterion for evaluating the practicality of microneedles is the length of time they must be worn. Delivery of a given dose may take anywhere from a few minutes to a few hours, depending on the design and intended use of the microneedles product [102–104]. Patients may become resistant to the effective usage of microneedles if the wearing duration is too long. Besides, microneedle insertion pressure may be decreased by vibration [105] and an impact-insertion applicator can facilitate an efficient and reproducible application of highly dense microneedle array [75]. Microneedles were built with an attached applicator to modulate the insertion force, mode, and velocity [26, 32]. Yet, the applicator may make microneedle application less hassle-free than it otherwise would be. In order to facilitate the insertion process, microneedles should have a simple and inexpensive molded portion connected to the backside of the needles [106].

14.3.2.4 Case Studies of Microneedles Acceptability

Results from a survey of the general public and a group of healthcare professionals showed that both groups were positive about the potential of microneedles. While this research reflects the views of a representative sample of the general public and medical practitioners, general attitudes will differ from group to group and rely on various factors such as education level, access to counseling, individual experience, and others [84]. The acceptability of microneedle patches for minimally assisted self-administration of influenza vaccine has been demonstrated in first-in-humans research [10]. Using concepts from the theory of reasoned action, Norman and colleagues assessed patients' perceptions of microneedles as a painless delivery system. The researchers surveyed people in Atlanta, Georgia, USA, on their perspectives toward receiving seasonal flu vaccine by intramuscular injection

(IM), microneedles patch, or no vaccination. Perceived adverse effects of microneedles insertion and injections, as well as participants' impressions of the acceptability of the microneedle patch by physicians, family, and friends, were also measured. Statistical results indicated that switching to a self-applied microneedle patch from an IM injection may increase the immunization rate from 44% to 65%. Among those who are routinely vaccinated, 51% favored the microneedles application over the injection, and among those who had never been vaccinated, 30% would be open to it. The majority of respondents (64%) also said they would prefer to self-vaccinate using microneedles. The proper use of microneedles was also a concern for 84% of the research participants [10]. A few people who tried to insert microneedles into their skin with only their thumbs ended up having to use more force than anticipated. However, success rates significantly increased when a cheap snap-based device was used as an applicator. Based on these findings, it seems that the self-administration of vaccinations using microneedles in conjunction with a simple device producing insertion-force feedback is a successful strategy [10, 12]. Though a wide range of individuals participated in the trial, it remains unclear whether or not patients of advanced age or those with impaired physical capacity will be able to self-administer the flu vaccine using microneedles. One may dispute that patients who are too feeble to apply the patch themselves would undoubtedly have a caregiver who would perform that task for them.

Positive patient reactions to microneedles and an improvement in vaccination rate were confirmed in a phase III investigation of Intanza®. Patients (1,679 subjects) filled out a validated questionnaire on their thoughts and experiences with intradermal influenza vaccination. Ninety-five percent were receptive to being revaccinated, and 96% said they were pleased or extremely satisfied with the microneedles-based injection method. Supporting these results were post-release surveys conducted in the Czech Republic, Australia, Argentina, and Turkey. Regarding prescriber satisfaction, 85% of prescribers in Australia and Argentina reported being content or highly satisfied, whereas, in Turkey and the Czech Republic, that number soared to 95% [10]. Researchers also reported encouraging results when asking children how they felt about using microneedles instead of hypodermic needles for drawing blood samples [46]. Microneedle-assisted monitoring as a substitute to the blood sampling method was well-received in another research polling children and parents of premature infants [107].

Interestingly, the MicronJet® microneedle technology was not regarded as superior to the traditional syringe in research that evaluated parents' perceptions of administering several immunizations in a single visit [108]. This method is similar to other vaccine delivery systems in that it employs four hollow silicon microneedles with a length of 0.6 mm and is connected to a typical syringe barrel. This layout may explain the lower acceptance found in this research. Patients have been found to effectively insert microneedles into their skin after guidance given by pharmacist consultation and a patient information leaflet [87]. A "dosing indication" has also been constructed to reassure patients of a successful application [109]. This might be especially helpful for the elderly, whose physical abilities and manual dexterity may diminish due to age [110]. Using hollow microneedles, researchers in another study examined the effectiveness of influenza vaccination when given by a healthcare practitioner against when given by the patients themselves. Forty-two percent liked the procedure they had experienced, 42% were neutral, and 16% chose the other way when given a choice between self-administration and delivery by a healthcare practitioner [111]. Healthcare providers' and patients' perspectives on microneedles as a drug delivery method were studied by Birchall and colleagues [88]. Focus groups were arranged with members of the general public and medical staff. The microneedle technique was deemed "excellent for children" in all seven focus groups. The results of the qualitative focus groups were subsequently confirmed by means of questionnaires.

While all members of the general public and 74% of medical practitioners were enthusiastic about microneedles technology, 26% of the healthcare professionals were ambivalent. Ninety-two percent of the general public thought microneedles might be used to deliver children's medication. Potential benefits of this technique include less discomfort and minimal tissue injury. However, issues have been raised about the delivery's efficacy, associated cost, the possibility of infection, the wide range in skin thickness among persons, and the delayed onset of effect. Eighty-eight percent of respondents said they would be comfortable self-administering the microneedles if given specific instructions, but just 25% expected to be able to buy the microneedles from a pharmacy for home use. As another point, if given a choice between a hypodermic needle injection and microneedles, 96% of subjects would choose the former if the injection was found to be more efficient. Both medical experts and members of the general public agreed in this survey that an indication was required to ensure that the correct dose was given to the patient by microneedles. Patients also seem to favor microneedle designs that provide feedback on proper application, such as a "click" sound. Most of the individuals who participated in this study acknowledged the potential benefits of utilizing microneedles, such as decreased discomfort, lower tissue damage, minimal infection risk, reduced needlestick injury, ease of self-administration, and possible application in children, needle-phobic people, and those with diabetes [88].

In another research, investigators in Northern Ireland, UK, interviewed 16 parents to get their viewpoint on microneedles technology as a tool for drawing blood and skin interstitial fluid from infants [98]. Parents were receptive to microneedles because of the reduced pain, ease of administration, and the resemblance to a sticking plaster. Mooney et al. (2014) conducted a focus group study with 86 children and revealed that microneedles are more acceptable to children than traditional hypodermic needles when used for sampling procedures. Unsurprisingly, the children questioned favored noninvasive microneedles-based techniques for drawing blood samples [46]. Children's perspectives on microneedles for drug administration were also addressed via focus groups with 66 children aged 9–15, of whom 14 were receiving medicine for chronic conditions. Children's positive reactions to microneedles have been attributed to their lessened discomfort, self-application possibility, and novelty compared to more conventional difficult-to-swallow pill forms. The same research also collected perspectives from pediatricians and the general public on microneedles technology for pediatric drug delivery. The general public (93.6% of participants) and pediatricians (85.9% of survey participants) considered microneedles a promising drug delivery method. However, they acknowledged the necessity for a dosage indication and an applicator to provide confidence that the microneedle system had been applied correctly. In particular, pediatricians perceived microneedles as having great potential for administering analgesics, vaccines, and antiemetics to children. Ninety-two percent of pediatricians highlighted pain reduction as the primary potential benefit of microneedles, followed by ease of application in children with needle phobia (86.9%), ease of administration compared to hypodermic needles (71.8%), controlled drug delivery (69.6%), and decreased bleeding (66.5%). However, the pediatricians who took part in this research also recognized possible drawbacks of this technology, including allergies or skin irritations (72.8%), a high price (66%), a potential reduction in precision in the drug delivery (61.3%), and misapplication of the microneedles (46.1%). The general public is more likely than pediatricians to choose microneedles over oral administration, but both groups are in agreement that microneedles are preferable when it comes to injecting the drug into children. Compared to pediatricians, the general public is more enthusiastic about the potential of microneedles as drug delivery systems. It is possible that pediatricians and other medical experts are more skeptical of the microneedles technology because of their extensive training and medical expertise [45]. Focus groups were also used in research conducted by Zosano Pharma to gauge interest in their coated microneedles patch for the release of parathyroid hormone to manage osteoporosis. The device includes an applicator to make microneedles insertion more manageable. There were 288 postmenopausal women participants with osteoporosis who participated in the focus groups; 93% of them found the concept of the microneedles patch highly appealing, and 90% found it simple to apply. Eighty-two percent of the participants used the Zosano Pharma patch's built-in applicator to apply the patch successfully on their first try. These findings highlight the significance of providing patients with counseling and explanatory leaflets before using microneedles devices. In another investigation, hydrogel-forming swelling microneedles were used with a pressure-indicating sensor film as a cheap and easy way to validate successful microneedles application *in vivo*. Pressurex-micro Green 1 sensor film, for example, changes its coloration in response to pressures greater than 20 N/cm^2. Patient compliance and acceptability may improve due to the method's visual feedback confirming proper microneedles application [109]. Self-administration of microneedles in healthy subjects without the aid of an applicator was studied in 2014 research by Donnelly and colleagues. Patients were given either a patient information sheet or individual pharmacy counseling on how to use the microneedles device. After proper training and instruction, it was demonstrated that hydrogel-forming microneedles could be self-applied effectively and reliably without the need for an applicator [87].

14.4 Manufacturing and Regulatory Issues

14.4.1 Manufacturing Issues

Given the novelty of microneedles technology, it would be necessary to set up dedicated facilities capable of producing them in large quantities [10]. Precision manufacturing using micro-production methods like micromachining and nanoprocessing would be required to make microneedles. Precision machining, extrusion, casting, and shaping of microneedles are all essential processes that must be enabled for microneedles production. While a sizable initial investment is required to set up these procedures, the manufacturing costs are anticipated to be on par with or lower than those of injectable products [6] after the initial setup period. The prospect for large-scale microneedles production is in high demand due to the recent growth in the use of microneedles and the scarcity of commercial microneedles goods. According to Bhatnagar et al., an improved understanding of production materials and chemistry will aid organizations in reaching their financial targets, allowing them to scale up production [112] and enhance revenues. To fabricate a single array of microneedles, most existing techniques of manufacture necessitate a number of stages [113]. Removing this barrier would pave the way for studies that might one day lead to a decrease in the number of steps required to produce microneedles. Microneedle devices are fabricated in small quantities, with a lot of manual work, during the early phases of development. This is adequate for most preclinical and clinical studies in phase I. The production process has to be more automated, spacious, and controlled as phase II clinical investigations are rapidly approaching in the development process. By the end of phase III clinical trials, supplies will have reached their highest level of automation, along with enhanced capabilities and improved process control [60]. Raw material accessibility, component complexity, production steps, and the feasibility of using current manufacturing processes all are factors that should determine the optimal product design. Moreover, the volume and cost goals of production should be included in the product's design. There will be substantial technical, infrastructural, and aseptic processing hurdles associated with the scaling up of processes to manufacture cGMP-compliant products. To ensure the efficacy, safety, and purity of a therapeutic agent or the reliability and performance of a device product, manufacturers must use excellent manufacturing procedures that are suitable for the development stage. Products that use microneedles to administer an active ingredient must meet the standards for both the drug and the medical device. When working with microneedle products [114], achieving content uniformity of 85–115% of the intended minute dose might be difficult. When it comes to coated microneedles, for instance, the key to the technology's success will be increasing coating effectiveness and scaling up the production processes [60]. Multiple predictive computational models have been employed to enhance the efficiency of manufacturing processes [115–117], and these methods may be adapted to the production of microneedles. Interestingly, high-resolution, inexpensive, and rapid production are only some of the benefits offered by additive manufacturing [118, 119]. Since the device dimensions and formulation can be altered with very few postprocessing steps, fabricating a microneedle array with a 3D printer has clear advantages over more traditional ways of producing such an array. When first attempted, the cost-effectiveness and turnaround time of laboratory-based techniques might be problematic, making them impractical for large production [120]. The requirements for quality assurance, quality control, and good manufacturing practice all have an immediate and direct effect on the cycle time. Microneedle categorization will also have an impact on these recommendations. The 2003 severe acute respiratory syndrome (SARS) pandemic, the 2009 H1N1 swine flu pandemic, the outbreaks of Avian influenza A(H5N1) and A(H7N9), the 2014 Ebola crisis, and the 2020 COVID-19 pandemic are all examples of catastrophic events where a fast turnaround was necessary due to an urgent demand for effective products [39, 120]. The requirement for mass production of microneedles exacerbates these problems because of the additional resources needed to solve the complications that arise when manufacturing biopharmaceuticals to work in tandem with and contained within microneedles. Critical design issues linked to large-scale manufacturing will also need to be addressed to facilitate the mass production of microneedle patches. These include setting up and maintaining environmental controls (temperature and humidity) and managing the logistics of chemistry, manufacturing, and control processes.

14.4.1.1 Specific Manufacturing Issues

There is a significant difficulty in reliably producing a large number of microneedle arrays with a high degree of structural integrity. Maintaining strict control over the molding process is essential for achieving the desired level of pattern accuracy and repeatability. It is possible to construct a histogram of the typical microneedle length over a certain number of arrays taken randomly from a given manufacturing batch. The relative standard deviation of the mean microneedle length was subsequently determined for the sample set of microneedle arrays [60].

The selection of materials for the microneedles and array substrate is crucial. Microneedle materials might range from polymers to glass to silicon and metals. Materials utilized in the production of pharmaceutical products must be traced as far back as feasible in the supply chain so that appropriate processing, cleaning conditions, and sufficient supervision can be maintained at every production stage. For aseptic manufacturing of products requiring sterility [60], procedures should be developed with adequate environmental controls once materials have been acquired. The microneedles' materials also factor heavily toward their regulatory approval or clearance. Historically, metals like stainless steel have been used in healthcare settings. The regulatory process for using such materials will be much simplified in comparison to using unapproved materials [2]. Early in the development cycle, a device design must adhere to limits such as the materials requirements and risk assessments in conformance with ISO 10993. In light of the importance of using only nontoxic, nonirritant, nonallergenic materials in the production of polymeric materials, there is a concerted effort to ensure that microneedles meet all of these criteria. Concerns about the material's safety and biocompatibility take precedence. Using biocompatible materials speeds up the development process and saves a lot of money, but switching to entirely new materials takes much more effort and resources. ISO 10993–1:2018 is a consensus standard used often to determine what level of biocompatibility is considered reasonable. Dissolving microneedles must be made from a material that will not break down in storage, will not cause skin irritation, and will not leave behind a polymeric material that builds up on the skin. Both solid and hollow microneedles must be sufficiently robust to not break during the application and to not break in the skin after removal. There must be a strategy to mass-produce microneedles without compromising quality, stability, or cost. Microneedles made from an innovative material (liquid crystal polymer) are strong enough to pierce the skin, yet bend rather than fracture under high mechanical pressure (250 N). This material lends itself to precise molding at a low cost on a mass-production scale. In terms of fracture resistance, a microneedle array made of liquid crystal polymer performed exceptionally well [60].

For any therapy intervention to be successful, dose uniformity and consistency are essential. A mold must be capable of being filled with a certain quantity of drug formulation and then dried into a microneedle structure. The drug formulation must be coated on the solid microneedles uniformly and consistently for coated microneedles. The hollow microneedle system relies on a precision-engineered injector to accurately administer the drug through hollow microneedles. To prevent leakage, fluid pressurization of the drug reservoir must initiate immediately after microneedle application. This will reduce the void volume in the fluid flow channel. Achieving dosing precision after varying storage conditions necessitates an injector that is designed to deliver sufficient injection pressure. In addition, a more consistent manufacturing process may be attained by using automation, such as using robots to carry out certain tasks in the production process. Coated microneedles generally seem to possess consistency throughout an array because the coated formulation is confined to the top half of each microneedle, owing to the coating process's reproducibility and reliability. This consistency is thought to assist in the coated microneedles' capacity to deliver the medication to the skin. The drug amount on each microneedle array is found to be uniform due to the controlled coating procedure. To enhance the manufacturing capacity and improve the process control to ensure the quality of the finished product, automation in all production steps has to be essentially improved, such as micromolding, dimensions measurement, mechanical evaluation, arrangement of microneedles into the patch, and coating process [60].

The stability of the therapeutic agent is another critical factor to consider while developing a drug product. Drug products may need to be kept in a cold chain throughout transportation and storage at distribution facilities, pharmacies, and patients' homes, depending on their stability and shelf life. Transdermal delivery of biotherapeutics and vaccines using microneedles has several promising benefits, including the possibility of increased stability. For vaccine producers, ensuring a consistent supply chain is a primary concern. Concerns about the acceptability of the finished vaccine patch product may be highlighted throughout the supply chain review, as is the case with all vaccine production processes. Acceptability concerns with a rubella vaccine product, including a porcine-based ingredient, negatively impacted the vaccination coverage in Indonesia, while vaccines with bovine-related components may not be suitable in some regions [91]. Unlike the commercially available PTH(1–34) liquid injectable product, which must be stored in the refrigerator for long-term stability [121], the parathyroid hormone (1–34)-coated microneedle device has an 18-month shelf life at room temperature (25°C). Similarly, trivalent influenza vaccine-coated microneedle arrays were frozen and thawed three times. Flu hemagglutinin (HA) antigen-coated arrays were frozen at –15°C for at least 24 h before being slowly thawed for 3 h at room temperature (about 25°C). After three freeze-thaw cycles, the reactivity of all three types of influenza antigen was still at around 85–90%. The antigen bioactivity was not significantly altered, as the 10–15% reactivity reduction found in the research was stated to be within the variation of the analysis [122].

14.4.1.2 *Microneedles Sterilization*

Microneedle sterilization has been considered a crucial aspect of microneedle safety. If sterilization is necessary, the strategy implemented is critical since typical methods (dry heat, steam sterilization, gamma or microwave radiation, ethylene oxide) may have a detrimental effect on the microneedle structure and the active component they carry. It will be costly for manufacturers to sterilize and aseptically produce pharmaceutical products. Undoubtedly, it will be necessary to give significant attention to the logistics of mass-producing microneedle devices for the public at large. Many alternative methods exist today for fabricating microneedles; these methods vary significantly from those used to manufacture more traditional dosage forms. Microneedles, especially those that are coated or micromolded, may necessitate several processes during production. Microneedles made of silicon often need to be produced in a clean environment. This means that any pharmaceutical or medical device company trying to commercialize microneedle products would likely need to invest heavily to design, develop, and refine a cost-effective and reliable process for producing microneedles in large quantities. In addition, typical quality control techniques will need modification. Interestingly, there are currently DermaRoller® devices on the market that employ solid microneedles to treat various skin issues. Despite widespread use, the supplier does not advise sterilizing DermaRoller® devices used for self-skin care in between each usage. The sole suggested cleaning method is to rinse the roller head in hot water, dry it, and then spray it with roller cleaner. In addition, producers have recorded no adverse effects thus far [123]. However, it is advised that the microneedle devices be sterilized before use due to the priority given to patient safety and the fact that microneedles are sharp structures. Using disposable microneedles products (with a reusable applicator) that are both sterile and tamper-proof may be a workable solution to the issues outlined earlier [84].

The amount of bioburden control necessary during clinical development should be determined after the manufacturer has conducted a risk assessment. For microneedles to be safe and effective without triggering an immune response or infection, they may not be required to be manufactured in a sterile environment. However, several investigations have already focused on evaluating microneedle sterilization processes in anticipation of the prospective requirement for sterilization that may be demanded by regulatory agencies [55]. The sterilization of microneedles is a topic that has received a comparatively modest amount of academic investigation. Raw materials and manufacturing equipment should be sterilized to reduce the risk of contamination from personnel or the surrounding environment. Filtration of air and water, cleaning, and microbiological monitoring of buildings, machinery, and materials all are vital manufacturing activities. The production process may also include a final sterilizing step [124]. Exposure to ultraviolet light, radiation, or ethylene oxide, as well as the inclusion of certain preservatives, all are promising approaches for sterilizing microneedles [125]. Sterilization of metal microneedles is relatively simple, although many pharmaceuticals administered via microneedles are sensitive to standard sterilization processes such as moist and dry heat and gamma irradiation. Consequently, the product's efficacy may be drastically diminished upon sterilization [55]. Designing sterile manufacturing techniques, such as aseptic production or terminal sterilization, early in the development phase is essential when a product requires to be sterile. Aseptic manufacture has been demonstrated in previous research to provide sterility without compromising the effectiveness of the device or medication. Although this technique is employed for drug–device combinations, it is not often favored owing to its high production costs [126]. Aseptic manufacturing will be cumbersome and challenging to implement if mass production is envisaged. Production is strictly controlled, and clean conditions and stringent operating procedures are required for aseptic processing, significantly increasing the production's expense and complication. Sterilization methods, including moist heat, microwave heat, or gamma radiation [127], would be excellent for aseptic production. However, these sterilizing strategies may contaminate the delivery system by damaging the microneedles or drug payloads. To choose the most suitable sterilization technique for each microneedles–drug combination, it is necessary to consider the effects these processes may have on the microneedles' physicochemical properties [55] or the encapsulated therapeutic agents [128, 129]. In particular, gamma irradiation degraded the model protein and changed its structure and the drug release kinetics from dissolving microneedles, while wet and dry heat sterilization ruined all formulations. The inclusion of silver nanoparticles into dissolving microneedles formulation has been proposed as a viable alternative to the sterilizing procedure. When applied to a skin site, the nanosized silver in the microneedle array may function as a powerful antibacterial agent, preventing any possible infection [130]. Terminal sterilization following microneedle production is theoretically feasible, but the sterilization technique must be compatible with the materials used to make microneedles and ensure the drug stability. To realize the objective of delivering sterile microneedles products to target customers, the finished packing may undergo terminal sterilization by conventional and customary techniques such as gamma irradiation or ethylene oxide [131]. While research on terminal sterilization of vaccine-loaded microneedles patches is still in its infancy, it has been observed that irradiating a microneedle patch carrying a peptide molecule using electron beams and gamma rays causes unacceptable changes to the product [128]. Terminal sterilization, where the product is sterilized after it is made and packed [55], is an option for certain products. However, aseptic handling [128] is necessary for many drugs and biomolecules since their activity is compromised during the sterilizing procedure. Remarkably, the physicochemical characteristics and release kinetics of both small and large molecules were undisturbed by gamma irradiation in hydrogel-forming microneedles made from super-swelling polymeric materials [55]. Besides, immersion in 70% ethanol for 30 min was effective in sterilizing silicon microneedles [25].

Several investigations have been conducted to study the effect of sterilization on the properties and quality of microneedles. McCrudden and colleagues investigated the impact of sterilizing methods on microneedle characteristics and drug payload [55]. These methods included steam sterilization, dry heat sterilization, and gamma radiation. The researchers observed that gamma irradiation (25 kGy) substantially lowered loaded drug quantity (ovalbumin and ibuprofen) in dissolving microneedles and the lyophilized drug reservoir while having no effect on the physical attributes or capacity of the unloaded microneedles to transport the drugs across neonatal porcine skin [55]. Hydrogel-forming microneedles also consistently had endotoxin levels lower than the 20 endotoxin units/device threshold set by the US Food and Drug Administration. Low endotoxin levels and the lack of microbiological contamination indicate that these microneedles provide a negligible hazard to human health if applied properly [55]. Hydrogel-forming swelling microneedles displayed no sign of microbial development even after being stored at a humidity level of 86%. Furthermore, *E. coli* did not proliferate in crosslinked microneedles, demonstrating the lack of a microbial colony [52]. Likewise, gamma radiation-based terminal sterilization provided microneedles completely free of microorganisms [55]. This indicates that, unlike hypodermic needles, microneedles lower the possibility of infection and confine any microbes to the epidermis rather than allowing them to penetrate the deeper dermis layers [94]. The use of microneedles to create microchannels in the stratum corneum has been shown to have a negligible effect on microbial penetration [50, 51]. Research by Donnelly and coworkers reveals that microorganisms, including *Candida albicans*, *Pseudomonas aeruginosa*, and *Staphylococcus* epidermidis, are capable of entering the skin tissue via microneedles-created channels. Nevertheless, no microbes are able to penetrate far into the viable epidermis, and the microbial load is markedly lower for microneedle insertion than for conventional hypodermic needles [50].

14.4.1.3 Manufacturing Costs and Market Incentives

Most pharmaceutical companies will have to foresee a realistic expectation of retrieving the substantial costs associated with conducting any late-stage clinical studies to showcase the product's efficacy necessary to justify approval of a new product before they decide to invest in commercializing the product. Microneedle patch production for existing pharmaceuticals may merely demand bridging research in comparison to the development of new drugs; however, it could also result in modifications in formulation or dosage, which may eventually necessitate substantial and costly regulatory amendments. As it is, there seem to be little economic incentives for innovation in regard to existing low-cost, well-established medications. Some approvals have been around for quite a long time, and the thought of revising safety profiles or altering manufacturing processes to meet updated regulatory requirements raises concerns about the significant costs and possible risks [132]. If a single producer holds a large portion of a certain market, other companies may be incentivized to enter the field with innovative new products for the competition [91].

Much attention has been paid to the mass production and commercialization of microneedle patches for vaccination. Advancement toward clinical deployment of microneedle patches for immunization has been relatively gradual, reflecting current commercial incentives, despite significant progressions in microneedle technology and fundamental research. A key hurdle is the absence of an anticipated acceptable return on investment for vaccine producers to develop marginal progress in vaccine delivery platforms and for inexpensive, traditional vaccines in particular [133, 134]. Vaccine development will inevitably rely on external financial incentives owing to the unavailability of competitiveness that would generate economic incentives for vaccine patch producers [91]. The structure of the vaccination market, which consists of a limited number of suppliers and major purchasers, alters the financial incentives and contributes to market segmentation. In particular, market segmentation results in multi-dose vaccinations with lower prices for developing countries and single-dose vaccines with premium prices for developed countries. Established market incentives are highly advantageous in developed nations, with some benefits for innovation deriving from the prospect to obtain a substantial market share for advanced and novel products. Influenza vaccine microneedles patches are on track to become the very first possible vaccine patch to reach phase III clinical trial. Furthermore, as the composition of seasonal influenza vaccine is altered every year, there is potential for the whole population to require yearly injection of seasonal influenza vaccine, making a flu vaccination patch a highly promising vaccine patch with great market value. Financial projections for vaccination patches do not presently justify the expenditures required for approved vaccine patches to arrive on the market shortly, according to the current state of vaccine patch technology and conversations with important stakeholders [132]. Manufacturers' interest in developing novel vaccines for use in developing countries will depend on their level of previous expertise with such products. Public–private collaborations and other incentives, including national or international financing, will likely be necessary to promote the development and application of vaccination patches in developing regions. The public–private alliances may draw in funding that balance the costs and risks of doing so, which is especially helpful for low-margin goods or niche markets. In this light, investors may have some impact on when exactly vaccination patches hit shelves. There may be no necessity for public–private cooperation in the markets of developed countries if adequate private finance is already in place and the market is competitive. Vaccination patches may allow a product to stand out from the crowd, which would be a massive bonus in the commercial arena. The development of vaccination patches might benefit significantly from national research funding. While general financing methods for the patch technology could help answer some common issues, specialized funding for vaccination patches is more likely to address the fundamental immunobiological problems that arise from particular vaccines [91].

The manufacturing method has to be low-cost and consistent, in addition to being authorized by the appropriate regulatory bodies. Microneedle technologies are most often used for vaccination; thus, it is crucial that they can be mass-produced in the hundreds of thousands, if not millions, of patches in a short time. Since the manufacturing processes are adapted from conventional microchip production in the microelectronics sector, silicon microneedles may unquestionably be manufactured in such large numbers. Unfortunately, the present coating techniques are not scalable. The centrifugation processes used in micromolding techniques for polymeric microneedles are obviously not scalable. For this reason, companies like Corium, LTS, and Rodan + Fields have developed proprietary manufacturing processes for mass-producing polymeric microneedles [94].

14.4.1.4 Manufacturing Issues with Microneedle Types

To fabricate coated microneedles, it is essential to prepare coating formulations that uniformly coat the needles' tips without wasting a lot of drug-loaded formulation on the array substrate, and that can retain their shape and functionality for the duration of the product's shelf life. Excipients are often used in coating formulations because they assist in keeping the drug contained on the microneedles' surface rather than the array substrate. They also aid in keeping the coating droplets in place on the microneedles even after being stored for an extended period. Coating solid microneedles with a drug require a formulation that keeps the drug chemically and physically stable and allows the coated drug to be released from the microneedles and into the skin tissue after the skin insertion of the microneedle array. To accurately predict the wear time of a microneedle system, formulation and product design must account for how quickly the drug would be released from the array of needles. Wear times for coated microneedles are usually brief, in the range of 5–30 min, in contrast to more conventional transdermal patches, intended to give drug administration over the duration of hours or days. Drug release from coated microneedles depends on the properties of the drug and formulation, both of which should be evaluated throughout the preclinical phase [60].

Dissolving microneedles require a polymeric matrix sufficiently robust to construct microneedles that can pierce the skin and preserve their physical integrity during insertion while possessing the desired dissolution profile to release the drug payload into the skin tissue. The tip bore of hollow microneedles may get clogged, and they are often less sturdy than solid microneedles. Because of these limitations, needle design and insertion techniques must be carefully considered. In addition, due to the lessened potential for leakage, a single hollow microneedle may be chosen over arrays of multiple hollow microneedles. Hollow microneedle arrays, nevertheless, may be preferable over single hollow microneedles due to the greater quantity of drug that could be delivered if each individual microneedle on the array comes with its own drug reservoir [135]. Multiple criteria, such as drug content, excipients, pH, tonicity, dose volume, and formulation viscosity, must be considered when developing a safe and efficient drug formulation for intradermal delivery. The formulation must also be sterile and devoid of pyrogens. Early in the development process, the formulation should be tested for its mechanical and biological effects on the skin. Administration of viscous fluids may require much longer than expected since the speed of intradermal injection is inversely related to formulation viscosity. Injection needles must be sufficiently robust to retain their structure throughout the insertion process and long enough to remain underneath the epidermis layer during the fluid injection. A tight seal between the needle and the skin is necessary during intradermal drug administration using hollow microneedles at high pressure. The drug formulation will seep out onto the skin surface rather than stay in the skin if the seal is compromised [60].

14.4.1.5 Supply Chain, Storage, and Disposal Issues

Microneedles offer several advantages during storage and transportation. Since microneedles patches are much more compact than a vaccination vial and needle-syringe system, they may be easier to store and distribute. Once integrated into a patch, a microneedle array of this size might have a representative volume of around 1 cm^3 [135, 136]. Vaccines might be packaged as microneedle patches, which would drastically reduce their bulk during transportation, storage, and disposal [13]. However, packing the product (perhaps in multi-dose packages) would still increase its overall size. In addition, the threat of subsequent disease transmission and needlestick injuries is reduced since microneedles are designed for single use and readily disposable (depending primarily on the type); they do not necessitate specific sharps waste disposal and do not call for medical equipment reuse. Nowadays, it is not uncommon to find vaccines in vials suitable for more than one dose. By opening a fresh vial when there are not enough patients to utilize the full vial, vaccines may be squandered, or a patient may not get the vaccination if the device is not used properly. Microneedles are convenient since they do not require reconstitution and are compact (unless they have a large applicator). Moreover, microneedles may be cheaper to ship, store, and dispose of than injectables [20].

Transporting vaccines and other biologicals that need continual refrigeration may be challenging. This is a major issue, particularly for developing nations, since it raises both complexity and expense [10]. A substantial amount of money might be saved by using microneedles since they are not required to be stored in a cold chain. Vaccines are stored in a dry state within microneedle patches, and they may be rendered thermostable with the addition of appropriate excipients. If microneedle patches could be properly stabilized and stored at ambient conditions, the necessity for a cold chain may be eliminated. If only moderate thermostability is obtained, microneedle patches might be refrigerated at crucial distribution centers, but taken out of the cold chain during shipping, storage at village clinics, or mass immunization campaigns [13]. The stability at high temperatures of microneedle patches used to administer influenza vaccine has been the subject of numerous studies. In a recent investigation, researchers found that some formulations may be stored for at least six months at 25°C and at least a few weeks at 40°C [137]. There have been studies on the thermostability of microneedle patches containing adenovirus and measles vaccines, which have been demonstrated to be stable for at least four months at 25°C and to lose less than tenfold efficacy after four months of storage at 40°C [138, 139]. Comparable to malaria test kits, polymeric microneedles may be hygroscopic and susceptible to elevated temperatures, necessitating the usage of specific packaging and the inclusion of desiccants to prevent moisture absorption. This, in turn, would drive up packing costs [140]. Microneedle devices will need packaging for storage and transportation. Efficient product labeling and healthcare professional counseling may only be able to govern patient handling to a small extent. The packaging of a drug or other therapeutic agents is only as effective as its ability to withstand typical handling and storage conditions without being damaged or tampered with.

14.4.2 Regulatory Issues of Microneedles

14.4.2.1 Introduction of Microneedles Regulatory Issues

Drug products would have to comply with stringent regulations and pharmacopoeial criteria before they could be made available to the general public. The final price tag [120] will be significantly affected by the product's complexity and the amount of time needed to fulfill regulatory requirements. Since microneedles penetrate and disrupt the skin's protective barrier, they raise a number of unique scientific and regulatory concerns that must be solved before they can be approved. Microneedles will face less resistance to regulatory approval if they are treated as a novel dosage form rather than a subset of the established transdermal drug delivery systems [113]. No universally recognized regulatory requirements exist at this time for genuine microneedles products. The microneedle patch system lacks explicit instructions and formal guidelines in the United States. Unfortunately, there are now no true microneedles items available; hence there are no established standards and regulations for them. This introduces new layers of complexity into large-scale production, which necessitates universally acceptable benchmarks for evaluating product quality. This is a substantial stumbling block to commercializing microneedle products [120]. To ensure patient safety, regulatory agencies may need more assurances than only cGMP production [55]. While there are regulations for traditional transdermal patches, they only apply to the skin's surface; since microneedles enter the skin, they raise new questions about their safety and efficacy. Therefore, changes must be made to how microneedles are approved and regulated to deal with the unique challenges they provide. A novel dosage form [24] may be required for microneedles classification. It would be necessary to get answers to a variety of questions, and the way they were resolved would affect how much the finished product would cost. The Food and Drug Administration (FDA) has released guidelines clarifying the criteria for classifying a microneedle product as a medical device, depending on its intended application. A microneedle system is regarded to be a medical device if it is used "in the diagnosis of disease or other conditions, or the cure, mitigation, treatment, or prevention of disease" or if it is employed "to affect the structure or any function of the body of man." It will be necessary to deal with regulatory requirements, including over-the-counter practices, the legitimacy of self-vaccination for children and healthcare personnel, and the associated documentation [10]. A feedback mechanism or indication is beneficial since patients may not be sure they got the correct dose [9, 31]. This feedback system has the potential to improve immunization record-keeping as well. Since microneedles puncture the skin, there is a potential for infection; thus, regulatory criteria should account for microbiological criteria and other critical safety considerations. The production process will be significantly more expensive if aseptic manufacturing is required to ensure that low bioburden criteria are fulfilled.

Microneedles have already shown their effectiveness in the administration of biomacromolecules; thus, the number of possible applications is only going to grow. The first-to-market microneedle drug delivery systems will substantially impact the regulatory requirements; early industry advocates of the technology will have the opportunity to set the bar for quality that subsequent microneedle products must satisfy [120]. The appropriate authorities must also approve the pharmaceuticals that will be administered by microneedle patch before they can be used. Therefore, the first commercialized microneedle patch is highly anticipated, and it is expected that further products will be introduced after regulatory guidance is established for their production and usage [141]. The standard for future generations of microneedle monitoring or diagnostic products may be determined by the regulatory requirements imposed on the first items of their kind to arrive on the market [85]. Industries and researchers interested in adopting microneedle technology would benefit significantly from standardized recommendations for the use of established methods of manufacture, assessment, test requirements for approval, and quality control. In 2017, the Food and Drug Administration published "Regulatory Considerations for Microneedling Devices" to simplify the process of manufacturing microneedles as medical devices. Since then, Norman et al. have published an article about this subject, "Scientific Considerations for microneedle Products: Product Development, Manufacturing, and Quality Control" [142]. The FDA has held technical seminars on microneedle devices where scientists have examined the requirements for microneedle systems [60, 142]. Biopharmaceutics, nonclinical applications, mechanical properties, stability, sterility, and patient usage all have received expanded attention. Individual manufacturers would benefit significantly from an additional direction, such as the establishment of international consensus guidelines and standards [120, 132]. This would permit trade-offs on product features that are less important while still achieving the most crucial objectives. There is currently no microneedles-based vaccination product available on the market that regulatory agencies have given the green light on. They also disclosed the evidence required for approving these items, such as aseptic microneedle production or the use of terminal sterilizing processes [127]. One example is that silicon microneedles production necessitates a clean room environment, which is one of many factors to consider. The advantages for patients and manufacturers will be substantial after regulatory barriers are cleared, and production processes are established, optimized, and validated to current good manufacturing practice standards [143].

14.4.2.2 Category of Microneedles

Inevitably, regulatory agencies will classify microneedles according to the existing information and intended use. This means that microneedles devices may one day be classified as drug delivery systems, consumer goods, or medical devices. Whether the finished product has to be terminally sterilized, manufactured under an aseptic environment, or merely demonstrated to have a low bioburden may depend on how the microneedles are classified [55]. For solid microneedles in which the drug is coated onto the needles, the drug administration is frequently facilitated by an applicator. The applicator would get market authorization in the NDA or BLA of the combination product due to its distinctive features with respect to its utilization of the coated microneedle array. Since the applicator will be included in the same package as the coated microneedle patch, this combination product will most likely fall under subcategory 3.2(e)(2). The patch containing the microneedles may be considered a 3.2(e)(1) product, although solid microneedles are more effective when they come with an applicator to ensure effective drug delivery [60]. The FDA considers injection devices to be Class II medical devices, meaning a 510 K application is required for clearance if the new device is "essentially comparable" to the already marketed device. Combination devices also include hollow microneedles; however, those that necessitate a microneedle device for drug administration may be classified as 3.2(e) (1) or 3.2(e)(2), depending on the finished products before being presented to the market. Some producers of hollow microneedles may choose to construct the complete product in their production facility, creating the device ready for use by the patients or health professionals upon opening the packaging. To qualify as a 3.2(e)(1) or single integrated product, the drug and device components must be intended for delivery to the end user as a single unit [60]. Dissolving microneedles are similar to existing dissolving or disintegrating pharmaceutical products since they are also constructed from a drug-loaded polymeric matrix [55]. Microneedles that form hydrogel swelling structures or are made of metal may be used for drug administration and could be removed intact from the skin; hence they may be categorized with other parenteral drugs or medical devices. But it is possible that they could all fall under the category of "drug product." When a company wants to mass manufacture a product, knowing which quality criteria the product must meet becomes crucial [120].

14.4.2.3 Quality System for Microneedles

14.4.2.3.1 Introduction of Quality System

The development of microneedle technology includes several research fields, such as chemistry, toxicology, biopharmaceutics, skin physiology, materials science, human factors, and mechanical engineering. To ensure that the relevant factors are examined at a crucial time throughout the development process, all of these studies are supported by a quality management system used for drug–device combination products [60]. The ICH Harmonized Tripartite Guidelines might be combined with other standards to provide a unified set of tests and requirements for new drug products and parenteral drug products that could be used for microneedles. Specific quality criteria within the framework of Good Manufacturing Practice are required for large-scale microneedle production.

It is challenging to evaluate the microneedles' performance due to the absence of standardized testing and equipment used to verify physical qualities and insertion capacity. For microneedles products to enter the commercial market, a Pharmaceutical Quality System that includes Good Manufacturing Practices and Quality Risk Management [120] must be developed and properly executed. Production parameters, in-process assessment, document review, product specification compliance, and a visual inspection of the finished product are some of the aspects that should be considered in a comprehensive evaluation [120].

Quality control tests for microneedles are purely conjectural without knowledge of their categorization and requirements specification. Microneedles need to be able to puncture the skin, penetrate deep enough, and come out without significantly damaging the tissue. When employed, dissolving microneedles must rapidly and completely release their drug payload. For drugs to be delivered successfully, hollow microneedles must be kept "open" throughout the injection process. Hydrogel-forming microneedles must expand to the desired size before delivering the drug to the skin. Microneedles must not cause any damage or injuries to the patient. The United States Food and Drug Administration (FDA) has released a draft guidance on "microneedling" for cosmetic use, and PATH provided a fact sheet depicting an initiative for facilitating the advancement of microneedles for drug delivery, both of which raise interesting points irrespective of the ongoing controversies about microneedles production and acceptability. The pricing of microneedles products will be affected by the stringent quality controls and pharmacopeial regulations that must be met throughout the production. Within the context of a suitable quality system for these drug–device combinations, data packages must be produced for all domains used in the production of the product. Detailed assessment of each product component and key interactions are required for product development and data package creation. Recent research and reviews highlighted important factors that impact design options while fabricating microneedles [12, 144]. These assessments offer an opportunity to identify desired product features and develop quality target product profiles so that prospective users may make suggestions on their preferences for various product aspects [91].

Microneedle delivery systems fall within the purview of the current Good Manufacturing Practice system as outlined in 21 CFR 4 in the United States since they are drug–device combination products. In other parts of the world, cGMP systems might be classified based on the individual or combined properties of the product used to administer the drug. By picking a fundamental set of criteria from one of the primary cGMP systems and incorporating the 21 CFR 4 defined features of the other cGMP systems, cGMP in the United States may take a simplified approach, combining the criteria of drug cGMP contained in 21 CFR 210/211 and device cGMP listed in 21 CFR 820. Since cGMP regulations include all of these product categories, they must be considered during the design phase of microneedle delivery systems (21 CFR 820.30). Combination product developers must take precautions beyond those generally used to ensure the safety of each component. This calls for a characterization of the interaction between the drug component and the packed device [60]. Elements of primary packaging that aid in drug delivery must also be defined in light of primary packaging standards for appropriateness, compatibility, safety, performance, and functionality.

When applicable, it is necessary to account for the typical range of variations in analyses and production. The skin model is a critical factor for technology, formulation, and drug delivery when developing a microneedle system. In the initial stages of product development, it is crucial to evaluate the relevance of various animal models as a surrogate for human testing. When considering *in vivo* skin models, the preclinical species is a viable solution because of its skin's physiology, its manageability, and its surface area [145]. Physiologically and in terms of skin structure, porcine skin is favored over other species [146]. Furthermore, research is being conducted to create artificial membranes and other skin models that could be valuable for testing the insertion of microneedle arrays and other crucial attributes of microneedle products [147, 148]. Since skin cannot be utilized for quality control testing, it is essential that model membranes be able to mimic skin's structure [39]. However, the development of a standardized release and dissolution test from dissolving microneedle arrays, similar to those widely accessible for conventional dosage forms, is a critical component that has been largely neglected in the field [149]. Biological tissue has been frequently employed in the release study in the scientific literature [150]. Nevertheless, quality control tests cannot be carried out on biological tissue since they cannot be standardized. Hence, following the microneedle array application, drug penetration through the skin must be mimicked by an artificial membrane [120].

14.4.2.3.2 Considerations of Quality System

ICH Quality Guidelines have been reported to provide valuable suggestions for constructing chemistry, manufacturing, and controls (CMC) data packages of microneedle products [60]. The International Conference on Harmonization (ICH) Q6A guidance was adopted to establish a set of quality attributes universal to all microneedles, as revealed by Lutton and colleagues. Accordingly, tests for dissolution, disintegration, friability, dosage uniformity, stability, water content, microbial limits, sterility, particulate matter, antimicrobial preservative content, extractable, system functionality, and osmolarity will presumably be conducted on microneedles during production (Table 14.1). In addition, microneedle delivery systems may be evaluated on a case-by-case basis, following the technical standards outlined in ISO 11608 [60].

TABLE 14.1

ICH Quality Guidance for Data Packages of Microneedle Products

ICH Quality Guidance	Guidance Title	Scope of Guideline	Relevance to Microneedle Products
ICH Q1 A(R2)	Stability Testing: New Drug Substances and Products	Guidelines for stability study protocol include temperature, humidity, and testing time	Design a stability procedure to determine the shelf life of microneedle products
B	Photostability of New Drug Substances and Products	Evaluation technique for light sensitivity; an appendix to the primary stability guideline	Product-specific application
C	New Dosage Forms	New dosage form stability guidelines for the same active ingredient in a different product category; an appendix to the primary stability guideline	Using an active pharmaceutical ingredient in a prior dosage form may lead to a reduced stability database for submission
D	Bracketing and Matrixing Designs	Standards for bracketing and matrix designs in reduced stability testing	Pull point matrices may lessen the required testing, but they can also increase the risk associated with predicting when a product will expire if it comes in more than one strength

TABLE 14.1 *(Continued)*

ICH Quality Guidance for Data Packages of Microneedle Products

ICH Quality Guidance	Guidance Title	Scope of Guideline	Relevance to Microneedle Products
E	Evaluation of Stability Data	Analysis of stability data and shelf life prediction using statistical methods	The guideline is relevant and practical
ICH Q3	**Impurities:**		
A(R2)	New Drug Substances	Limits for reporting, identification, and qualification	Conforms to the same minimum levels as other dosage types
B(R2)	New Drug Products	Interaction-generated degradation products	Similar to various dosage forms in terms of interactions between active pharmaceutical ingredients, excipients, and primary packaging components
C(R7)	Guideline for Residual Solvents	Limits on the level of residual solvents in drug product	Similar to other dosage forms, a heavy reliance on active pharmaceutical ingredients and excipients
D(R2)	Guideline for Elemental Impurities	Permitted daily exposures and limits for elemental impurities in drug products (oral, parenteral, inhalation, cutaneous, and transdermal routes)	
ICH Q6	**Specifications: Test Procedures and Acceptance Criteria:**		
A	New Drug Substances and New Drug Products: Chemical Substances	Procedure for choosing tests and defining specifications	Provides recommendations for determining required specifications
B	Biotechnological/ Biological Products	Justify and establish specifications for proteins and polypeptides	Specifications as an element to control product quality
ICH Q8(R2)	Pharmaceutical Development	Module 3.2.P.2: Quality by Design (QbD) in pharmaceutical development	Uniquely specify quality target product profile and critical quality attributes for microneedle products, as with other dosage forms

Researchers have also given scientific arguments for establishing a well-defined Quality Target Product Profile (QTPP) at an early stage of product development, together with the associated process parameters. Recognizing and accounting for potential changes in the optimal target product profile between developed and developing nations, as well as across various pharmaceutical molecules, is a crucial step in the development process (Table 14.2) [12, 132]. To be used in clinical settings, microneedles must meet what regulatory authorities perceive as potential concerns and prospective criteria from a regulatory viewpoint [127]. To meet the requirements of both drugs and medical devices, it may be essential to use data packages to support the proper chemistry, manufacturing, and control (CMC) of microneedles products. It is beneficial to determine whether the requirements of USP <3> chapter, Topical and Transdermal Products, apply to the desired microneedles product. The specific USP <3> criteria relevant to the particular product must be identified via in-depth research. USP <3> describes a variety of tests, such as the peel adhesion test, the release liner peel test, and the tack test. For the microneedle patch, conducting a case-by-case analysis of the method's suitability and specifications is crucial. Several universal, standardized quality

TABLE 14.2

Quality Considerations for Microneedle Products

Product Quality Tests	Relevance to Microneedle Products
Description	Applicable
Identification	Applicable
Assay	Applicable, depending on the specific product and analytical method
Impurities and degradation products	Applicable, depending on the specific product and analytical method
Water content	Applicable, depending on the specific formulation. If applicable, a water content measurement should be performed. For hygroscopic microneedles, this test is a requirement. Information about the product's sensitivity to water or hydration might be used to support the acceptance criteria. A loss-on-drying approach may be sufficient in certain situations; however, a specialized detection method for water (such as Karl Fischer titration) is desirable [120]
Microbial limits	Unless the product's components have been examined before production and the manufacturing method has been validated to provide no considerable risk of microbial contamination or growth, testing the microbiological limit of the finished product is recommended. This test is especially useful for microneedles due to the requirement for a sterile or minimal bioburden product. While most parenteral injectables fall into the former, certain polymeric microneedles do not promote microbial growth [120]
Antimicrobial preservative content	Applicable for multiple-dose parenteral products but irrelevant for single-dose microneedle patches. The use of an antibacterial preservative seems inappropriate for microneedles products [120]
Antioxidant content	Applicable, depending on specific drug formulations
Sterility	The necessity for sterilization, aseptic processing, or just a minimal bioburden [85] in the finished product has to be considered. Microneedles devices are not officially categorized as sterile or non-sterile items; instead, they may be aseptically produced or terminally sterilized, depending on the regulations [55]. A minimal bioburden may be adequate if the system possesses intrinsic and verifiable antimicrobial properties. However, the view of regulatory agencies on whether or not microneedles must be sterile is unknown [94]. Due to the potential for infection, microneedles must meet stringent safety standards in terms of bioburden or sterility and packaging. This has implications for how microneedle products are developed, manufactured, and marketed. The Food and Drug Administration (FDA) recommends that sterilization be planned as early as feasible in the development phase. The necessity for sterility in a microneedle depends on its intended use, the kind of tissue it will be inserted into, how long it will be kept in place, and the type of patients it will be used on
pH	May be irrelevant, depending on the specific product
Particle size	Probably irrelevant, microneedles formulations are generally a solution. Applicable only if particle-based formulations are injected into the skin via hollow microneedles, coated onto solid microneedles, or loaded into the polymeric matrix of dissolving or swelling microneedles
Microneedle design: density, arrangement, and geometry	Skin penetration of microneedles relies heavily on their optimal geometry. Optimizing the microneedles in terms of their length, arrangement, sharpness, and penetration rate is crucial. Microneedle penetration depth is affected by a number of factors beyond their length, including their geometry (i.e., base size, tip radius, base-to-tip ratio, and needle-to-needle spacing), materials, and arrangement on the array [152, 153]. If the mechanical strength is high enough, a sharper tip will penetrate farther than a blunt one [154, 155]. Specific microneedles' geometries should be developed to pierce the skin to the required depth. The appropriate drug quantity cannot be administered without a sufficient number of microneedles. An optimal formulation for dissolving microneedles balances drug payloads,

TABLE 14.2 *(Continued)*

Quality Considerations for Microneedle Products

Product Quality Tests	Relevance to Microneedle Products
	microneedle count, geometry, and drug delivery efficiency. Because of the "bed of nails" effect, microneedles may not be able to penetrate deeply enough if they are too densely packed. Multiple hollow microneedles, rather than a single needle, may deliver large volumes of liquid formulation into the skin. Intradermal injections may employ high injection pressure, a large number of microneedles, and a specific needle configuration to overcome the dermal resistance to injection flow and inject a significant volume of fluid [60]
Dissolution	It may also be desirable to develop a dissolution test that could differentiate the formulation changes or process factors that substantially impact product dissolution or when another component of the specification does not manage such changes. This might be significant for techniques like photopolymerization and crosslinking in which the microneedles undergo significant structural modifications [120]
Disintegration	Disintegration testing is most useful when a correlation to dissolution has been identified or when disintegration has been demonstrated to be more discriminatory than dissolution. This evaluation may include testing microneedles' dissolving in the skin and releasing the drug payload [120]
Mechanical testing/ Hardness/Friability	For microneedles to function properly, they need to have characteristics like resistance to breakage and a high required force for deformation. There has to be mechanical testing of microneedles to ensure they are sufficiently robust to puncture the skin but not so fragile that they break off within. As users may insert needles with a spectrum of forces and they cannot "calibrate" their applied force, insertion tests to assure users can manually insert the needles effectively, verification of microneedles penetration, and evaluations to ensure skin integrity returns to original status after microneedles treatment are all necessary. Microneedles undergo a wide range of pressures during insertion, withdrawal, storage, and transportation. Therefore, it is vital to assess its mechanical qualities, including its sharpness, static loading, linear buckling, and shear representation. Microneedle bending, buckling, and baseplate breakage are the most prevalent types of mechanical failures, and they may reduce drug efficacy, induce local adverse effects, and ultimately cause failed treatment. The stability of any pharmaceutical ingredient contained in a microneedle system depends on its capacity to maintain its intrinsic form and strength and resist moisture uptake during storage [120].
Content uniformity: between products, among the needles in a microneedle system, and within individual needles	Content uniformity could be evaluated on the entire array or from individual microneedles on the array, depending on how the system is configured. All traditional transdermal patch products require this type of testing. Dissolving, coated, and hydrogel-forming microneedles require relatively consistent drug content, whereas solid and hollow microneedle systems do not. Understanding how the drug is distributed on a single microneedle is critical, especially for dissolving and coated microneedles, as only a portion of the needle may penetrate the skin. Only the drug load on the inserted portion is delivered. Particularly difficult is the process of consistently coating microneedles. The coating layer's uniformity and smoothness depend on several parameters, including formulation rheological characteristics and surface tension, needle geometry, needle roughness, and dimensions [102]. Environmental factors, including humidity, temperature, and airflow, heavily influence the quality of the coated layer
Particulate matter	This test evaluates the solution's clarity and the absence of subvisible particles. Suitable for hollow microneedles with a liquid formulation
Extractables and leachables	Eliminating this test is generally allowed if development and stability data indicate that extractables are typically below the limits that are established to be acceptable and safe. More research is required if the packaging or formulation is altered [120]
Functionality testing of delivery systems	A functioning test for microneedles is to determine how effectively they penetrate skin over time during the product's shelf life [120]

(Continued)

TABLE 14.2 *(Continued)*

Quality Considerations for Microneedle Products

Product Quality Tests	Relevance to Microneedle Products
Osmolarity	It is essential to monitor the osmolarity of a product carefully whenever its tonicity is stated on the label. For microneedle-based systems, this will be irrelevant [120]
Packaging	The packing must be secure, preventing any moisture from entering the product. Patients can quickly and easily access the product they need without risking injury to their skin during product removal from the packaging
Potential for microneedles reapplication	It is possible to reinsert the skin after removing certain types of microneedles from the skin. Self-inactivating microneedles, including dissolving and hydrogel-forming microneedles, are favorable
Disposal procedures	Nonbiodegradable microneedles may provide a health risk. The disposal process has to take into account environmental factors
Deposition of microneedles material into the skin	Risks are associated with dissolving and coated microneedles intended to treat chronic diseases. A change in product application location is necessary. The potential for short-term and long-term side effects must be clarified
Ease and reproducibility of microneedles application	The device has to be user-friendly so that patients may use it as intended without too much difficulty. The microneedle array may be applied to the skin by hand or using an applicator. The viscoelasticity of skin dramatically reduces the depth of microneedles penetration achieved by hand application. Furthermore, hand application may lead to substantial variability in drug delivery due to differences in skin thickness and the force with which people would apply. The microneedle array may be inserted into the skin at a consistent rate using a force-based or spring-driven applicator. The fundamental function of an applicator is to reliably deliver the entire quantity of drug to the intended site of action
Confirmation of microneedles insertion	Necessary to provide evidence of proper dosing and administration. Helpful in giving patients confidence that they are using the product properly
Potential immunological effects	Microneedles' repeated puncturing of the skin raises the possibility of an immune response. Provide indications of immunological safety
Stability	Any stability issue linked with the product in the marketed package may be detected by a continual program to evaluate the stability of the product after marketing. The ongoing stability strategy ensures that the product is, and will continue to be, stable under the specified storage conditions for the duration of its labeled shelf life [120]. Both the microneedles and the drug must be stable for the products to be stable in their entirety. Needles are evaluated in terms of deformation and durability, whereas drugs loaded in microneedles may have concerns with crystallinity, particle size, and polymorphism. Coated microneedles also face the challenge of formulation displacement. Another major issue with coated microneedles is the delamination of the coated layer from the microneedles' surface during application [59]. Since the drugs are dissolved in the excipient matrix, the stability of dissolving microneedles is complicated. The stability of the drug throughout production and storage depends on the drug-excipient compatibility. The microneedles must be safe to be deposited into the skin, sufficiently robust to penetrate the skin without fracture, and stable enough to maintain their mechanical strength throughout transportation and storage without losing the encapsulated drug [1]
Biocompatibility	To ensure products are safe for human use, biocompatibility evaluation of the materials in their finished and in-process stages is essential. User-contact parts of microneedles devices were tested for cytotoxicity, irritation, sensitization, acute systemic toxicity, and material-mediated pyrogenicity to determine their biocompatibility. USP and the National Toxicology Program offer testing protocols to evaluate acute systemic toxicity and materials-related pyrogenicity. Biocompatibility testing based on skin-exposure times:

TABLE 14.2 *(Continued)*

Quality Considerations for Microneedle Products

Product Quality Tests	Relevance to Microneedle Products		
	Skin-contact Duration	*Recommended Testing*	*Factors*
	Limited (≤24 h)	Cytotoxicity Sensitization Irritation or intracutaneous reactivity	Acute systemic toxicity Material-related pyrogenicity Chemical characterization of extracted material
	Prolonged (>24 h, ≤30 days)	Cytotoxicity Sensitization Irritation or intracutaneous reactivity	Acute systemic toxicity Material-related pyrogenicity Chemical characterization of extracted material Subacute/subchronic systemic toxicity Implantation
	Chronic, repeated wearing (>30 days)	Cytotoxicity Sensitization Irritation or intracutaneous reactivity Genotoxicity Subacute/subchronic systemic toxicity	Acute systemic toxicity Material-related pyrogenicity Chemical characterization of extracted material Subacute/subchronic systemic toxicity Implantation Chronic toxicity Carcinogenicity
Skin penetration	Microneedles must be able to pierce the skin without fracturing and leaving debris behind. Transepidermal water loss [156, 157], skin electrical resistance [26], and post-insertion staining are the most popular qualitative methods used to evaluate skin penetration. Skin features, including surface nonuniformity and viscoelasticity, as well as needle geometry and mechanical robustness, significantly impact the insertion force and depth of microneedles penetration into the skin. The insertion force for microneedles must always be greater than the microneedles' fracture/breaking force [1]		
Penetration depth	Microneedle product development necessitates measuring the depth of penetration since reliable and reproducible penetration is a crucial quality attribute of microneedles [120]. Histology, confocal microscopy, optical coherence tomography, fluorescence microscopy, X-ray computed tomography, and high-speed X-ray imaging are some methods that might be used to determine the penetration depth. Microneedle geometries and dimensions (needle length, base size, tip radius, base-to-tip ratio, needle-to-needle distance), microneedle material, and insertion force were all reported to significantly impact penetration depth. Accurate measures of penetration depth may greatly aid the development of microneedle arrays and applicators. Applicator design may be adjusted and optimized for maximum drug delivery by monitoring microneedles penetration depth throughout the development process [60]		
Endotoxin	Regulatory agencies have not reported limits of allowable endotoxin exposure that are particular to microneedles		

(Continued)

TABLE 14.2 *(Continued)*

Quality Considerations for Microneedle Products

Product Quality Tests	Relevance to Microneedle Products
Mode of use of microneedles	Several design selections are made based on how a microneedle will be applied. If a topical formulation is applied after microneedles insertion and removal, it will be necessary to provide a positioning or marker mechanism that helps the user locate the formulation over the microneedles-pretreated region. Due to their small loading capacity, coated or dissolving microneedles can only be used with very potent drugs. Dissolution kinetics and the amount of drug that remained on used microneedles or delivered into the skin must be studied and optimized during formulation development. Constraints on injection pressure and volume are important factors to consider while designing hollow microneedles [158]
Microneedle array adhesion	After being inserted into the skin, microneedles must stay there for the duration of drug delivery. Microneedles may be secured using medical adhesive [60]. Kept in the skin, microneedle arrays only last approximately a week before being dislodged by natural processes, including sloughing dead skin, sweating, and physical movement. Human clinical studies are necessary to assess the adhesive wear qualities of the product [158] since *in vitro* and animal models of adhesion have poor prediction capacities
Irritation, sensitization, and immune response	Special toxicity testing for skin irritation is conducted on an animal model of microneedle devices prior to human clinical studies. Irritation and sensitization are investigated as part of the safety examination in clinical trials and separate human investigations undertaken throughout clinical development. It is of interest to understand whether or not patients have any adverse effects from repeated microneedle usage in the form of an immunological response to the drug, excipients, or microneedle materials
Skin healing	After a disruption in the skin's protective barrier is recognized, the body immediately turns to repair the injury and close up the pores [159]. The skin's ability to heal quickly is a positive attribute for short-term microneedle systems like coated or dissolving microneedles or intradermal injection. Hence, the possibility of developing an infection and experiencing skin irritation is lower. However, the skin's ability to heal close the channels, reducing delivery, for applications that need extended periods of contact, such as skin pretreatment before patch application or continuous drug administration via hollow needles. The rate at which the channels close is affected by several factors, including needle size, subject age, occlusive conditions, and the composition of the formulation in contact with the skin
User-device interface	It is standard procedure to perform numerous rounds of formative human factors testing on the user-device interface. It is important that the delivery system's dimensions, geometries, and weight be suitable for the intended user. The Food and Drug Administration (FDA) offers practical references for considering these aspects on a delivery system–specific basis and in terms of general principles. It is crucial that a microneedle system be set up so that the user may apply it safely and efficiently with as few steps as possible [60]. Human factors studies examine each user task associated with using the microneedle system. These tasks involve taking the microneedle system out of the package, preparing the system for the application, delivering the dose, removing the system from the delivery site, and eventually having the product discarded. There are both visual and audible indicators that let the user know when the injection is finished. All microneedle systems need concise and unambiguous instructions. The most effective microneedle system will have a user-friendly layout that makes it easy for anybody to use. The early hazard and risk analysis may help improve the functionality of the microneedle system. An in-depth analysis is performed on each process and function to identify possible errors and implement appropriate corrective actions. Preventing injuries caused by sharp objects is a typical focus of risk assessments. The shorter needles and lower reuse possibility of certain microneedle systems may allow for the reduction or elimination of sharp injury–protective measures. After conducting a risk assessment and any necessary modification, the microneedle system is evaluated in a formative human factors study. Subjects

TABLE 14.2 *(Continued)*

Quality Considerations for Microneedle Products

Product Quality Tests	Relevance to Microneedle Products
	perform a mock administration while reading and following specific instructions. User defects may be detected during the tasks like setting up the system, locating it, activating it, and removing it. Skin adhesion, application locations, application duration, and application frequency are other aspects that may be assessed. During the study, researchers observe and record user behavior and input, assess the findings, and use hazard/risk analysis to rectify any major design issues. These findings enable additional improvements to the microneedle device and associated protocols. The delivery system is assessed in a summative human factors validation study after a risk analysis, redesigning, and subsequent formative trials. This may proceed alongside or independent of ongoing formulation development, preclinical studies, and human clinical investigations. Finally, the human factors methods, assessment, and outcomes of successful validation testing indicate that the users can operate the delivery system as intended [60].

control testing might be helpful in characterizing and comparing the mechanical strength and insertion capability of microneedles [120]. Automatic quality management at each step of the manufacturing process is essential for the mass production of microneedles. A drug product must be approved for release for human use after meeting stringent regulatory and pharmacopoeial requirements. Since pharmacopoeial criteria are generated from the tests that the regulatory agencies accept as part of a manufacturer's filed dossier, no such standards will be developed for microneedles products until a variety of microneedles products are commercialized. The most important concerns for future microneedles development are the optimization and validation of the technology, as well as the addressing of regulatory questions, such as long-term safety and sterility criteria [151]. Time delays associated with regulatory processing, licensing, and compliance, as well as the complexity of batch manufacturing, quality control, packaging, labeling, and storage, necessitate investments of resources on the part of manufacturers. If only partial information is accessible when the application is submitted, it is possible that the acceptance criteria will need to be altered. The acceptance criteria must logically center on the product's safety and efficacy. Similarly, novel analytical methods are always being developed, and current technologies are constantly being improved. As microneedles continue to advance toward commercialization, it will be necessary to employ such technologies where they are thought to provide an extra layer of quality assurance or when they are warranted [120]. It is important to realize, nevertheless, that qualification and validation criteria require a reevaluation of any changes made to established production processes or the development of new methods. Justification for each technique and acceptance criteria should be provided in the first proposal for a specification. The justification has to reference the necessary development findings, pharmacopoeial guidelines (if available), test results for drug substances and products used in toxicological and clinical investigations, and findings from accelerated and long-term stability testing. It is also essential to account for a range of variability that is relevant for both the production and the analytical processes. The applicant has to justify unconventional procedures. This rationale has to be based on information gleaned through the production of the novel pharmaceutical product. Theoretical limits for a particular process or acceptance criteria may factor into this justification [120].

When developing an applicator for use with a microneedle system, it is crucial to comply with several guidelines (Table 14.3). A phased approach is adopted because certain device

TABLE 14.3

Possible Standards for Microneedle Applicator

Factors	Guidelines	Phase of Development
Materials	USP Class VI for plastics Biocompatibility (ISO 10993–1)	Before phase I
Human factors	Applying Human Factors and Usability Engineering to Optimize Medical Device Design (Guidance for Industry and FDA Staff) IEC 62366–1: Medical devices	Phased approach; summative before or during phase III
Applicator packaging	Standard Practice for Performance Testing of Shipping Containers and Systems (ASTM D4169–16)	Phased approach
Sterility	Sterilization of Health Care Products—Radiation (ISO 11137) Packaging for Terminally Sterilized Medical Devices (ISO 11607)	Phased approach
Device performance	Needle-based Injection Systems for Medical Use (ISO 11608)	Phase III

elements may be considered in the early design stage but not confirmed until later in the development of the combination product.

14.5 Microneedles in Clinical Trials

14.5.1 Overview of Microneedles Applications in Clinical Trials

The capability for microneedle-mediated delivery of a wide variety of therapeutic agents, including small molecules, macromolecules, and vaccines, has been demonstrated in multiple proof-of-concept trials, but no pharmaceutical products employing microneedle delivery technology have yet been approved. Many clinical studies have been conducted using microneedle systems [61]. Clinical trials have shown the efficacy of microneedles in the treatment of a variety of skin conditions (including scarring, wrinkles, alopecia, acne keratosis, and warts), as well as the administration of a variety of medications. Studies using a microneedles patch span a wide range of topics, from the effectiveness of microneedles patches compared to hypodermic needles for drug delivery to diagnostic and monitoring.

Searching for "microneedles" in October 2022 on ClinicalTrials.gov returns 138 results, of which 88 are already completed trials from all over the world. The most typical types of research are intradermal vaccination, diabetes, dermatology, and anesthesia. Only four research have progressed to phase IV trials, and one of them is investigating intradermal administration of the flu vaccine. Irritation of the eye (uveitis) and swelling of the retina (macular edema) account for seven of the trials, of which two are complete [39]. It has been noted that there have been many studies conducted on healthy subjects, two of which are now complete. Many studies have examined the efficacy of microneedles in delivering vaccines, particularly influenza [143]. While researchers have mainly employed hollow microneedles in their investigations, dissolving microneedles is beginning to gain popularity. Although most microneedles clinical studies are still in their preliminary phase I/II, most have been focused on insulin administration or influenza vaccination. Vaccine delivery utilizing microneedle technology is the subject of 12 completed and 2 ongoing clinical investigations. In the majority of these studies, vaccines are delivered by hollow microneedles (Soluvia®, MicronJet®), while a few studies employ a dissolving microneedle patch. Varicella-zoster, polio, and influenza vaccines are all in the trial phase at the moment.

It is critical to fulfilling the ethical requirements of clinical trials. Investigators and sponsors have an obligation to conform to ethical guidelines for the safety of trial participants. Clinical procedures, the Institutional Review Board (IRB) approval (institutional review boards), and informed consent from research patients to ensure they understand the potential consequences of participating in the study are necessary to meet ethical standards. Registration in a clinical trials registry is an ethical duty to ensure complete disclosure of clinical data for studies of drugs or biologics beyond phase I or medical device studies beyond feasibility studies. Financial disclosure of possible conflicts of interest is required for clinical research aimed at regulatory submission.

Manufacturers always provide regulatory agencies with evidence that they have implemented measures to ensure the benefits of human clinical trials outweigh the risks. In the United States, applications for medical devices are known as investigational device exemptions (IDEs), whereas those for pharmaceuticals or vaccines are known as an investigational new drug (IND). Nonclinical safety evaluations, production process management, design controls, risk management, a clinical protocol, and informed consent approved by an IRB constitute the submission for medical devices. Submission of justification to an IRB may allow studies evaluating the use of microneedles as devices without active ingredients to be classified as nonsignificant risk studies (NSR). If NSR status is granted, the IDE does not need to be submitted to the FDA, and the Sponsor is responsible for documenting any abbreviated IDE procedures [158]. Microneedle products require IND submission before human clinical studies, in addition to animal studies on drug absorption and pharmacokinetics or immune response, localized toxicity results on skin irritation, and a chemistry, manufacturing, and controls (CMC) assessment demonstrating assurance over the formulation, potency, and purity of the product [160]. In the process of developing medical devices and drug–device combination systems, the phase of "design control" is a vital step. A design and development strategy, design inputs, design outputs, design validation testing, and design reviews are important steps in preparing for clinical investigations. Parameters or criteria for the product's performance (i.e., drug levels, sensor sensitivity), dimensions and geometries (i.e., needle length), and safety (i.e., biocompatibility, bioburden) all constitute design inputs. *In vitro* and animal studies aim to verify a design by showing that it produces the desired results. To ensure the safety and functionality of the clinical product for use on human participants, the findings of design validation testing are reviewed before human clinical studies. Moreover, risk management is carried out to ensure that sufficient measures are taken to protect the subjects. To confirm that the product works as intended, it must undergo design validation, which includes both clinical investigations and human factors research [158].

There are generally three phases of clinical development for pharmaceuticals and vaccines. Microneedle delivery of the medication in a limited number of healthy participants is evaluated in phase I trials for both safety and pharmacokinetics/immune reaction. Phase II trials involve a larger sample size of the intended population and identify a dosing range for medication effectiveness or vaccination immunological response. Phase III trials verify the finished formulation and product design for a broader patient group to ensure safety and efficacy. Clinical trials for medical devices generally consist of two phases: an initial feasibility or pilot study conducted on a limited population utilizing prototypes of the device and a subsequent pivotal study conducted on a larger target population, employing the finalized device design [158].

Several challenges of microneedles in clinical trials have been reported. Clinical studies that used microneedles as a medical device were somewhat sluggish since they required approval for each item of microneedles separately, in contrast to the rapidly growing microneedles industry [61]. Clinical trials did not necessarily mirror the progress gained in the industry. Many different technologies that address specific clinical needs have been reported within the microneedles industry's technical sector, including material application [161], dose control technologies [162], microneedles application utilizing 3D print [163], mass manufacturing employing micromolding technique [164], and a feedback mechanism regarding application method, duration, and quantitative drug delivery [88]. Standardized good manufacturing practice (GMP) infrastructure for medical devices and an effective mass manufacturing technology for microneedles may necessitate more work. Specifically, clinical investigations with more stringent production management and control are required to achieve satisfactory results in conditions calling for repeated regular usage with a small delivery dose. The clinical research protocol must include comprehensive documentation of each of these procedures. This issue may be solved by creating standard operating procedures for using microneedles in human studies. Considering factors like how to appropriately apply microneedles from the viewpoint of the users is crucial for optimizing microneedle efficacy and ensuring safety [61].

14.5.2 Microneedle Applications in Clinical Trials

Extensive preclinical and clinical studies have been performed to investigate the safety and effectiveness of microneedles in various cosmeceutical, diagnostic, and therapeutic settings. Microneedles have been the focus of clinical research for the administration of vaccines and insulin throughout the last decade. Microneedle derma rollers, a form of solid microneedles, have been demonstrated to be the most desirable option in clinical studies for cosmeceutical purposes. Transdermal delivery using microneedles and nanoparticles is still in the early stages of research. Glucose monitoring studies with a hydrogel microneedles patch have also been initiated.

14.5.2.1 Cosmetic Applications

Physical skin disruption, using rollers or arrays of solid microneedles, is required for cosmetic microneedles to reduce wrinkles, acne scars, and stretch marks [165]. Microneedles or skin pretreatments are also used for aesthetic purposes, and they help cosmetic active ingredients such as collagen creams and vitamin C penetrate the skin more efficiently [86]. Class I devices ((k)-exempt) generally pose the least risk to users, and several cosmetic devices fall into this category. Needles on Class I medical devices must be shorter than 0.3 mm in length, and advertising for these products is prohibited from making any therapeutic values. Previously, there have been few regulatory hurdles for cosmetic applications, but in 2015, the FDA released a warning notice to multiple manufacturers, stating, "at this time, the safe ranges of needle lengths, penetration depths, and speeds of the device are unknown; therefore, FDA has safety concerns regarding the potential for the needles to damage vessels and nerves." Researchers have employed microneedles for aesthetic skin care and the treatment of scars and wrinkles. Microneedles were more successful than the control group in each of the 19 clinical investigations (Table 14.4). One wrinkle research, however, reported that a superficial dermal insertion was superior to microneedles for clinical evaluation of infraorbital wrinkles [166].

TABLE 14.4

Clinical Studies of Microneedle Applications in the Cosmetic Field

CT No.	Clinical Trial	Condition and Diseases	Drug and Device	Phase	Location	Status
NCT02174393	Microneedling plus the universal peel for acne scarring	Acne scarring	Solid (MicroPen)	NA	Bergen Dermatology, Englewood Cliffs (NJ, USA)	Completed
NCT02207738	Comparison of efficacy between fractional microneedling radiofrequency and bipolar radiofrequency for acne scar	Acne scarring	Solid (microneedling radiofrequency device)	NA	Seoul National University, College of Medicine, Seoul (Korea)	Completed
NCT02025088	Comparison of treatments for atrophic acne scars	Acne scarring	Solid (derma roller)	NA	Hospital de Clínicas de Porto Alegre (Brazil)	Unknown
NCT02660320	Comparison of the efficacy of microholes versus laser-assisted dermabrasion for repigmenting in vitiligo skin	Vitiligo-macular depigmentation	Solid (derma roller)	NA	CHU de Nice, CH Creteil, CHU de Bordeaux (France)	Completed
NCT02962180	Transplantation of basal cell layer suspension using Derma-rolling system in vitiligo	Vitiligo	Solid (derma roller)	NA	Ibn Sina University Hospital (Morocco)	Unknown
NCT02368626	Safety and efficacy of the EndyMed Pro system using RF microneedles fractional skin remodeling	Aging	Solid (EndyMed Pro™ RF microneedles)	NA	NA	Unknown
NCT02154503	Evaluating the efficacy of microneedling in the treatment of androgenetic alopecia	Androgenetic alopecia	Solid (microneedling)	I	The Skin Care Centre (Canada)	Unknown
NCT02489994	Performance of the ePrime System for cellulite	Cellulite	Solid (ePrime Syneron Candela)	NA	Bowes Leyda, David Goldberg, Macrene Alexiades, Girish Munavalli (USA)	Unknown
NCT01257763	Tolerability study of the application of a 3M microstructured transdermal system	Healthy	Solid (transdermal microchannel skin system)	I	Northwestern University Feinberg School of Medicine (USA)	Completed
NCT02497846	Teosyal® PureSense redensity [I] injection using MicronJet® needle in the treatment of crow's feet wrinkles	Crow's feet wrinkle	Hollow (MicronJet™)	IV	Docteur Micheels (Switzerland)	Completed

(Continued)

TABLE 14.4 (Continued)

Clinical Studies of Microneedle Applications in the Cosmetic Field

CT No.	Clinical Trial	Condition and Diseases	Drug and Device	Phase	Location	Status
NCT03380845	Comparison of 1,550-nm laser and fractional radiofrequency microneedle for the treatment of acne scars in ethnic skin	Acne scars	Device: Fraxel Restore Device: Fractora	NA	Massachusetts General Hospital (USA)	Completed
IRCT2014101519543N1	Treatment of stria alba by microneedle radiofrequency device	Stria alba	Device: RF microneedle	NA	Vice Chancellor for Research, Isfahan University of Medical Sciences (Iran)	NA
NCT03426098	Secret Micro-Needle Fractional RF System® for the treatment of facial wrinkles	Aging wrinkle	Device: secret microneedle fractional RF system	NA	West Dermatology Research Center (USA)	Unknown
NCT02660320	Comparison of the efficacy of microholes versus laser-assisted dermabrasion for repigmenting in vitiligo skin dermabrasion	Vitiligo—Macular Depigmentation	Device: Dermabrasion	NA	CHU de Nice, CH Creteil, CHU de Bordeaux (France)	Completed
NCT03390439	Treatment of atrophic striae with percutaneous collagen induction therapy versus fractional non-ablative laser	Striae distensae	Device: Nd: YAP 1,340-nm laser Device: microneedling	NA	Ana Paula Naspolini, Porto Alegre (Brazil)	Completed
NCT02962180	Transplantation of basal cell layer suspension using derma-rolling system in vitiligo	Vitiligo	Device: dermabrasion with derma roller	NA	Ibn Sina University Hospital (Morocco)	Unknown
NCT03409965	Lutronic Infini and LaseMD systems in combination treatment	Face and neck wrinkles, texture, pigmentation	Device: dermabrasion with derma roller	NA	Moradi M.D., The Aesthetic Clinique (USA)	Completed
NCT05108272	Comparison of cosmetic and functional outcome of silicone sheeting and microneedling on hypertrophic scars	Hypertrophic scar	Microneedling Percutaneous collagen induction	NA	Foundation University, FFH (Pakistan)	Recruiting

NA: not applicable; RF: radiofrequency

14.5.2.2 Prevention, Monitoring, and Diagnosis

Without causing any pain or irritation, microneedles can be employed to withdraw the skin's interstitial fluid, which is equivalent to plasma and has comparable levels of several chemicals (Table 14.5) [34]. Hydrogel-forming microneedles for caffeine and glucose [33] and hollow microneedles for glucose monitoring [167] have shown the ability to collect skin fluid from human participants for offline analysis. Interstitial fluid sampled using hollow microneedles and connected to an *in situ* electrochemical sensor has been reported in clinical investigations to be able to quantify blood glucose in diabetic patients continuously for three days [168]. Microneedle-assisted glucose monitoring has received much attention as a potential solution to effective insulin therapy for diabetic patients. An interstitial glucose monitoring sensor built on a solid microneedle array has been shown to be feasible in a pilot investigation including both healthy subjects and individuals with type 1 diabetes [169]. The results demonstrated that currents produced by amperometric sensors are clinically appropriate for monitoring blood glucose levels. The successful application of a microneedle patch for tracking beta-lactam antibiotics was revealed in a clinical study, suggesting that this minimally invasive technique has the potential for therapeutic

TABLE 14.5

Clinical Studies of Microneedles-based Diagnosis

NCT No.	Clinical Trial	Condition and Diseases	Drug and Device	Phase	Location	Status
NCT02682056	Glucose measurement using microneedle patches (GUMP)	Diabetes (diagnosis)	Device: hydrogel-forming microneedle patch Device: IV catheter Device: lancet	NA	Children's Healthcare of Atlanta, Emory Children's Center (USA)	Completed
NCT03332628	Racial/ethnic differences in microneedle response	Healthy	Device: microneedle HA patch	NA	University of Iowa (USA)	Completed
NCT03847610	Minimally invasive sensing of beta-lactam antibiotics (MISBL)	Healthy volunteers	Drug: phenoxymethyl penicillin Device: microneedle array	I	NIHR Imperial CRF (UK)	Completed
NCT03795402	Analysis of noninvasively collected microneedle device samples from mild plaque psoriasis for use in transcriptomics profiling	Psoriasis vulgaris	Device: microneedle device microneedles as a sampling device	Cohort, prospective	Innovaderm Research, Inc. (Canada)	Completed

(Continued)

TABLE 14.5 *(Continued)*

Clinical Studies of Microneedles-based Diagnosis

NCT No.	Clinical Trial	Condition and Diseases	Drug and Device	Phase	Location	Status
NCT01611844	Optimization of tuberculosis intradermal skin test (TB Dermatest)	Healthy volunteers	Device: microneedle BD 1.5 mm 30G Drug: Tubertest® Device: Lancet 26G × 16 mm Drug: Tubertest® Hollow (BD Research Catheter)	NA	Unité de Recherche Clinique en Immunologie Lyon Sud (URCI-LS) (France)	Completed
NCT01628484	Physiological study to determine allergic skin activity after different skin preparation	Birch pollen allergy	Other: Prick lancet Other: tape stripping Other: microneedles (3M, sMTS)	I	University Hospital Zurich (Switzerland)	Completed

drug monitoring [170]. Similar results to those derived from *in vivo* blood and microdialysis samples were reported when employing the microneedle monitoring device. The analysis of skin biomarkers is another promising diagnostic application for microneedle technology. Local skin disorders, including atopic dermatitis, melanoma, infectious skin diseases, and psoriasis, are frequently associated with systemic and internal conditions like Alzheimer's disease, breast cancer, cardiovascular disease, and diabetes [171, 172]. Early in 2010, researchers conducted a clinical study employing microneedles of 1.5 mm in length to track tuberculosis (TB) and skin allergies [171]. Unfortunately, it does not seem that BD offers microneedle solutions for TB testing. Successful TB skin screening using chitin microneedles in guinea pigs was disclosed in 2014 [173]. But thus far, no reports of using microneedles in human practice have been documented. Microneedles used in a recent clinical study demonstrated efficacy and safety for TB skin tests on par with those achieved with traditional needles [174].

14.5.2.3 Vaccination

Vaccines delivered intradermally have been shown to elicit stronger immune responses than traditional methods (Table 14.6) [43]. However, injecting a vaccine accurately and repeatedly into the intradermal tissue with a conventional needle and syringe requires a trained health professional. Thus, dissolving and solid microneedles have been the subject of extensive research for their potential to be used in the administration of vaccines. These include vaccines for influenza, measles, human papilloma virus, hepatitis B, hepatitis C, West Nile and chikungunya, diphtheria, and Bacillus Calmette–Guerin [60]. Fluzone® intradermal influenza vaccine and rabies vaccination [86] employ the Becton Dickinson Soluvia™ Micro Injection system, which consists of a single 1.5-mm stainless steel hollow microneedle connected to a conventional syringe. The NanoPass™ MicronJet 600™ is a set of three silicon microneedles that are 600 µm long and designed to fit into a traditional

TABLE 14.6

Clinical Studies for Microneedles-based Vaccination

NCT No.	Clinical Trial	Condition and Diseases	Drug and Device	Phase	Location	Status
NCT02438423	Inactivated influenza vaccine delivered by microneedle patch or by hypodermic needle	Influenza	Biological: inactivated influenza vaccine using a microneedle patch	I	The Hope Clinic (USA)	Completed
NCT01049490	Dose sparing intradermal S-OIV H1N1 influenza vaccination device	Influenza infection	Influenza S-OIV H1N1 vaccination MicronJet 600™	NA	The University of Hong Kong, Queen Mary Hospital (China)	Completed
NCT00558649	A pilot study to evaluate the safety and immunogenicity of low-dose flu vaccines	Influenza, human	MicronJet device Influenza flu vaccine (Fluarix®)	NA	NA	Completed
NCT01304563	2010/2011 Trivalent influenza vaccination	Influenza	MicronJet™ Influenza TIV 2010/2011 influenza vaccine	NA	The University of Hong Kong, Queen Mary Hospital (China)	Completed
NCT01707602	Routes of immunization and flu immune responses	Influenza	Microneedle injection Influenza Intanza®	I and II	GH Cochin—Broca—Hôtel-Dieu CIC BT505 (France)	Completed
NCT01368796	Comparison of four influenza vaccines in seniors	Influenza vaccine	Influenza Agriflu®, Fluad®, Intanza®, Vaxigrip® BD microneedle injection	IV	University of British Columbia (Canada)	Completed
NCT00258934	Immunogenicity study of the influenza vaccine in adults	Orthomyxoviridae infections Influenza	Inactivated, split-virion influenza vaccine Inactivated, split-virion, influenza virus	II	Sanofi Pasteur (Belgium, Germany, Switzerland)	Completed
NCT00383526	Study of inactivated, split-virion influenza vaccine compared with the reference vaccine Vaxigrip® in the elderly	Orthomyxoviridae infection Influenza Myxovirus infection	Inactivated, split-virion influenza vaccine	III	Sanofi Pasteur (Belgium, Germany, Switzerland)	Completed

(Continued)

TABLE 14.6 (Continued)

Clinical Studies for Microneedles-based Vaccination

NCT No.	Clinical Trial	Condition and Diseases	Drug and Device	Phase	Location	Status
NCT00296829	Immunogenicity of two dosages of inactivated, split-virion influenza vaccine given by an alternate route in the elderly	Orthomyxoviridae infection Influenza Myxovirus infection	Inactivated, split-virion influenza vaccine	II	Sanofi Pasteur (Belgium, Germany, Switzerland)	Completed
NCT00606359	Immunogenicity of the inactivated split-virion influenza vaccine in renal transplant subjects	Influenza Orthomyxoviridae infections	BD Soluvia ™ Influenza (in renal transplant patients) Influenza vaccine	II	Lyon (France)	Completed
NCT0558649	A pilot study to evaluate the safety and immunogenicity of low-dose flu vaccines	Influenza, human	MicronJet™ Influenza Fluarix®	NA	NanoPass Technologies Ltd.	Completed
NCT01737710	Atopic Dermatitis Research Network (ADRN) influenza vaccine study	Dermatitis, atopic	Fluzone® intradermal Influenza quadrivalent influenza vaccine	NA	National Jewish Health, Northwestern University, Boston Children's Hospital, University of Rochester Medical Center, Oregon Health & Science University (USA)	Completed
NCT01813604	Immunogenicity of inactivated and live polio vaccines	Poliomyelitis	Hollow (MicronJet 600™)	III	Mirpur Health Clinic (Bangladesh)	Completed
NCT01686503	Intradermal versus intramuscular polio vaccine booster in HIV-infected subjects	Polio immunity	Hollow (MicronJet 600™)	II	C3ID Clinic, Eastern Virginia Medical School (USA)	Completed
NCT02329457	Varicella-zoster virus (VZV) vaccine for hematopoietic stem cell transplantation	Varicella-zoster infection	Hollow (microneedle syringe)	II/III	Ivan Hung (Hong Kong)	Completed
NCT03207763	Microneedle patch study in healthy infants/young children	Vaccination skin absorption	Dissolving microneedles	NA	Emory Children's Center (USA)	Completed

NA: not applicable.

syringe. The Food and Drug Administration has granted its approval for the product to be used in the United States, and it has also been issued the CE mark. Human clinical trials have used NanoPass microneedle devices for the administration of vaccines against seasonal strains of influenza [175], herpes zoster [176], and polio in infant populations [177] and tuberculin skin testing [174]. In clinical research, rabies vaccines were administered with the assistance of BD 34 G hollow microneedles, which are manufactured and distributed by BD Medical-Pharmaceutical Systems [178]. Testing of dissolving microneedles for influenza vaccination has also progressed to the clinical trial stage [103].

14.5.2.4 Delivery of Macromolecules

Biologics have been tested in human subjects in clinical trials, including insulin and glucagon for diabetes, parathyroid hormone-related protein analogues for postmenopausal osteoporosis [71, 179, 180], and aflibercept and acetonide for diabetic macular edema (Table 14.7). The application of a microneedle delivery system is most likely to improve the intradermal delivery of insulin. Clinical studies using pulled microneedles to administer insulin were conducted by Gupta and collaborators [80, 81], and a clinical investigation using stainless steel microneedles for insulin delivery was conducted by Pettis and coworkers [181, 182]. Clinical investigations with type 1 diabetics have shown that the microneedle device is less invasive and may have a quicker onset of effect [82]. A clinical study for individuals with type 2 diabetes employing microneedles produced superior pharmacokinetic results—a fast effect of insulin owing to a lesser duration to achieve T_{max}, avoidance of late hypoglycemic effects due to a reasonably consistent insulin concentration in the blood, and minimal intersubject variation in T_{max} as compared to subcutaneous insulin injection. According to the pharmacokinetic profile, insulin administered through the microneedle device was superior to insulin injected subcutaneously for preventing postprandial glucose increases in individuals with type 2 diabetes. BD currently provides 4-, 5-, and 6-mm pen needles for insulin administration as a substitute to subcutaneous injections [80]; therefore, the Soluvia BD system with 1.5-mm microneedles seems to be discontinued. Subcutaneous insulin administration in individuals with diabetes is advised using 4-mm pen needles and 6-mm syringes [183, 184]. Research into the pharmacokinetics and route of insulin delivery has demonstrated that intradermal administration results in quicker absorption than subcutaneous injection [81, 185, 186]. In the phase I clinical trial employing hollow microneedles, 3M investigators compared the efficacy of intradermal administration to that of the commercially available subcutaneous autoinjector for delivery of HUMIRA® [60]. The findings show that a therapeutic dose of a macromolecule (144 kDa) may be delivered effectively through 3M's hollow microneedle system. Studies with microneedles are also being conducted to deliver drugs to treat postmenopausal osteoporosis. Teriparatide, the 1–34 amino acid peptide analogue of the parathyroid hormone, and abaloparatide are two anabolic drugs for osteoporosis that are now on the market. Clinical studies of microneedle devices, including these two medications, are now ongoing [187]. In 2009, a phase II clinical trial was conducted employing microneedles to administer recombinant human parathyroid hormone 1–34 teriparatide (PTH, 4.1 kDa). The study lasted six months and included randomization, multicenter administration, blinding, and multiple dosing [188]. Findings showed that 40 μg of PTH administered by solid titanium microneedles was able to effectively deliver PTH, on par with a 20 μg injected Forteo. The transdermal microneedle formulation of parathyroid hormone 1–34 (PTH) ZP-PTH was devised by Zosano Pharma Corporation [179]. The product utilizes arrays of titanium microneedles manufactured using photochemical etching. Dissolving microneedle PTH formulation has been revealed by Corium to have completed phase II clinical trial.

TABLE 14.7

Clinical Studies of Microneedle-mediated Delivery of Macromolecules

NCT No.	Clinical Trial	Condition & diseases	Drug & device	Phase	Location	Status
NCT00837512	Insulin delivery using microneedles in type 1 diabetes	Type 1 diabetes mellitus	Device: hollow microneedle (1 mm) Device: subcutaneous (SC) insulin catheter	II and III	Emory University (USA)	Completed
NCT02837094	Enhanced Epidermal Antigen-specific Immunotherapy Trial-1 (EE-ASI-1)	Type 1 diabetes	Drug: C19-A3 GNP (MicronJet 600)	I	Cardiff University	Unknown
NCT02329457	VZV vaccine for hematopoietic stem cell transplantation (VZIDST)	Varicella-zoster infection	Biological: Zostavax	II and III	The University of Hong Kong	Completed
NCT03274674	Use of injectable-platelet-rich-fibrin (I-PRF) to thicken gingival phenotype	Periodontoclasia Gingiva; Injury condition Blood clot Gingiva disorder	Other: I-PRF	NA	Bezmialem Vakif University (Turkey)	Completed
NCT00602914	A pilot study to assess the safety, PK, and PD of insulin injected via MicronJet or conventional needles	Diabetes mellitus	Device: MicronJet Device: conventional needle (NanoPass microneedle)	Early phase I	NanoPass Technologies Ltd.	Completed
NCT02459938	Safety and efficacy of ZP-glucagon to injectable glucagon for hypoglycemia	Hypoglycemia	Solid/metal (drug-coated titanium microneedles) Zosano microneedle patch	I	Nucleus Network (Australia)	Completed
NCT00489918	Dose-ranging study—macroflux parathyroid hormone (PTH) in postmenopausal women with osteoporosis	Osteoporosis	Drug: Teriparatide (Zosano Pharma)	II	Zosano Pharma Corporation	Completed
NCT02478879	A study to determine the patient preference between Zosano Pharma parathyroid hormone (ZP-PTH) patch and the Forteo pen	Postmenopausal osteoporosis	Coated titanium (ZP-PTH microneedle patch)	I	Covance Daytona Beach Clinical Research Unit (USA)	Completed

NCT01674621	Phase II study of BA058 (abaloparatide) transdermal delivery in postmenopausal women with osteoporosis	Postmenopausal osteoporosis	Drug; BA058 placebo Drug; BA058 TD (50, 100, 150 μg) Drug; BA058 injection (80 μg) (TD: Coated 3M microstructured transdermal system (MTS), 250 μm, 316 microprojections)	II	Radius Health, Inc.	Completed
NCT03360903	Adalimumab microneedles in healthy volunteers	Pain injection site	Biological: Adalimumab ID or SC Biological: Adalimumab SC Other: Saline ID or SC (3M hMTS, 1,500 μm, 12 needles)	I and II	Centre for Human Drug Research (Netherlands)	Completed
NCT03054480	Fractional microneedle radiofrequency and I botulinum toxin A for primary axillary hyperhidrosis	Primary axillary hyperhidrosis	Device: fractional microneedle radiofrequency Drug; botulinum toxin type A	NA	Thep Chalermchai, Mae Fah Luang, University Hospital	Completed
NCT03126786	Suprachoroidal CLS-TA with intravitreal aflibercept versus aflibercept alone in subject with diabetic macular edema	Diabetic macular edema	IVT aflibercept, Sham SC, SC CLS-TA	II	Clearside Biomedical, Inc.	Completed
NCT03203174	The use of microneedles with topical botulinum toxin for the treatment of palmar hyperhidrosis	Hyperhidrosis	Solid (Sham microneedle) Botulinum toxin type A	I	University of California, Davis	Completed
NCT01684956	Pharmacokinetic comparison of intradermal versus subcutaneous insulin and glucagon delivery in type 1 diabetes	Type 1 diabetes	Hollow (MicronJet™)	II	Massachusetts General Hospital (USA)	Unknown

(Continued)

TABLE 14.7 (Continued)

Clinical Studies of Microneedle-mediated Delivery of Macromolecules

NCT No.	Clinical Trial	Condition & diseases	Drug & device	Phase	Location	Status
NCT01557907	Multi-day (3) in-patient evaluation of intradermal versus subcutaneous basal and bolus insulin infusion	Diabetes	Hollow (BD Research Catheter)	I/II	Profil Institut fur Stoffwechselfforschung GmbH (Germany)	Completed
NCT01120444	Study of the effects on blood glucose following intradermal and subcutaneous dosing of insulin in diabetic patients	Diabetes	Hollow (BD research catheter)	I/II	Profil Institute of Clinical Research (Germany)	Completed
NCT01061216	Pharmacokinetics/dynamics of basal (continuous) insulin infusion administered either intradermally or subcutaneously	Diabetes mellitus, type 1/2	Hollow (BD Research Catheter)	I/II	Profil Institut fur Stoffwechselfforschung GmbH (Germany)	Completed
NCT00553488	Feasibility study of the effect of intradermal insulin injection on blood glucose levels after eating	Diabetes mellitus, type 1	BD Research Catheter (34G × 1.5 mm needle) Insulin	II	Profil Institut fur Stoffwechselfforschung GmbH (Germany)	Completed

NA: not applicable.

14.5.2.5 Delivery of Small Molecules

Microneedles have been used extensively to enhance the transdermal and intradermal delivery of small molecules in several clinical trials (Table 14.8). One of the first clinical trials of a microneedle delivery system included the systemic delivery of naltrexone [189]. Several further clinical trials involving the administration of local anesthetics by microneedles have also been conducted. Li and coworkers employed solid microneedles from Nanomed Devices for the dermal administration of dyclonine [190], whereas Gupta and collaborators used pulled hollow microneedles for the dermal delivery of lidocaine [191]. Transdermal delivery of naltrexone was also performed by Wermeling et al. using solid microneedles [189]. Anesthesia for ambulatory individuals should have a quick onset of effect, low discomfort, low cost, and be easily administered by the patients. Lidocaine was administered to the forearm of participants using 500-μm-long hollow microneedles in a clinical investigation and found to be significantly less painful and as efficient as lidocaine injection using a conventional hypodermic needle [191]. Perhaps most notably, the microneedle device was favored over the hypodermic needle by 77% of the study's participants. Rapid and sustained effects have been reported in clinical trials utilizing coated or dissolving microneedles for lidocaine administration [15, 153, 192]. Migraine treatment with zolmitriptan has been the subject of several ongoing clinical studies using microneedle technologies. Coated microneedles, for instance, have shown a T_{max} value equivalent to that achieved by subcutaneous injections of sumatriptan, with the additional benefits of faster absorption and fewer metabolites than oral administration [193]. Migraine headaches that are particularly difficult to treat responded favorably to zolmitriptan delivered by an adhesive dermally applied microarray, according to a phase IIa/III clinical study [194, 195]. According to a March 2019 report, a study examining the microneedles' long-term toxicity was performed [196]. A microneedle device for the delivery of zolmitriptan has been given conditional approval by the Food and Drug Administration. Triamcinolone acetonide is also being tested in a clinical study for the treatment of noninfectious uveitis [197]. When triamcinolone was injected into the suprachoroidal region of rabbits, it was shown to have a 12-fold greater effect on the retina, sclera, and choroid than intravitreal injections, while having a far lesser impact on the lens and anterior segment. Uveitis may be treated with corticosteroids, and Clearside Biomedical has successfully employed a single microneedle to achieve this goal [197].

14.6 Microneedles Products on the Market

14.6.1 Factors Driving Microneedles into the Market

It has only been recently that microneedles technology has been swiftly transitioning from the research to commercial development phases (Table 14.9). Large-scale manufacturing efforts have been undertaken in the field of microneedle systems. Numerous microneedle-based products are now in various design and development stages at multiple companies (Fig. 14.2). It comes as a surprise that so few microneedle products have made it to the market. In reality, some may not consider the currently available commercial microneedles products to be the best possible microneedles products, nor do they represent the original, broader perspective for microneedles in their purest form: simple products that

TABLE 14.8

Clinical Studies of Microneedle-mediated Delivery of Small Molecules

NCT No.	Clinical Trial	Condition and Diseases	Drug and Device	Phase	Location	Status
NCT02955576	Microneedle patch for psoriatic plaques	Psoriasis Administration, topical	Dissolving microneedle (microneedle-HA patch)	NA	St. Vincent's Hospital (Korea)	Unknown
NCT02192021	Microneedle array—doxorubicin in patients with cutaneous T-cell lymphoma (CTCL)	Cutaneous T-cell lymphoma	Device: microneedle array—doxorubicin	1	University of Pittsburgh Medical Center (USA)	Recruiting
NCT02952001	Extension study of patients with noninfectious uveitis who participated in CLS1001–301	Uveitis Uveitis, posterior Uveitis, anterior Uveitis, intermediate Panuveitis	Drug: 4 mg CLS-TA suprachoroidal injection Drug: Sham procedure	NA	Clearside Biomedical, Inc.	Completed
NCT01812837	The use of microneedles in photodynamic therapy	Actinic keratosis	Device: microneedle Drug: aminolevulinic acid Radiation: blue light	NA	University of California, Davis (USA)	Completed
NCT01789320	Safety study of suprachoroidal triamcinolone acetonide via microneedle to treat uveitis	Uveitis, intermediate uveitis, posterior uveitis, panuveitis, noninfectious uveitis	Triamcinolone acetonide (Triesence®) Hollow microneedle Single microneedle (SCS Microinjector®)	I and II	Clearside Biomedical, Inc.	Completed
NCT02594644	The use of microneedles to expedite treatment time in photodynamic therapy	Keratosis, actinic	Solid (microneedle roller) Solid/metal (stainless steel)	NA	University of California, Davis	Completed
NCT02262110	Microneedle lesion preparation prior to aminolevulinic acid photodynamic therapy (ALA-PDT) for AK on the face	Actinic keratosis	Drug: ALA Drug: topical solution vehicle Device: IBL 10 mW Procedure: microneedle lesion preparation Device: IBL 20 mW	2	DUSA Pharmaceuticals, Inc.	Completed
NCT02745392	Safety and efficacy of ZP-zolmitriptan intracutaneous microneedle systems for the acute treatment of migraine	Acute migraine	Solid/metal (drug-coated titanium microneedles) Adhesive dermally applied microarray (ADAM) by Zosano	II/III	Zosano Pharma Corporation	Completed

NCT number	Title	Condition	Device/Drug	Phase	Sponsor	Status
NCT03646188	Dose escalation trial to evaluate dose limiting toxicity/maximum tolerated dose of microneedle arrays containing doxorubicin (D-MNA) in basal cell carcinoma (BCC)	Basal cell carcinoma	Drug: placebo-containing MNA; Drug: 25 µg doxorubicin-containing MNA; Drug: 50 µg doxorubicin-containing MNA; Drug: 100 µg doxorubicin-containing MNA; Drug: 200 µg doxorubicin-containing MNA	I	SkinJect, Inc.	Terminated
NCT03847610	Minimally invasive sensing of beta-lactam antibiotics	Healthy volunteers	Drug: phenoxymethyl penicillin; Device: microneedle array	I	Imperial College London	Completed
NCT03097315	Suprachoroidal injection of CLS-TA in patients with noninfectious uveitis	Uveitis, posterior uveitis, anterior uveitis, intermediate panuveitis	Drug: 4 mg CLS-TA suprachoroidal injection	III	Clearside Biomedical, Inc.	Completed
NCT04053140	Closed-loop control of penicillin delivery	Healthy volunteers	Device: microneedle array; Device: microneedle array and closed-loop control of penicillin delivery; Drug: penicillin G_1200 mg; Drug: penicillin G_2400 mg; Drug: penicillin G_600 mg/h	I	Imperial College London	Recruiting
NCT02596750	The effect of microneedle pretreatment on topical anesthesia	Pain	Device: microneedle roller; Device: Sham microneedle roller	NA	University of California Davis (USA)	Completed
NCT00539084	A study to assess the safety and efficacy of a microneedle device for local anesthesia	Local anesthesia intradermal injections	Hollow (MicronJet™)	NA	NanoPass Technologies Ltd.	Completed
NCT02995057	Safety demonstration of microneedle insertion	Allergic reaction to nickel	Device: gold- or silver-coated, or uncoated nickel microneedles	NA	University of British Columbia (Canada)	Completed
NCT03415373	Clinical evaluation of healthy subjects receiving intradermal saline using the microneedle adapter (Model UAR-2S)	Intradermal injection	Device: microneedle adapter (Model UAR-2S); Device: hypodermic needle + syringe	NA	inVentiv Health Clinique (Canada)	Completed
NCT03282227	A study to evaluate the long-term safety of M207 in the acute treatment of migraine (ADAM)	Migraine	Solid/metal (drug-coated titanium microneedles); Adhesive dermally applied microarray by Zosano	III	Zosano Pharma Corporation	Completed
NCT04393168	Proof-of-concept study of LymphMonitor 1.0 to assess the lymphatic vessel function	Lymphedema Secondary lymphedema	Hollow/silicon microneedles MicronJet600® Combination product: lymphatic clearance measurement	I	University Hospital Zurich (Switzerland)	Completed

NA: not applicable.

TABLE 14.9

Microneedle Delivery Systems for Commercialization

Product Name	Company/Manufacturer	Description	Application
Dermapen	Dermaroller GmbH	An electric motor unit with a spring that punches skin at a rate of 412–700 cycles per minute is loaded onto a pen-shaped device with an array of 12 solid microneedles	Acne, scars, skin lesions, wrinkles, stretch marks, and hair loss are some of the skin issues that benefit from this system
Darmaroller®	White Lotus Beauty	Cylindrical assembly with 192 solid titanium microneedles (0.5 mm in length)	Prevalent use in cosmetics and skincare. This product could effectively treat acne, stretch marks, and alopecia. Efficient at increasing drug permeation (minoxidil, hyaluronic acid, etc.)
Derma stamp	White Lotus Beauty	A device with 40 solid needles and an electric motor that moves back and forth in a stamping motion	Scar, age spots, varicella scar, and wrinkle treatment by collagen induction therapy
DermaFrac	Dermafrac Co.	A miniature solid microneedles roller made of stainless steel, fitted with an electric power supply and instrument for serum infusion, including light-emitting gadgets	Signs of aging, such as wrinkles, hyperpigmentation, acne, and an uneven skin tone
Onvax	Becton Dickinson	Microneedles made of silicon or plastic mounted on a handheld applicator	Intradermal vaccine delivery
LiteClear	Nanomed Skincare	Silicon solid microneedles pen for skin pretreatment	Treatment of acne and skin blemishes
h-patch	Valeritas	Solid microneedles	Basal and bolus delivery of insulin
Beauty Mouse	Dermaroller GmbH	Numerous microchannels for improved drug permeation are created by the combination of three 50 mm rollers and 480 solid microneedles	Making the skin more receptive to anti-cellulite treatments
NanoCare	NanoPass, Inc.	A portable tool of solid microneedles for skin regeneration and amplifying the aesthetic effects of topical products	Cosmetic use
Adminstamp	AdminMed	An array of solid microneedles (1,400 µm in length, arranged on a 1 cm² circular substrate), connected to the applicator with six stainless steel screws	Excellent skin sensation and aesthetics complement enhanced transdermal drug delivery

TABLE 14.9 *(Continued)*

Microneedle Delivery Systems for Commercialization

Product Name	Company/ Manufacturer	Description	Application
MacroFlux™	Zosano Pharma	Metal solid microneedle array with a coating layer of PTH on titanium microneedles (340 µm long)	Treatment of osteoporosis Transdermal delivery of peptides and vaccines
ZP Patch	Zosano Pharma	Solid microneedles	Transdermal drug delivery
Nanopatch™	Vaxxas	An array of thousands of coated silicon microneedles	Polio vaccine Fluvax®
3M coated microstructured transdermal system	3M	Coated microneedles with an applicator 250, 500, and 700 µm in needle length. 316 needles on an array	Transdermal delivery of drugs and vaccines
3M hollow microstructured transdermal system	3M	12 hollow microneedles (1,500 µm long) on an array	Cancer vaccine (PAN-301-1) Transdermal delivery of liquid formulations with various viscosities
Fluarix	NanoPass, Inc. Sanofi Pasture, Inc.	Three hollow microneedles (600 µm long) attached to a syringe	Quadrivalent inactivated influenza vaccine
Pandemrix	NanoPass, Inc. GSK	Three hollow microneedles (600 µm long) attached to a syringe	H1N1 pandemic influenza
MicronJet™	NanoPass Technologies Ltd. Sanofi Pasture, Inc.	Four silicon hollow microneedles (450 µm long) affixed to the tip of a plastic adapter and a syringe	Intradermal vaccine delivery (influenza, polio, varicella-zoster, cancers, hepatitis B, COVID-19)
MicronJet 600	NanoPass Technologies Ltd. Sanofi Pasture, Inc.	Three silicon hollow microneedles (600 µm long) attached to a syringe	Intradermal delivery of polio, zoster, and influenza vaccines and insulin
Fluzone	Sanofi Pasteur, Inc. Becton Dickinson	A hand-prefilled syringe gun unit injects 1.5 mL vaccine solution by a microinjector via hollow microneedles	Quadrivalent inactivated "split virus" influenza vaccine
Soluvia™	Sanofi-Aventis Becton Dickinson	A prefilled syringe attached to a hollow microneedle (1.5 mm long)	Influenza vaccine Intradermal delivery of drugs and vaccines
Microinfusor	Becton Dickinson	An electrical pump is attached to a patch of hollow microneedles to provide a hands-free drug delivery device (capacity 0.2–15 mL)	Influenza vaccine, insulin, and highly viscous formulations of biomolecules
Nanoject	Debiotech	Hollow microneedles patch (300–1,000 µm long) with side holes, made by MEMS technology	Intradermal drug delivery Injection of diagnostic fluid
Micro-Trans	Valeritas, Inc.	Metal or biodegradable polymer-based hollow microneedles	Intradermal drug delivery independent of drug size, structure, charge, or skin properties

(Continued)

TABLE 14.9 *(Continued)*

Microneedle Delivery Systems for Commercialization

Product Name	Company/ Manufacturer	Description	Application
IDflu®/Intanza®	Sanofi-Aventis Becton Dickinson	A hollow microneedle (1.5 mm long) connected to a needle shielding system for intradermal injection of 0.1 mL volume	Intradermal influenza vaccination
AdminPen	AdminMed/ NanoBioSciences	43 stainless steel hollow microneedles (1,100 μm long) on a 1 cm² circular array connected to a conventional syringe	Transdermal delivery of liquid formulations of vaccines and drugs
Debioject™	Debiotech	Injections of up to 0.5 mL may be made in only a few seconds using a single or multiple hollow silicon microneedles with a length ranging from 350 μm to 900 μm and side-shielded delivery apertures	Intradermal delivery of Pasteur® rabies vaccine
Drugmat®	Theraject, Inc.	Sumatriptan-loaded dissolving microneedles patch made from a sugar polysaccharide	Treatment of migraine
Vaxmat®	Theraject, Inc.	Sumatriptan-loaded dissolving microneedles patch made from trehalose and sodium carboxymethyl cellulose	Treatment of migraine
MicroCor®	Corium International, Inc.	PTH(1–34)-loaded dissolving microneedles patch (200 μm long)	Treatment of osteoporosis
MicroHyala®	CosMED Pharmaceutical Co. Ltd.	Dissolving microneedles patch made of biocompatible hyaluronic acid	Wrinkle treatment . Influenza vaccine delivery
Microneedle patch	Micron Biomedical, Inc.	Dissolving microneedles (650 μm long, 100 microneedles on an array)	Inactivated rotavirus Flu vaccination
Kindeva hollow microstructured transdermal system	3M	Hollow microneedles (1,500 μm long) on a 1 cm² array for the intradermal injection of 0.5–2 mL liquid formulation of various viscosities	Delivery of cancer vaccines
Hollow microneedle system	Flugen	An array of six hollow polymeric microneedles, each with three ports	Influenza vaccine delivery
Vaxipatch™	Verndari	Stainless steel microneedle (600 μm long)	Intradermal delivery of live attenuated measles, influenza, COVID-19 vaccine

TABLE 14.9 *(Continued)*

Microneedle Delivery Systems for Commercialization

Product Name	Company/ Manufacturer	Description	Application
Dissolving Micropile Chip	BioSerenTach, Inc.	Dissolving microneedles (500 µm long, 100–300 microneedles on 1 cm² array)	Transdermal delivery of insulin
Sofusa®	Sorrento therapeutics	Nanotopographical imprinted coated microneedles	Immuno-oncology
BetaConnect™	Bayer HealthCare Pharmaceuticals, Inc.	An electronic auto-injector to inject a volume of 0.25–1 mL	Transdermal delivery of Betaseron® (interferon beta-1b)
SCS microinjector®	Clearside Biomedical, Inc.	30-gauge hollow microneedle (700–800 µm long)	Inject drug solution (i.e., triamcinolone acetonide) into the suprachoroidal region
I'm Fill Needle Patch	Karatica Co., Ltd.	An array of 400 dissolving microneedles	Hyaluronic acid, acetyl hexapeptide-8 moisturizing, antiaging effects for cosmetic purposes
Royal skin hyaluronic acid micropatch	Junmok International Co., Ltd.	Dissolving microneedles (500–750 µm long)	Hyaluronic acid, lactose moisturizing, antiaging effects for cosmetic use
Acropass	Raphas Co., Ltd.	Dissolving microneedles (350 µm long)	Hyaluronic acid, epidermal growth factor moisturizing, antiaging
Neo Basic HA Fill Micro Patch	Nissha Co., Ltd.	An array of 3,600 dissolving microneedles	Hyaluronic acid-based skincare
ADAM	Zosano Pharma	Zolmitriptan-coated titanium solid microneedles (500 µm long)	Treatment of acute migraine
Micropatch™	Nemaura pharma, Ltd.	Drug coated on microneedles' surface with a frustoconical-shaped pellet	Intradermal delivery of vaccines
V-Go®	Valeritas, Inc.	30G hypodermic floating needle (300 µm needle diameter)	Basal-bolus insulin treatment
Memspatch Insulin microneedle Device (IMD)	Nemaura Pharma, Ltd.	Shallow hollow microneedles with skin penetration of 2–4 mm	Transdermal insulin delivery
Trevyent™	SteadyMed, Ltd.	Drug infusion pump system	Treprostinil injection for the treatment of pulmonary arterial hypertension
Enable Smart enFuse™	Enable Injections, Inc.	Deliver therapeutics at a low pressure, in response to the pressure in the subcutaneous tissue, using a reservoir and pump	Infusion of liquid drug formulations
SkinPen Precision System	Bellus Medical	14 hollow microneedles (1.5 mm long) with 11 settings for the needle length ranging from 0.5 to 2.5 mm	Skin rejuvenation Treatment of wrinkles and acne scars
Exceed microneedling device	MT. DERM GmbH	A pen-type device with six microneedles (1.5 mm long) in a square arrangement	Repair and restore aging skin

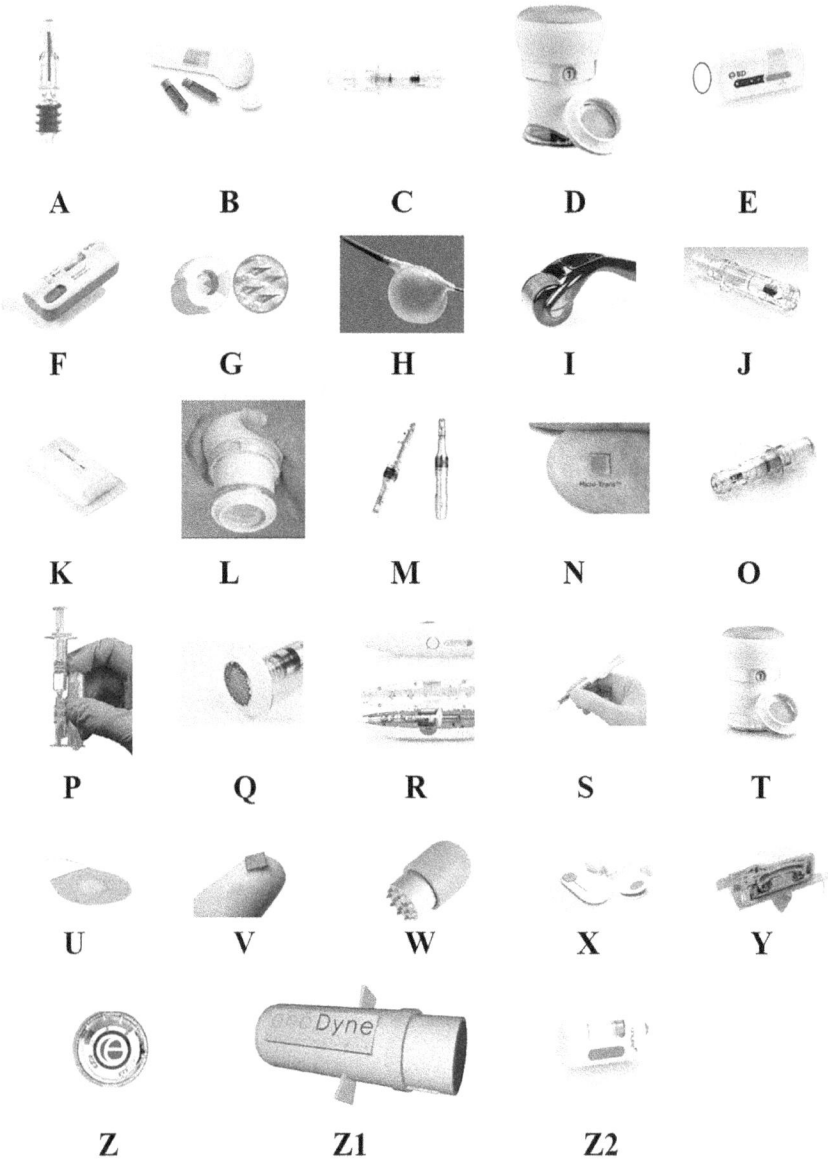

FIGURE 14.2
Current microneedle products for drug delivery or therapeutic use. (A) MicronJet™ 600 from NanoPass Technologies Ltd. (B) 3M™ Hollow Microstructured Transdermal System® from 3M. (C) BD Soluvia™ from Becton Dickenson. (D) Qtrypta™ from Zosano Pharma. (E) SCS Microinjector® from Clearside Biomedical, Inc. (F) BD Microinfusor patch injector from Becton Dickenson. (G) MicroCor® from Corium, Inc. (H) Bullfrog® micro-infusion device from Mercator MedSystems, Inc. (I) Dermaroller®. (J) Fluzone® from Sanofi Pasteur, Inc. (K) V-Go® from Valeritas, Inc. (L) Macroflux® from Zosano Pharma. (M) Dr. Pen Ultima A6 Microneedling Pen from Dr. Pen. (N) Micro-Trans™ from Valeritas. (O) Intanza® from Sanofi Pasteur, Inc. (P) Debioject™ from Debiotech. (Q) AdminPen™ from NanoBioSciences. (R) BetaConnect™ from Bayer HealthCare Pharmaceuticals, Inc. (S) SCS Microinjector from Clearside Biomedical, Inc. (T) ZP Patch Technology transdermal microprojection delivery system from Zosano Pharma. (U) Microneedle Patch from Micron Biomedical, Inc. (V) Nanopatch™ from Vaxxas. (W) Micropatch™ from Nemaura Pharma, Ltd. (X) Memspatch insulin microneedle device (IMD) from Nemaura Pharma, Ltd. (Y) Trevyent™ from SteadyMed, Ltd. (Z) Enable Smart enFuse™ from Enable Injections, Inc. (Z1) Hero Patch from anoDyne nanotech. (Z2) Imperium from Unilife. Images reprinted with permission from respective sources.

may be used in patch type, easily, noninvasively, inexpensively, and mandating no specialized training or waste disposal units. Each kind of medication should have its dedicated microneedle-based system for effective drug administration, which would include the drug itself, a stable formulation, suitable microneedles, and a reliable microneedle applicator [135]. However, there are presently no microneedle-based drug delivery systems that are available for commercial acquisition on the market. The demand for properly manufactured microneedles in large quantities is undeniable. Unfortunately, this has not yet been effectively leveraged because of the difficulties in scaling up manufacturing. Neither the present state of research nor the desirable goals are reflected in the microneedle products available on the market. Not all goods labeled "microneedles" are smaller than a standard hypodermic needle. In addition to the currently available Soluvia™, over 24 microneedles products are now in development. Microneedle delivery systems are typically offered as patches rather than syringe systems. Only a limited number of microneedle devices are commercially available; the vast majority are still undergoing testing in human subjects. Several microneedle products have been developed and launched on the market. MicronJet 600™, Debioject™, Betaconnect™, and Soluvia™ are just a few examples of FDA-approved microneedles injection devices. Controlling the penetration depth or injection rate is possible using a pen-type injection device that incorporates a standard syringe into an injector. Disposable units made up of a hollow microneedle and a regular commercial syringe may be the first designed injection device for noninvasive intradermal injections. Disposable microneedles devices, such as the MicronJet 600™ from NanoPass Technologies Ltd., the Debioject™ from Debiotech, and the AdminPen™ from NanoBiosciences, may be attached to the tips of syringes.

Since its introduction as a method of aesthetic therapy, microneedling has been around for more than a decade. Skin is often punctured with a roller or microneedling device, and a topical product is applied to the treated area. Initially, microneedles were employed to enhance skin texture by stimulating collagen synthesis in response to microneedles-induced injuries. Wrinkles, acne, skin lesions, and scars are conditions that may benefit greatly from microneedling treatment. Hyaluronic acid dissolving microneedles is another kind of microneedles that is gaining favor in cosmetics. Many people turn to injectable hyaluronic acid to smooth out wrinkles and fine lines [198]. There are only a few numbers of intradermal systems available for the delivery of pharmaceuticals and vaccines. Although numerous products are in the late phase of clinical studies [18], Intanza/IDflu was the first intradermal influenza vaccine to be approved in Europe, Australia, Canada, and the United States. Several of Zosano Pharma's drugs, including ZP-PTH for the treatment of severe osteoporosis and M203 for the treatment of migraine, are now in either phase II or III of clinical trials. In the absence of a commercially viable microneedles-based drug delivery product, only microneedles devices for drug administration are presently available [113, 199]. In any case, a selected few businesses have obtained Good Manufacturing Practice (GMP) manufacturing licenses to produce microneedle patches. Both LTS Lohmann Therapie-Systeme AG and Corium, Inc., fall under this category. There are now just a handful of papers out there on diagnosing using microneedle devices. Microneedles allow for the extraction of limited sample quantities, which may be used for processing or included in a diagnostic system.

The development of more efficient methods for fabricating microneedles is crucial in the widespread use of these products. After a decade of study, the manufacturing of microneedles may be mass-produced and even outsourced. The ability to apply microneedles technology to a wide variety of conditions is a critical factor in the rapid commercialization of this technology (Table 14.10).

TABLE 14.10

Features of Different Microneedle Designs [136]

Microneedle Design	Simple Design and Manufacturing	Simple Application by Patients	Maximum Drug-delivered Dose	Drug Delivery Control
Microneedle pretreatment	++++	+++	+++	++
Microneedle patch	++	++++	+	++
Microneedles with reservoir patch	+++	++++	++	+++
Hollow microneedles	+	+	++++	++++

Many pharmaceutical companies and research laboratories have shown a lot of interest in microneedles-based product development (fabrication and manufacturing techniques), including 3M, Corium, Zosano Pharma, Alza Corporation, Becton-Dickinson Technologies, Valeritas, Vaxxas, microneedle Therapy System, NanoPass Technologies, Quadmedicine, Lohmann Therapie-Systeme (LTS), and others. Several organizations have taken preliminary measures to explore the possibility of large-scale production of microneedles; for instance, LTS is actively engaging in scale-up of the microneedles production systems. The most critical concerns for the development of microneedles are the optimization and validation of these technologies and addressing regulatory queries, such as long-term safety and sterility criteria [151].

14.6.2 Microneedles Products on the Market

Soluvia® and Micronjet®, the first microneedle-based products to arrive on the market, are made of metal and silicon, respectively.

1. For vaccination, Becton-Dickinson Technologies developed and patented the first commercially available microneedles product, Soluvia®, a prefillable microinjection system that employs a very short hollow stainless steel needle for intradermal drug delivery. A 1.5-mm-long, 30-gauge stainless steel needle is built into the BD Soluvia® device, which is a glass prefillable spring-based syringe. More than 700 participants and 3,500 injections were employed in BD's clinical studies to reveal BD Soluvia™'s safety and convenience [200]. Moreover, BD clinical testing demonstrated that the microneedles were hardly detectable while entering the skin and successfully administered the drug into the intradermal layer across a wide range of subjects' gender, race, and weight [201]. IDFlu®, Intanza®, and Fluzone® are the brand names under which Sanofi Pasteur has sold its intradermal influenza vaccine injection. Intradermal microinjection was pioneered with the launch of Intanza® [202]. In 2009, Sanofi Pasteur introduced the world's first dermal-targeting influenza vaccine, Intanza® [200]. This included two doses of the influenza vaccine Intanza® administered intradermally with microneedles: 9 µg for people aged 18–59 and 15 µg for persons aged 60 and over. Many clinical trials have shown that the advantages of Intanza outweigh its risks, yet the marketing authorization holder has requested that the product be removed from the European Union market as of 2018. After receiving approval in 2011, Fluzone Intradermal® reported revenues of $8.05 billion in 2013 and $6.23 billion during

the first three quarters of 2014. A single dosage of this product costs $15.5 in the United States, while the cost of the standard Fluzone® vaccine is $12.04. [94]. The price of an influenza vaccine administered through a microneedles patch is predicted to be comparable to that of an intramuscular injection. Furthermore, there will be preliminary expenditures connected with the production process setup for microneedles. A pharmacy's stocking, marketing, and documentation charges for an influenza vaccine were estimated to bring the total cost of self-vaccination to around $5.50 (range of 4.60–11.70) in 2012 [16].

2. MiconJet, manufactured by the Israeli firm NanoPass Technologies, is a silicon-based, hollow microneedles device approved for intradermal injection. It is used for the administration of vaccines. It is a disposable microneedle device with four hollow silicon microneedles that are all less than 500 µm in length and affixed to a plastic device that may be used with any regular syringe to inject drugs and vaccines that are safe for intradermal injection. MicronJet has been shown to induce a comparable or superior immunogenicity response as the conventional vaccination while giving just 20% of the dose [203]. Clinical experiments using MicronJet® technology have shown that intradermal administration of local anesthetics, insulin, and influenza vaccine is efficacious, safe, and noninvasive. Using the MicronJet® and a standard needle, the researchers compared the pharmacokinetics and pharmacodynamics of glucose and insulin injections in phase I clinical study published in 2009. NanoPass Technologies' MicronJet® gained FDA approval in February 2010. By 2022 and 2030, sales of MicronJet® vaccination systems are projected to reach $37.4 million and $132.1 million, respectively. The company designed MicronJet 600® as a novel device model [175] to enhance device performance, specifically the insertion method. Yonsei University conducted a clinical trial in 2019 to compare the safety and immunogenicity of Bacillus Calmette–Guerin injections administered using the MicronJet 600® device versus those administered with a traditional needle. The FDA has approved the MicronJet 600® delivery system for intradermal injections of any material or medication authorized for intradermal administration [50, 204]. There have been clinical studies of the MicronJet 600® delivery system for the H1N1 pandemic influenza vaccine (Pandemrix®), poliomyelitis, and polio immunity, and the quadrivalent inactivated influenza vaccine (Fluarix®) [1]. Hollow and measuring 600 µm in length, MicronJet 600® is a pyramid-shaped microneedle designed for intradermal injections. Both the 510(k) clearance from the FDA and the CE mark have been awarded to the MicronJet 600®. The FDA is reviewing phase II clinical studies of the MicronJet 600® for allergy, cancer immunotherapy, and varicella-zoster vaccine delivery. Improved immunological response to full dosage of intramuscular Fluzone® has been observed using MicronJet 600® with just 4–40% of the intramuscular dose [176, 205, 206].

3. The SCS microinjector®, manufactured by Clearside Biomedical, Inc., is a 30-gauge hollow microneedle with a range of needle lengths of less than 1.2 mm intended for single usage. To produce the SCS microinjector, a stainless steel needle of 33G was laser-shaped and electropolished to the finished product [207]. The drug formulation is injected into the suprachoroidal region, allowing the drug to diffuse across the posterior segment of the eye. For disorders linked with macular edema, this microinjector is suitable for drug delivery to the choroid and retina.

4. Micro-Trans™ microneedle Array Patch (Valeritas) allows for dermal drug delivery regardless of the drug's size, structure, charge, or the properties of the patient's

skin. To provide a noninvasive drug delivery, the arrays are designed to only reach the superficial layers of skin.

5. The MicroCor® microneedles delivery system from Corium, Inc., is a novel, single-step, user-friendly, needle-free device for the transdermal delivery of drugs and vaccines. These microneedles are biodegradable and dissolvable upon penetration into the skin, releasing the drug for local or systemic administration. The technology incorporates the active ingredients directly into the arrays. The microneedles may be up to 200 µm in length, allowing for excellent flexibility in the skin penetration depth (from stratum corneum to dermis layer) and administration duration (from bolus to sustained drug delivery). Although the safety and effectiveness of MicroCor® products have not yet been validated, the business successfully showed the capacity to integrate a wide variety of molecules into the MicroCor® system. This innovative technology has facilitated the delivery of large molecules, including peptides, proteins, and vaccines, via the skin. It also allows for small molecules to permeate the skin more rapidly. The business plans to invest between $15 and $18 million to increase the manufacturing capacity for MicroCor®. Clinical assessment of the MicroCor PTH(1–34) product for the management of osteoporosis has been completed at phase IIa.

6. Multiple preclinical investigations researching the transdermal delivery of proteins, peptides, and vaccines using 3M's microstructured transdermal system (MTS) using either solid (sMTS) or hollow microneedles (hMTS) have exhibited promising results. sMTS was utilized effectively in phase I and II clinical investigations, and currently, hollow MTS is accessible for use during trials. The 3M sMTS systems have the capability to provide a one-of-a-kind pharmacokinetic profile since it improves the delivery efficiency of certain medications and vaccines, leading to a faster onset of action. Coated microneedles are utilized in the 3M sMTS product to transport water-soluble, polar, and ionic compounds through the skin. Using this technology, drugs have been effectively delivered into the skin, with local anesthetic taking effect rapidly [15]. The insertion of 250-µm-long microneedle patches into hairless guinea pig skin was effective, penetrating to a depth of 120 µm and delivering 60–70% of the naloxone hydrochloride loaded on the sMTS [208]. In 2019, Radius Health, Inc., conducted a phase III clinical study of an abaloparatide-coated sMTS system for the treatment of osteoporosis in postmenopausal women. To transdermally administer vaccines and hormones, 3M is currently researching the effectiveness of a hollow microstructured transdermal system (hMTS) in tandem with an applicator. hMTS of 500–900 µm in length has been investigated for the administration of human growth hormone at a bioavailability comparable to that achieved with a standard hypodermic syringe. Disposable units of the 3M hMTS may be fitted into a specially designed applicator. There have recently been models with an array of 12 hollow microneedles, each roughly 1,500 µm in length, on a circular substrate 1 cm^2 in size. The molded polymeric microneedles are attached to a spring-loaded applicator and a reservoir for fluids. With an injection period of around 1–5 min, the hMTS system can administer pharmaceutical formulations like Cimzia®, Monoclonal AB, and protein, which require roughly 0.5–2 mL. The immunological response to hMTS intradermal injection was superior to intramuscular administration [209]. According to the 3M human tolerability research, the hMTS system can deliver roughly 2 mL of the drug solution within 2 min [210]. Moreover, in 2017, Panacea Pharmaceuticals, Inc.,

conducted an FDA phase I clinical research for intradermal injection of PAN-301–1: HAAH nanoparticle therapeutic vaccine utilizing a 3M hMTS system. Besides, a microneedle array with 351 microneedles/cm^2 (650 μm in length) is used in the 3M microchannel skin system as a pretreatment for the skin before dermatological procedures [15].

7. The primary objective of the Zosano patch was to improve the administration of protein, peptides, vaccines, and other biologics. The designers' goal behind the array of coated titanium microneedles is bolus drug delivery into the skin. A reusable application device is included with the microneedles patch. With the use of Alza's Macroflux® technology, Zosano Pharma carried out a pivotal phase III clinical investigation. As a means of administering parathyroid hormone for treating severe postmenopausal osteoporosis, the researchers used a drug-coated titanium microneedle patch. Highly promising and extensive phase II outcomes indicate an excellent possibility of a successful phase III trial. Macroflux® is used to increase the bioavailability and efficacy of biopharmaceuticals by the controlled, consistent delivery of these molecules without causing the patient undue pain. The Macroflux® system utilizes an array of drug-coated titanium microneedles arranged on an area of 8 cm^2 with around 300 microprojections/cm^2. It was reported that the drug-coated microneedles could pass through the stratum corneum and release the drug payload into the microcapillaries. Studies have indicated that the patch allowed for consistent penetration depth over the whole skin-treated area to an average depth of 100 μm [211]. Zosano Pharma has included a crucial applicator in this device. This applicator has been designed with the convenience of senior people in mind, applying a steady and painless force. Positive results were also obtained in focus study groups with patients (288 postmenopausal women with osteoporosis in the age of 60–85). Ninety-three percent of patients stated they liked the patch design "very well," and 90% said it was simple to use; furthermore, 82% of patients could apply the patch properly the first time without assistance. It seems that including the applicator device increased patient acceptance and confidence in the device. Currently, under investigation by the FDA, Qtrypta™ (zolmitriptan intracutaneous microneedle device) was developed by Zosano Pharma Corporation for the acute treatment of migraine in adults. The adhesive dermally applied microarray (ADAM) patch technology was designed by Zosano Pharma Corp. ADAM is adhered to the skin in a bandage-like way through the ZP-applicator. The therapeutic effect of ADAM in the phase I clinical study was three times greater than the oral delivery of zolmitriptan for the treatment of migraines [193]. A phase III clinical study has since been performed.

8. Imperium, manufactured by Unilife, is the first disposable, prefilled, multi-day insulin patch pump. Due to its similarity to an insulin pen, the device comes prefilled and preassembled, making its usage as simple as following three basic steps to initiate subcutaneous insulin infusion. Users may obtain a bolus dose whenever they choose by pressing a button. Bluetooth Low Energy and other wireless communication technologies are possible additions to Imperium that allow integration with smartphone applications that serve as reminders and status updates for patients.

9. Prefilled and disposable, the anoDyne system is indeed the size of a thumb and designed to administer insulin. It may be self-administered in practically any location with little to no discomfort. There are also dosage indications that are

color-coded for convenience. After being pressed into the skin, the minuscule needle retracts and locks into place, making it impossible to reuse.

10. The Daytona MT Dermal Roller, developed by Daytona Pharmaceutical Laboratory, is a portable roller with solid microneedles that may be used to treat various skin and hair issues. A dermal roller, like the Daytona MT, may promote collagen production and help make skin defects less noticeable. Dermaroller® is a cylindrical assembly of 192 titanium microneedles of 0.5 mm in length for use with topical creams and serums for skin treatment. The FDA has provided its mark of approval for it to be used in cosmetics. The FDA has cleared the patented MTS Roller™ as a safe and effective therapeutic adjunct. The device was designed for aesthetic purposes, making it a good option for the noninvasive, non-ablative treatment of issues, including hyperpigmentation, aging, and scarring (acne, surgical). Evidence from clinical trials shows that the device is superior to ablative therapies like dermabrasion and laser resurfacing for reducing the appearance of scars and wrinkles and is as efficient as non-ablative methods.

11. The AdminPen™ injection device uses a microneedle array technology termed AdminPatch. The AdminPen™ is an array of planar microneedles with a rectangular base and a tapered needle tip, and it has a needle length of 500–1,400 µm. These solid microneedles open a channel via which the injected medication may penetrate the skin. The AdminPatch is equipped with a fluidic connection of the AdminPen™ device, which is linked externally to a liquid drug reservoir by means of a simple, inexpensive molded plastic portion affixed to its rear side. Almost any syringe with a luer lock connection could work with this device. Several vaccines, liquid drug formulations, cosmeceuticals, and hair growth stimulants may now be administered with more efficiency and less discomfort owing to the AdminPen™ device. Microfabrication technology is employed to produce these devices because this technique reduces production costs. The AdminPen™ is manufactured using electrochemical machining, electrical discharge machining, and other processes [212].

12. Microinfusor® (Becton Dickinson Technologies) is a drug delivery device that uses a hollow microneedle to provide medication through intradermal injections. It is possible to provide many therapeutic drugs by the subcutaneous route with a volume range of 0.2–15 mL, and the administration period may range from around a few seconds to several minutes. The automated device may be used in clinical settings or at home to administer large quantities of very viscous drug formulations without the need for human intervention. Intradermal delivery of an influenza vaccine with Microinfusor® has been shown to be just as effective as intramuscular administration in preclinical experiments [213].

13. h-Patch™ is a disposable controlled delivery product for subcutaneous drug administration that is both easy to use and flexible, allowing for either point-of-care fill or prefilled fluids for lyophilized pharmaceuticals to be used in conjunction with conventional filling procedures [202].

14. Bullfrog® Micro-Infusion Device is an innovative microneedle-based device designed by Mercator MedSystems, Inc., to administer therapeutic drugs by injection into adventitial regions. A balloon-encased microneedle is located at the end of the device. The FDA has granted 510(k) approval for the commercialization of this product, and it carries the CE mark.

15. Microdermics has developed microelectromechanical systems (MEMS)-based metal hollow microneedles and manufactured a disposable unit prototype that can be attached to a standard syringe. They used their proprietary system to showcase innovative multi-injection adaptors and customized kits. Microdermics has been producing and packaging pharmaceuticals under an arrangement with Vetter, a contract development and manufacturing organization, since 2017 [214].

16. The BetaConnect™ electronic auto-injector, manufactured by Bayer HealthCare, is a pen-type injection device with a very long and thin needle that allows the user to customize the injection's depth and duration. Betaseron®, which is employed to treat relapsing-remitting multiple sclerosis, is delivered by BetaConnect™. With its FDA-approved smartphone application myBETAapp™, a user may adjust the injection volume from 0.25 mL to 1 mL of the drug solution at a penetration depth of 8–12 mm. BetaConnect™ was used in a patient satisfaction survey by Bayer HealthCare. Adjusting the injection's depth and speed resulted in improved user satisfaction with using a standard syringe [215]. Furthermore, the Food and Drug Administration (FDA) approved BetaConnect™ by Bayer HealthCare as the first and only electronic auto-injector in 2015 [214].

17. Hollow microneedles device, Debioject™, measuring 350–900 µm in length, is capable of infusing drug solutions into the skin dermis utilizing the poke-and-flow method. Debioject™ was produced with the use of photolithography and deep silicon etching techniques [216]. In the same vein as other microneedles devices on the market, Debioject™ has received the CE mark of approval. Intradermal rabies vaccination with Rabique Pasteur® at 20% of the usual intramuscular dose was the subject of an FDA phase I clinical investigation utilizing Debioject™ in 2015. Debioject™-based vaccination against rabies generated a comparable humoral immune response to full-dose intramuscular injection with traditional hypodermic needles [217].

18. Painlessly and patch-free, the JUVIC Microlancer device discharges solid insulin microneedles directly into the skin [218]. The microneedles in this spring-loaded device are cone-shaped and solid and injected into the skin tissue. Microneedles, typically 600 µm in length with a 252 µm base radius, may be delivered to a depth of 50–100 µm in a period of 50–100 ms [214].

19. The microneedle Patch, developed by Micron Biomedical, is a bandage-like product that transports dermal immune system cells into the skin to promote the epidermis' immune response. The Micron Biomedical Microneedle Patch was shown to be safe and to elicit an immune response as effectively as a flu vaccine in a phase I clinical study.

20. Nanopatch™ is an innovative coated microneedles product developed and marketed by Vaxxas in collaboration with the World Health Organization for vaccine administration that allows for the activation of the skin's immune system. The Nanopatch™ comprises around 20,000 vaccine-coated microneedles arranged on a 1 cm² area. With the use of Nanopatch™, the immunogenicity of Fluvax® was improved in a mouse model, while the vaccine's efficiency was enhanced despite the use of a considerably lower dose. Presently, clinical studies of the Nanopatch™ are being conducted for the Australian New Zealand Clinical Trials Registry [214]. Polio vaccine delivery experiments using Nanopatch™ have been undertaken to complete preclinical research and comply with good manufacturing standards (GMP).

21. Micropatch™ is a solid dosage delivery device designed and manufactured by Nemaura Pharma, Ltd. Micropatch™ can deliver a consistent drug dose under the skin because the medications are coated on the needle's surface with a frustoconical-shaped pellet. Using a micropress, a freeze-dried vaccine and excipients are compressed to the pellet's final dimensions [214].

21. V-Go®, a simple and disposable needles-based device for the administration of basal-bolus insulin treatment, was developed by Valeritas, Inc., and received FDA 510(k) clearance. Patients with type 2 diabetes may manage their glucose levels with the aid of the V-Go® device, which uses a 30-G hypodermic floating needle to administer insulin at the push of a button without the need for batteries or complex programming [219].

22. Memspatch® insulin microneedle device (Nemaura Pharma, Ltd.) is an injector that slides the operational component to inject insulin, alleviating patients' concerns about needle discomfort. Recent clinical research found that compared to alternative pen injectors, patients using Memspatch® experienced significantly less discomfort while injecting their insulin for type 2 diabetes [214].

23. SteadyMed, Ltd. has designed a drug infusion pump system. To deliver a sterile liquid drug formulation, the Trevyent™ from SteadyMed, Ltd. is outfitted with an ECell® that expands on its own and presses a piston, causing the main container to collapse. SteadyMed, Ltd. must comply with a request from the Food and Drug Administration to resubmit its new drug application for Trevyent™ for the treatment of pulmonary arterial hypertension [214].

24. The Enable Smart enFuse™ system, manufactured by Enable Injections, Inc., offers a feature that lets the user suspend the injection at any moment. It can hold different drug quantities depending on the reservoir capacity. With the Smart enFuse™'s built-in reconstitution filling mechanism, users can easily mix, reconstitute, and transfer lyophilized formulations or combine two liquid formulations into a single one.

25. Microdemics's Prefill Patch: Microdermics has devised a needle patch device (branded Prefilled Patch) that, when affixed to the skin, alleviates discomfort during injection and enhances the patient's satisfaction and response to therapy. Dose-sparing intradermal vaccine administration is achieved by the use of these devices, which contain varying quantities of drug [214].

14.7 Future of Microneedles

14.7.1 Promising Future of Microneedles

Although microneedle devices have the potential to advance significantly in the fields of pharmaceuticals, immunization, and disease treatment, they are still a relatively new technology that has not been thoroughly explored. Microneedles of varying designs have been demonstrated to be effective for intradermal and transdermal delivery of drugs, biomolecules, vaccines, and cosmetic substances; therefore, it is expected that the industry effort in the development of microneedle products will increase. In addition, cutting-edge uses for microneedle technology will emerge. To ensure the therapeutic safety of microneedles, further study into their efficacy and features, as well as the polymeric materials employed in their manufacturing, is required. Thus, advances in this technology will lead to the creation of new devices that are less expensive, smaller, noninvasive, more acceptable, and more convenient for the administration of a wide variety of biopharmaceuticals, likely resulting in lower doses and fewer adverse effects [202].

Vaccination using microneedles requires extensive translation of preclinical investigations into clinical trials and the development of commercial manufacturing capable of mass-producing microneedles at an affordable price. It is expected that the commercial feasibility of an influenza vaccine patch will become apparent within the next decade, and the efforts to design vaccine patches as a delivery platform will advance during this time. The resources provided to support various work streams by various parties will determine the progress [91]. As the number of human clinical studies increases, more microneedles are expected to reach the commercial market. Microneedles-based vaccine products will be the first to hit major markets, setting the scene for safety, effectiveness, and the public's perspective on the technology. Microneedle vaccination is predicted to replace traditional immunization, leading to higher vaccination coverage and, perhaps, a decrease in infectious diseases, particularly in developing nations. Success with microneedles is most likely to be observed in the vaccination sector before the technology is introduced to the market for chronic diseases [6]. The success of microneedles in the future depends on their long-term safety, manufacturing processes, and compliance with standardized GMP criteria. Marketing techniques will also be crucial in capturing as much of the market share as possible in comparison to more established and well-liked traditional delivery methods. As the first drug-loading microneedles product has the potential to reach commercialization, it emerges that several pharmaceutical firms are willing to defer microneedles development until its success becomes evident, as the difficult and expensive manufacturing of microneedles, as well as several application-associated concerns, can impede their clinical translation. In the future, a decrease in both price and number of steps required to fabricate a microneedles product is anticipated, attributable to developments in micromachining and 3D printing technology.

The eventual successful development of microneedle delivery systems and monitoring devices will rely not only on their capability to fulfill their intended purpose but also on their general acceptance among healthcare practitioners (e.g., physicians, nurses, and pharmacists) and patients. It is crucial to alter the mindset by demonstrating that microneedles provide much more than just serving as a basic vaccine delivery platform. Significant progress has been achieved in the elimination of the necessity for conventional needles and syringes in the treatment of illnesses, including HIV, diabetes, Alzheimer's, and cancers, primarily owing to the development of microneedles. When it comes to transdermal drug delivery, several different microneedle kinds and designs have been demonstrated to be effective in lab and animal studies. The spectrum of medications that might theoretically be delivered into and across the skin has been considerably expanded. As the number of novel molecules of biological origin continues to rise, this will be of growing importance and increase the significance of the transdermal delivery field. Microneedles' emerging application in biofluid extraction for drugs or endogenous analyte assessment is intriguing [220, 221]. It is undeniable that there is a lot of room for growth in this industry, with the potential for microneedle monitoring devices to be sent directly to patients' homes and then sent back to a lab for examination. With further refinement, a microneedles sampling device may be employed in viral testing, which would be essential in the battle against future pandemics. Due to the lowered regulatory requirements, pharmaceutical manufacturers may be prepared to initially invest in such devices since the design of the microneedle might be CE certified as medical equipment rather than a drug product [39]. With the advent of next-generation smart-microneedle systems, it will be possible to construct a closed-loop responsive device in which a microneedles delivery system will deliver a therapeutic agent in response to signals supplied by a microneedle monitoring component. If current technology trends continue, the microneedle system may soon replace conventional dosage forms and monitoring equipment for pharmaceuticals [126]. Coronavirus (COVID-19) has had a global effect, and a microneedles-based strategy is a promising option for combating the pandemic. To lessen the number of unreliable COVID-19 test results, Chen and colleagues developed oropharyngeal swabs equipped with microneedles [222]. This idea allows physicians to quickly and easily separate positive and negative samples by efficiently trapping the virus. Now that a vaccine against COVID-19 is on the market, it would be possible to deliver the vaccine using microneedles and have it administered by the public at large [223].

Therefore, a significant paradigm change in the area of drug delivery is envisaged via the application of microneedle systems, notably in the administration of therapeutic agents historically unreachable in conventional drug delivery methods [202]. This innovative technology is expected to pave the way for the next generation of transdermal delivery systems, which will benefit patients and doctors. There is a demand for more research into the design and development of methods that would allow for a low-cost, efficient way for microneedle mass manufacturing, as well as addressing any regulatory issues regarding the usage of microneedle devices. With the fast growth of cutting-edge new information fueling technological progress, the future of the microneedle industry seems to be exceptionally bright. It is anticipated that developments in microneedle-based technology will eventually lead to better illness prevention, diagnosis, and control and therefore contribute to an enhancement in the quality of life for patients all over the world.

14.7.2 Areas of Improvement

The technological difficulties and dose restrictions of most microneedle systems, as well as the more complicated regulatory process for advanced designs, provide the greatest obstacle to the advancement of microneedles [224]. Several obstacles, such as discomfort, microbial contamination, and the administration of therapeutically sufficient quantity of medications, must be overcome before these microneedles may find broad clinical usage. Additionally, there is a restriction on the maximum drug loading quantity, inadequate mechanical strength, inconsistent drug delivery, and a restricted selection of materials [225]. It seems that vaccines and other potent pharmaceuticals that only require to be administered in small doses will be the ones to get therapeutically effective dosing. The delivery of biotechnology-derived macromolecules also presents some challenges. This is because of the large molecular weight and hydrophilicity of these molecules, which makes it difficult to transfer them through the skin [3]. Future research should focus on enhancing the acceptability of microneedle systems, conducting clinical studies on the immunogenicity and safety of self-vaccination, scaling up production, and reducing the number of failed insertion attempts for microneedle patches. Several vaccines have shown superior efficacy with microneedles treatment in animal studies, but this has not yet been demonstrated in humans. The processes linked with enhanced immunogenicity need to be further elucidated. The projected supply chain simplification results from reduced product dimensions and improved product thermostability. However, the exact level of thermostability and the actual effect on healthcare systems have not been revealed. Dissolving microneedles are anticipated to significantly reduce the hazard of sharp wastes. While microneedles eliminate one concern related to hypodermic needles, they may have other issues that will not be known until they are used by a wide range of individuals in various settings and cultural contexts. Microneedles-based vaccination has the potential to reduce vaccine waste and eliminate the requirement for vaccine reconstitution; however, these advantages may come with unforeseen effects. Microneedles' usage as a channel-creating skin pretreatment is directly proportional to the number of open microchannels they provide. The time it takes for the channels to close after being punctured by microneedles might vary depending on the skin type and properties. It has come to light in recent years that people of various races and ethnicities have varying microchannel closure times, with darker skin taking longer to close. These results suggest that further investigation into the safety and effectiveness of microneedles in a wide range of human populations is required [226]. In a clinical setting, microneedles must meet strict human safety criteria. Evaluations of microneedles' pharmacokinetics and pharmacodynamics are also necessary to ensure their safety and effectiveness. Microneedles made from silicon and other polymers have been criticized for lacking the required mechanical strength to penetrate human skin. An optimal solution involves making microneedles with high fracture and low insertion forces. Moreover, the two-step process of applying microneedles (first porating the skin and then applying a patch) may be a nuisance. There should be a reasonable balance between increased penetration and minimal discomfort [3]. Questions were raised about the product's efficacy, the availability of methods to verify effective drug delivery (i.e., a visual dose indicator), the duration it takes for the drug to take effect, the price of the system, and the likelihood of accidental, inappropriate, or injurious use. There must be a way to certify that the microneedle was successfully inserted into each patient and that the procedure was performed correctly. Aside from the possibility of infection, issues with injecting minute quantities and variations in skin thickness across patients also worried medical professionals [84]. Microneedle-based delivery systems being accidentally applied to the same location, which may result in altered microchannel closure kinetics, increased infection risk from a larger disruption, unexpected flux values, or interference from extended hydration.

There will be new difficulties in mass-producing microneedles when the technology moves from the laboratory to the marketplace. Because microneedles are so distinct from existing drug delivery systems, new production equipment will need to be installed. The production of high-quality microneedles on a constant basis is a major problem in the microneedle manufacturing industry because of its complexity and specialization [6]. Furthermore, microneedles must be protected from humidity and bacteria by being sealed in airtight packages. Still up in the air is how much making microneedles will set back, which opens the door for innovations that might reduce that price. Microneedle vaccination has the potential to reduce costs by balancing the prices of products and vaccine delivery, which can be predicted using models, but the actual cost will depend on the vaccine and the usage situation. The price of microneedles products might be drastically lowered by the development of terminal sterilizing procedures that negate the necessity for aseptic manufacture [13]. The production cost of microneedles is predicted to rise dramatically if aseptic manufacturing procedures or final sterilizing methods are required. Initial capital expenditure is needed due to the need for specialized industrial machines, various manufacturing procedures, and a clean room facility. Furthermore, quality control testing for microneedles (such as geometry, mechanical strength, and *in vitro/in vivo* correlation) currently does not have clear regulatory standards.

Regulatory concerns, industry cost, and user-friendliness are all issues that need to be addressed [85]. Novel vaccination patches must demonstrate safety and efficacy compared to currently available vaccines and fulfill non-inferiority criteria before they can enter the commercial market [91]. Safety issues such as anaphylaxis and syncope, along with legal issues like proper waste disposal, mailing of biologicals, over-the-counter regulation, compensation for vaccination injuries, and the acceptability of self-vaccination among children and healthcare professionals, must be resolved before regulatory approval can be granted. Finding acceptable methods of recording self-administered immunizations and reimbursing patients is also essential [10].

Historically, many unsuccessful products have been created because their developers ignored the interests of the final consumer. In light of this, it is incredibly necessary that the viewpoints and suggestions of patients be respected and treated seriously. It deems essential to measure the level of acceptability among healthcare practitioners and other stakeholders since a self-administered microneedle system would constitute a significant change in the healthcare system. Painless microneedles have been found to reduce needle fear and increase patient compliance [75, 88]. Since missed doses could be reduced significantly, the use of microneedles in drug delivery can potentially lessen the requirement for readmission to the hospital. Needle reuse, needlestick injuries, and the requirement for specialized sharps disposal may be mitigated by the utilization of dissolving and hydrogel-forming microneedles. This means that the enormous advantages may outweigh the early scale-up investment spent by the industry on the patients and the healthcare professionals. Although early research suggests that microneedles may be properly administered by less qualified persons, including patients themselves, more comprehensive evaluation and superior microneedle designs are required to ensure effective vaccine administration. There is also the risk of unexpected drug delivery to healthy subjects from patients' fallen patches, or a modified drug delivery profile owing to heat exposure from an external source, a more extended patch wearing time, inadvertent ingestion with serious consequences, an accidental prick during removal from the package, and device usage under unstudied conditions. To achieve acceptability from healthcare providers, patients, and, most crucially, regulatory agencies, it is most likely that an application device and a "dosage indicator" will be contained within the microneedle product "package," with the array of microneedles being disposable while the applicator and dosing indicator being reusable. Patients will also want reassurance that the microneedle device was correctly applied to their skin. This is particularly true in the event of a worldwide pandemic or bioterrorism attack, when the use of self-administered microneedles may be required.

References

[1] Lee KJ, Jeong SS, Roh DH, et al. A practical guide to the development of microneedle systems—in clinical trials or on the market. Int J Pharm. 2020;573:118778.

[2] Donnelly RF, Raj Singh TR, Woolfson AD. Microneedle-based drug delivery systems: microfabrication, drug delivery, and safety. Drug Deliv. 2010;17:187–207.

[3] Ita K. Transdermal delivery of drugs with microneedles—potential and challenges. Pharmaceutics. 2015;7:90–105.

[4] Yang M, Zahn JD. Microneedle insertion force reduction using vibratory actuation. Biomed Microdevices. 2004;6:177–182.

[5] Azmana M, Mahmood S, Hilles AR, et al. Transdermal drug delivery system through polymeric microneedle: a recent update. J Drug Deliv Sci Technol. 2020;60:101877.

[6] Richter-Johnson J, Kumar P, Choonara YE, et al. Therapeutic applications and pharmacoeconomics of microneedle technology. Expert Rev Pharmacoecon Outcomes Res. 2018;18:359–369.

[7] Adhikari BB, Goodson JL, Chu SY, et al. Assessing the potential cost-effectiveness of microneedle patches in childhood measles vaccination programs: the case for further research and development. Drugs RD. 2016;16:327–338.

[8] Lee BY, Bartsch SM, Mvundura M, et al. An economic model assessing the value of microneedle patch delivery of the seasonal influenza vaccine. Vaccine. 2015;33:4727–4736.

[9] Lim D-J, Vines JB, Park H, et al. Microneedles: a versatile strategy for transdermal delivery of biological molecules. Int J Biol Macromol. 2018;110:30–38.

[10] Norman JJ, Arya JM, McClain MA, et al. Microneedle patches: usability and acceptability for self-vaccination against influenza. Vaccine. 2014;32:1856–1862.

[11] Quinn HL, Bonham L, Hughes CM, et al. Design of a dissolving microneedle platform for transdermal delivery of a fixed-dose combination of cardiovascular drugs. J Pharm Sci. 2015;104:3490–3500.

[12] Prausnitz MR. Engineering microneedle patches for vaccination and drug delivery to skin. Annu Rev Chem Biomol Eng. 2017;8:177–200.

[13] Arya J, Prausnitz MR. Microneedle patches for vaccination in developing countries. J Control Release. 2016;240:135–141.

[14] Schmier J, Ogden K, Nickman N, et al. Costs of providing infusion therapy for rheumatoid arthritis in a hospital-based infusion center setting. Clin Ther. 2017;39:1600–1617.

[15] Zhang Y, Brown K, Siebenaler K, et al. Development of lidocaine-coated microneedle product for rapid, safe, and prolonged local analgesic action. Pharm Res. 2012;29:170–177.

[16] Prosser LA, O'Brien MA, Molinari N-AM, et al. Non-traditional settings for influenza vaccination of adults. Pharmacoeconomics. 2008;26:163–178.

[17] Adhikari BB. Microneedle patch measles vaccine reduces costs. Pharmaco Economics Outcomes News. 2016;764:26–22.

[18] Bariya SH, Gohel MC, Mehta TA, et al. Microneedles: an emerging transdermal drug delivery system. J Pharm Pharmacol. 2012;64:11–29.

[19] Rouphael NG, Paine M, Mosley R, et al. The safety, immunogenicity, and acceptability of inactivated influenza vaccine delivered by microneedle patch (TIV-MNP 2015): a randomised, partly blinded, placebo-controlled, phase 1 trial. The Lancet. 2017;390:649–658.

[20] Prausnitz MR, Mitragotri S, Langer R. Current status and future potential of transdermal drug delivery. Nat Rev Drug Discov. 2004;3:115–124.

[21] Bediz B, Korkmaz E, Khilwani R, et al. Dissolvable microneedle arrays for intradermal delivery of biologics: fabrication and application. Pharm Res. 2014;31:117–135.

[22] Park J-H, Prausnitz MR. Analysis of mechanical failure of polymer microneedles by axial force. J Korean Phys Soc. 2010;56:1223.

[23] Gittard SD, Chen B, Xu H, et al. The effects of geometry on skin penetration and failure of polymer microneedles. J Adhes Sci Technol. 2013;27:227–243.

[24] Larrañeta E, McCrudden MT, Courtenay AJ, et al. Microneedles: a new frontier in nanomedicine delivery. Pharm Res. 2016;33:1055–1073.

[25] O'Mahony C. Structural characterization and in-vivo reliability evaluation of silicon microneedles. Biomed Microdevices. 2014;16:333–343.

[26] Davis SP, Landis BJ, Adams ZH, et al. Insertion of microneedles into skin: measurement and prediction of insertion force and needle fracture force. J Biomech. 2004;37:1155–1163.

[27] Martanto W, Moore JS, Couse T, et al. Mechanism of fluid infusion during microneedle insertion and retraction. J Control Release. 2006;112:357–361.

[28] Martanto W, Moore JS, Kashlan O, et al. Microinfusion using hollow microneedles. Pharm Res. 2006;23:104–113.

[29] Martanto W, Baisch SM, Costner EA, et al. Fluid dynamics in conically tapered microneedles. AIChE J. 2005;51:1599–1607.

[30] Quinn HL, Larrañeta E, Donnelly RF. Dissolving microneedles: safety considerations and future perspectives. Ther Deliv. 2016;7:283–285.

[31] Jeong H-R, Lee H-S, Choi I-J, et al. Considerations in the use of microneedles: pain, convenience, anxiety and safety. J Drug Target. 2017;25:29–40.

[32] Palakurthi NK, Correa ZM, Augsburger JJ, et al. Toxicity of a biodegradable microneedle implant loaded with methotrexate as a sustained release device in normal rabbit eye: a pilot study. J Ocul Pharmacol Ther. 2011;27:151–156.

[33] Caffarel-Salvador E, Brady AJ, Eltayib E, et al. Hydrogel-forming microneedle arrays allow detection of drugs and glucose in vivo: potential for use in diagnosis and therapeutic drug monitoring. PLoS One. 2015;10:e0145644.

[34] Romanyuk AV, Zvezdin VN, Samant P, et al. Collection of analytes from microneedle patches. Anal Chem. 2014;86:10520–10523.

[35] Galvin O, Srivastava A, Carroll O, et al. A sustained release formulation of novel quininib-hyaluronan microneedles inhibits angiogenesis and retinal vascular permeability in vivo. J Control Release. 2016;233:198–207.

[36] Ye Y, Yu J, Wang C, et al. Microneedles integrated with pancreatic cells and synthetic glucose-signal amplifiers for smart insulin delivery. Adv Mater. 2016;28:3115–3121.

[37] Yu J, Zhang Y, Ye Y, et al. Microneedle-array patches loaded with hypoxia-sensitive vesicles provide fast glucose-responsive insulin delivery. Proc Natl Acad Sci. 2015;112:8260–8265.

[38] McCrudden MTC, Alkilani AZ, McCrudden CM, et al. Design and physicochemical characterisation of novel dissolving polymeric microneedle arrays for transdermal delivery of high dose, low molecular weight drugs. J Control Release. 2014;180:71–80.

[39] Kirkby M, Hutton AR, Donnelly RF. Microneedle mediated transdermal delivery of protein, peptide and antibody based therapeutics: current status and future considerations. Pharm Res. 2020;37:1–18.

[40] Jani P, Manseta P, Patel S. Pharmaceutical approaches related to systemic delivery of protein and peptide drugs: an overview. Int J Pharm Sci Rev Res. 2012;12:42–52.

[41] Sauerborn M, Brinks V, Jiskoot W, et al. Immunological mechanism underlying the immune response to recombinant human protein therapeutics. Trends Pharmacol Sci. 2010;31:53–59.

[42] Huang C-M. Topical vaccination: the skin as a unique portal to adaptive immune responses. Semin Immunopathol. 2007;29:71–80.

[43] Lambert PH, Laurent PE. Intradermal vaccine delivery: will new delivery systems transform vaccine administration? Vaccine. 2008;26:3197–3208.

[44] Kettwich SC, Sibbitt WL, Brandt JR, et al. Needle phobia and stress-reducing medical devices in pediatric and adult chemotherapy patients. J Pediatr Oncol Nurs. 2007;24:20–28.

[45] Caffarel-Salvador E, Tuan-Mahmood T-M, McElnay JC, et al. Potential of hydrogel-forming and dissolving microneedles for use in paediatric populations. Int J Pharm. 2015;489:158–169.

[46] Mooney K, McElnay JC, Donnelly RF. Children's views on microneedle use as an alternative to blood sampling for patient monitoring. Int J Pharm Pract. 2014;22:335–344.

[47] Gill HS, Prausnitz MR. Does needle size matter? J Diabetes Sci Technol. 2007;1:725–729.

[48] Chege M, McConville A, Davis J. Microneedle drug delivery systems: appraising opportunities for improving safety and assessing areas of concern. J Chem Health Saf [Internet] [cited 2016 Aug 13]; Available from: www.sciencedirect.com/science/article/pii/S1871553216300238.

[49] Marshall S, Sahm LJ, Moore AC. Microneedle technology for immunisation: perception, acceptability and suitability for paediatric use. Vaccine. 2016;34:723–734.

[50] Donnelly RF, Singh TRR, Tunney MM, et al. Microneedle arrays allow lower microbial penetration than hypodermic needles in vitro. Pharm Res. 2009;26:2513–2522.

[51] Li W-Z, Huo M-R, Zhou J-P, et al. Super-short solid silicon microneedles for transdermal drug delivery applications. Int J Pharm. 2010;389:122–129.

[52] Donnelly RF, Singh TRR, Alkilani AZ, et al. Hydrogel-forming microneedle arrays exhibit antimicrobial properties: potential for enhanced patient safety. Int J Pharm. 2013;451:76–91.

[53] McCrudden MTC, Torrisi BM, Al-Zahrani S, et al. Laser-engineered dissolving microneedle arrays for protein delivery: potential for enhanced intradermal vaccination. J Pharm Pharmacol. 2015;67:409–425.

[54] Donnelly RF. Clinical translation and industrial development of microneedle-based products. microneedles drug vaccine Deliv patient Monit. John Wiley & Sons, Ltd; 2018. p. 307–322. [Internet] [cited 2022 Nov 8]. Available from: https://onlinelibrary.wiley.com/doi/abs/10.1002/9781119305101.ch11.

[55] McCrudden MTC, Alkilani AZ, Courtenay AJ, et al. Considerations in the sterile manufacture of polymeric microneedle arrays. Drug Deliv Transl Res. 2015;5:3–14.

[56] Al-Zahrani S, Zaric M, McCrudden C, et al. Microneedle-mediated vaccine delivery: harnessing cutaneous immunobiology to improve efficacy. Expert Opin Drug Deliv. 2012;9:541–550.

[57] Beisson F, Aoubala M, Marull S, et al. Use of the tape stripping technique for directly quantifying esterase activities in human stratum corneum. Anal Biochem. 2001;290:179–185.

[58] Baek C, Han M, Min J, et al. Local transdermal delivery of phenylephrine to the anal sphincter muscle using microneedles. J Control Release. 2011;154:138–147.

[59] Gupta J, Gill HS, Andrews SN, et al. Kinetics of skin resealing after insertion of microneedles in human subjects. J Control Release. 2011;154:148–155.

[60] Ghosh TK. Dermal drug delivery: from innovation to production. Florida: CRC Press; 2020.

[61] Jeong S-Y, Park J-H, Lee Y-S, et al. The current status of clinical research involving microneedles: a systematic review. Pharmaceutics. 2020;12:1113.

[62] Soltani-Arabshahi R, Wong JW, Duffy KL, et al. Facial allergic granulomatous reaction and systemic hypersensitivity associated with microneedle therapy for skin rejuvenation. JAMA Dermatol. 2014;150:68–72.

[63] Chow AY, Pardue MT, Chow VY, et al. Implantation of silicon chip microphotodiode arrays into the cat subretinal space. IEEE Trans Neural Syst Rehabil Eng. 2001;9:86–95.

[64] Bal SM, Caussin J, Pavel S, et al. In vivo assessment of safety of microneedle arrays in human skin. Eur J Pharm Sci. 2008;35:193–202.

[65] Kaushik S, Hord AH, Denson DD, et al. Lack of pain associated with microfabricated microneedles. Anesth Analg. 2001;92:502–504.

[66] Noh Y-W, Kim T-H, Baek J-S, et al. In vitro characterization of the invasiveness of polymer microneedle against skin. Int J Pharm. 2010;397:201–205.

[67] Hoesly FJ, Borovicka J, Gordon J, et al. Safety of a novel microneedle device applied to facial skin: a subject-and rater-blinded, sham-controlled, randomized trial. Arch Dermatol. 2012;148:711–717.

[68] Matsuo K, Yokota Y, Zhai Y, et al. Corrigendum to "A low-invasive and effective transcutaneous immunization system using a novel dissolving microneedle array for soluble and particulate antigens" [J. Control. Release 161 (2012) 10–17]. J Control Release. 2014;184:9.

[69] Lee JW, Choi S-O, Felner EI, et al. Dissolving microneedle patch for transdermal delivery of human growth hormone. Small. 2011;7:531–539.

[70] Katsumi H, Liu S, Tanaka Y, et al. Development of a novel self-dissolving microneedle array of alendronate, a nitrogen-containing bisphosphonate: evaluation of transdermal absorption, safety, and pharmacological effects after application in rats. J Pharm Sci. 2012;101:3230–3238.

[71] Cosman F, Lane NE, Bolognese MA, et al. Effect of transdermal teriparatide administration on bone mineral density in postmenopausal women. J Clin Endocrinol Metab. 2010;95:151–158.

[72] Vicente-Perez EM, Larrañeta E, McCrudden MT, et al. Repeat application of microneedles does not alter skin appearance or barrier function and causes no measurable disturbance of serum biomarkers of infection, inflammation or immunity in mice in vivo. Eur J Pharm Biopharm. 2017;117:400–407.

[73] Shah V, Taddio A, Rieder MJ, et al. Effectiveness and tolerability of pharmacologic and combined interventions for reducing injection pain during routine childhood immunizations: systematic review and meta-analyses. Clin Ther. 2009;31:S104–S151.

[74] Taddio A, Appleton M, Bortolussi R, et al. Reducing the pain of childhood vaccination: an evidence-based clinical practice guideline. CMAJ. 2010;182:E843–E855.

[75] Gill HS, Denson DD, Burris BA, et al. Effect of microneedle design on pain in human volunteers. Clin J Pain. 2008;24:585–594.

[76] Sezgin B, Ozel B, Bulam H, et al. The effect of microneedle thickness on pain during minimally invasive facial procedures: a clinical study. Aesthetic Surg J Am Soc Aesthetic Plast Surg. 2014;34:757–765.

[77] Gupta J, Park SS, Bondy B, et al. Infusion pressure and pain during microneedle injection into skin of human subjects. Biomaterials. 2011;32:6823–6831.

[78] Kolli CS. Microneedles: bench to bedside. Ther Deliv. 2015;6:1081–1088.

[79] Haq MI, Smith E, John DN, et al. Clinical administration of microneedles: skin puncture, pain and sensation. Biomed Microdevices. 2009;11:35–47.

[80] Gupta J, Felner EI, Prausnitz MR. Minimally invasive insulin delivery in subjects with type 1 diabetes using hollow microneedles. Diabetes Technol Ther. 2009;11:329–337.

[81] Gupta J, Felner EI, Prausnitz MR. Rapid pharmacokinetics of intradermal insulin administered using microneedles in type 1 diabetes subjects. Diabetes Technol Ther. 2011;13:451–456.

[82] Norman JJ, Brown MR, Raviele NA, et al. Faster pharmacokinetics and increased patient acceptance of intradermal insulin delivery using a single hollow microneedle in children and adolescents with type 1 diabetes. Pediatr Diabetes. 2013;14:459–465.

[83] Ayala GX, Elder JP. Qualitative methods to ensure acceptability of behavioral and social interventions to the target population. J Public Health Dent. 2011;71:S69–S79.

[84] Sachdeva VK, Banga A. Microneedles and their applications. Recent Pat Drug Deliv Formul. 2011;5:95–132.

[85] Donnelly RF, Mooney K, Caffarel-Salvador E, et al. Microneedle-mediated minimally invasive patient monitoring. Ther Drug Monit. 2014;36:10–17.

[86] Kalluri H, Choi S-O, Guo XD, et al. Evaluation of microneedles in human subjects. In: Dragicevic NI, Maibach H, editors. Percutaneous penetration enhancers physical methods penetration enhancers. Berlin and Heidelberg: Springer; 2017. p. 325–340. [Internet] [cited 2022 Nov 8]. Available from: https://doi.org/10.1007/978-3-662-53273-7_20.

[87] Donnelly RF, Moffatt K, Alkilani AZ, et al. Hydrogel-forming microneedle arrays can be effectively inserted in skin by self-application: a pilot study centred on pharmacist intervention and a patient information leaflet. Pharm Res. 2014;31:1989–1999.

[88] Birchall JC, Clemo R, Anstey A, et al. Microneedles in clinical practice–an exploratory study into the opinions of healthcare professionals and the public. Pharm Res. 2011;28:95–106.

[89] Griffin P, Elliott S, Krauer K, et al. Safety, acceptability and tolerability of uncoated and excipient-coated high density silicon micro-projection array patches in human subjects. Vaccine. 2017;35:6676–6684.

[90] Guillermet E, Alfa DA, Phuong Mai LT, et al. End-user acceptability study of the nanopatch™; a microarray patch (MAP) for child immunization in low and middle-income countries. Vaccine. 2019;37:4435–4443.

[91] Badizadegan K, Goodson JL, Rota PA, et al. The potential role of using vaccine patches to induce immunity: platform and pathways to innovation and commercialization. Expert Rev Vaccines. 2020;19:175–194.

[92] Grohskopf LA, Sokolow LZ, Fry AM, et al. Update: ACIP recommendations for the use of quadrivalent live attenuated influenza vaccine (LAIV4)—United States, 2018–19 influenza season. Morb Mortal Wkly Rep. 2018;67:643.

[93] Ripolin A, Quinn J, Larrañeta E, et al. Successful application of large microneedle patches by human volunteers. Int J Pharm. 2017;521:92–101.

[94] Caffarel-Salvador E, Donnelly RF. Transdermal drug delivery mediated by microneedle arrays: innovations and barriers to success. Curr Pharm Des. 2016;22:1105–1117.

[95] Mooney K, McElnay JC, Donnelly RF. Paediatricians' opinions of microneedle-mediated monitoring: a key stage in the translation of microneedle technology from laboratory into clinical practice. Drug Deliv Transl Res. 2015;5:346–359.

[96] Arnou R, Frank M, Hagel T, et al. Willingness to vaccinate or get vaccinated with an intradermal seasonal influenza vaccine: a survey of general practitioners and the general public in France and Germany. Adv Ther. 2011;28:555–565.

[97] Dhont PA, Albert A, Brenders P, et al. Acceptability of Intanza® 15 µg intradermal influenza vaccine in Belgium during the 2010–2011 influenza season. Adv Ther. 2012;29:562–577.

[98] Mooney K, McElnay JC, Donnelly RF. Parents' perceptions of microneedle-mediated monitoring as an alternative to blood sampling in the monitoring of their infants. Int J Pharm Pract. 2015;23:429–438.

[99] Donnelly RF, Singh TRR, Morrow DI, et al. Microneedle-mediated transdermal and intradermal drug delivery. New Jersey: John Wiley & Sons; 2012.

[100] Li XJ, Zhou Y. Microfluidic devices for biomedical applications. Cambridge: Woodhead Publishing; 2021.

[101] Bhat-Schelbert K, Lin CJ, Matambanadzo A, et al. Barriers to and facilitators of child influenza vaccine–perspectives from parents, teens, marketing and healthcare professionals. Vaccine. 2012;30:2448–2452.

[102] Gill HS, Prausnitz MR. Coated microneedles for transdermal delivery. J Control Release. 2007;117:227–237.

[103] Hirobe S, Azukizawa H, Hanafusa T, et al. Clinical study and stability assessment of a novel transcutaneous influenza vaccination using a dissolving microneedle patch. Biomaterials. 2015;57:50–58.

[104] Lee K, Lee CY, Jung H. Dissolving microneedles for transdermal drug administration prepared by stepwise controlled drawing of maltose. Biomaterials. 2011;32:3134–3140.

[105] Aoyagi S, Izumi H, Fukuda M. Biodegradable polymer needle with various tip angles and consideration on insertion mechanism of mosquito's proboscis. Sens Actuators Phys. 2008;143:20–28.

[106] Vadim, Yuzhakov V. The AdminPenTM microneedle device for painless & convenient drug delivery. Drug Deliv Technol May. 2010;10.

[107] Mooney K, McElnay JC, Donnelly RF. A qualitative assessment of the views of children and parents of premature babies on microneedle-mediated monitoring as a potential alternative to blood sampling. Int J Pharm Pract. 2012;20:21–22.

[108] Kaaijk P, Kleijne DE, Knol MJ, et al. Parents' attitude toward multiple vaccinations at a single visit with alternative delivery methods. Hum Vaccines Immunother. 2014;10:2483–2489.

[109] Vicente-Pérez EM, Quinn HL, McAlister F, et al. The use of a pressure-indicating sensor film to provide feedback upon hydrogel-forming microneedle array self-application in vivo. Pharm Res. 2016;33:3072–3080.

[110] Quinn HL, Hughes CM, Donnelly RF. In vivo and qualitative studies investigating the translational potential of microneedles for use in the older population. Drug Deliv Transl Res. 2018;8:307–316.

[111] Coleman BL, McGeer AJ, Halperin SA, et al. A randomized control trial comparing immunogenicity, safety, and preference for self- versus nurse-administered intradermal influenza vaccine. Vaccine. 2012;30:6287–6293.

[112] Bhatnagar S, Gadeela PR, Thathireddy P, et al. Microneedle-based drug delivery: materials of construction. J Chem Sci. 2019;131:1–28.

[113] Larrañeta E, Lutton REM, Woolfson AD, et al. Microneedle arrays as transdermal and intradermal drug delivery systems: materials science, manufacture and commercial development. Mater Sci Eng R Rep. 2016;104:1–32.

[114] Ameri M, Fan SC, Maa Y-F. Parathyroid hormone PTH(1–34) formulation that enables uniform coating on a novel transdermal microprojection delivery system. Pharm Res. 2010;27:303–313.

[115] Akter T, Desai S. Developing a predictive model for nanoimprint lithography using artificial neural networks. Mater Des. 2018;160:836–848.

[116] Desai S, Bidanda B, Lovell MR. Material and process selection in product design using decision-making technique (AHP). Eur J Ind Eng. 2012;6:322–346.

[117] Elhoone H, Zhang T, Anwar M, et al. Cyber-based design for additive manufacturing using artificial neural networks for industry 4.0. Int J Prod Res. 2020;58:2841–2861.

[118] Ogunsanya M, Isichei J, Parupelli SK, et al. In-situ droplet monitoring of inkjet 3D printing process using image analysis and machine learning models. Procedia Manuf. 2021;53:427–434.

[119] Tofail SAM, Koumoulos EP, Bandyopadhyay A, et al. Additive manufacturing: scientific and technological challenges, market uptake and opportunities. Mater Today. 2018;21:22–37.

[120] Lutton REM, Moore J, Larrañeta E, et al. Microneedle characterisation: the need for universal acceptance criteria and GMP specifications when moving towards commercialisation. Drug Deliv Transl Res. 2015;5:313–331.

[121] Ameri M, Daddona PE, Maa Y-F. Demonstrated solid-state stability of parathyroid hormone PTH (1–34) coated on a novel transdermal microprojection delivery system. Pharm Res. 2009;26:2454–2463.

[122] Kommareddy S, Baudner BC, Bonificio A, et al. Influenza subunit vaccine coated microneedle patches elicit comparable immune responses to intramuscular injection in guinea pigs. Vaccine. 2013;31:3435–3441.

[123] Prausnitz MR, Mikszta JA, Cormier M, et al. Microneedle-based vaccines. In: Walter Orenstein, Richard W. Compans, editors. Vaccines for pandemic influenza. New York: Springer; 2009. p. 369–393.

[124] Aulton ME, Taylor K. Aulton's pharmaceutics: the design and manufacture of medicines. Amsterdam, NL: Elsevier Health Sciences; 2013.

[125] Cai B, Xia W, Bredenberg S, et al. Bioceramic microneedles with flexible and self-swelling substrate. Eur J Pharm Biopharm. 2015;94:404–410.

[126] Cahill EM, O'Cearbhaill ED. Toward biofunctional microneedles for stimulus responsive drug delivery. Bioconjug Chem. 2015;26:1289–1296.

[127] Hassan M. Regulatory considerations and commercialization of 3D printed MN mediate vaccine delivery. Dhaka: Brac University; 2020.

[128] Ameri M, Wang X, Maa Y-F. Effect of irradiation on parathyroid hormone PTH(1–34) coated on a novel transdermal microprojection delivery system to produce a sterile product-adhesive compatibility. J Pharm Sci. 2010;99:2123–2134.

[129] Lee S, Lee S, Song KB. Effect of gamma-irradiation on the physicochemical properties of porcine and bovine blood plasma proteins. Food Chem. 2003;82:521–526.

[130] García LEG, MacGregor MN, Visalakshan RM, et al. Self-sterilizing antibacterial silver-loaded microneedles. Chem Commun. 2019;55:171–174.

[131] Prausnitz MR, Allen MG, Gujral I-J. Microneedle drug delivery device. Google Patents; 2003. [Internet] [cited 2016 Aug 23]. Available from: www.google.com/patents/US6611707.

[132] Peyraud N, Zehrung D, Jarrahian C, et al. Potential use of microarray patches for vaccine delivery in low- and middle- income countries. Vaccine. 2019;37:4427–4434.

[133] Butler D. Translational research: crossing the valley of death. Nature. 2008;453:840–842.

[134] O'Brien KL, Binka F, Marsh K, et al. Mind the gap: jumping from vaccine licensure to routine use. The Lancet. 2016;387:1887–1889.

[135] van der Maaden K, Jiskoot W, Bouwstra J. Microneedle technologies for (trans)dermal drug and vaccine delivery. J Control Release. 2012;161:645–655.

[136] Kim Y-C, Park J-H, Prausnitz MR. Microneedles for drug and vaccine delivery. Adv Drug Deliv Rev. 2012;64:1547–1568.

[137] Mistilis MJ, Bommarius AS, Prausnitz MR. Development of a thermostable microneedle patch for influenza vaccination. J Pharm Sci. 2015;104:740–749.

[138] Bachy V, Hervouet C, Becker PD, et al. Langerin negative dendritic cells promote potent CD8+ T-cell priming by skin delivery of live adenovirus vaccine microneedle arrays. Proc Natl Acad Sci. 2013;110:3041–3046.

[139] Edens C, Collins ML, Goodson JL, et al. A microneedle patch containing measles vaccine is immunogenic in non-human primates. Vaccine. 2015;33:4712–4718.

[140] Barbé B, Gillet P, Beelaert G, et al. Assessment of desiccants and their instructions for use in rapid diagnostic tests. Malar J. 2012;11:326.

[141] Watkinson AC, Kearney M-C, Quinn HL, et al. Future of the transdermal drug delivery market–have we barely touched the surface? Expert Opin Drug Deliv. 2016;13:523–532.

[142] Norman JJ, Strasinger C. Scientific considerations for microneedle drug products: product development, manufacturing, and quality control. 4th Int Conf Microneedles. 2016.

[143] Donnelly R, Douroumis D. Microneedles for drug and vaccine delivery and patient monitoring. Drug Deliv Transl Res. 2015;5:311–312.

[144] Jacoby E, Jarrahian C, Hull HF, et al. Opportunities and challenges in delivering influenza vaccine by microneedle patch. Vaccine. 2015;33:4699–4704.

[145] Barbero AM, Frasch HF. Pig and guinea pig skin as surrogates for human in vitro penetration studies: a quantitative review. Toxicol In Vitro. 2009;23:1–13.

[146] Simon GA, Maibach HI. The pig as an experimental animal model of percutaneous permeation in man: qualitative and quantitative observations—an overview. Skin Pharmacol Physiol. 2000;13:229–234.

[147] Koelmans WW, Krishnamoorthy G, Heskamp A, et al. Microneedle characterization using a double-layer skin simulant. Mech Eng Res. 2013;3:51.

[148] Larrañeta E, Moore J, Vicente-Pérez EM, et al. A proposed model membrane and test method for microneedle insertion studies. Int J Pharm. 2014;472:65–73.

[149] Siewert M, Dressman J, Brown CK, et al. FIP/AAPS guidelines to dissolution/in vitro release testing of novel/special dosage forms. AAPS PharmSciTech. 2003;4:43–52.

[150] Garland MJ, Migalska K, Tuan-Mahmood T-M, et al. Influence of skin model on in vitro performance of drug-loaded soluble microneedle arrays. Int J Pharm. 2012;434:80–89.

[151] Donnelly RF, Woolfson AD. Patient safety and beyond: what should we expect from microneedle arrays in the transdermal delivery arena? Ther Deliv. 2014;5:653–662.

[152] Donnelly RF, Majithiya R, Singh TRR, et al. Design, optimization and characterisation of polymeric microneedle arrays prepared by a novel laser-based micromoulding technique. Pharm Res. 2011;28:41–57.

[153] Kochhar JS, Lim WXS, Zou S, et al. Microneedle integrated transdermal patch for fast onset and sustained delivery of lidocaine. Mol Pharm. 2013;10:4272–4280.

[154] Khanna P, Luongo K, Strom JA, et al. Sharpening of hollow silicon microneedles to reduce skin penetration force. J Micromechanics Microengineering. 2010;20:045011.

[155] Olatunji O, Das DB, Garland MJ, et al. Influence of array interspacing on the force required for successful microneedle skin penetration: theoretical and practical approaches. J Pharm Sci. 2013;102:1209–1221.

[156] Sivamani RK, Stoeber B, Liepmann D, et al. Microneedle penetration and injection past the stratum corneum in humans. J Dermatol Treat. 2009;20:156–159.

[157] Verbaan FJ, Bal SM, van den Berg DJ, et al. Assembled microneedle arrays enhance the transport of compounds varying over a large range of molecular weight across human dermatomed skin. J Control Release. 2007;117:238–245.

[158] Stoeber B, Sivamani RK, Maibach HI. Microneedling in clinical practice. Boca Raton, Florida: CRC Press; 2020.

[159] Kalluri H, Banga AK. Formation and closure of microchannels in skin following microporation. Pharm Res. 2011;28:82–94.

[160] Prausnitz MR. Microneedles for transdermal drug delivery. Adv Drug Deliv Rev. 2004;56:581–587.

[161] Singh P, Carrier A, Chen Y, et al. Polymeric microneedles for controlled transdermal drug delivery. J Control Release. 2019;315:97–113.

[162] Jayaneththi VR, Aw K, Sharma M, et al. Controlled transdermal drug delivery using a wireless magnetic microneedle patch: preclinical device development. Sens Actuators B Chem. 2019;297:126708.

[163] Economidou SN, Lamprou DA, Douroumis D. 3D printing applications for transdermal drug delivery. Int J Pharm. 2018;544:415–424.

[164] Qiu ZJ, Ma Z, Gao S. Effects of process parameters on the molding quality of the micro-needle array. IOP Conf Ser Mater Sci Eng. IOP Publishing; 2016. p. 012014.

[165] Majid I. Microneedling therapy in atrophic facial scars: an objective assessment. J Cutan Aesthetic Surg. 2009;2:26.

[166] Lu W, Wu P, Zhang Z, et al. Curative effects of microneedle fractional radiofrequency system on skin laxity in Asian patients: a prospective, double-blind, randomized, controlled face-split study. J Cosmet Laser Ther. 2017;19:83–88.

[167] Wang PM, Cornwell M, Prausnitz MR. Minimally invasive extraction of dermal interstitial fluid for glucose monitoring using microneedles. Diabetes Technol Ther. 2005;7:131–141.

[168] Jina A, Tierney MJ, Tamada JA, et al. Design, development, and evaluation of a novel microneedle array-based continuous glucose monitor. J Diabetes Sci Technol. 2014;8:483–487.

[169] Sharma S, El-Laboudi A, Reddy M, et al. A pilot study in humans of microneedle sensor arrays for continuous glucose monitoring. Anal Methods. 2018;10:2088–2095.

[170] Gowers SAN, Freeman DME, Rawson TM, et al. Development of a minimally invasive microneedle-based sensor for continuous monitoring of β-lactam antibiotic concentrations in vivo. ACS Sens. 2019;4:1072–1080.

[171] Paliwal S, Hwang BH, Tsai KY, et al. Diagnostic opportunities based on skin biomarkers. Eur J Pharm Sci. 2013;50:546–556.

[172] Portugal-Cohen M, Horev L, Ruffer C, et al. Non-invasive skin biomarkers quantification of psoriasis and atopic dermatitis: cytokines, antioxidants and psoriatic skin auto-fluorescence. Biomed Pharmacother. 2012;66:293–299.

[173] Jin J, Reese V, Coler R, et al. Chitin microneedles for an easy-to-use tuberculosis skin test. Adv Healthc Mater. 2014;3:349–353.

[174] Lee H-J, Choi H-J, Kim D-R, et al. Safety and efficacy of tuberculin skin testing with microneedle MicronJet600™ in healthy adults. Int J Tuberc Lung Dis. 2016;20:500–504.

[175] Levin Y, Kochba E, Hung I, et al. Intradermal vaccination using the novel microneedle device MicronJet600: past, present, and future. Hum Vaccines Immunother. 2015;11:991–997.

[176] Beals CR, Railkar RA, Schaeffer AK, et al. Immune response and reactogenicity of intradermal administration versus subcutaneous administration of varicella-zoster virus vaccine: an exploratory, randomised, partly blinded trial. Lancet Infect Dis. 2016;16:915–922.

[177] Anand A, Zaman K, Estívariz CF, et al. Early priming with inactivated poliovirus vaccine (IPV) and intradermal fractional dose IPV administered by a microneedle device: a randomized controlled trial. Vaccine. 2015;33:6816–6822.

[178] Laurent PE, Bourhy H, Fantino M, et al. Safety and efficacy of novel dermal and epidermal microneedle delivery systems for rabies vaccination in healthy adults. Vaccine. 2010;28:5850–5856.

[179] Daddona PE, Matriano JA, Mandema J, et al. Parathyroid hormone (1–34)-coated microneedle patch system: clinical pharmacokinetics and pharmacodynamics for treatment of osteoporosis. Pharm Res. 2011;28:159–165.

[180] Naito C, Katsumi H, Suzuki T, et al. Self-dissolving microneedle arrays for transdermal absorption enhancement of human parathyroid hormone (1–34). Pharmaceutics. 2018;10:215.

[181] Pettis RJ, Ginsberg B, Hirsch L, et al. Intradermal microneedle delivery of insulin lispro achieves faster insulin absorption and insulin action than subcutaneous injection. Diabetes Technol Ther. 2011;13:435–442.

[182] Pettis RJ, Hirsch L, Kapitza C, et al. Microneedle-based intradermal versus subcutaneous administration of regular human insulin or insulin lispro: pharmacokinetics and postprandial glycemic excursions in patients with type 1 diabetes. Diabetes Technol Ther. 2011;13:443–450.

[183] Bergenstal RM, Strock ES, Peremislov D, et al. Safety and efficacy of insulin therapy delivered via a 4mm pen needle in obese patients with diabetes. Mayo Clin Proc. 2015;90:329–338.

[184] Frid AH, Kreugel G, Grassi G, et al. New insulin delivery recommendations. Mayo Clin Proc. 2016;91:1231–1255.

[185] Kochba E, Levin Y, Raz I, et al. Improved insulin pharmacokinetics using a novel microneedle device for intradermal delivery in patients with type 2 diabetes. Diabetes Technol Ther. 2016;18:525–531.

[186] Rini CJ, McVey E, Sutter D, et al. Intradermal insulin infusion achieves faster insulin action than subcutaneous infusion for 3-day wear. Drug Deliv Transl Res. 2015;5:332–345.

[187] Tella SH, Kommalapati A, Correa R. Profile of abaloparatide and its potential in the treatment of postmenopausal osteoporosis. Cureus. 2017;9. [Internet] [cited 2022 Nov 8]. Available from: www.cureus.com/articles/6792-profile-of-abaloparatide-and-its-potential-in-the-treatment-of-postmenopausal-osteoporosis.

[188] Ita K. Transdermal delivery of drugs with microneedles: strategies and outcomes. J Drug Deliv Sci Technol. 2015;29:16–23.

[189] Wermeling DP, Banks SL, Hudson DA, et al. Microneedles permit transdermal delivery of a skin-impermeant medication to humans. Proc Natl Acad Sci. 2008;105:2058–2063.

[190] Li X, Zhao R, Qin Z, et al. Microneedle pretreatment improves efficacy of cutaneous topical anesthesia. Am J Emerg Med. 2010;28:130–134.

[191] Gupta J, Denson DD, Felner EI, et al. Rapid local anesthesia in humans using minimally invasive microneedles. Clin J Pain. 2012;28:129–135.

[192] Baek S-H, Shin J-H, Kim Y-C. Drug-coated microneedles for rapid and painless local anesthesia. Biomed Microdevices. 2017;19:2.

[193] Kellerman DJ, Ameri M, Tepper SJ. Rapid systemic delivery of zolmitriptan using an adhesive dermally applied microarray. Pain Manag. 2017;7:559–567.

[194] Spierings EL, Brandes JL, Kudrow DB, et al. Randomized, double-blind, placebo-controlled, parallel-group, multi-center study of the safety and efficacy of ADAM zolmitriptan for the acute treatment of migraine. Cephalalgia. 2018;38:215–224.

[195] Tepper SJ, Dodick DW, Schmidt PC, et al. Efficacy of ADAM zolmitriptan for the acute treatment of difficult-to-treat migraine headaches. Headache J Head Face Pain. 2019;59:509–517.

[196] Kolluru C, Williams M, Chae J, et al. Recruitment and collection of dermal interstitial fluid using a microneedle patch. Adv Healthc Mater. 2019;8:1801262.

[197] Goldstein DA, Do D, Noronha G, et al. Suprachoroidal corticosteroid administration: a novel route for local treatment of noninfectious uveitis. Transl Vis Sci Technol. 2016;5:14.

[198] Sunil D, Savita Y, Rishu S. Microneedling for acne scars in Asian skin type: an effective low cost treatment modality. J Cosmet Dermatol. 2014;13. [Internet] [cited 2022 Oct 11]. Available from: https://pubmed.ncbi.nlm.nih.gov/25196684/.

[199] Ogundele M, Okafor HK. Transdermal drug delivery: microneedles, their fabrication and current trends in delivery methods. J Pharm Res Int. 2017;18:1–14.

[200] Laurent PE, Bonnet S, Alchas P, et al. Evaluation of the clinical performance of a new intradermal vaccine administration technique and associated delivery system. Vaccine. 2007;25:8833–8842.

[201] Laurent A, Mistretta F, Bottigioli D, et al. Echographic measurement of skin thickness in adults by high frequency ultrasound to assess the appropriate microneedle length for intradermal delivery of vaccines. Vaccine. 2007;25:6423–6430.

[202] Indermun S, Luttge R, Choonara YE, et al. Current advances in the fabrication of microneedles for transdermal delivery. J Control Release. 2014;185:130–138.

[203] Kis EE, Winter G, Myschik J. Devices for intradermal vaccination. Vaccine. 2012;30:523–538.

[204] Donnelly RF, Singh TRR, Garland MJ, et al. Hydrogel-forming microneedle arrays for enhanced transdermal drug delivery. Adv Funct Mater. 2012;22:4879–4890.

[205] Burton SA, Ng C-Y, Simmers R, et al. Rapid intradermal delivery of liquid formulations using a hollow microstructured array. Pharm Res. 2011;28:31–40.

[206] Hung IFN, Levin Y, To KKW, et al. Dose sparing intradermal trivalent influenza (2010/2011) vaccination overcomes reduced immunogenicity of the 2009 H1N1 strain. Vaccine. 2012;30:6427–6435.

[207] Kim YC, Edelhauser HF, Prausnitz MR. Targeted delivery of antiglaucoma drugs to the supraciliary space using microneedles. Invest Ophthalmol Vis Sci. 2014;55:7387–7397.

[208] Banga AK. Transdermal and intradermal delivery of therapeutic agents: application of physical technologies. Boca Raton, Florida: CRC Press; 2011.

[209] Fuller S, Lebowitz M, Stewart S, et al. Enhanced immunogenicity of a nanoparticle therapeutic cancer vaccine targeting HAAH delivered intradermally using 3M's hollow microstructured transdermal system (hMTS). J Immunother Cancer. 2015;3:P433.

[210] Dick LA, Paul S. Innovative drug delivery technology to meet evolving need of biologics & small moledules. Ondrugdelivery Mag. 2019;56:4–6.

[211] Matriano JA, Cormier M, Johnson J, et al. Macroflux® microprojection array patch technology: a new and efficient approach for intracutaneous immunization. Pharm Res. 2002;19:63–70.

[212] Hegde NR, Kaveri SV, Bayry J. Recent advances in the administration of vaccines for infectious diseases: microneedles as painless delivery devices for mass vaccination. Drug Discov Today. 2011;16:1061–1068.

[213] Alarcon JB, Hartley AW, Harvey NG, et al. Preclinical evaluation of microneedle technology for intradermal delivery of influenza vaccines. Clin Vaccine Immunol. 2007;14:375–381.

[214] Lee K, Park SH, Lee JY, et al. Commercialized microneedles. Microneedling Clin Pract. 2020;91–108.

[215] Ziemssen T, Sylvester L, Rametta M, et al. Patient satisfaction with the new interferon beta-1b autoinjector (BETACONNECT™). Neurol Ther. 2015;4:125–136.

[216] Kendall MA, Chong Y-F, Cock A. The mechanical properties of the skin epidermis in relation to targeted gene and drug delivery. Biomaterials. 2007;28:4968–4977.

[217] Vescovo P, Rettby N, Ramaniraka N, et al. Safety, tolerability and efficacy of intradermal rabies immunization with DebioJect™. Vaccine. 2017;35:1782–1788.

[218] Jung HI, Lahiji SF. Painless and patchless shooting microstructure. 2020. [Internet] [cited 2022 Nov 8]. Available from: https://patents.google.com/patent/US10737081B2/en.

[219] Kapitza C, Fein S, Heinemann L, et al. Basal—prandial insulin delivery in type 2 diabetes mellitus via the V-Go™: a novel continuous subcutaneous infusion device. J Diabetes Sci Technol. 2008;2:40–46.

[220] Samant PP, Prausnitz MR. Mechanisms of sampling interstitial fluid from skin using a microneedle patch. Proc Natl Acad Sci. 2018;115:4583–4588.

[221] Xue P, Zhang L, Xu Z, et al. Blood sampling using microneedles as a minimally invasive platform for biomedical diagnostics. Appl Mater Today. 2018;13:144–157.

[222] Chen W, Cai B, Geng Z, et al. Reducing false negatives in COVID-19 testing by using microneedle-based oropharyngeal swabs. Matter. 2020;3:1589–1600.

[223] Aldawood FK, Andar A, Desai S. A comprehensive review of microneedles: types, materials, processes, characterizations and applications. Polymers. 2021;13:2815.

[224] Vrdoljak A. Review of recent literature on microneedle vaccine delivery technologies. Vaccine Dev Ther. 2013;3:47–55.

[225] Liu S, Jin M, Quan Y, et al. Transdermal delivery of relatively high molecular weight drugs using novel self-dissolving microneedle arrays fabricated from hyaluronic acid and their characteristics and safety after application to the skin. Eur J Pharm Biopharm. 2014;86:267–276.

[226] Ogunjimi AT, Carr J, Lawson C, et al. Micropore closure time is longer following microneedle application to skin of color. Sci Rep. 2020;10:18963.

Index

For Product Safety Concerns and Information please contact our EU
representative GPSR@taylorandfrancis.com
Taylor & Francis Verlag GmbH, Kaufingerstraße 24, 80331 München, Germany

www.ingramcontent.com/pod-product-compliance
Lightning Source LLC
Chambersburg PA
CBHW082104220326
41598CB00066BA/5251

* 9 7 8 1 0 3 2 5 1 4 0 8 6 *